Vitamin C in Health and Disease

Vitamin C in Health and Disease

Special Issue Editors

Anitra C. Carr
Jens Lykkesfeldt

MDPI • Basel • Beijing • Wuhan • Barcelona • Belgrade

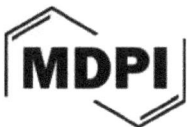

MDPI

Special Issue Editors
Anitra C. Carr
University of Otago
New Zealand

Jens Lykkesfeldt
University of Copenhagen
Denmark

Editorial Office
MDPI
St. Alban-Anlage 66
Basel, Switzerland

This is a reprint of articles from the Special Issue published online in the open access journal *Nutrients* (ISSN 2072-6643) in 2017 (available at: http://www.mdpi.com/journal/nutrients/special_issues/ vitamin_c_health_disease)

For citation purposes, cite each article independently as indicated on the article page online and as indicated below:

LastName, A.A.; LastName, B.B.; LastName, C.C. Article Title. *Journal Name* **Year**, *Article Number*, Page Range.

ISBN 978-3-03897-029-3 (Pbk)
ISBN 978-3-03897-030-9 (PDF)

Contents

About the Special Issue Editors

Anitra C. Carr, Dr., is a Sir Charles Hercus Health Research Fellow and Principal Investigator at the University of Otago, Christchurch, New Zealand. Dr. Carr is particularly interested in the role of micronutrients in human health and disease and has spent much of her research career investigating the antioxidant and health effects of vitamin C. From 1998–2001, she carried out an American Heart Association Postdoctoral Fellowship at the Linus Pauling Institute, Oregon State University, Corvallis, USA, under the mentorship of the eminent vitamin C researcher, Prof. Balz Frei. Whilst there, she produced a number of high impact publications on vitamin C in human health and disease. More recently, Dr. Carr has been carrying out human intervention studies investigating the bioavailability and potential health effects of both oral and intravenous vitamin C, particularly its roles in cancer and infection.

Jens Lykkesfeldt, Dr., received his MSc (organic chemistry; 1989) and his PhD (biochemistry; 1992) from the Technical University of Denmark. From 1993–1995, he was a postdoc at the Department of Pharmacology, University of Copenhagen, Denmark and from 1996–1998 visiting scientist at the Department of Molecular and Cell Biology, University of California, Berkeley, USA. In 1998, he became an associate professor in pharmacology at the University of Copenhagen. He defended his DSc degree in medicine in 2005 with a thesis on smoking and vitamin C. In 2008, he was appointed professor at the University of Copenhagen and, in 2009, professor and chair in experimental pharmacology and toxicology, which is his current position. Dr. Lykkesfeldt's research interests include the roles of oxidative stress and antioxidants in neurogenesis, chronic diseases and aging. He has published about 100 scientific papers on vitamin C.

Preface to "Vitamin C in Health and Disease"

Vitamin C is a ubiquitous water-soluble electron donor in living organisms and an essential nutrient in man. Having both specific and unspecific biological functions, it has been widely accepted as the most important hydrophilic antioxidant but also as a specific cofactor in enzymatic reactions or as a regulatory molecule. Far beyond the long accepted role in collagen biosynthesis, new functions of vitamin C in human health are continually being unravelled. This improved mechanistic understanding is starting to provide rationales explaining the extensive epidemiological literature that, for decades, has consistently shown strong associations between poor vitamin C status in human populations and increased morbidity and mortality.

The present volume encompasses both original research and literature reviews authored by experts in the field. Covering a wide range of topics including the role and function of vitamin C in infection and immunity, cardiovascular, skin and renal health, as well as cognition, neurodegeneration and aging, this book provides a valuable update on present developments in the field of vitamin C in health and disease.

Despite decades of scientific advances in understanding the role of vitamin C in human health, the various global and governmental health authorities show very little consensus in their recommended daily dietary intake of vitamin C that ranges from 40 to about 200 mg/day. One primary challenge in determining the daily requirement for optimum health is the lack of established dose-response relationships for vitamin C. This volume also presents emerging strategies to determine vitamin C requirements and presents new evidence of associations between poor vitamin C status and diabetes.

Vitamin C continues to surprise and fascinate researchers around the world as we expand our knowledge of this simple yet important carbohydrate. We hope this volume will inspire new investigations into the ever expanding biology of vitamin C.

Anitra C. Carr, Jens Lykkesfeldt
Special Issue Editors

nutrients

MDPI

Review
Vitamin C and Infections

Harri Hemilä

Department of Public Health, University of Helsinki, Helsinki FI-00014, Finland; harri.hemila@helsinki.fi;
Tel.: +358-41-532-9987

Received: 31 January 2017; Accepted: 15 March 2017; Published: 29 March 2017

Abstract: In the early literature, vitamin C deficiency was associated with pneumonia. After its identification, a number of studies investigated the effects of vitamin C on diverse infections. A total of 148 animal studies indicated that vitamin C may alleviate or prevent infections caused by bacteria, viruses, and protozoa. The most extensively studied human infection is the common cold. Vitamin C administration does not decrease the average incidence of colds in the general population, yet it halved the number of colds in physically active people. Regularly administered vitamin C has shortened the duration of colds, indicating a biological effect. However, the role of vitamin C in common cold treatment is unclear. Two controlled trials found a statistically significant dose–response, for the duration of common cold symptoms, with up to 6–8 g/day of vitamin C. Thus, the negative findings of some therapeutic common cold studies might be explained by the low doses of 3–4 g/day of vitamin C. Three controlled trials found that vitamin C prevented pneumonia. Two controlled trials found a treatment benefit of vitamin C for pneumonia patients. One controlled trial reported treatment benefits for tetanus patients. The effects of vitamin C against infections should be investigated further.

Keywords: ascorbic acid; bacteria; bacterial toxins; common cold; herpes zoster; pneumonia; protozoa; respiratory tract infections; viruses; tetanus

1. Early History on Vitamin C and Infections

Vitamin C was identified in the early twentieth century in the search for a substance, the deficiency of which would cause scurvy [1,2]. Scurvy was associated with pneumonia in the early literature, which implies that the factor that cured scurvy might also have an effect on pneumonia.

Alfred Hess (1920) summarized a series of autopsy findings as follows: "pneumonia, lobular or lobar, is one of the most frequent complications (of scurvy) and causes of death" and "secondary pneumonias, usually broncho-pneumonic in type, are of common occurrence and in many (scurvy) epidemics constitute the prevailing cause of death" [3]. He later commented that in "infantile scurvy ... a lack of the antiscorbutic factor (vitamin C) which leads to scurvy, at the same time predisposes to infections (particularly of the respiratory tract) ... Similar susceptibility to infections goes hand in hand with adult scurvy" [4]. In the early 1900s, Casimir Funk, who coined the word "vitamin", noted that an epidemic of pneumonia in the Sudan disappeared when antiscorbutic (vitamin C-containing) treatment was given to the numerous cases of scurvy that appeared at about the same time [5].

The great majority of mammals synthesize vitamin C in their bodies, but primates and the guinea pig cannot. Therefore, the guinea pig is a useful animal model on which to study vitamin C deficiency. Bacteria were often found in histological sections of scorbutic guinea pigs, so much so that some early authors assumed that scurvy might be an infectious disease. However, Hess (1920) concluded that such results merely showed that the tissues of scorbutic animals frequently harbor bacteria, and "there is no doubt that the invasion of the blood-stream does occur readily in the course of scurvy, but this takes place generally after the disease has developed and must be regarded as a secondary phenomenon and therefore unessential from an etiological standpoint. Indeed one of the striking and important symptoms of scurvy is the marked susceptibility to infection" [3]. When summarizing autopsy findings of experimental scurvy in the guinea pig, Hess also noted that "Pneumonia is met with very frequently and constitutes a common terminal infection".

Vitamin C was considered as an explanation for scurvy, which was regarded as a disease of the connective tissues, since many of the symptoms such as poor wound healing implied crucial effects on the connective tissues. Therefore, the mainstream view in medicine regarded vitamin C as a vitamin that safeguards the integrity of connective tissues [6]. The implications of the earlier research by Hess and others were superseded. This historical background might explain the current lack of interest in the effects of vitamin C on infections, even though firm evidence that vitamin C influences infections has been available for decades.

Early literature on vitamin C and infections was reviewed by Clausen (1934), Robertson (1934), and Perla and Marmorston (1937) [5,7,8]. Those reviews are thorough descriptions of the large number of early studies on the topic of this review. Scanned versions of those reviews and English translations of many non-English papers cited in this review are available at the home page of this author [9]. The book on scurvy by Hess (1920) is available in a digitized format [3].

2. Biology Relevant to the Effects of Vitamin C on Infections

Evidence-based medicine (EBM) emphasizes that in the evaluation of treatments researchers should focus primarily on clinically relevant outcomes, and little weight should be put on biological explanations. Therefore, this review focuses on infections and not on the immune system. Immune system effects are surrogates for clinical effects and there are numerous cases when surrogates had poor correlations with clinically relevant outcomes [10]. Nevertheless, biology provides a useful background when we consider the plausibility of vitamin C to influence infections.

2.1. Dose–Concentration Relationship

The vitamin C level in plasma of people in good health becomes saturated at about 70 µmol/L when the intake is about 0.2 g/day [11]. On the other hand, when vitamin C intake is below 0.1 g/day, there is a steep relationship between plasma vitamin C level and the dose of the vitamin. Clinical scurvy may appear when the plasma concentration falls below 11 µmol/L, which corresponds to an intake of less than 0.01 g/day [12–14]. Thus, when healthy people have a dietary intake of about 0.2 g/day of vitamin C, there is usually no reason to expect a response to vitamin C supplementation. This does not apply universally because certain studies have shown the benefits of supplementation, even though the baseline intake was as high as 0.5 g/day (see below). If the initial vitamin C intake is lower than about 0.1 g/day, effects of vitamin C supplementation may be expected on the basis of the dose–concentration curve. Nevertheless, this argument does not apply to patients with infections since their vitamin C metabolism is altered and they have decreased vitamin C levels (see below).

2.2. Infections Increase Oxidative Stress

Vitamin C is an antioxidant. Therefore, any effects of vitamin C may be most prominent under conditions when oxidative stress is elevated. Many infections lead to the activation of phagocytes, which release oxidizing agents referred to as reactive oxygen species (ROS). These play a role in the processes that lead to the deactivation of viruses and the killing of bacteria [15]. However, many of the ROS appear to be harmful to the host cells, and in some cases they seem to play a role in the pathogenesis of infections [16,17]. Vitamin C is an efficient water-soluble antioxidant and may protect host cells against the actions of ROS released by phagocytes. Phagocytes have a specific transport system by which the oxidized form of vitamin C (dehydroascorbic acid) is imported into the cell where it is converted into the reduced form of vitamin C [18,19].

Influenza A infection in mice resulted in a decrease in vitamin C concentration in bronchoalveolar lavage fluid, which was concomitant with an increase in dehydroascorbic acid, the oxidized form of vitamin C [20], and in vitamin C deficiency influenza led to greater lung pathology [21]. Respiratory syncytial virus decreased the expression of antioxidant enzymes thereby increasing oxidative damage [22]. Bacterial toxins have also led to the loss of vitamin C from many tissues in animal studies [1] (p. 6).

Increased ROS production during the immune response to pathogens can explain the decrease in vitamin C levels seen in several infections. There is evidence that plasma, leukocyte and urinary vitamin C levels decrease in the common cold and in other infections [1,23]. Hume and Weyers (1973) reported that vitamin C levels in leukocytes halved when subjects contracted a cold and returned to the original level one week after recovery [24]. Vitamin C levels are also decreased by pneumonia [25–28].

Decreases in vitamin C levels during various infections imply that vitamin C administration might have a treatment effect on many patients with infections. There is no reason to assume that the saturation of plasma or leukocyte vitamin C levels during infections is reached by the 0.2 g/day intake of vitamin C that applies to healthy people (see above). In particular, Hume and Weyers (1973) showed that supplementation at the level of 0.2 g/day was insufficient to normalize leukocyte vitamin C levels in common cold patients, but when 6 g/day of vitamin C was administered, the decline in leukocyte vitamin C induced by the common cold was essentially abolished [24].

2.3. Vigorous Physical Activity Increases Oxidative Stress

Heavy physical stress leads to the elevation of oxidative stress [29]. Therefore, responses to vitamin C might be observed when people are particularly active physically. Electron spin resonance studies have shown that vitamin C administration decreased the levels of free radicals generated during exercise [30] and vitamin C administration attenuated the increases in oxidative stress markers caused by exercise [31]. Therefore, vitamin C supplementation might have beneficial effects on people who are under physical stress. In such cases there is no reason to assume that 0.2 g/day of vitamin C might lead to maximal effects of the vitamin. Direct evidence of benefits of vitamin C supplementation to physically active people was found in three randomized trials in which 0.5 to 2 g/day of vitamin C prevented exercise-induced bronchoconstriction [32,33].

2.4. Vitamin C May Protect against Stress Caused by Cold and Hot Environments

Studies in animals and humans have indicated that vitamin C may protect against stress caused by cold and hot environments [34–37]. Some common cold studies with positive results investigated physically active participants in cold environments and other studies investigated marathon runners in South Africa (see below). Therefore, the effects of vitamin C in the protection against cold or heat stress might also be relevant when explaining the benefits in those studies.

2.5. Marginally Low Vitamin C Status Might Lead to Benefits of Supplementation

It seems evident that any effects of vitamin C supplementation may be more prominent when the baseline vitamin C level is particularly low. As noted above, a profound vitamin C deficiency was associated with pneumonia in the early literature. It seems plausible that less severe vitamin C deficiency, which may be called "marginal vitamin C deficiency", can also be associated with increased risk and severity of infections, although the effects may be less pronounced than those caused by scurvy.

Low vitamin C levels are not just of historical relevance. Cases of scurvy in hospitals have been described in several recent case reports [38,39]. One survey estimated that about 10% of hospitalized elderly patients had scurvy [40]. Surveys have also shown that plasma vitamin C levels below 11 μmol/L were found for 14% of males and 10% of females in the USA, 19% of males and 13% of females in India, 40% of elderly people living in institutions in the UK, 23% of children and 39% of women in Mexico, and 79%–93% of men in Western Russia. Moreover, 45% of a cohort of pregnant women in rural India had plasma vitamin C levels below 4 μmol/L and the mean plasma vitamin C level fell to 10 μmol/L in a cohort of pregnant or lactating women in Gambian villages in the rainy season [41].

The mean vitamin C intake in adults in the USA has been about 0.10 g/day, but 10% of the population has had intake levels of less than 0.04 g/day [14]. Thus, if low intake levels of vitamin C have adverse effects on the incidence and severity of infections, this may be important also in population groups in western countries, and not just in developing countries.

2.6. Vitamin C Has Effects on the Immune System

Vitamin C levels in white blood cells are tens of times higher than in plasma, which may indicate functional roles of the vitamin in these immune system cells. Vitamin C has been shown to affect the functions of phagocytes, production of interferon, replication of viruses, and maturation of T-lymphocytes, etc. in laboratory studies [1,23,42–44]. Some of the effects of vitamin C on the immune system may be non-specific and in some cases other antioxidants had similar effects.

2.7. The Diverse Biochemical, Physiological, and Psychological Effects of Vitamin C

Biochemistry textbooks usually mention the role of vitamin C in collagen hydroxylation. However, the survival time of vitamin C deficient guinea pigs was extended by carnitine [45] and by glutathione [46], which indicates that scurvy is not solely explained by defects in collagen hydroxylation, and it is not clear whether hydroxylation is important at all in explaining scurvy [6]. Vitamin C participates in the enzymatic synthesis of dopamine, carnitine, a number of neuroendocrine peptides, etc. [6,47–50]. Vitamin C is also a powerful antioxidant, as mentioned above.

Experimentally induced vitamin C deficiency leads to depression and fatigue [11,51]. Recently, vitamin C was reported to improve the mood of acutely hospitalized patients [52,53]. Such effects cannot be explained by collagen metabolism, and vitamin C effects on the immune system are not plausible explanations either. Instead, the effects of vitamin C on the neuroendocrine system or carnitine metabolism might explain such effects. Thus, if vitamin C has beneficial effects on patients with infections, that does not unambiguously indicate that these effects are mediated by the immune system per se.

2.8. The Effects of Antioxidants against Infections May Be Heterogeneous

It is quite a common assumption that the effects of vitamins are uniform. Thus, if there is benefit, it is often assumed that the same benefit applies to all people. However, it seems much more likely that the effects of vitamins, including vitamin C, vary between people depending on biology and their lifestyle. Thus, it is possible that there are benefits (or harms) restricted to special conditions or to particular people. In the case of vitamin E, there is very strong evidence for the heterogeneity in its effects on pneumonia [54,55] and on the common cold [56]. Although the factors modifying the effects of vitamin E cannot be extrapolated to vitamin C, it seems probable that there is comparable heterogeneity in the effects of vitamin C.

3. Infections in Animals

Early research showed that severe deficiency of vitamin C increased the incidence and severity of infections in guinea pigs. Hemilä (2006) carried out a systematic search of animal studies on vitamin C and infections and analyzed their findings [1], which are summarized in Tables 1–3 and discussed below.

3.1. Studies with Diets Containing Vitamin C

Many early studies with guinea pigs did not examine the effect of pure vitamin C. Instead, "vitamin-C-deficient groups" were fed diets that contained only small amounts of vitamin C, whereas the "vitamin C group" was administered oranges or other foods that contained high levels of vitamin C. The findings of studies on guinea pigs with tuberculosis and other bacterial infections are shown in Table 1.

Assuming that vitamin C containing foods do not influence infections, by pure chance only, one positive result at the level of $p < 0.01$ would be expected for a group of 100 studies. However,

20 of the reported 28 studies found significant benefits from feeding diets rich in vitamin C (Table 1). Although these findings are consistent with the notion that low vitamin C intake may increase the susceptibility to and the severity of infections, other substances in fruit and vegetables might also contribute to this effect, thus confounding the differences between the study groups.

As one example of Table 1 studies, McConkey (1936) reported that the administration of tuberculous sputum to 16 guinea pigs that were vitamin C deficient led to intestinal tuberculosis to 15 of them, but none of the five guinea pigs that were administered tomato juice as a source of vitamin C suffered from intestinal tuberculosis [57] (pp. 507–508).

Table 1. Effect of vitamin-C-rich foods on infections in guinea pigs.

Infection	No. of Studies	No. of Studies with Benefit in Any Infectious Disease Outcome with $p \leq 0.01$
All	28	20
Tuberculosis (TB)	11	7
Bacterial infection (non-TB) [a]	15	11
Diphtheria toxin	2	2

One group of guinea pigs was administered a vitamin-C-poor diet, and the other group was administered oranges, cabbage, etc. as supplements to the vitamin-C-poor diet. Based on Appendix 3 in Hemilä (2006) [1] (pp. 119–121). See Supplementary file 1 of this review for the list of the studies. p(1-tail) is used in this table. [a] Bacterial infections included pneumococcus, group C streptococcus, *Staphylococcus*, and *Salmonella typhimurium*.

3.2. Studies with Pure Vitamin C

Table 2 summarizes the animal studies in which pure vitamin C was administered to the "vitamin C" group. Overall, 148 animal studies had been published by 2005.

Out of the 148 studies, over half found a significant benefit, $p < 0.01$, for at least one infectious disease outcome. Furthermore, over a third of the studies found a benefit at the level of $p < 0.001$ [1]. Of the 100 studies with mammals, 58 found a significant benefit, $p < 0.01$, from vitamin C on some infectious disease outcome.

A benefit of vitamin C against infections was found in all animal groups. Although rats and mice synthesize vitamin C in their bodies, half or more of the studies with these species found significant benefits of additional vitamin C. This implies that rats and mice do not necessarily synthesize sufficient amounts of vitamin C to reach optimal levels that prevent or curtail infections. In addition to mammals, vitamin C protected against infections in several studies with birds and fishes.

Vitamin C was found to be beneficial against various groups of infectious agents including bacteria, viruses, *Candida albicans*, and protozoa (Table 2). Over half ($n = 97$) of all the studies evaluated the effect of vitamin C on bacterial infections or bacterial toxins, and 55 out of those studies found significant benefits of vitamin C ($p < 0.01$). Studies in which animals were administered diphtheria toxin, tetanus toxin, or endotoxin are also relevant, because these toxins are essential components in the pathogenesis of the bacterial infections. Over half of the studies on viruses, *Candida albicans* and protozoa also reported significant benefits ($p < 0.01$).

Table 3 shows the distribution of infections in studies that reported decreases in mortality caused by infections ($p < 0.001$). It is apparent that vitamin C reduced mortality in all etiological groups.

As one example of the studies in Tables 2 and 3, Dey (1966) reported that five rats administered twice the minimal lethal dose of tetanus toxin all died, whereas 25 rats administered vitamin C either before or after the same dose of toxin all lived [58].

In addition to the animal studies yielding quantitative data on the effect of vitamin C on infections in Tables 1–3, a few studies reported interesting findings of vitamin C effects against infections in studies without control groups [1] (p. 9). For example, two case-series suggested therapeutic benefit of vitamin C on dogs afflicted by the canine distemper virus. Belfield (1967) described a series of 10 dogs that appeared to benefit from 1–2 g/day of intravenous vitamin C over three days [59]. Leveque (1969) noted that usually only 5%–10% of dogs recovered from canine distemper with signs of central nervous system (CNS) disturbance. He became interested in Belfield's report and in a series of 16 dogs showing CNS disturbance that were treated with vitamin C, the proportion of dogs that recovered was 44% (95% CI: 20%–70%; based on 7/16) [60].

Table 2. Effect of pure vitamin C on infectious disease outcomes in animal studies.

Category	No. of Studies in the Category	No. of Studies with Benefit in Any Infectious Disease Outcome with $p \leq 0.01$
All studies	148	86
Time of publication		
Published in 1935–1949	40	20
Published in 1950–1989	48	32
Published in 1990–2005	60	34
Animal species		
Monkey	13	4
Guinea pig	36	21
Cow, sheep, rabbit	10	8
Cat	1	1
Rat	15	10
Gerbil, hamster	7	5
Mouse	18	9
Mammals [a]	100	58
Birds	13	8
Fish	35	20
Etiological agent		
Tuberculosis (TB)	8	3
Bacteria (non-TB)	70	36
Bacterial toxins	19	16
Virus	22	12
Candida albicans	6	4
Protozoa	23	15

A shorter version of this table was published in Hemilä (2006) [1] (p. 8). This table is based on data collected and analyzed in Appendix 2 of [1] (pp. 105–118). See Supplementary file 1 of this review for the list of the studies and their characteristics. p(1-tail) is used in this table. [a] The mammals category combines all the mammal species from the rows above.

Table 3. Infectious agents in studies in which vitamin C decreased the mortality of mammals by $p \leq 0.025$.

All Studies	29
Tuberculosis (TB)	6
Bacteria (non-TB) [a]	7
Bacterial toxin [b]	6
Virus (rabies)	1
Candida albicans	2
Protozoa [c]	7

Table 3 is restricted to mortality as the outcome, and to studies in which the effect of vitamin C on mortality was statistically significant. See Supplementary file 1 of this review for a list of the studies in which vitamin C decreased mortality by $p \leq 0.025$ (1-tail). In comparison, Table 2 includes studies with all infectious disease outcomes, such as incidence without the animals dying, and various forms of severity of infectious diseases. [a] Bacterial infections included pneumococcus and β-hemolytic streptococci; [b] Bacterial toxins included diphtheria toxin, tetanus toxin, endotoxin, and a set of clostridial toxins; [c] Protozoa infections include *Entamoeba histolytica*, *Leishmania donovani*, *Toxoplasma gondii*, and *Trypanosoma brucei*.

3.3. Implications of the Animal Studies

Many of the studies on vitamin C and infections summarized in Table 2 are old. However, it is unlikely that administering a specified dose of pure vitamin C and evaluating clinical outcomes of infections, such as mortality, will have changed meaningfully since those early days. Furthermore, 60 studies were published in the 1990s or later, and half of these later reports also found significant benefits of vitamin C on at least one infectious disease outcome.

The studies on guinea pigs are most interesting since that species is dependent on dietary vitamin C as are humans. Infections in guinea pigs against which vitamin C was significantly beneficial included *Mycobacterium tuberculosis*, β-hemolytic streptococci, *Fusobacterium necrophorum*, diphtheria toxin, *Entamoeba histolytica*, *Trypanosoma brucei*, and *Candica albicans* [1].

Some of the 148 studies in Table 2 were small and did not have sufficient statistical power to test whether vitamin C and control groups might differ. However, this problem cannot explain the large number of reported significant benefits. In contrast, inclusion of studies with a low statistical power biases the findings towards the opposite direction, leading to false negative findings.

Mortality and severity of infections in animals are definitive outcomes. In this respect, the animal studies with actual infections are much more relevant to humans than studies on laboratory determinations of the human immune system.

Given the universal nature of the effect of vitamin C against infections in diverse animal species as seen in Table 2, it seems obvious that vitamin C also has influences on infections in humans. It seems unlikely that human beings qualitatively differ from all of the animal species that have been used in the experiments listed in Table 2. Nevertheless, it is not clear to what degree the animal studies can be extrapolated to human subjects.

The fundamental question in human beings is not whether vitamin C affects the susceptibility to and severity of infections. Instead, the relevant questions are the following: What are the population groups who might benefit from higher vitamin C intakes? What is the dose-dependency relation between intake and the effects on infections? How does the optimal level of intake differ between healthy people and patients with infections?

4. The Common Cold

The term "the common cold" does not refer to any precisely defined disease, yet the set of symptoms that is called "the common cold" is personally familiar to practically everybody [61]. Typically the symptoms consist of nasal discharge, sore throat, cough, with or without fever. Young children typically have half a dozen colds per year, and the incidence decreases with age so that elderly people have colds about once per year [62]. The common cold is the leading cause of acute morbidity and of visits to a physician in high-income countries, and a major cause of absenteeism from work and school. The economic burden of the common cold is comparable to that of hypertension or stroke [63].

The most relevant definition of the common cold is based on the symptoms; thus the "common cold" does not always entail a viral etiology. Although the majority of common cold episodes are caused by respiratory viruses, similar symptoms are also caused by certain bacterial infections and by some non-infectious causes such as allergic and mechanical irritation. The cough and sore throat after running a marathon does not necessarily imply a viral etiology, although some researchers have assumed so. It is still reasonable to use the term the "common cold" in such a context on the grounds of the symptom-based definition.

4.1. Vitamin C and the Common Cold

Interest in the effects of vitamin C on the common cold originated soon after purified vitamin C became available. The first controlled trials on vitamin C were carried out as early as the 1940s. For example, in the 1950s, a British study examined the clinical effects of vitamin C deprivation, and reported that "the geometric mean duration of colds was 6.4 days in vitamin C-deprived subjects and 3.3 days in non-deprived subjects", and the authors concluded that the absence of vitamin C tended to cause colds to last longer [12].

Figure 1 shows the number of participants in placebo-controlled studies in which ≥1 g/day of vitamin C was administered. It also illustrates the main time points of the history of vitamin C and the common cold.

In 1970, Linus Pauling, a Nobel laureate in chemistry and also a Nobel Peace Prize winner, wrote a book on vitamin C and the common cold [64]. He also published two meta-analyses, which were among the earliest meta-analyses in medicine [65,66]. Pauling identified four placebo-controlled studies from which he calculated that there was strong evidence that vitamin C decreased the "integrated morbidity" of colds ($p = 0.00002$ [65]). By integrated morbidity, Pauling meant the total burden of the common cold: the combination of the incidence and duration of colds. In his analysis, Pauling put the greatest weight on the study by Ritzel (1961), which was a randomized controlled trial (RCT) with double-blinded placebo control and the subjects were schoolchildren in a skiing camp in the Swiss Alps [67]. Ritzel's study was methodologically the best of the four and used the highest dose of vitamin C, 1 g/day, and therefore Pauling concluded that gram doses of vitamin C would be beneficial against colds [64–66].

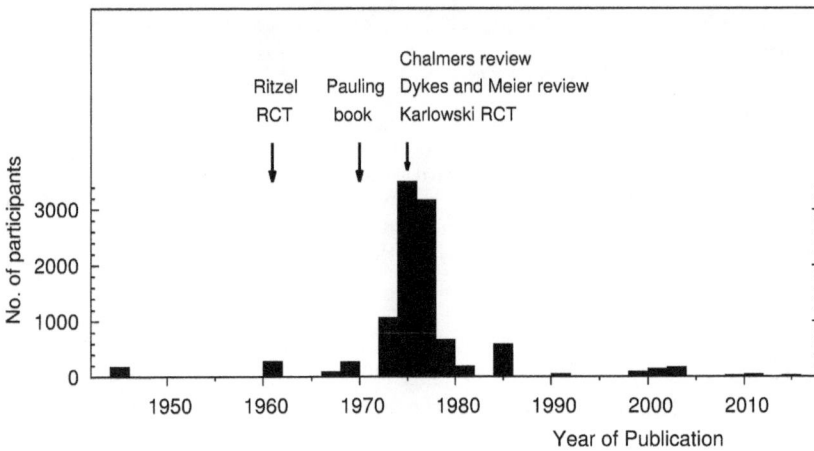

Figure 1. The numbers of participants in the placebo-controlled trials for which ≥1 g/day of vitamin C was administered. The numbers of participants in studies published over two consecutive years are combined and plotted for the first of the two years. This figure is based on data collected by Hemilä and Chalker (2013) [68,69]. See Supplementary file 1 of this review for the list of the studies. RCT, randomized controlled trial.

The activity of Pauling, in turn, led to a great upsurge in interest in vitamin C among lay people and also in academic circles in the early 1970s. From 1972 to 1979, in that eight-year period, 29 placebo-controlled studies were published, which amounted to a total of 8409 participants (Figure 1) [68,69]. Thus, the mean number of participants per study was 290.

In the interval from 1972 to 1975, five placebo-controlled trials were published that used ≥2 g/day of vitamin C. Those five studies were published after Pauling's book and therefore they formally tested Pauling's hypothesis. A meta-analysis by Hemilä (1996) showed that there was very strong evidence from the five studies that colds were shorter or less severe in the vitamin C groups ($p = 10^{-5}$), and therefore those studies corroborated Pauling's hypothesis that vitamin C was indeed effective against colds [70].

After the mid-1970s, however, interest in the topic plummeted so much so that during the 30-year period from 1985 to 2014, only 11 placebo-controlled trials comprising just 538 participants in total were published, with a mean of 49 participants per study (Figure 1). Thus, the number of studies published after 1985 is much lower than during the 1970s. In addition, the few recent studies are much smaller than the trials published in the 1970s. Therefore, the great majority of the data on vitamin C and the common cold that are currently available originated within the decade after the publication of Pauling's book.

This sudden lack of interest after the middle of the 1970s can be explained by three papers published in the same year by Chalmers (1975), Karlowski et al. (1975), and Dykes and Meier (1975) [71–73] (Figure 1). Few trials were started after 1975, which indicates the great impact of these three papers. First, the findings of the placebo controlled studies will be summarized, and then difficulties in the interpretation of common cold studies will be considered, and finally problems in the three papers that were published in 1975 will be discussed.

4.2. Vitamin C Does Not Decrease the Average Incidence of Colds in the General Community

Table 4 summarizes the findings of the studies on vitamin C and the common cold in the Cochrane review by Hemilä and Chalker (2013) [68,69]. Regularly administered vitamin C has not decreased the average number of colds among the general population (Table 4). Another meta-analysis combined the findings of the six largest trials that had used ≥ 1 g/day of vitamin C and calculated that there was no difference in the vitamin and placebo groups with RR = 0.99 (95% CI 0.93, 1.04) [74,75].

Table 4. Effects of regular vitamin C on the incidence and duration of the common cold [a].

Outcome Participants	No. of Studies	No. of Participants	Effect of Vitamin C (95% CI)	*p*
Incidence of colds [b]				
General population	24	10,708	−3% (−6% to 0%)	
People under heavy short-term physical stress	5	598	−52% (−65% to −36%)	10^{-6}
Duration of colds		No. of colds		
All studies (≥ 0.2 g/day)	31	9745	−9.4% (−13% to −6%)	10^{-7}
Adults (≥ 1 g/day)	13	7095	−8% (−12% to −4%)	10^{-4}
Children (≥ 1 g/day)	10	1532	−18% (−27% to −9%)	10^{-5}
Severity of colds		No. of colds		
All studies	16	7209	−0.12 (−0.17 to −0.07) [c]	10^{-6}

This table summarizes the main findings of the Cochrane review by Hemilä and Chalker (2013) [68,69]. [a] Regular supplementation of vitamin C means that vitamin C was administered each day over the whole study period. Duration and severity of colds indicates the effects on colds that occurred during the study; [b] Incidence indicates here the number of participants who had ≥ 1 cold during the study; [c] The unit in this comparison is the standard deviation. Thus −0.12 means that symptoms were decreased by 0.12 times the SD of the outcome.

Thus, there is no justification for "ordinary people" to take vitamin C regularly in order to prevent colds. However, this conclusion does not mean that regular vitamin C supplementation is ineffective for all people. There is strong evidence that vitamin C decreases the incidence of colds under special conditions and/or among certain population groups.

4.3. Vitamin C May Decrease Common Cold Incidence in Special Conditions

Vitamin C halved the incidence of colds in five RCTs during which the participants were under heavy short-term physical activity (Table 4) [68,76]. Three of the studies used marathon runners in South Africa as subjects, whereas one study used Canadian military personnel on winter exercise, and the fifth study was on schoolchildren in a skiing camp in the Swiss Alps, i.e., the Ritzel (1961) trial [67]. Thus, three studies were conducted under conditions of a hot environment and profound physical stress and the other two were carried out under cold environments and physical stress (see Section 2.4).

Another group in which vitamin C has prevented colds is British men [74,75,77]. Four trials found that vitamin C decreased the incidence of colds by 30%, and in another set of four trials, the proportion of men who had recurrent common cold infections during the study decreased by a mean of 46%. All these studies were carried out in the 1970s or earlier, and according to surveys, the intake of vitamin C in the United Kingdom was low when the studies were carried out, 0.03 to 0.06 g/day, and three of the U.K. trials specifically estimated that the dietary vitamin C intake was between 0.015

to 0.05 g/day [74]. In particular, Baird (1979) administered only 0.08 g/day of vitamin C yet they observed 37% lower incidence of colds in the vitamin C group, indicating that it was the "marginal deficiency" and not a high dose that explained the benefit [77,78].

In addition, the levels of vitamin C are usually lower in men than in women, which may explain the benefit for British males, in comparison to no apparent effect in British females. Evidently, the dietary vitamin C intake in the United Kingdom has increased since the 1970s, and therefore these studies do not indicate that vitamin C supplementation would necessarily influence colds in ordinary British men nowadays. However, if low dietary vitamin C intake increases the risk of respiratory infections, then that may be currently relevant in other contexts, since there are still many population groups that have low intakes of vitamin C. A recent small study in the USA by Johnston (2014) was restricted to 28 males with marginally low vitamin C levels, mean 30 μmol/L, and found a decrease in common cold incidence, RR = 0.55 (95% CI: 0.33–0.94; $p = 0.04$) [79], which may also be explained by the low vitamin C levels.

4.4. Vitamin C Might Protect against the Common Cold in a Restricted Subgroup of the General Community

Although vitamin C has not influenced the average common cold incidence in the general community trials (Table 4), some of them found that there was a subgroup of people who had obtained benefits from vitamin C. In a Canadian trial, Anderson (1972) [80] reported that in the vitamin C group there were 10 percentage points more participants with no "days confined to house" because of colds (57% vs. 47%; $p = 0.01$, [1] (p. 44)). Thus, one in 10 benefited from vitamin C in this outcome. In a trial with Navajo schoolchildren, Coulehan (1974) [81] found that in the vitamin C group there were 16 percentage points more children who were "never ill on active surveillance by a medically trained clerk or the school nurse" (44% vs. 29%; $p < 0.001$; [1] (p. 44)). A more recent study in the UK by van Straten (2002) reported that vitamin C decreased the number of participants who had recurrent colds by 17 percentage points [82] (19% vs. 2%; $p < 0.001$, [1] (p. 47)). Thus, the statistical evidence of benefit for a restricted subgroup in these three trials is strong.

4.5. Vitamin C Shortens and Alleviates the Common Cold

The effect of vitamin C on the duration and severity of the common cold has been studied in regular supplementation trials and in therapeutic trials. Regular supplementation means that vitamin C was administered each day over the whole study period, and the outcome is the duration and severity of colds that occurred during the study. Therapeutic vitamin C trial means that vitamin C administration was started only after the first common cold symptoms had occurred and the duration of colds were then recorded.

In regular supplementation studies, ≥0.2 g/day of vitamin C decreased the duration of colds by 9% (Table 4). When the dosage was ≥1 g/day of vitamin C, the mean duration of colds was shortened by 8% in adults and by 18% in children. Vitamin C also significantly alleviated the severity of the colds.

Therapeutic studies have hitherto not shown consistent benefit from vitamin C. However, therapeutic trials are more complex to conduct and interpret than regular supplementation trials. If the timing of the initiation of supplementation or the duration of supplementation influences the extent of the benefit, false negative findings may result from inappropriate study protocols. For example, four therapeutic studies used only 2–3 days of 2–4 g/day vitamin C supplementation, whereas the mean duration of colds in these studies was about a week. None of these studies detected any benefit from vitamin C [68,83]. On the other hand, Anderson (1974) [84] found that 8 g/day on the first day only reduced the duration of colds significantly (Figure 2). In addition, in a five-day therapeutic trial, Anderson (1975) [85] reported a 25% reduction in "days spent indoors per subject" because of illness ($p = 0.048$) in the vitamin C group (1 to 1.5 g/day) [1] (p. 48). Finally, none of the therapeutic studies investigated children, although the effect of regular vitamin C has been greater in children (Table 4). Thus, although the regular supplementation trials unambiguously show that vitamin C shortens and alleviates the common cold, there is no consistent evidence that therapeutic supplementation is effective.

4.6. Possible Differences in the Effects of Vitamin C between Subgroups

The regular supplementation study by Anderson (1972) is one of the largest that has been carried out [80]. They found that the proportion of participants who were not confined to the house decreased by 10 percentage points in the vitamin C group. In addition, they found that per episode the days confined to the house was 21% shorter in the vitamin C group. Together these combine to a 30% reduction in the days confined to the house per person ($p = 0.001$). Such a large effect gives statistical power for subgroup comparisons.

Anderson (1972) reported that vitamin C decreased total days confined to house by 46% in participants who had contact with young children, but just by 17% in participants who did not have contact with young children (Table 5). Anderson (1972) also reported that vitamin C decreased total days confined to house by 43% in participants who usually had two or more colds per winter, but just by 13% in participants who usually had zero to one cold per winter (Table 5).

In a study with adolescent competitive swimmers, Constantini (2011) found a significant difference between males and females in the effect of vitamin C, whereby the vitamin halved the duration and severity of colds in males but had no effect on females [86]. In a study with British students, Baird (1979) also found a significant difference between males and females, but the outcome was the incidence of colds (Table 5).

Carr (1981) found that vitamin C had a beneficial effect on the duration of colds for twins living separately, but not for twins living together [87]. This subgroup difference might be explained by swapping of tablets by twins living together, which was not possible for twins living separately.

The significant within-trial differences in the effect of vitamin C on the common cold indicate that there is no universal effect of vitamin C valid over the whole population. Instead, the size of the vitamin C effect seems to depend on various characteristics of people (see Section 2.8).

Table 5. Possible differences in the effects of vitamin C on the common cold between subgroups.

Study	Subgroup	Effect of Vitamin C	Outcome	Test of Subgroup Differences (*p*)
Anderson (1972) [80]	Contact with young children No contact with young children	−46% −17%	total days confined to house	0.036
Anderson (1972) [80]	Usually ≥2 colds per winter Usually 0–1 colds per winter	−43% −13%	total days confined to house	0.033
Constantini (2011) [86]	Male adolescent competitive swimmers Female adolescent competitive swimmers	−47% +16%	duration of colds	0.003
Baird (1979) [78]	Male students in UK Female students in UK	−37% +24%	incidence of colds	0.0001
Carr (1981) [87]	Twins living separately Twins living together	−35% +1%	duration of colds	0.035

Calculation of the subgroup differences for the Anderson (1972) and the Carr (1981) studies is described in Supplementary file 2. The interactions in the Constantini (2011) and Baird (1979) trials were calculated in [77,86]. *p*(2-tail) is used in this table.

4.7. Dose Dependency of Vitamin C Supplementation Effect

An earlier meta-analysis of dose-dependency calculated that on average 1 g/day of vitamin C shortened the duration of colds in adults on average by 6% and in children by 17%; and ≥2 g/day vitamin C shortened the duration of colds in adults by 21% and in children by 26% [83]. Thus, higher doses were associated with greater effects. In addition, children weigh less than adults and the greater effects in children may be explained by a greater dose per weight. Nevertheless, such a comparison suffers from numerous simultaneous differences between the trials. The most valid examination of dose–response is within a single study so that the virus distribution is similar in each trial arm and the outcome definition is identical.

Coulehan (1974) [81] administered 1 g/day to children and observed a 12% reduction in common cold duration, and in parallel they administered 2 g/day to other children and observed a 29% reduction in cold duration. Although the point estimates suggest a dose–response, the study was small and the 95% CIs overlap widely [68,83].

In a 2 × 2 design, Karlowski (1975) [72] randomized participants to 3 g/day regular vitamin C and to 3 g/day vitamin C treatment for five days when the participant caught a cold. Thus, one study arm was administered placebo, the second was administered regular vitamin C, the third therapeutic, and the fourth arm was administered regular + therapeutic vitamin C (i.e., 6 g/day). The four arms of the Karlowski trial are shown in Figure 2A. The 95% CIs show the comparisons with the placebo group. The test for trend for a linear regression model gives $p = 0.018$.

Anderson (1974) [84] randomized participants to a placebo and two vitamin C treatment arms which were administered vitamin C only on the first day of the cold. One treatment arm (arm #7) was given 4 g/day of, and another (arm #8) was given 8 g/day. These arms are compared with the placebo arm #4 in Figure 2B. The 95% CIs show the comparisons with the placebo group. The test for trend in a linear regression model gives $p = 0.013$.

Finally, some case reports have proposed that vitamin C doses should be over 15 g/day for the best treatment of colds [88,89]. Thus, it is possible that the doses used in most of the therapeutic studies, up to just 6–8 g/day, have not been sufficiently high to properly test the effects of vitamin C that might be achievable.

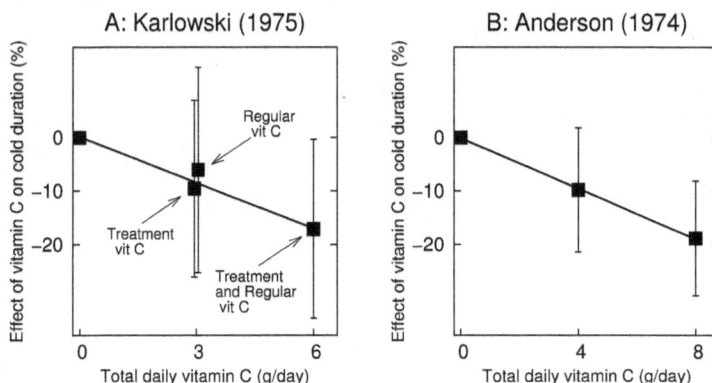

Figure 2. (A) Dose–response relationship in the Karlowski (1975) trial. The placebo arm is located at 0 g/day, the 3 g/day regular vitamin C and the 3 g/day treatment vitamin C arms are in the middle and the regular + treatment arm is at 6 g/day [72]. The 95% CIs are shown for the comparison against the placebo arm. With inverse-variance weighing, test for trend in a linear model gives $p(\text{2-tail}) = 0.018$. The addition of the linear vitamin C effect to the statistical model containing a uniform vitamin C effect improved the regression model by $p = 0.002$. Previously, analysis of variance for trend calculated $p = 0.040$ for the linear trend [83]; **(B)** Dose–response relationship in the Anderson (1974) trial. The placebo arm #4 is located at 0 g/day, vitamin C treatment arm #7 at 4 g/day and vitamin C treatment arm #8 at 8 g/day [84]. In the Anderson (1974) trial, vitamin C was administered only on the first day of the common cold. The 95% CIs are shown for the comparison against the placebo arm. With inverse-variance weighing, test for trend in a linear model gives $p(\text{2-tail}) = 0.013$. See Supplementary file 2 for the calculation of the trend for both studies.

4.8. Vitamin C and Complications of the Common Cold

Given the strong evidence that regularly administered vitamin C shortens and alleviates common cold symptoms, it seems plausible that vitamin C might also alleviate complications of the common cold. One frequent complication is the exacerbation of asthma [90].

A systematic review identified three studies that provided information on the potential pulmonary effects of vitamin C in sufferers of common cold–induced asthma [91]. A trial conducted in Nigeria studied asthmatic patients whose asthma exacerbations resulted from respiratory infections. A vitamin C dose of 1 g/day decreased the occurrence of severe and moderate asthma attacks by 89% [92]. Another study on patients who had infection-related asthma reported that 5 g/day vitamin C decreased the prevalence of bronchial hypersensitivity to histamine by 52 percentage points [93]. A third study found that the administration of a single dose of 1 g vitamin C to non-asthmatic common cold patients decreased bronchial sensitivity in a histamine challenge test [94].

It has also been proposed that vitamin C might prevent sinusitis and otitis media [95,96], but to our knowledge there are no data from controlled studies.

A further complication of viral respiratory infections is pneumonia; this is discussed in the section on pneumonia.

5. Problems in the Interpretation: Non-Comparability of the Vitamin C and Common Cold Trials

5.1. Vitamin C Doses in Vitamin C and Control Groups

One great problem in the interpretation of vitamin C trials arises from the fundamental difference between vitamin C and ordinary drugs such as antibiotics. In a trial of an ordinary drug, the control group is not given the drug, which simplifies the interpretation of the findings. In contrast, it is impossible to select control subjects who have zero vitamin C intake and no vitamin C in their system. Thus, all vitamin C trials de facto compare two different vitamin C levels. The lower dose is obtained from the diet, and it has varied considerably among the controlled studies. In addition, the vitamin C supplement doses given to the vitamin C groups have also varied extensively. Finally, the placebo group in some trials was also given extra vitamin C, which further confuses the comparisons. Therefore, the comparison of different vitamin C studies and the generalization of their findings is complicated. As an illustration of these problems, Table 6 shows examples of the variations in vitamin C doses that were used in the common cold trials.

There are 10- to 30-fold differences in the vitamin C intake in the diet of the control groups of the Baird (1979) [78], the Glazebrook (1942) [97], and the Sabiston (1974) [98] trials compared with the Peters (1993) [99] trial, yet all of them are labeled "control groups" of vitamin C trials (Table 6). Evidently, we should not expect similar effects of supplemental vitamin C in such dissimilar studies. Usually the dietary intake of vitamin C is not estimated and therefore cannot be taken into account when comparing studies.

Vitamin C was administered to the placebo group in some studies. For example, Carr (1981) [87] administered 0.07 g/day and some other studies administered 0.01 to 0.05 g/day to the control subjects. This was done to refute the notion that any possible effects of high doses were due to the treatment of marginal deficiencies. Such reasoning does not seem sound, since there are population groups for which ordinary dietary vitamin C intake is particularly low and it would be important to know whether vitamin C supplementation might be beneficial for them. Thus, marginal vitamin C deficiency is also an important issue. The administration of vitamin C to the control group biases the possible effects of vitamin C supplementation downwards.

Finally, there are up to a 240-fold difference between the lowest and highest vitamin C supplementary dose used in the common cold trials, yet the dosage is often ignored. For example, in his influential review (see Figure 1), Chalmers (1975) [71] presented data from the following studies in the same table: Karlowski (1975) study administered up to 6 g/day of vitamin C to their subjects [72], whereas the Cowan (1942) study administered only 0.025 g/day as the lowest dose [100]. Chalmers

(1975) did not list the vitamin C dosages in his table and therefore his readers were unable to consider whether the comparison of such different studies was reasonable or not. Still, Chalmers' review has been widely cited as evidence that vitamin C is not effective against colds [1] (pp. 36–38).

Finally, combinations of the above variations lead to paradoxes. The "vitamin C group" of the Baird (1979) study received about 0.05 g/day of vitamin C from food and 0.08 g/day from supplements, which amounted to 0.13 g/day of total vitamin C [78]. In contrast, the "placebo group" in the study by Peters (1994) received about four times as much, 0.5 g/day, of vitamin C from their usual diet [99]. Furthermore, Baird (1979) administered 0.08 g/day of vitamin C to their vitamin C group [78], whereas Carr (1981) administered 0.07 g/day vitamin C to their placebo group [87]. Thus, the dosages of vitamin C were essentially the same, but the groups were on the opposite sides in the evaluation of vitamin C effects.

High dietary vitamin C intake, and vitamin C supplementation of the placebo group, cannot lead to false positive findings about the efficacy of vitamin C against colds. In contrast, they can lead to false negative findings or estimates biased towards the null effect.

Table 6. Variations in vitamin C dose in the control and vitamin C groups.

Trial Country, Participants	Vitamin C Level (g/Day)		
	Dietary Intake Level in the Control Group	Supplement to the Control Group [a]	Supplement to the Vitamin C Group
Cowan (1942) [100] USA, schoolchildren	?		0.025–0.05
Baird (1979) [78] UK, students	0.05		0.08
Glazebrook (1942) [97] UK, boarding school boys	0.015		0.05–0.3
Peters (1993) [99] South Africa, marathon runners	0.5		0.6
Sabiston (1974) [98] Canada, military recruits	0.04		1
Carr (1981) [87] Australia, twins	?	0.07	1
Karlowski (1975) [72] USA, NIH employees	b		3–6

Modified from Table 12 from Hemilä (2006) [1] (p. 34). [a] In addition to Carr (1981), a few studies administered 0.01 to 0.05 g/day of vitamin C to the placebo group, but they are not listed here; [b] In the 1970s, the average vitamin C intake in the USA was approximately 0.1 g/day. The participants of the Karlowski (1975) study were employees of the National Institutes of Health and therefore their mean dietary intake of vitamin C probably was higher than the national average, but intake of vitamin C was not estimated.

5.2. Non-Compliance of Participants

Carr (1981) studied twins, some of whom lived together, whereas others lived apart [87]. Vitamin C had a significant effect on the duration and severity of colds in twins living apart, but no effect in twins living together (Table 5). Furthermore, the duration of colds among twins living together (5.4 days in vitamin C and placebo groups) was in the middle of the duration of colds among the vitamin C group (4.9 days) and placebo group (7.5 days) of twins living apart. An evident explanation for such a difference between twins living together and twins living apart, is that twins who lived together exchanged their tablets to some extent, whereas the twins who lived apart could not do so. Two studies on children found an increase in vitamin C levels in the plasma of boys and in the urine of boys of the placebo (sic) groups [81,101], which indicates tablet swapping among the children on vitamin C and placebo. Thus, non-compliance may have confounded the results and the true effects of vitamin C might be greater than those reported.

5.3. Implications of the Common Cold Studies

Given the great variations in the vitamin C dosage levels in the vitamin C and control groups, and the apparent problem of non-compliance in some studies, it is obvious that the comparison of different "vitamin C trials" can be complicated. The generalization of the findings of any particular trial is limited irrespective of its methodological quality and statistical power. However, the large variations in vitamin C levels in the vitamin C and control groups, and the non-compliance in some studies, both predispose against a false positive differences between the study groups. In contrast, they make it more difficult to detect true differences, and therefore the findings on common cold duration and severity shown in Table 4 may be biased downwards and might camouflage even stronger true effects.

6. Evaporation of Interest in Vitamin C and the Common Cold after 1975

Given the strong evidence from studies published before 1970 that vitamin C has beneficial effects against the common cold [65], and from the ≥2 g/day vitamin C studies published between 1972 and 1975 [70], it is puzzling that the interest in vitamin C and the common cold collapsed after 1975 so that few small trials on vitamin C and the common cold have been conducted thereafter (Figure 1).

This sudden loss of interest can be explained by the publication of the three highly important papers in 1975 (Figure 1). These papers are particularly influential because of their authors and the publication forums. Two of the papers were published in *JAMA* [72,73], and the third paper was published in the *American Journal of Medicine* [71]. Both of these journals are highly influential medical journals with extensive circulations. Two of the papers were authored by Thomas Chalmers [71,72], who was a highly respected and influential pioneer of RCTs [1,102,103], and the third paper was authored by Paul Meier [73], who was a highly influential statistician, e.g., one of the authors of the widely used Kaplan–Meier method [1,104,105].

Karlowski, Chalmers, et al. (1975) [72] published the results of a RCT in *JAMA*, in which 6 g/day of vitamin C significantly shortened the duration of colds (Figure 2A). However, these authors claimed that the observed benefit was not caused by the physiological effects of vitamin C, but by the placebo effect. However, the "placebo-effect explanation" was shown afterwards to be erroneous. For example, Karlowski et al. had excluded 42% of common cold episodes from the subgroup analysis that was the basis for their conclusion, without giving any explanation of why so many participants were excluded. The numerous problems of the placebo explanation are detailed in a critique by Hemilä [1,106,107]. Chalmers wrote a response [108], but did not answer the specific issues raised [109].

In the same year (1975), Chalmers published a review of the vitamin C and common cold studies. He pooled the results of seven studies and calculated that vitamin C would shorten colds only by 0.11 (SE 0.24) days [71]. Such a small difference has no clinical importance and the SE indicates that it is simply explained by random variation. However, there were errors in the extraction of data, studies that used very low doses of vitamin C (down to 0.025 g/day) were included, and there were errors in the calculations [1,110]. Pauling had proposed that vitamin C doses should be ≥1 g/day. When Hemilä and Herman (1995) included only those studies that had used ≥1 g/day of vitamin C and extracted data correctly, they calculated that colds were 0.93 (SE 0.22) days shorter, which is over eight times that calculated by Chalmers, and highly significant ($p = 0.01$) [110].

The third paper was a review published in *JAMA* by Michael Dykes and Paul Meier (1975). They analyzed selected studies and concluded that there was no convincing evidence that vitamin C has effects on colds [73]. However, they did not calculate the estimates of the effect nor any *p*-values, and many comments in their analysis were misleading. Pauling wrote a manuscript in which he commented upon the review by Dykes and Meier and submitted it to *JAMA*. Pauling stated afterwards that his paper was rejected even after he twice made revisions to meet the suggestions of the referees and the manuscript was finally published in a minor journal [111,112]. The rejection of Pauling's papers was strange since the readers of *JAMA* were effectively prevented from seeing the other side of an important controversy. There were also other problems that were not pointed out by Pauling; see [1,70].

Although the three papers have serious biases, they have been used singly or in the combinations of two as references in nutritional recommendations, in medical textbooks, in texts on infectious diseases and on nutrition, when the authors claimed that vitamin C had been shown to be ineffective for colds [1] (pp. 21–23, 36–38, 42–45). The American Medical Association, for example, officially stated that "One of the most widely misused vitamins is ascorbic acid. There is no reliable evidence that large doses of ascorbic acid prevent colds or shorten their duration" [113], a statement that was based entirely on Chalmers's 1975 review.

These three papers are the most manifest explanation for the collapse in the interest in vitamin C and the common cold after 1975, despite the strong evidence that had emerged by that time that ≥2 g/day vitamin C shortens and alleviates colds [70].

7. Pneumonia

Pneumonia is the most common severe infection, which is usually caused by bacteria and viruses.

As recounted at the beginning of this review, the association between frank vitamin C deficiency and pneumonia was noted by Alfred Hess and other early authors, when the chemical identity of vitamin C was not yet known. Vitamin C was purified in the early 1930s and soon thereafter a few German and U.S. physicians proposed that vitamin C might be beneficial in the treatment of pneumonia. For example, Gander and Niederberger (1936) concluded from a series of 15 cases that "the general condition is always favorably influenced (by vitamin C) to a noticeable extent, as is the convalescence, which proceeds better and more quickly than in cases of pneumonia, which are not treated with vitamin C" [114] and other German physicians also claimed benefits of vitamin C [115,116]. Translations of these papers are available [9]. Case reports from the USA also suggested that vitamin C was beneficial against pneumonia [117–119].

A Cochrane review on vitamin C and pneumonia identified three controlled trials that reported the number of pneumonia cases in participants who were administered vitamin C and two therapeutic trials in which pneumonia patients were given vitamin C [27,28].

7.1. Vitamin C and the Incidence of Pneumonia

Table 7 shows the findings of the three vitamin C and pneumonia trials. Each of them found a ≥80% lower incidence of pneumonia for their vitamin C group [27,28,120].

Glazebrook (1942) studied male students (15–20 years) in a boarding school in Scotland during World War II [97]. No formal placebo was used; however, 0.05 to 0.3 g/day of vitamin C was added to the morning cocoa and to an evening glass of milk in the kitchen. Thus, the placebo effect does not seem to be a relevant concern in the dining hall. The ordinary diet of the schoolboys contained only 0.015 g/day vitamin C so that their intake was particularly low.

Kimbarowski (1967) studied the effect of 0.3 g/day of vitamin C on military recruits who had been hospitalized because of influenza type-A in the former Soviet Union [121]. Thus, these pneumonia cases were complications of the viral respiratory infection. Vitamin C also shortened the mean stay in hospital for pneumonia treatment (9 vs. 12 days).

The latest of the three pneumonia prevention trials was carried out during a two-month recruit training period with U.S. Marine recruits by Pitt (1979) [122]. The dose of vitamin C was 2 g/day. This was a randomized double-blind placebo-controlled trial, whereas the two earlier studies were not.

The findings of the three studies are consistent with the notion that the level of vitamin C intake may influence the risk of pneumonia. However, all the three studies were carried out using special participants under particular conditions, and their findings cannot be generalized to the ordinary current Western population. Dietary vitamin C intake was particularly low in the oldest study, and may also have been low in the second study. Thus, the benefit of vitamin C supplementation may be explained by the correction of marginal deficiency in these two older studies. However, in the study by Pitt (1979), the baseline plasma level of vitamin C, 57 μmol/L, corresponds to the dietary vitamin C intake of about 0.1 g/day [11]. Furthermore, although the dose of 2 g/day was high, the plasma level of vitamin C increased only by 36% for the vitamin C group. This also indicates that the basal dietary intake vitamin C was high. Thus, treating marginal vitamin C deficiency is not a reasonable explanation for that latest study.

It is also worth noting that two of these trials used military recruits, and the third used young males who were accommodated in a boarding school [123]. Therefore, the exposure to viruses and bacteria causing pneumonia may have been much higher compared to children and young adults living at home. In each of the three trials, the incidence of pneumonia in the control group was very high when compared with the incidence in the ordinary population [124,125]. A high incidence of pneumonia has been reported in military recruits [126], but the incidence of pneumonia has been even higher in some child populations of the developing countries [127] (Table 7).

It seems reasonable to consider that these three studies observed a true effect of vitamin C against pneumonia in their specific circumstances. However, these findings should not be extrapolated to different circumstances. It would seem worthwhile to examine the effect of vitamin C in population groups that have a high incidence of pneumonia concomitantly with a low intake of vitamin C [27,41].

Table 7. Effect of vitamin C on the incidence of pneumonia.

Study	Pneumonia Cases/Total		p [a]	Incidence of Pneumonia in the Control Group (1/1000 Person-Years)
	Vitamin C	Control		
Glazebrook (1942) [97]	0/335	17/1100	0.006	30
Kimbarowski (1967) [121]	2/114	10/112	0.022	9% [b]
Pitt (1979) [122]	1/331	7/343	0.009	120
	Incidence of pneumonia in selected populations:			
Merchant (2004) [124]	Middle-aged males in the USA			3
Hemilä (2004) [125]	Middle-aged males in Finland			5
Pazzaglia (1983) [126]	Military recruits in the USA			60
Paynter (2010) [127]	Children in developing countries, up to			400

Modified from Hemilä (2006) [1] (p. 51). [a] Mid-p (1-tail); combined test for all three sets of data: $p = 0.00002$ [120]; [b] 9% of the hospitalized influenza A patients contracted pneumonia.

7.2. Vitamin C in the Treatment of Pneumonia

Two studies have reported on the therapeutic effect of vitamin C for pneumonia patients [27,28].

Hunt (1994) carried out a randomized, double-blind placebo controlled trial with elderly people in the UK (mean age 81 years), who were hospitalized because of acute bronchitis or pneumonia [26]. The mean plasma vitamin C level at baseline was 23 μmol/L and one third of the patients had a vitamin C level of just ≤11 μmol/L. There was a significant difference in the effect of 0.2 g/day of vitamin C between patients who were more ill and those who were less ill when admitted to the hospital. Vitamin C reduced the respiratory symptom score in the more ill patients but not in their less ill counterparts. There were also six deaths during the study, all among the more ill participants: five in the placebo group, but only one in the vitamin C group.

Mochalkin (1970) examined the effect of vitamin C on pneumonia patients in the former Soviet Union [25]. Although a placebo was not administered to the control group, two different doses of vitamin C were used and the observed difference between the low and high dosage cannot be explained by the placebo effect. The high-dose regime administered on average twice the quantity of vitamin C of the low dose, but both of them were related to the dosage of antibiotics so that the low dose vitamin C ranged from 0.25 to 0.8 g/day, and the high dose ranged from 0.5 to 1.6 g/day. The duration of hospital stay in the control group (no vitamin C supplementation) was 23.7 days. In the low dose vitamin C group the hospital stay was 19% shorter and in the high dose vitamin C group it was 36% shorter. A benefit was also reported on the normalization of chest X-ray, temperature, and erythrocyte sedimentation rate.

Although both of these therapeutic studies give support to the old case reports stating that vitamin C is beneficial for pneumonia patients, the findings cannot be directly generalized to typical pneumonia patients of Western countries.

8. Tetanus

Tetanus is a disease caused by the toxin of *Clostridium tetani*, which may contaminate wounds. An early case report claimed that vitamin C was beneficial against tetanus in an unvaccinated six-year-old boy in the USA [128]. A Cochrane review identified one controlled trial in which the effect of vitamin C on tetanus patients was examined [129,130].

Jahan (1984) studied the effect of 1 g/day of intravenous vitamin C on tetanus patients in Bangladesh [131]. In children aged one to 12 years, there were no deaths in the vitamin C group, whereas there were 23 deaths in the control group ($p = 10^{-9}$) [1] (p. 17). In tetanus patients aged 13 to 30 years, there were 10 deaths in the vitamin C group compared with 19 deaths in the control group ($p = 0.03$). The significant difference between the above-described age groups may be caused by the difference in the body weights of the patients. In the young children the same dose of vitamin C corresponds to a substantially higher dose per unit of weight. Although there were methodological weaknesses in the trial, they are unlikely explanations for the dramatic difference in the younger participants [129].

9. Other Infections

The effect of vitamin C supplementation on the common cold has been most extensively studied. One important reason for extensive research on vitamin C and the common cold seems to be the wide publicity given to it by Pauling [1,132]. Probably some researchers wanted to show that Pauling was either right or wrong, whereas others just wanted to study a topic about which a Nobel Prize winner had put his credibility on the line. Another reason for the large number of studies on the common cold is that it is a non-severe ubiquitous infection, and it is very easy to find common cold patients in schools and work places. It is much more difficult to study more serious infections.

The three infections discussed above, the common cold, pneumonia, and tetanus, were selected on the basis that the effects of vitamin C have been evaluated in Cochrane reviews, which entails a thorough literature search and a careful analysis of the identified trials. However, the selection of these three infections does not imply that the effects of vitamin C are limited to them.

Table 2 indicates that vitamin C may have effects on various infections caused by viruses, bacteria, *Candida albicans* and protozoa. Vitamin C might have similar effects in humans. However, it also seems evident that the role of additional vitamin C depends on various factors such as the initial dietary intake level, other nutritional status, the exposure level to pathogens, the level of exercise and temperature stress, etc.

Three extensive searches of the older literature on vitamin C and infections have been published, and they give an extensive list of references, but none of these publications gave a balanced discussion of the findings [133–135]. A few studies on the possible effects of vitamin C on other infections are outlined below, but this selection is not systematic.

Terezhalmy (1978) [136] used a double-blind placebo-controlled RCT and found that the duration of pain caused by herpes labialis was shortened by 51%, from 3.5 to 1.3 days ($p = 10^{-8}$), when patients were administered 1 g/day of vitamin C together with bioflavonoids [1] (pp. 15–17). Furthermore, when vitamin C treatment was initiated within 24 hours of the onset of the symptoms, only six out of 26 patients (23%) developed herpes vesicles, whereas with later initiation of vitamin C, eight out of 12 patients (67%) developed vesicles ($p = 0.003$ in the test of interaction). Vitamin C was administered with bioflavonoids, so the study was not specific to vitamin C, but there is no compelling evidence to indicate that bioflavonoids affect infections.

Herpes zoster (reactivation of varicella zoster virus) can cause long lasting post-herpetic neuralgia (PHN). Chen (2009) found that patients with PHN had significantly lower plasma vitamin C plasma than healthy volunteers, and their RCT showed that vitamin C administration significantly decreased the pain level of PHN [137]. A number of other reports have also suggested that vitamin C may be effective against the pain caused by herpes zoster [138–142].

Patrone (1982) and Levy (1996) reported that vitamin C administration was beneficial to patients who had recurrent infections, mainly of the skin [143,144]. Many of the patients had impaired neutrophil functions and therefore the findings cannot be generalized to the ordinary population.

Galley (1997) reported that vitamin C increased the cardiac index in patients with septic shock [145]. Pleiner (2002) reported that intravenous vitamin C administration preserved vascular reactivity to acetylcholine in study participants who had been experimentally administered *Escherichia coli* endotoxin [146].

It seems unlikely that the effects of vitamin C on herpetic pain, cardiac index and the vascular system are mediated through effects on the immune system. Such effects are probably caused by other mechanisms instead. The question of the possible benefits of vitamin C against infections is therefore not just a question about the immune system effects of the vitamin, as was discussed earlier in this review (see Section 2.7).

Some physicians used vitamin C for a large set of infectious disease patients and described their experiences in case reports that are worth reading [89,147].

10. Observational Studies on Vitamin C and Infections

Cohort studies on vitamins are often unreliable because diet is strongly associated with numerous lifestyle factors that cannot be fully adjusted for in statistical models. Therefore, there may always remain an unknown level of residual confounding [148]. The main source of vitamin C in the diet is fruit, and high dietary vitamin C intake essentially always means a high fruit intake [149]. Thus, any substantial correlations between vitamin C intake and infections could also reflect some other substances in fruit. Only two observational studies are commented upon in this section.

Merchant (2004) studied men whose ages ranged from 40 to 75 years in the USA and found no association between their vitamin C intake and community-acquired pneumonia [124]. These males were U.S. health professionals; thus they were of a population that has a great interest in factors that affect health. The incidence of pneumonia was only three cases per 1000 person-years (Table 7). The median vitamin C intake of the lowest quintile was 0.095 g/day and of the highest quintile it was 1.1 g/day. In contrast, the overall median of the adult U.S. population is about 0.1 g/day, and 10% of the U.S. population has an intake level of less than 0.04 g/day [14]. Thus, Merchant and colleagues' cohort study indicates that increasing the vitamin C intake upwards from the median level in the USA will not lead to any further decline in the already low pneumonia incidence among male health professionals. However, the study is uninformative about whether decreasing vitamin C level downwards from 0.1 g/day might increase pneumonia risk, or about whether vitamin C might have effects in populations that have particularly high incidences of pneumonia (Table 7). Even though we must be cautious about interpreting observational studies, it seems that biological differences, rather than methodological differences, are most reasonable explanations for the divergence between the findings in the Merchant et al. cohort study and the three controlled trials shown in Table 7.

A cohort analysis of Finnish male smokers that is part of the Alpha-Tocopherol Beta-Carotene Cancer prevention (ATBC) Study found a significant inverse association between dietary vitamin C intake and tuberculosis risk in participants who were not administered vitamin E supplements [150,151]. The highest quartile had the median dietary vitamin C intake level of 0.15 g/day, whereas the lowest quartile had an intake level of only 0.052 g/day. The adjusted risk of tuberculosis in the lowest vitamin C intake quartile was 150% higher than that of the highest intake quartile. This is consistent with the animal studies that found that low vitamin C intake increases the susceptibility to, and severity of, tuberculosis (Tables 1–3).

11. Potentially Harmful Interactions between Vitamins C and E

Vitamin C and vitamin E are both antioxidants and they protect against ROS. Therefore, these substances are of parallel interest as water-soluble vitamin C regenerates the lipid-soluble vitamin E in vitro [152]. Dietary vitamin C intake modified the effect of vitamin E on mortality in the ATBC Study, which indicates that these substances may also have clinically important interactions [153]. However, the major sources of the vitamin C in this subgroup were fruit, vegetables and berries and other substances in these foods might also have explained the modification of the vitamin E effect. Such a possibility was refuted by calculating the residual intake of fruit, vegetables and berries, and showing that the residual did not modify the effect of vitamin E. Vitamin C was thus indicated as the specific modifying factor. A similar approach was used to show that vitamin C specifically modified the effect of vitamin E on pneumonia [154].

Two subgroups of the ATBC Study were identified in which the combination of high dietary vitamin C intake and vitamin E supplementation increased the risk of pneumonia by 248% and 1350% when compared with high vitamin C intake without vitamin E (Table 8). In the former subgroup, one extra case of pneumonia was caused for every 13 participants and in the latter subgroup, for every 28 participants. In both subgroups, the residual intake of fruit, vegetables and berries did not modify the effect of vitamin E, indicating specificity of vitamin C. The total number of participants in the ATBC Study was 29,133 and in that respect the identified subgroups were relatively small and at 1081 individuals only amounted to 4% of all the ATBC participants. However, in these two subgroups the harm arising from the combination of vitamins C and E was substantial [154].

Another subgroup analysis of the ATBC Study found that the combination of high vitamin C intake together with vitamin E supplementation increased the risk of tuberculosis in heavy smokers by 125% compared with high vitamin C alone subgroup (Table 8). Thus, one extra case of tuberculosis arose in every 240 participants who had high intakes of vitamins C and E [150,151].

ROS have been implicated in the pathogenesis of diverse diseases, including infections. Antioxidants have been assumed to be beneficial since they react with ROS. However, given the suggestions that people should take vitamins C and E to improve their immune system, the subgroup findings in Table 8 are somewhat alarming. Nevertheless, the harm in the three subgroups is limited to the combination of vitamins C and E. This author does not know of any findings that indicate that similar doses of vitamin C alone might cause harm.

Table 8. Increase in pneumonia and tuberculosis risk with the combination of vitamins C and E.

Infection, ATBC Study Subgroup	No. of Participants	Effect of Vitamin E RR (95% CI)	Test of Interaction p	NNH
Pneumonia Body weight < 60 kg who started smoking at ≤20 years Dietary vitamin C				
<median	467	0.98 (0.48 to 2.0)	0.026	
≥median (75 mg/day)	468	3.48 (1.61 to 7.5)		13
Pneumonia Body weight ≥ 100 kg who started smoking at ≤20 years Dietary vitamin C				
<median	613	1.37 (0.46 to 4.0)	0.019	
≥median (95 mg/day)	613	14.5 (1.84 to 114)		28
Tuberculosis Smoking ≥ 20 cigarettes/day Dietary vitamin C				
<median	9073	0.82 (0.50 to 1.33)	0.011 [a]	
≥median (90 mg/day)	8172	2.25 (1.19 to 4.23)		240

Subgroups of the ATBC Study in which vitamin C increased the risk of pneumonia and tuberculosis [150,151,154]. ATBC Study, Alpha-Tocopherol Beta-Carotene Cancer prevention Study. NNH, number needed to harm: how many people in the particular subgroup need to be exposed to the treatment to cause harm to one person. RR, relative risk. [a] Interaction test was calculated for this review.

12. Misconceptions and Prejudices about Vitamin C and Infections

In the first half of the 20th century, a large number of papers were published in the medical literature on vitamin C and infections and several physicians were enthusiastic about vitamin C. The topic was not dismissed because of large-scale controlled trials showing that vitamin C was ineffective. Instead, many rather large trials found benefits of vitamin C. There seem to be four particular reasons why the interest in vitamin C and infections disappeared.

First, antibiotics were introduced in the mid-20th century. They have specific and sometimes very dramatic effects on bacterial infections and therefore are much more rational first line drugs for patients with serious infections than vitamin C. Secondly, vitamin C was identified as the explanation for scurvy, which was considered a disease of the connective tissues. Evidently it seemed irrational to consider that a substance that "only" participates in collagen metabolism might also have effects on infections. However, the biochemistry and actions of vitamin C are complex and not limited to collagen metabolism. Thirdly, the three papers published in 1975 appeared to herald the loss of interest in vitamin C and the common cold (Figure 1) and it seems likely that they increased the negative attitude towards vitamin C for other infections as well. Fourthly, "if a treatment bypasses the medical establishment and is sold directly to the public ... the temptation in the medical community is to accept uncritically the first bad news that comes along" [155].

The belief that vitamin C is "ineffective" has been widely spread. For example, a survey of general practitioners in the Netherlands revealed that 47% of respondents considered that homeopathy is efficacious for the treatment of the common cold, whereas only 20% of those respondents considered that vitamin C was [156]. Prejudices against vitamin C are not limited to the common cold. Richards compared the attitudes and arguments of physicians to three putative cancer medicines, 5-fluorouracil, interferon and vitamin C, and documented unambiguous bias against vitamin C [157–159]. Goodwin and Tangum gave several examples to support the conclusion that there has been a systematic bias against the concept that vitamins may yield benefits in levels higher than the minimum needed to avoid the classic deficiency diseases [160].

The use of vitamin C for preventing and treating colds falls into the category of alternative medicine under the classifications used by the National Institutes of Health in the USA and of the Cochrane collaboration. However, such categorization does not reflect the level of evidence for vitamin C, but reflects the low level of acceptance amongst the medical community, and may further amplify the inertia and prejudices against vitamin C [161].

13. Conclusions

From a large series of animal studies we may conclude that vitamin C plays a role in preventing, shortening, and alleviating diverse infections. It seems evident that vitamin C has similar effects in humans. Controlled studies have shown that vitamin C shortens and alleviates the common cold and prevents colds under specific conditions and in restricted population subgroups. Five controlled trials found significant effects of vitamin C against pneumonia. There is some evidence that vitamin C may also have effects on other infections, but there is a paucity of such data. The practical importance and optimally efficacious doses of vitamin C for preventing and treating infections are unknown. Vitamin C is safe and costs only pennies per gram, and therefore even modest effects may be worth exploiting.

Supplementary Materials: The following are available online at http://www.mdpi.com/2072-6643/9/4/339/s1, Supplementary file 1 and Supplementary file 2.

Acknowledgments: No external funding. Parts of this review were published as earlier versions in the dissertation by Hemilä (2006) [1]. Links to translations of the non-English papers cited in this review and many other references are available at [9].

Conflicts of Interest: The author declares no conflict of interest.

References

1. Hemilä, H. Do vitamins C and E affect Respiratory Infections? Ph.D. Thesis, University of Helsinki, Helsinki, Finland, 2006. Available online: https://hdl.handle.net/10138/20335 (accessed on 17 March 2017).
2. Carpenter, K.J. *The History of Scurvy and Vitamin C*; Cambridge University Press: Cambridge, UK, 1986.
3. Hess, A.F. *Scurvy: Past and Present*; Lippincott: Philadelphia, PA, USA, 1920. Available online: http://chla.library.cornell.edu (accessed on 17 March 2017).
4. Hess, A.F. Diet, nutrition and infection. *N. Engl. J. Med.* **1932**, *207*, 637–648. [CrossRef]
5. Robertson, E.C. The vitamins and resistance to infection: Vitamin C. *Medicine* **1934**, *13*, 190–206. [CrossRef]
6. Englard, S.; Seifter, S. The biochemical functions of ascorbic acid. *Annu. Rev. Nutr.* **1986**, *6*, 365–406. [PubMed]
7. Clausen, S.W. The influence of nutrition upon resistance to infection. *Physiol. Rev.* **1934**, *14*, 309–350.
8. Perla, D.; Marmorston, J. Role of vitamin C in resistance. Parts I and II. *Arch. Pathol.* **1937**, *23*, 543–575, 683–712.
9. Hemilä, H. Vitamin C and Infections. Available online: http://www.mv.helsinki.fi/home/hemila/N2017 (accessed on 17 March 2017).
10. De Gruttola, V.; Fleming, T.; Lin, D.Y.; Coombs, R. Validating surrogate markers—Are we being naive? *J. Infect. Dis.* **1997**, *175*, 237–246. [CrossRef] [PubMed]
11. Levine, M.; Conry-Cantilena, C.; Wang, Y.; Welch, R.W.; Washko, P.W.; Dhariwal, K.R.; Park, J.B.; Lazarev, A.; Graumlich, J.F.; King, J.; et al. Vitamin C pharmacokinetics in healthy volunteers: Evidence for a recommended dietary allowance. *Proc. Natl. Acad. Sci. USA* **1996**, *93*, 3704–3709. [CrossRef] [PubMed]
12. Bartley, W.; Krebs, H.A.; O'Brien, J.R.P. *Vitamin C Requirement of Human Adults*; A Report by the Vitamin C Subcommittee of the Accessory Food Factors Committee; Her Majesty's Stationery Office (HMSO): London, UK, 1953.
13. Hodges, R.E.; Hood, J.; Canham, J.E.; Sauberlich, H.E.; Baker, E.M. Clinical manifestations of ascorbic acid deficiency in man. *Am. J. Clin. Nutr.* **1971**, *24*, 432–443. [PubMed]
14. Food and Nutrition Board. *Food and Nutrition Board, Institute of Medicine: Dietary Reference Intakes for Vitamin C, Vitamin E, Selenium and Carotenoids*; National Academy Press: Washington, DC, USA, 2000; pp. 95–185.
15. Segal, A.W. How neutrophils kill microbes. *Annu. Rev. Immunol.* **2005**, *23*, 197–223. [CrossRef] [PubMed]
16. Akaike, T. Role of free radicals in viral pathogenesis and mutation. *Rev. Med. Virol.* **2001**, *11*, 87–101. [CrossRef] [PubMed]
17. Peterhans, E. Oxidants and antioxidants in viral diseases. *J. Nutr.* **1997**, *127*, 962S–965S. [PubMed]
18. Wang, Y.; Russo, T.A.; Kwon, O.; Chanock, S.; Rumsey, S.C.; Levine, M. Ascorbate recycling in human neutrophils: Induction by bacteria. *Proc. Natl. Acad. Sci. USA* **1997**, *94*, 13816–13819. [CrossRef] [PubMed]
19. Nualart, F.J.; Rivas, C.I.; Montecinos, V.P.; Godoy, A.S.; Guaiquil, V.H.; Golde, D.W.; Vera, J.C. Recycling of vitamin C by a bystander effect. *J. Biol. Chem.* **2003**, *278*, 10128–10133. [CrossRef] [PubMed]
20. Buffinton, G.D.; Christen, S.; Peterhans, E.; Stocker, R. Oxidative stress in lungs of mice infected with influenza A virus. *Free Radic. Res. Commun.* **1992**, *16*, 99–110. [CrossRef] [PubMed]
21. Li, W.; Maeda, N.; Beck, A. Vitamin C deficiency increases the lung pathology of influenza virus-infected gulo−/− mice. *J. Nutr.* **2006**, *136*, 2611–2616. [PubMed]
22. Hosakote, Y.M.; Jantzi, P.D.; Esham, D.L.; Spratt, H.; Kurosky, A.; Casola, A.; Garofalo, R.P. Viral-mediated inhibition of antioxidant enzymes contributes to the pathogenesis of severe respiratory syncytial virus bronchiolitis. *Am. J. Respir. Crit. Care Med.* **2011**, *183*, 1550–1560. [CrossRef] [PubMed]
23. Hemilä, H. Vitamin C and the common cold. *Br. J. Nutr.* **1992**, *67*, 3–16. [CrossRef] [PubMed]
24. Hume, R.; Weyers, E. Changes in leucocyte ascorbic acid during the common cold. *Scott. Med. J.* **1973**, *18*, 3–7. [CrossRef] [PubMed]
25. Mochalkin, N.I. Ascorbic acid in the complex therapy of acute pneumonia. *Voenno-Meditsinskii Zhurnal* **1970**, *9*, 17–21. (In Russian). [PubMed]
26. Hunt, C.; Chakravorty, N.K.; Annan, G.; Habibzadeh, N.; Schorah, C.J. The clinical effects of vitamin C supplementation in elderly hospitalised patients with acute respiratory infections. *Int. J. Vitam. Nutr. Res.* **1994**, *64*, 212–219. [PubMed]
27. Hemilä, H.; Louhiala, P. Vitamin C for preventing and treating pneumonia. *Cochrane Database Syst. Rev.* **2013**, *8*, CD005532.

28. Hemilä, H.; Louhiala, P. Vitamin C for Preventing and Treating Pneumonia. Available online: http://www.mv.helsinki.fi/home/hemila/CP (accessed on 17 March 2017).

29. Powers, S.K.; Jackson, M.J. Exercise-induced oxidative stress: Cellular mechanisms and impact on muscle force production. *Physiol. Rev.* **2008**, *88*, 1243–1276. [CrossRef] [PubMed]

30. Ashton, T.; Young, I.S.; Peters, J.R.; Jones, E.; Jackson, S.K.; Davies, B.; Rowlands, C.C. Electron spin resonance spectroscopy, exercise, and oxidative stress: An ascorbic acid intervention study. *J. Appl. Physiol.* **1999**, *87*, 2032–2036. [PubMed]

31. Mullins, A.L.; van Rosendal, S.P.; Briskey, D.R.; Fassett, R.G.; Wilson, G.R.; Coombes, J.S. Variability in oxidative stress biomarkers following a maximal exercise test. *Biomarkers* **2013**, *18*, 446–454. [CrossRef] [PubMed]

32. Hemilä, H. Vitamin C may alleviate exercise-induced bronchoconstriction: A meta-analysis. *BMJ Open* **2013**, *3*, e002416. [CrossRef] [PubMed]

33. Hemilä, H. The effect of vitamin C on bronchoconstriction and respiratory symptoms caused by exercise: A review and statistical analysis. *Allergy Asthma Clin. Immunol.* **2014**, *10*, 58. [CrossRef] [PubMed]

34. LeBlanc, J.; Stewart, M.; Marier, G.; Whillans, M.G. Studies on acclimatization and on the effect of ascorbic acid in men exposed to cold. *Can. J. Biochem. Physiol.* **1954**, *32*, 407–427. [CrossRef] [PubMed]

35. Dugal, L.P. Vitamin C in relation to cold temperature tolerance. *Ann. N. Y. Acad. Sci.* **1961**, *92*, 307–317. [CrossRef] [PubMed]

36. Strydom, N.B.; Kotze, H.F.; van der Walt, W.H.; Rogers, G.G. Effect of ascorbic acid on rate of heat acclimatization. *J. Appl. Physiol.* **1976**, *41*, 202–205. [PubMed]

37. Chang, C.Y.; Chen, J.Y.; Chen, S.H.; Cheng, T.J.; Lin, M.T.; Hu, M.L. Therapeutic treatment with ascorbate rescues mice from heat stroke-induced death by attenuating systemic inflammatory response and hypothalamic neuronal damage. *Free Radic. Biol. Med.* **2016**, *93*, 84–93. [CrossRef] [PubMed]

38. Holley, A.D.; Osland, E.; Barnes, J.; Krishnan, A.; Fraser, J.F. Scurvy: Historically a plague of the sailor that remains a consideration in the modern intensive care unit. *Intern. Med. J.* **2011**, *41*, 283–285. [CrossRef] [PubMed]

39. Smith, A.; Di Primio, G.; Humphrey-Murto, S. Scurvy in the developed world. *Can. Med. Assoc. J.* **2011**, *183*, E752–E752. [CrossRef] [PubMed]

40. Raynaud-Simon, A.; Cohen-Bittan, J.; Gouronnec, A.; Pautas, E.; Senet, P.; Verny, M.; Boddaert, J. Scurvy in hospitalized elderly patients. *J. Nutr. Health Aging* **2010**, *14*, 407–410. [PubMed]

41. Hemilä, H.; Louhiala, P. Vitamin C may affect lung infections. *J. R. Soc. Med.* **2007**, *100*, 495–498. [CrossRef] [PubMed]

42. Beisel, W.R. Single nutrients and immunity: Vitamin C. *Am. J. Clin. Nutr.* **1982**, *35*, 423–428, 460–461.

43. Webb, A.L.; Villamor, E. Update: Effects of antioxidant and non-antioxidant vitamin supplementation on immune function. *Nutr. Rev.* **2007**, *65*, 181–217. [CrossRef] [PubMed]

44. Manning, J.; Mitchell, B.; Appadurai, D.A.; Shakya, A.; Pierce, L.J.; Wang, H.; Nganga, V.; Swanson, P.C.; May, J.M.; Tantin, D.; et al. Vitamin C promotes maturation of T-cells. *Antioxid. Redox Signal.* **2013**, *19*, 2054–2067. [PubMed]

45. Jones, E.; Hughes, R.E. Influence of oral carnitine on the body weight and survival time of avitaminotic-C guinea pigs. *Nutr. Rep. Int.* **1982**, *25*, 201–204.

46. Mårtensson, J.; Han, J.; Griffith, O.W.; Meister, A. Glutathione ester delays the onset of scurvy in ascorbate-deficient guinea pigs. *Proc. Natl. Acad. Sci. USA* **1993**, *90*, 317–321. [CrossRef] [PubMed]

47. Padh, H. Cellular functions of ascorbic acid. *Biochem. Cell Biol.* **1990**, *68*, 1166–1173. [CrossRef] [PubMed]

48. Rebouche, C.J. Ascorbic acid and carnitine biosynthesis. *Am. J. Clin. Nutr.* **1991**, *54*, 1147S–1152S. [PubMed]

49. Rice, M.E. Ascorbate regulation and its neuroprotective role in the brain. *Trends Neurol. Sci.* **2000**, *23*, 209–216.

50. May, J.M.; Harrison, F.E. Role of vitamin C in the function of the vascular endothelium. *Antioxid. Redox Signal.* **2013**, *19*, 2068–2083. [CrossRef] [PubMed]

51. Kinsman, R.A.; Hood, J. Some behavioral effects of ascorbic acid deficiency. *Am. J. Clin. Nutr.* **1971**, *24*, 455–464. [PubMed]

52. Zhang, M.; Robitaille, L.; Eintracht, S.; Hoffer, L.J. Vitamin C provision improves mood in acutely hospitalized patients. *Nutrition* **2011**, *27*, 530–533. [CrossRef] [PubMed]

53. Wang, Y.; Liu, X.J.; Robitaille, L.; Eintracht, S.; MacNamara, E.; Hoffer, L.J. Effects of vitamin C and vitamin D administration on mood and distress in acutely hospitalized patients. *Am. J. Clin. Nutr.* **2013**, *98*, 705–711. [CrossRef] [PubMed]

54. Hemilä, H.; Kaprio, J. Subgroup analysis of large trials can guide further research: A case study of vitamin E and pneumonia. *Clin. Epidemiol.* **2011**, *3*, 51–59. [CrossRef] [PubMed]

55. Hemilä, H. Vitamin E and the risk of pneumonia: Using the I^2-statistic to quantify heterogeneity within a controlled trial. *Br. J. Nutr.* **2016**, *116*, 1530–1536. [CrossRef] [PubMed]

56. Hemilä, H.; Virtamo, J.; Albanes, D.; Kaprio, J. The effect of vitamin E on common cold incidence is modified by age, smoking and residential neighborhood. *J. Am. Coll. Nutr.* **2006**, *25*, 332–339. [CrossRef] [PubMed]

57. McConkey, M.; Smith, D.T. The relation of vitamin C deficiency to intestinal tuberculosis in the guinea pig. *J. Exp. Med.* **1933**, *58*, 503–517. [CrossRef] [PubMed]

58. Dey, P.K. Efficacy of vitamin C in counteracting tetanus toxin toxicity. *Naturwissenschaften* **1966**, *53*, 310. [CrossRef] [PubMed]

59. Belfield, W.O. Vitamin C in treatment of canine and feline distemper complex. *Vet. Med. Small Anim. Clin.* **1967**, *62*, 345–348. [PubMed]

60. Leveque, J.I. Ascorbic acid in treatment of the canine distemper complex. *Vet. Med. Small Anim. Clin.* **1969**, *64*, 997–1001. [PubMed]

61. Eccles, R. Is the common cold a clinical entity or a cultural concept? *Rhinology* **2013**, *51*, 3–8. [PubMed]

62. Monto, A.S.; Ullman, B.M. Acute respiratory illness in an American community: The Tecumseh Study. *JAMA* **1974**, *227*, 164–169. [PubMed]

63. Fendrick, A.M.; Monto, A.S.; Nightengale, B.; Sarnes, M. The economic burden of non-influenza-related viral respiratory tract infection in the United States. *Arch. Int. Med.* **2003**, *163*, 487–494. [CrossRef]

64. Pauling, L. *Vitamin C and the Common Cold*; Freeman: San Francisco, CA, USA, 1970.

65. Pauling, L. The significance of the evidence about ascorbic acid and the common cold. *Proc. Natl. Acad. Sci. USA* **1971**, *68*, 2678–2681. [CrossRef] [PubMed]

66. Pauling, L. Ascorbic acid and the common cold. *Am. J. Clin. Nutr.* **1971**, *24*, 1294–1299. [CrossRef] [PubMed]

67. Ritzel, G. Critical analysis of the role of vitamin C in the treatment of the common cold. *Helv. Med. Acta* **1961**, *28*, 63–68. (In German). [PubMed]

68. Hemilä, H.; Chalker, E. Vitamin C for preventing and treating the common cold. *Cochrane Database Syst. Rev.* **2013**, *1*, CD000980.

69. Hemilä, H.; Chalker, E. Vitamin C for Preventing and Treating the Common Cold. Available online: http://www.mv.helsinki.fi/home/hemila/CC (accessed on 17 March 2017).

70. Hemilä, H. Vitamin C supplementation and common cold symptoms: Problems with inaccurate reviews. *Nutrition* **1996**, *12*, 804–809. [CrossRef]

71. Chalmers, T.C. Effects of ascorbic acid on the common cold: An evaluation of the evidence. *Am. J. Med.* **1975**, *58*, 532–536. [CrossRef]

72. Karlowski, T.R.; Chalmers, T.C.; Frenkel, L.D.; Kapikian, A.Z.; Lewis, T.L.; Lynch, J.M. Ascorbic acid for the common cold: A prophylactic and therapeutic trial. *JAMA* **1975**, *231*, 1038–1042. [PubMed]

73. Dykes, M.H.M.; Meier, P. Ascorbic acid and the common cold: Evaluation of its efficacy and toxicity. *JAMA* **1975**, *231*, 1073–1079. [CrossRef] [PubMed]

74. Hemilä, H. Vitamin C intake and susceptibility to the common cold. *Br. J. Nutr.* **1997**, *77*, 59–72. [CrossRef] [PubMed]

75. Bates, C.J.; Schorah, C.J.; Hemilä, H. Vitamin C intake and susceptibility to the common cold: Invited comments and Reply. *Br. J. Nutr.* **1997**, *78*, 857–866. [PubMed]

76. Hemilä, H. Vitamin C and common cold incidence: A review of studies with subjects under heavy physical stress. *Int. J. Sports Med.* **1996**, *17*, 379–383. [CrossRef] [PubMed]

77. Hemilä, H. Vitamin C and sex differences in respiratory tract infections. *Respir. Med.* **2008**, *102*, 625–626. [CrossRef] [PubMed]

78. Baird, I.M.; Hughes, R.E.; Wilson, H.K.; Davies, J.E.; Howard, A.N. The effects of ascorbic acid and flavonoids on the occurrence of symptoms normally associated with the common cold. *Am. J. Clin. Nutr.* **1979**, *32*, 1686–1690. [PubMed]

79. Johnston, C.S.; Barkyoumb, G.M.; Schumacher, S.S. Vitamin C supplementation slightly improves physical activity levels and reduces cold incidence in men with marginal vitamin C status: A randomized controlled trial. *Nutrients* **2014**, *6*, 2572–2583. [CrossRef] [PubMed]

80. Anderson, T.W.; Reid, D.B.W.; Beaton, G.H. Vitamin C and the common cold: A double-blind trial. *Can. Med. Assoc. J.* **1972**, *107*, 503–508. [PubMed]

81. Coulehan, J.L.; Reisinger, K.S.; Rogers, K.D.; Bradley, D.W. Vitamin C prophylaxis in a boarding school. *N. Engl. J. Med.* **1974**, *290*, 6–10. [CrossRef] [PubMed]

82. Van Straten, M.; Josling, P. Preventing the common cold with a vitamin C supplement: A double-blind, placebo-controlled survey. *Adv. Ther.* **2002**, *19*, 151–159. [CrossRef] [PubMed]

83. Hemilä, H. Vitamin C supplementation and common cold symptoms: Factors affecting the magnitude of the benefit. *Med. Hypotheses* **1999**, *52*, 171–178. [PubMed]

84. Anderson, T.W.; Suranyi, G.; Beaton, G.H. The effect on winter illness of large doses of vitamin C. *Can. Med. Assoc. J.* **1974**, *111*, 31–36. [PubMed]

85. Anderson, T.W.; Beaton, G.H.; Corey, P.N.; Spero, L. Winter illness and vitamin C: The effect of relatively low doses. *Can. Med. Assoc. J.* **1975**, *112*, 823–826. [PubMed]

86. Constantini, N.W.; Dubnov-Raz, G.; Eyal, B.B.; Berry, E.M.; Cohen, A.H.; Hemilä, H. The effect of vitamin C on upper respiratory infections in adolescent swimmers: A randomized trial. *Eur. J. Pediatr.* **2011**, *170*, 59–63. [CrossRef] [PubMed]

87. Carr, A.B.; Einstein, R.; Lai, Y.C.; Martin, N.G.; Starmer, G.A. Vitamin C and the common cold: A second MZ co-twin control study. *Acta Genet. Med. Gemellol.* **1981**, *30*, 249–255. [CrossRef] [PubMed]

88. Bee, D.M. The vitamin C controversy. *Postgrad. Med.* **1980**, *67*, 64. [CrossRef] [PubMed]

89. Cathcart, R.F. Vitamin, C.; titrating to bowel tolerance, anascorbemia, and acute induced scurvy. *Med. Hypotheses* **1981**, *7*, 1359–1376. [CrossRef]

90. Gern, J.E. The ABCs of rhinoviruses, wheezing, and asthma. *J. Virol.* **2010**, *84*, 7418–7426. [CrossRef] [PubMed]

91. Hemilä, H. Vitamin C and common cold-induced asthma: A systematic review and statistical analysis. *Allergy Asthma Clin. Immunol.* **2013**, *9*, 46. [CrossRef] [PubMed]

92. Anah, C.O.; Jarike, L.N.; Baig, H.A. High dose ascorbic acid in Nigerian asthmatics. *Trop. Geogr. Med.* **1980**, *32*, 132–137. [PubMed]

93. Schertling, M.; Winsel, K.; Müller, S.; Henning, R.; Meiske, W.; Slapke, J. Action of ascorbic acid on clinical course of infection related bronchial asthma and on reactive oxygen metabolites by BAL cells. *Z. Klin. Med.* **1990**, *45*, 1770–1774. (In German).

94. Bucca, C.; Rolla, G.; Arossa, W.; Caria, E.; Elia, C.; Nebiolo, F.; Baldi, S. Effect of ascorbic acid on increased bronchial responsiveness during upper airway infection. *Respiration* **1989**, *55*, 214–219. [CrossRef] [PubMed]

95. Miegl, H. Acute upper respiratory tract infection and its treatment with vitamin C. *Wien. Med. Wochenschr.* **1957**, *107*, 989–992. (In German). [PubMed]

96. Miegl, H. About the use of vitamin C in otorhinolaryngology. *Wien. Med. Wochenschr.* **1958**, *108*, 859–864. (In German) [PubMed]

97. Glazebrook, A.J.; Thomson, S. The administration of vitamin C in a large institution and its effect on general health and resistance to infection. *J. Hyg.* **1942**, *42*, 1–19. [CrossRef] [PubMed]

98. Sabiston, B.H.; Radomski, M.W. *Health Problems and Vitamin C in Canadian Northern Military Operations*; DCIEM Report No. 74-R-1012; Defence and Civil Institute of Environmental Medicine: Downsview, ON, Canada, 1974.

99. Peters, E.M.; Goetzsche, J.M.; Grobbelaar, B.; Noakes, T.D. Vitamin C supplementation reduces the incidence of postrace symptoms of upper-respiratory-tract infection in ultramarathon runners. *Am. J. Clin. Nutr.* **1993**, *57*, 170–174. [PubMed]

100. Cowan, D.W.; Diehl, H.S.; Baker, A.B. Vitamins for the prevention of colds. *JAMA* **1942**, *120*, 1268–1271. [CrossRef]

101. Miller, J.Z.; Nance, W.E.; Norton, J.A.; Wolen, R.L.; Griffith, R.S.; Rose, R.J. Therapeutic effect of vitamin C: A co-twin control study. *JAMA* **1977**, *237*, 248–251. [CrossRef] [PubMed]

102. Liberati, A. Thomas C Chalmers. *Lancet* **1996**, *347*, 188. [CrossRef]

103. Dickersin, K. Thomas Clark Chalmers. *JAMA* **1996**, *276*, 656–657. [CrossRef]

104. Pincock, S. Paul Meier. *Lancet* **2011**, *378*, 978. [CrossRef]

105. Betts, K. Paul Meier: A man behind the method. *Am. J. Public Health* **2012**, *102*, 2026–2029. [CrossRef] [PubMed]

106. Hemilä, H. Vitamin, C.; the placebo effect, and the common cold: A case study of how preconceptions influence the analysis of results. *J. Clin. Epidemiol.* **1996**, *49*, 1079–1084.

107. Hemilä, H. Analysis of clinical data with breached blindness. *Stat. Med.* **2006**, *25*, 1434–1437. [CrossRef] [PubMed]

108. Chalmers, T.C. Dissent to the preceding article by H. Hemilä. *J. Clin. Epidemiol.* **1996**, *49*, 1085. [CrossRef]

109. Hemilä, H. To the dissent by Thomas Chalmers. *J. Clin. Epidemiol.* **1996**, *49*, 1087. [CrossRef]

110. Hemilä, H.; Herman, Z.S. Vitamin C and the common cold: A retrospective analysis of Chalmers' review. *J. Am. Coll. Nutr.* **1995**, *14*, 116–123. [CrossRef] [PubMed]

111. Pauling, L. Ascorbic acid and the common cold: Evaluation of its efficacy and toxicity. Part I. *Med. Tribune* **1976**, *17*, 18–19. [CrossRef] [PubMed]

112. Pauling, L. Ascorbic acid and the common cold. Part II. *Med. Tribune* **1976**, *17*, 37–38.

113. Council of Scientific Affairs, American Medical Association. Vitamin preparations as dietary supplements and as therapeutic agents. *JAMA* **1987**, *257*, 1929–1936.

114. Gander, J.; Niederberger, W. Vitamin C in the treatment of pneumonia. *Münch. Med. Wochenschr.* **1936**, *83*, 2074–2077. (In German).

115. Bohnholtzer, E. Contribution to the question of pneumonia treatment with vitamin C. *Dtsch. Med. Wochenschr.* **1937**, *63*, 1001–1003. (In German). [CrossRef]

116. Hochwald, A. Vitamin C in the treatment of croupous pneumonia. *Dtsch. Med. Wochenschr.* **1937**, *63*, 182–184. (In German). [CrossRef]

117. Klenner, F.R. Virus pneumonia and its treatment with vitamin C. *South. Med. Surg.* **1948**, *110*, 36–38. [PubMed]

118. Klenner, F.R. Massive doses of vitamin C and the virus diseases. *South. Med. Surg.* **1951**, *113*, 101–107. [PubMed]

119. Dalton, W.L. Massive doses of vitamin C in the treatment of viral diseases. *J. Indiana State Med. Assoc.* **1962**, *55*, 1151–1154. [PubMed]

120. Hemilä, H. Vitamin C intake and susceptibility to pneumonia. *Pediatr. Infect. Dis. J.* **1997**, *16*, 836–837. [CrossRef] [PubMed]

121. Kimbarowski, J.A.; Mokrow, N.J. Colored precipitation reaction of the urine according to Kimbarowski as an index of the effect of ascorbic acid during treatment of viral influenza. *Dtsch. Gesundheitsw.* **1967**, *22*, 2413–2418. (In German). [PubMed]

122. Pitt, H.A.; Costrini, A.M. Vitamin C prophylaxis in marine recruits. *JAMA* **1979**, *241*, 908–911. [PubMed]

123. Hemilä, H. Vitamin C supplementation and respiratory infections: A systematic review. *Mil. Med.* **2004**, *169*, 920–925. [CrossRef] [PubMed]

124. Merchant, A.T.; Curhan, G.; Bendich, A.; Singh, V.N.; Willett, W.C.; Fawzi, W.W. Vitamin intake is not associated with community-acquired pneumonia in US men. *J. Nutr.* **2004**, *134*, 439–444. [PubMed]

125. Hemilä, H.; Virtamo, J.; Albanes, D.; Kaprio, J. Vitamin E and beta-carotene supplementation and hospital-treated pneumonia incidence in male smokers. *Chest* **2004**, *125*, 557–565. [CrossRef] [PubMed]

126. Pazzaglia, G.; Pasternack, M. Recent trends of pneumonia morbidity in US Naval personnel. *Mil. Med.* **1983**, *148*, 647–651. [PubMed]

127. Paynter, S.; Ware, R.S.; Weinstein, P.; Williams, G.; Sly, P.D. Childhood pneumonia: A neglected, climate-sensitive disease? *Lancet* **2010**, *376*, 1804–1805. [CrossRef]

128. Klenner, F.R. Recent discoveries in the treatment of lockjaw with vitamin C and tolserol. *Tri State Med. J.* **1954**, *2*, 7–11.

129. Hemilä, H.; Koivula, T. Vitamin C for preventing and treating tetanus. *Cochrane Database Syst. Rev.* **2013**, *11*, CD006665.

130. Hemilä, H.; Koivula, T. Vitamin C for Preventing and Treating Tetanus. Available online: http://www.mv. helsinki.fi/home/hemila/CT (accessed on 17 March 2017).

131. Jahan, K.; Ahmad, K.; Ali, M.A. Effect of ascorbic acid in the treatment of tetanus. *Bangladesh Med. Res. Counc. Bull.* **1984**, *10*, 24–28. [PubMed]

132. Hemilä, H. Vitamin C supplementation and the common cold—Was Linus Pauling right or wrong? *Int. J. Vitamin Nutr. Res.* **1997**, *67*, 329–335.

133. Stone, I. *The Healing Factor: Vitamin C against Disease*; Grosset Dunlap: New York, NY, USA, 1972.

134. Briggs, M. Vitamin C and infectious disease: A review of the literature and the results of a randomized, double-blind, prospective study over 8 years. In *Recent Vitamin Research*; Briggs, M.H., Ed.; CRC Press: Boca Raton, FL, USA, 1984; pp. 39–82.

135. Levy, T.E. *Vitamin C, Infectious Diseases, and Toxins*; Xlibris: Philadelphia, PA, USA, 2002.

136. Terezhalmy, G.T.; Bottomley, W.K.; Pelleu, G.B. The use of water-soluble bioflavonoid-ascorbic acid complex in the treatment of recurrent herpes labialis. *Oral Surg. Oral Med. Oral Pathol.* **1978**, *45*, 56–62. [CrossRef]

137. Chen, J.Y.; Chang, C.Y.; Feng, P.H.; Chu, C.C.; So, E.C.; Hu, M.L. Plasma vitamin C is lower in postherpetic neuralgia patients and administration of vitamin C reduces spontaneous pain but not brush-evoked pain. *Clin. J. Pain* **2009**, *25*, 562–569. [CrossRef] [PubMed]

138. Orient, J.M. Treating herpes zoster with vitamin C: Two case reports. *J. Am. Phys. Surg.* **2006**, *11*, 26–27.

139. Byun, S.H.; Jeon, Y. Administration of vitamin C in a patient with herpes zoster—A case report. *Korean J. Pain* **2011**, *24*, 108–111. [CrossRef] [PubMed]

140. Schencking, M.; Sandholzer, H.; Frese, T. Intravenous administration of vitamin C in the treatment of herpetic neuralgia: Two case reports. *Med. Sci. Monit.* **2010**, *16*, CS58–CS61. [PubMed]

141. Schencking, M.; Vollbracht, C.; Weiss, G.; Lebert, J.; Biller, A.; Goyvaerts, B.; Kraft, K. Intravenous vitamin C in the treatment of shingles: Results of a multicenter prospective cohort study. *Med. Sci. Monit.* **2012**, *18*, CR215–CR224. [PubMed]

142. Kim, M.S.; Kim, D.J.; Na, C.H.; Shin, B.S. A Study of Intravenous Administration of Vitamin C in the Treatment of Acute Herpetic Pain and Postherpetic Neuralgia. *Ann. Dermatol.* **2016**, *28*, 677–683. [CrossRef] [PubMed]

143. Patrone, F.; Dallegri, F.; Bonvini, E.; Minervini, F.; Sacchetti, C. Disorders of neutrophil function in children with recurrent pyogenic infections. *Med. Microbiol. Immunol.* **1982**, *171*, 113–122. [CrossRef] [PubMed]

144. Levy, R.; Shriker, O.; Porath, A.; Riesenberg, K.; Schlaeffer, F. Vitamin C for the treatment of recurrent furunculosis in patients with impaired neutrophil functions. *J. Infect. Dis.* **1996**, *173*, 1502–1505. [CrossRef] [PubMed]

145. Galley, H.F.; Howdle, P.D.; Walker, B.E.; Webster, N.R. The effects of intravenous antioxidants in patients with septic shock. *Free Radic. Biol. Med.* **1997**, *23*, 768–774. [CrossRef]

146. Pleiner, J.; Mittermayer, F.; Schaller, G.; MacAllister, R.J.; Wolzt, M. High doses of vitamin C reverse Escherichia coli endotoxin-induced hyporeactivity to acetylcholine in the human forearm. *Circulation* **2002**, *106*, 1460–1464. [CrossRef] [PubMed]

147. Klenner, F.R. Observations on the dose and administration of ascorbic acid when employed beyond the range of a vitamin in human pathology. *J. Appl. Nutr.* **1971**, *23*, 61–88.

148. Smith, G.D.; Lawlor, D.A.; Harbord, R.; Timpson, N.; Day, I.; Ebrahim, S. Clustered environments and randomized genes: A fundamental distinction between conventional and genetic epidemiology. *PLoS Med.* **2007**, *4*, e352. [CrossRef] [PubMed]

149. Block, G.; Norkus, E.; Hudes, M.; Mandel, S.; Helzlsouer, K. Which plasma antioxidants are most related to fruit and vegetable consumption? *Am. J. Epidemiol.* **2001**, *154*, 1113–1118. [CrossRef] [PubMed]

150. Hemilä, H.; Kaprio, J. Vitamin E supplementation may transiently increase tuberculosis risk in males who smoke heavily and have high dietary vitamin C intake. *Br. J. Nutr.* **2008**, *100*, 896–902. [CrossRef] [PubMed]

151. Hemilä, H.; Kaprio, J. Vitamin E supplementation may transiently increase tuberculosis risk in males who smoke heavily and have high dietary vitamin C intake—Reply by Hemilä & Kaprio. *Br. J. Nutr.* **2009**, *101*, 145–147.

152. Packer, J.E.; Slater, T.F.; Wilson, R.L. Direct observation of a free radical interaction between vitamin E and vitamin C. *Nature* **1979**, *278*, 737–738. [CrossRef] [PubMed]

153. Hemilä, H.; Kaprio, J. Modification of the effect of vitamin E supplementation on the mortality of male smokers by age and dietary vitamin C. *Am. J. Epidemiol.* **2009**, *169*, 946–953. [CrossRef] [PubMed]

154. Hemilä, H.; Kaprio, J. Vitamin E supplementation and pneumonia risk in males who initiated smoking at an early age: Effect modification by body weight and vitamin C. *Nutr. J.* **2008**, *7*, 33. [CrossRef] [PubMed]

155. Goodwin, J.S.; Goodwin, J.M. The tomato effect: Rejection of highly efficacious therapies. *JAMA* **1984**, *251*, 2387–2390. [CrossRef] [PubMed]

156. Knipschild, P.; Kleijnen, J.; Riet, G. Belief in the efficacy of alternative medicine among general practitioners in the Netherlands. *Soc. Sci. Med.* **1990**, *31*, 625–626. [CrossRef]

157. Richards, E. The politics of therapeutic evaluation: The vitamin C and cancer controversy. *Soc. Stud. Sci.* **1988**, *18*, 653–701. [CrossRef]
158. Richards, E. *Vitamin C and Cancer: Medicine or Politics?* St. Martins Press: New York, NY, USA, 1991.
159. Segerstråle, U. Vitamin C and cancer—Medicine or politics. *Science* **1992**, *255*, 613–615. [PubMed]
160. Goodwin, J.S.; Tangum, M.R. Battling quackery: Attitudes about micronutrient supplements in American Academic medicine. *Arch. Intern. Med.* **1998**, *158*, 2187–2191. [CrossRef] [PubMed]
161. Louhiala, P.; Hemilä, H. Can CAM treatments be evidence-based? *Focus Altern. Complement. Ther.* **2014**, *19*, 84–89. [CrossRef]

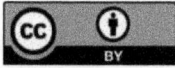

nutrients

MDPI

Review

Vitamin C and Immune Function

Anitra C. Carr [1],* and Silvia Maggini [2]

[1] Department of Pathology, University of Otago, Christchurch, P.O. Box 4345, Christchurch 8140, New Zealand
[2] Bayer Consumer Care Ltd., Peter-Merian-Strasse 84, 4002 Basel, Switzerland; silvia.maggini@bayer.com

Received: 21 September 2017; Accepted: 31 October 2017; Published: 3 November 2017

Abstract: Vitamin C is an essential micronutrient for humans, with pleiotropic functions related to its ability to donate electrons. It is a potent antioxidant and a cofactor for a family of biosynthetic and gene regulatory enzymes. Vitamin C contributes to immune defense by supporting various cellular functions of both the innate and adaptive immune system. Vitamin C supports epithelial barrier function against pathogens and promotes the oxidant scavenging activity of the skin, thereby potentially protecting against environmental oxidative stress. Vitamin C accumulates in phagocytic cells, such as neutrophils, and can enhance chemotaxis, phagocytosis, generation of reactive oxygen species, and ultimately microbial killing. It is also needed for apoptosis and clearance of the spent neutrophils from sites of infection by macrophages, thereby decreasing necrosis/NETosis and potential tissue damage. The role of vitamin C in lymphocytes is less clear, but it has been shown to enhance differentiation and proliferation of B- and T-cells, likely due to its gene regulating effects. Vitamin C deficiency results in impaired immunity and higher susceptibility to infections. In turn, infections significantly impact on vitamin C levels due to enhanced inflammation and metabolic requirements. Furthermore, supplementation with vitamin C appears to be able to both prevent and treat respiratory and systemic infections. Prophylactic prevention of infection requires dietary vitamin C intakes that provide at least adequate, if not saturating plasma levels (i.e., 100–200 mg/day), which optimize cell and tissue levels. In contrast, treatment of established infections requires significantly higher (gram) doses of the vitamin to compensate for the increased inflammatory response and metabolic demand.

Keywords: ascorbate; ascorbic acid; immunity; immune system; neutrophil function; microbial killing; lymphocytes; infection; vitamin C

1. Introduction

The immune system is a multifaceted and sophisticated network of specialized organs, tissues, cells, proteins, and chemicals, which has evolved in order to protect the host from a range of pathogens, such as bacteria, viruses, fungi, and parasites, as well as cancer cells [1]. It can be divided into epithelial barriers, and cellular and humoral constituents of either innate (non-specific) and acquired (specific) immunity [1]. These constituents interact in multiple and highly complex ways. More than half a century of research has shown vitamin C to be a crucial player in various aspects of the immune system, particularly immune cell function [2,3].

Vitamin C is an essential nutrient which cannot be synthesized by humans due to loss of a key enzyme in the biosynthetic pathway [4,5]. Severe vitamin C deficiency results in the potentially fatal disease scurvy [6]. Scurvy is characterized by weakening of collagenous structures, resulting in poor wound healing, and impaired immunity. Individuals with scurvy are highly susceptible to potentially fatal infections such as pneumonia [7]. In turn, infections can significantly impact on vitamin C levels due to enhanced inflammation and metabolic requirements. Early on, it was noted that scurvy often followed infectious epidemics in populations [7], and cases of scurvy have been reported following respiratory infection [8]. This is particularly apparent for individuals who are already malnourished.

Although the amount of vitamin C required to prevent scurvy is relatively low (i.e., ~10 mg/day) [9], the recommended dietary intakes for vitamin C are up to one hundred-fold higher than that for many other vitamins [10]. A diet that supplies 100–200 mg/day of vitamin C provides adequate to saturating plasma concentrations in healthy individuals and should cover general requirements for the reduction of chronic disease risk [11,12]. Due to the low storage capacity of the body for the water-soluble vitamin, a regular and adequate intake is required to prevent hypovitaminosis C. Epidemiological studies have indicated that hypovitaminosis C (plasma vitamin C < 23 μmol/L) is relatively common in Western populations, and vitamin C deficiency (<11 μmol/L) is the fourth leading nutrient deficiency in the United States [13,14]. There are several reasons why vitamin C dietary recommendations are not met, even in countries where food availability and supply would be expected to be sufficient. These include poor dietary habits, life-stages and/or lifestyles either limiting intakes or increasing micronutrient requirements (e.g., smoking and alcohol or drug abuse), various diseases, exposure to pollutants and smoke (both active and passive), and economic reasons (poor socioeconomic status and limited access to nutritious food) [15,16]. Even otherwise 'healthy' individuals in industrialized countries can be at risk due to lifestyle-related factors, such as those on a diet or eating an unbalanced diet, and people facing periods of excessive physical or psychological stress [15,16].

Vitamin C has a number of activities that could conceivably contribute to its immune-modulating effects. It is a highly effective antioxidant, due to its ability to readily donate electrons, thus protecting important biomolecules (proteins, lipids, carbohydrates, and nucleic acids) from damage by oxidants generated during normal cell metabolism and through exposure to toxins and pollutants (e.g., cigarette smoke) [17]. Vitamin C is also a cofactor for a family of biosynthetic and gene regulatory monooxygenase and dioxygenase enzymes [18,19]. The vitamin has long been known as a cofactor for the lysyl and prolyl hydroxylases required for stabilization of the tertiary structure of collagen, and is a cofactor for the two hydroxylases involved in carnitine biosynthesis, a molecule required for transport of fatty acids into mitochondria for generation of metabolic energy (Figure 1) [19].

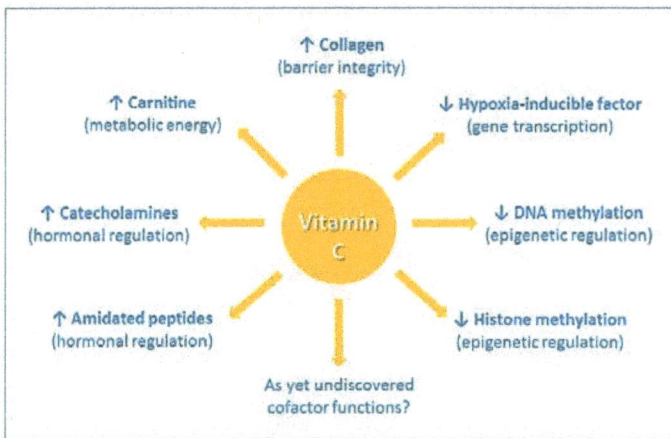

Figure 1. The enzyme cofactor activities of vitamin C. Vitamin C is a cofactor of a family of biosynthetic and gene regulatory monooxygenase and dioxygenase enzymes. These enzymes are involved in the synthesis of collagen, carnitine, catecholamine hormones, e.g., norepinephrine, and amidated peptide hormones, e.g., vasopressin. These enzymes also hydroxylate transcription factors, e.g., hypoxia-inducible factor 1α, and methylated DNA and histones, thus playing a role in gene transcription and epigenetic regulation. ↑ indicates an increase and ↓ indicates a decrease.

Vitamin C is also a cofactor for the hydroxylase enzymes involved in the synthesis of catecholamine hormones, e.g., norepinephrine, and amidated peptide hormones e.g., vasopressin, which are central to the cardiovascular response to severe infection [20]. Furthermore, research over the past 15 years or so has uncovered new roles for vitamin C in the regulation of gene transcription and cell signaling pathways through regulation of transcription factor activity and epigenetic marks (Figure 1) [21,22]. For example, the asparagyl and prolyl hydroylases required for the downregulation of the pleiotropic transcription factor hypoxia-inducible factor-1α (HIF-1α) utilize vitamin C as a cofactor [21]. Recent research has also indicated an important role for vitamin C in regulation of DNA and histone methylation by acting as a cofactor for enzymes which hydoxylate these epigenetic marks [22].

Our review explores the various roles of vitamin C in the immune system, including barrier integrity and leukocyte function, and discusses potential mechanisms of action. We discuss the relevance of the immune-modulating effects of vitamin C in the context of infections and conditions leading to vitamin C insufficiency.

2. Barrier Integrity and Wound Healing

The skin has numerous essential functions, the primary of which is to act as a barrier against external insults, including pathogens. The epidermal layer is highly cellular, comprising primarily keratinocytes, whilst the dermal layer comprises fibroblasts which secrete collagen fibers, the major component of the dermis [23]. Skin contains millimolar concentrations of vitamin C, with higher levels found in the epidermis than the dermis [24–26]. Vitamin C is actively accumulated into the epidermal and dermal cells via the two sodium-dependent vitamin C transporter (SVCT) isoforms 1 and 2 [27], suggesting that the vitamin has crucial functions within the skin. Clues to the role of vitamin C in the skin come from the symptoms of the vitamin C deficiency disease scurvy, which is characterized by bleeding gums, bruising, and impaired wound healing [28,29]. These symptoms are thought to be a result of the role of vitamin C as a co-factor for the prolyl and lysyl hydroxylase enzymes that stabilize the tertiary structure of collagen (Table 1) [30]. Further research has shown that vitamin C can also increase collagen gene expression in fibroblasts [31–35].

Table 1. Role of vitamin C in immune defense.

Immune System	Function of Vitamin C	Refs.
Epithelial barriers	Enhances collagen synthesis and stabilization	[30–35]
	Protects against ROS-induced damage [1]	[36–40]
	Enhances keratinocyte differentiation and lipid synthesis	[41–45]
	Enhances fibroblast proliferation and migration	[46,47]
	Shortens time to wound healing in patients	[48,49]
Phagocytes (neutrophils, macrophages)	Acts as an antioxidant/electron donor	[50–53]
	Enhances motility/chemotaxis	[54–63]
	Enhances phagocytosis and ROS generation	[64–71]
	Enhances microbial killing	[54,55,57,58,70,72]
	Facilitates apoptosis and clearance	[71,73,74]
	Decreases necrosis/NETosis	[73,75]
B- and T-lymphocytes	Enhances differentiation and proliferation	[62,63,76–82]
	Enhances antibody levels	[78,83–85]
Inflammatory mediators	Modulates cytokine production	[75,77,86–94]
	Decreases histamine levels	[56,61,95–101]

[1] ROS, reactive oxygen species; NET, neutrophil extracellular trap. Note that many of these studies comprised marginal or deficient vitamin C status at baseline. Supplementation in situations of adequate vitamin C status may not have comparable effects.

Vitamin C intervention studies in humans (using both dietary and gram doses of vitamin C) have shown enhanced vitamin C uptake into skin cells [26,36] and enhanced oxidant scavenging activity of the skin [36,37]. The elevated antioxidant status of the skin following vitamin C supplementation could potentially protect against oxidative stress induced by environmental pollutants [38,39]. The antioxidant effects of vitamin C are likely to be enhanced in combination with vitamin E [40,102].

Cell culture and preclinical studies have indicated that vitamin C can enhance epithelial barrier functions via a number of different mechanisms. Vitamin C supplementation of keratinocytes in culture enhances differentiation and barrier function via modulating signaling and biosynthetic pathways, with resultant elevations in barrier lipid synthesis [41–45]. Dysfunctional epithelial barrier function in the lungs of animals with serious infection can be restored by administration of vitamin C [74]. This was attributed to enhanced expression of tight junction proteins and prevention of cytoskeletal rearrangements.

Animal studies using the vitamin C-dependent Gulo knockout mouse indicated that deficiency did not affect the formation of collagen in the skin of unchallenged mice [103]; however, following full thickness excisional wounding there was significantly decreased collagen formation in vitamin C-deficient mice [46]. This finding is in agreement with an earlier study carried out with scorbutic guinea pigs [104]. Thus, vitamin C appears to be particularly essential during wound healing, also decreasing the expression of pro-inflammatory mediators and enhancing the expression of various wound healing mediators [46]. Fibroblast cell culture experiments have also indicated that vitamin C can alter gene expression profiles within dermal fibroblasts, promoting fibroblast proliferation and migration which is essential for tissue remodeling and wound healing [46,47]. Following surgery, patients require relatively high intakes of vitamin C in order to normalize their plasma vitamin C status (e.g., $\geq$500 mg/day) [105], and administration of antioxidant micronutrients, including vitamin C, to patients with disorders in wound healing can shorten the time to wound closure [48,49,106,107].

Leukocytes, particularly neutrophils and monocyte-derived macrophages, are major players in wound healing [108]. During the initial inflammatory stage, neutrophils migrate to the wound site in order to sterilize it via the release of reactive oxygen species (ROS) and antimicrobial proteins [109]. The neutrophils eventually undergo apoptosis and are cleared by macrophages, resulting in resolution of the inflammatory response. However, in chronic, non-healing wounds, such as those observed in diabetics, the neutrophils persist and instead undergo necrotic cell death which can perpetuate the inflammatory response and hinder wound healing [109,110]. Vitamin C is thought to influence several important aspects of neutrophil function: migration in response to inflammatory mediators (chemotaxis), phagocytosis and killing of microbes, and apoptosis and clearance by macrophages (see below).

3. Vitamin C and Leukocyte Function

Leukocytes, such as neutrophils and monocytes, actively accumulate vitamin C against a concentration gradient, resulting in values that are 50- to 100-fold higher than plasma concentrations [111–113]. These cells accumulate maximal vitamin C concentrations at dietary intakes of ~100 mg/day [114,115], although other body tissues likely require higher intakes for saturation [116,117]. Neutrophils accumulate vitamin C via SVCT2 and typically contain intracellular levels of at least 1 mM [111,118]. Following stimulation of their oxidative burst neutrophils can further increase their intracellular concentration of vitamin C through the non-specific uptake of the oxidized form, dehydroascorbate (DHA), via glucose transporters (GLUT) [118,119]. DHA is then rapidly reduced to ascorbate intracellularly, to give levels of about 10 mM [119]. It is believed that the accumulation of such high vitamin C concentrations indicates important functions within these cells.

Accumulation of millimolar concentrations of vitamin C into neutrophils, particularly following activation of their oxidative burst, is thought to protect these cells from oxidative damage [119]. Vitamin C is a potent water-soluble antioxidant that can scavenge numerous reactive oxidants and can also regenerate the important cellular and membrane antioxidants glutathione and vitamin E [120]. Upon phagocytosis or activation with soluble stimulants, vitamin C is depleted from neutrophils in an oxidant-dependent manner [50–53]. An alteration in the balance between oxidant generation and antioxidant defenses can lead to alterations in multiple signaling pathways, with the pro-inflammatory transcription factor nuclear factor κB (NFκB) playing a central role [121]. Oxidants can activate NFκB, which triggers a signaling cascade leading to continued synthesis of oxidative species and other inflammatory mediators [122,123]. Vitamin C has been shown to attenuate both oxidant generation and NFκB activation in dendritic cells in vitro, and NFκB activation in neutrophils isolated from septic Gulo knockout mice [75,124]. Thiol-containing proteins can be particularly sensitive to redox alterations within cells and are often central to the regulation of redox-related cell signaling pathways [125]. Vitamin C-dependent modulation of thiol-dependent cell signaling and gene expression pathways has been reported in T-cells [126,127].

Thus, vitamin C could modulate immune function through modulation of redox-sensitive cell signaling pathways or by directly protecting important cell structural components. For example, exposure of neutrophils to oxidants can inhibit motility of the cells, which is thought to be due to oxidation of membrane lipids and resultant effects on cell membrane fluidity [63]. Neutrophils contain high levels of polyunsaturated fatty acids in their plasma membranes, and thus improvements in neutrophil motility observed following vitamin C administration (see below) could conceivably be attributed to oxidant scavenging as well as regeneration of vitamin E [120].

3.1. Neutrophil Chemotaxis

Neutrophil infiltration into infected tissues is an early step in innate immunity. In response to pathogen- or host-derived inflammatory signals (e.g., *N*-formylmethionyl-leucyl-phenylalanine (fMLP), interleukin (IL)-8, leukotriene B4, and complement component C5a), marginated neutrophils literally swarm to the site of infection [128]. Migration of neutrophils in response to chemical stimuli is termed chemotaxis, while random migration is termed chemokinesis (Figure 2). Neutrophils express more than 30 different chemokine and chemoattractant receptors in order to sense and rapidly respond to tissue damage signals [128]. Early studies carried out in scorbutic guinea pigs indicated impaired leukocyte chemotactic response compared with leukocytes isolated from guinea pigs supplemented with adequate vitamin C in their diet (Table 1) [54–56,64]. These findings suggest that vitamin C deficiency may impact on the ability of phagocytes to migrate to sites of infection.

Patients with severe infection exhibit compromised neutrophil chemotactic ability [129–132]. This neutrophil 'paralysis' is believed to be partly due to enhanced levels of anti-inflammatory and immune-suppressive mediators (e.g., IL-4 and IL-10) during the compensatory anti-inflammatory response observed following initial hyper-stimulation of the immune system [133]. However, it is also possible that vitamin C depletion, which is prevalent during severe infection [20], may contribute. Studies in the 1980s and 1990s indicated that patients with recurrent infections had impaired leukocyte chemotaxis, which could be restored in response to supplementation with gram doses of vitamin C [57–60,65–67]. Furthermore, supplementation of neonates with suspected sepsis with 400 mg/day vitamin C dramatically improved neutrophil chemotaxis [134].

Recurrent infections can also result from genetic disorders of neutrophil function, such as chronic granulomatous disease (CGD), an immunodeficiency disease resulting in defective leukocyte generation of ROS [135], and Chediak-Higashi syndrome (CHS), a rare autosomal recessive disorder affecting vesicle trafficking [136]. Although vitamin C administration would not be expected to affect the underlying defects of these genetic disorders, it may support the function of redundant antimicrobial mechanisms in these cells. For example, patients with CGD showed improved leukocyte chemotaxis following supplementation with gram doses of vitamin C administered either enterally or parenterally [137–139]. This was associated with decreased infections and clinical improvement [137,138]. A mouse model of CHS showed improved neutrophil chemotaxis following vitamin C supplementation [140], and neutrophils isolated from two children with CHS showed improved chemotaxis following supplementation with 200–500 mg/day vitamin C [141,142], although this effect has not been observed in all cases [140,143]. The vitamin C-dependent enhancement of chemotaxis was thought to be mediated in part via effects on microtubule assembly [144,145], and more recent research has indicated that intracellular vitamin C can stabilize microtubules [146].

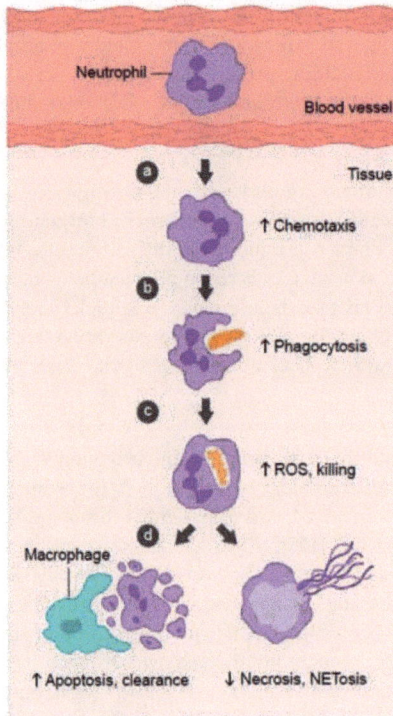

Figure 2. Role of vitamin C in phagocyte function. Vitamin C has been shown to: (**a**) enhance neutrophil migration in response to chemoattractants (chemotaxis), (**b**) enhance engulfment (phagocytosis) of microbes, and (**c**) stimulate reactive oxygen species (ROS) generation and killing of microbes. (**d**) Vitamin C supports caspase-dependent apoptosis, enhancing uptake and clearance by macrophages, and inhibits necrosis, including NETosis, thus supporting resolution of the inflammatory response and attenuating tissue damage.

Supplementation of healthy volunteers with dietary or gram doses of vitamin C has also been shown to enhance neutrophil chemotactic ability [61–63,147]. Johnston et al., proposed that the antihistamine effect of vitamin C correlated with enhanced chemotaxis [61]. In participants who had inadequate vitamin C status (i.e., <50 μM), supplementation with a dietary source of vitamin C (providing ~250 mg/day) resulted in a 20% increase in neutrophil chemotaxis [147]. Furthermore, supplementation of elderly women with 1 g/day vitamin C, in combination with vitamin E, enhanced neutrophil functions, including chemotaxis [148]. Thus, members of the general population may benefit from improved immune cell function through enhanced vitamin C intake, particularly if they have inadequate vitamin C status, which can be more prevalent in the elderly. However, it should be noted that it is not yet certain to what extent improved ex vivo leukocyte chemotaxis translates into improved in vivo immune function.

3.2. Phagocytosis and Microbial Killing

Once neutrophils have migrated to the site of infection, they proceed to engulf the invading pathogens (Figure 2). Various intracellular granules are mobilized and fuse with the phagosome, emptying their arsenal of antimicrobial peptides and proteins into the phagosome [149]. Components of the nicotinamide adenine dinucleotide phosphate (NADPH) oxidase assemble in the phagosomal membrane and generate superoxide, the first in a long line of ROS generated by neutrophils to kill pathogens. The enzyme superoxide dismutase converts superoxide to hydrogen peroxide, which can then be utilized to form the oxidant hypochlorous acid via the azurophilic granule enzyme myeloperoxidase [149]. Hypochlorous acid can further react with amines to form secondary oxidants known as chloramines. These various neutrophil-derived oxidants have different reactivities and specificities for biological targets, with protein thiol groups being particularly susceptible.

Neutrophils isolated from scorbutic guinea pigs exhibit a severely impaired ability to kill microbes [54,55,70], and studies have indicated impaired phagocytosis and/or ROS generation in neutrophils from scorbutic compared with ascorbate replete animals [68–70]. Generation of ROS by neutrophils from volunteers with inadequate vitamin C status can be enhanced by 20% following supplementation with a dietary source of vitamin C [147], and increases in both phagocytosis and oxidant generation were observed following supplementation of elderly participants with a combination of vitamins C and E [148]. Patients with recurrent infections [57,58,66,67,72], or the genetic conditions CGD or CHS [138,139,141,143,150], have impaired neutrophil bacterial killing and/or phagocytosis, which can be significantly improved following supplementation with gram doses of vitamin C, resulting in long lasting clinical improvement. A couple of studies, however, showed no improvement of ex vivo anti-fungal or anti-bacterial activity in neutrophils isolated from CGD or CHS patients supplemented with vitamin C [140,151]. The reason for these differences is not clear, although it may depend on the baseline vitamin C level of the patients, which is not assessed in most cases. Furthermore, different microbes have variable susceptibility to the oxidative and non-oxidative anti-microbial mechanisms of neutrophils. For example, *Staphylococcus aureus* is susceptible to oxidative mechanisms, whereas other microorganisms are more susceptible to non-oxidative mechanisms [152]. Therefore, the type of microbe used to assess the ex vivo neutrophil functions could influence the findings.

Patients with severe infection (sepsis) exhibit a decreased ability to phagocytose microbes and a diminished ability to generate ROS [153]. Decreased neutrophil phagocytosis was associated with enhanced patient mortality [154]. Interestingly, Stephan et al. [155] observed impaired neutrophil killing activity in critically ill patients prior to acquiring nosocomial infections, suggesting that critical illness itself, without prior infection, can also impair neutrophil function. This resulted in subsequent susceptibility to hospital-acquired infections. Impaired phagocytic and oxidant-generating capacity of leukocytes in patients with severe infection has been attributed to the compensatory anti-inflammatory response, resulting in enhanced levels of immunosuppressive mediators such as IL-10 [133], as well as to the hypoxic conditions of inflammatory sites, which diminishes substrate for ROS generation [156]. Another explanation is the larger numbers of immature neutrophils released from the bone marrow due to increased demands during severe infection. These immature 'band' cells have decreased functionality compared with differentiated neutrophils [157]. Thus, conflicting findings in severe infection could be due to variability in the total numbers of underactive immature neutrophils compared with activated fully-differentiated neutrophils [158,159]. Despite displaying an activated basal state, the mature neutrophils from patients with severe infection do not generate ROS to the same extent as healthy neutrophils following ex vivo stimulation [160]. The effect of vitamin C supplementation on phagocytosis, oxidant generation, and microbial killing by leukocytes from septic patients has not yet been explored.

3.3. Neutrophil Apoptosis and Clearance

Following microbial phagocytosis and killing, neutrophils undergo a process of programmed cell death called apoptosis [161]. This process facilitates subsequent phagocytosis and clearance of the spent neutrophils from sites of inflammation by macrophages, thus supporting resolution of inflammation and preventing excessive tissue damage (Figure 2). Caspases are key effector enzymes in the apoptotic process, culminating in phosphatidyl serine exposure, thus marking the cells for uptake and clearance by macrophages [162]. Interestingly, caspases are thiol-dependent enzymes, making them very sensitive to inactivation by ROS generated by activated neutrophils [163,164]. Thus, vitamin C may be expected to protect the oxidant-sensitive caspase-dependent apoptotic process following activation of neutrophils. In support of this premise, in vitro studies have shown that loading human neutrophils with vitamin C can enhance *Escherichia coli*-mediated apoptosis of the neutrophils (Table 1) [71]. Peritoneal neutrophils isolated from vitamin C-deficient Gulo mice exhibited attenuated apoptosis [75], and instead underwent necrotic cell death [73]. These vitamin C-deficient neutrophils were not phagocytosed by macrophages in vitro, and persisted at inflammatory loci in vivo [73]. Furthermore, administration of vitamin C to septic animals decreased the numbers of neutrophils in the lungs of these animals [74].

Numerous studies have reported attenuated neutrophil apoptosis in patients with severe infection compared with control participants [165–172]. The delayed apoptosis appears to be related to disease severity and is thought to be associated with enhanced tissue damage observed in patients with sepsis [173,174]. Immature 'band' neutrophils released during severe infection were also found to be resistant to apoptosis and had longer life spans [157]. Plasma from septic patients has been found to suppress apoptosis in healthy neutrophils, suggesting that pro-inflammatory cytokines were responsible for the increased in vivo survival of neutrophils during inflammatory conditions [165,174–176]. Interestingly, high-dose vitamin C administration has been shown to modulate cytokine levels in patients with cancer [177] and, although this has not yet been assessed in patients with severe infection, could conceivably be another mechanism by which vitamin C may modulate neutrophil function in these patients. To date, only one study has investigated the effect of vitamin C supplementation on neutrophil apoptosis in septic patients [178]. Intravenous supplementation of septic abdominal surgery patients with 450 mg/day vitamin C was found to decrease caspase-3 protein levels and, thus was presumed to have an anti-apoptotic effect on peripheral blood neutrophils. However, caspase activity and apoptosis of the neutrophils following activation was not assessed. Furthermore, circulating neutrophils may not reflect the activation status of neutrophils at inflammatory tissue loci. Clearly, more studies need to be undertaken to tease out the role of vitamin C in neutrophil apoptosis and clearance from inflammatory loci.

3.4. Neutrophil Necrosis and NETosis

Neutrophils that fail to undergo apoptosis instead undergo necrotic cell death (Figure 2). The subsequent release of toxic intracellular components, such as proteases, can cause extensive tissue damage [179,180]. One recently discovered form of neutrophil death has been termed NETosis. This results from the release of 'neutrophil extracellular traps' (NETs) comprising neutrophil DNA, histones, and enzymes [181]. Although NETs have been proposed to comprise a unique method of microbial killing [182,183], they have also been implicated in tissue damage and organ failure [184,185]. NET-associated histones can act as damage-associated molecular pattern proteins, activating the immune system and causing further damage [186]. Patients with sepsis, or who go on to develop sepsis, have significantly elevated levels of circulating cell-free DNA, which is thought to indicate NET formation [184,187].

Pre-clinical studies in vitamin C-deficient Gulo knockout mice indicated enhanced NETosis in the lungs of septic animals and increased circulating cell-free DNA [75]. The levels of these markers were attenuated in vitamin C sufficient animals or in deficient animals that were administered vitamin C (Table 1). The same investigators showed that in vitro supplementation of human neutrophils with vitamin C attenuated phorbol ester-induced NETosis [75]. Administration of gram doses of vitamin C to septic patients over four days, however, did not appear to decrease circulating cell-free DNA levels [188], although the duration of treatment may have been too short to see a sustained effect. It should be noted that cell-free DNA is not specific for neutrophil-derived DNA, as it may also derive from necrotic tissue; however, the association of neutrophil-specific proteins or enzymes, such as myeloperoxidase, with the DNA can potentially provide an indication of its source [184].

The transcription factor HIF-1α facilitates neutrophil survival at hypoxic loci through delaying apoptosis [189]. Interestingly, vitamin C is a cofactor for the iron-containing dioxygenase enzymes that regulate the levels and activity of HIF-1α [190]. These hydroxylase enzymes downregulate HIF-1α activity by facilitating degradation of constitutively expressed HIF-1α and decreasing binding of transcription coactivators. In vitamin C-deficient Gulo knockout mice, up-regulation of HIF-1α was observed under normoxic conditions, along with attenuated neutrophil apoptosis and clearance by macrophages [73]. HIF-1α has also been proposed as a regulator of NET generation by neutrophils [191], hence providing a potential mechanism by which vitamin C could downregulate NET generation by these cells [75].

3.5. Lymphocyte Function

Like phagocytes, B- and T-lymphocytes accumulate vitamin C to high levels via SVCT [192,193]. The role of vitamin C within these cells is less clear, although antioxidant protection has been suggested [194]. In vitro studies have indicated that incubation of vitamin C with lymphocytes promotes proliferation [76,77], resulting in enhanced antibody generation [78], and also provides resistance to various cell death stimuli [195]. Furthermore, vitamin C appears to have an important role in developmental differentiation and maturation of immature T-cells (Table 1) [76,79]. Similar proliferative and differentiation/maturation effects have been observed with mature and immature natural killer cells, respectively [196].

Early studies in guinea pigs showed enhanced mitotic activity of isolated peripheral blood lymphocytes following intraperitoneal vitamin C treatment, and enhanced humoral antibody levels during immunization [82–85]. Although one human intervention study has reported positive associations between antibody levels (immunoglobulin (Ig)M, (Ig)G, (Ig)A) and vitamin C supplementation [85], another has not [62]. Instead, Anderson and coworkers showed that oral and intravenous supplementation of low gram doses of vitamin C to children with asthma and healthy volunteers enhanced lymphocyte transformation, an ex vivo measure of mitogen-induced proliferation and enlargement of T-lymphocytes (Table 1) [62,63,81]. Administration of vitamin C to elderly people was also shown to enhance ex vivo lymphocyte proliferation [80], a finding confirmed using combinations of vitamin C with vitamins A and/or E [148,197]. Exposure to toxic chemicals can affect lymphocyte function, and both natural killer cell activity and lymphocyte blastogenic responses to T- and B-cell mitogens were restored to normal levels following vitamin C supplementation [198]. Although the human studies mentioned above are encouraging, it is apparent that more human intervention studies are needed to confirm these findings.

Recent research in wild-type and Gulo knockout mice indicated that parenteral administration of 200 mg/kg vitamin C modulated the immunosuppression of regulatory T-cells (Tregs) observed in sepsis [89]. Vitamin C administration enhanced Treg proliferation and inhibited the negative immunoregulation of Tregs by inhibiting the expression of specific transcription factors, antigens, and cytokines [89]. The mechanisms involved likely rely on the gene regulatory effects of vitamin C [79,89,199,200]. For example, recent research has implicated vitamin C in epigenetic regulation through its action as a cofactor for the iron-containing dioxygenases which hydroxylate methylated DNA and histones [22,201]. The ten-eleven translocation (TET) enzymes hydroxylate methylcytosine residues, which may act as epigenetic marks in their own right, and also facilitate removal of the methylated residues, an important process in epigenetic regulation [202]. Preliminary evidence indicates that vitamin C can regulate T-cell maturation via epigenetic mechanisms involving the TETs and histone demethylation [79,199,200]. It is likely that the cell signaling and gene regulatory functions of vitamin C, via regulation of transcription factors and epigenetic marks, play major roles in its immune-regulating functions.

3.6. Inflammatory Mediators

Cytokines are important cell signaling molecules secreted by a variety of immune cells, both innate and adaptive, in response to infection and inflammation [1]. They comprise a broad range of molecules, including chemokines, interferons (IFNs), ILs, lymphokines, and TNFs, which modulate both humoral and cell-based immune responses, and regulate the maturation, growth, and responsiveness of specific cell populations. Cytokines can elicit pro-inflammatory or anti-inflammatory responses, and vitamin C appears to modulate systemic and leukocyte-derived cytokines in a complex manner.

Incubation of vitamin C with peripheral blood lymphocytes decreased lipopolysaccharide (LPS)-induced generation of the pro-inflammatory cytokines TNF-α and IFN-γ, and increased anti-inflammatory IL-10 production, while having no effect on IL-1β levels [77]. Furthermore, in vitro addition of vitamin C to peripheral blood monocytes isolated from pneumonia patients decreased the generation of the pro-inflammatory cytokines TNF-α and IL-6 [86]. However, another study found that in vitro treatment of peripheral blood monocytes with vitamin C and/or vitamin E enhanced LPS-stimulated TNF-α generation, but did not affect IL-1β generation [87]. Furthermore, incubation of vitamin C with virus-infected human and murine fibroblasts enhanced generation of antiviral IFN [91–93]. Supplementation of healthy human volunteers with 1 g/day vitamin C (with and without vitamin E) was shown to enhance peripheral blood mononuclear cell-derived IL-10, IL-1, and TNF-α following stimulation with LPS [87,94]. Thus, the effect of vitamin C on cytokine generation appears to depend on the cell type and/or the inflammatory stimulant. Recent research has indicated that vitamin C treatment of microglia, resident myeloid-derived macrophages in the central nervous system, attenuates activation of the cells and synthesis of the pro-inflammatory cytokines TNF, IL-6, and IL-1β [90]. This is indicative of an anti-inflammatory phenotype.

Preclinical studies using Gluo knockout mice have highlighted the cytokine-modulating effects of vitamin C. Vitamin C-deficient Gulo knockout mice infected with influenza virus showed enhanced synthesis of the pro-inflammatory cytokines TNF-α and IL-1α/β in their lungs, and decreased production of the anti-viral cytokine IFN-α/β [88]. Administration of vitamin C to Gulo mice with polymicrobial peritonitis resulted in decreased synthesis of the pro-inflammatory cytokines TNF-α and IL-1β by isolated neutrophils [75]. Another study in septic Gulo mice administered 200 mg/kg parenteral vitamin C has shown decreased secretion of the inhibitory cytokines TGF-β and IL-10 by Tregs [89]. In this study, attenuated IL-4 secretion and augmented IFN-γ secretion was also observed, suggesting immune-modulating effects of vitamin C in sepsis. Overall, vitamin C appears to normalize cytokine generation, likely through its gene-regulating effects.

Histamine is an immune mediator produced by basophils, eosinophils, and mast cells during the immune response to pathogens and stress. Histamine stimulates vasodilation and increased capillary permeability, resulting in the classic allergic symptoms of runny nose and eyes. Studies using guinea pigs, a vitamin C-requiring animal model, have indicated that vitamin C depletion is associated with enhanced circulating histamine levels, and that supplementation of the animals with vitamin C resulted in decreased histamine levels [56,95–98]. Enhanced histamine generation was found to increase the utilization of vitamin C in these animals [96]. Consistent with the animal studies, human intervention studies with oral vitamin C (125 mg/day to 2 g/day) and intravenous vitamin C (7.5 g infusion) have reported decreased histamine levels [61,99–101], which was more apparent in patients with allergic compared with infectious diseases [101]. Although vitamin C has been proposed to 'detoxify' histamine [96,97], the precise mechanisms responsible for the in vivo decrease in histamine levels following vitamin C administration are currently unknown. Furthermore, effects of vitamin C supplementation on histamine levels are not observed in all studies [203].

4. Vitamin C Insufficiency Conditions

Numerous environmental and health conditions can have an impact on vitamin C status. In this section we discuss examples which also have a link with impaired immunity and increased susceptibility to infection. For example, exposure to air pollution containing oxidants, such as ozone and nitrogen dioxide, can upset the oxidant-antioxidant balance within the body and cause oxidative stress [204]. Oxidative stress can also occur if antioxidant defenses are impaired, which may be the case when vitamin C levels are insufficient [205]. Air pollution can damage respiratory tract lining fluid and increase the risk of respiratory disease, particularly in children and the elderly [204,206] who are at risk of both impaired immunity and vitamin C insufficiency [14,204]. Vitamin C is a free-radical scavenger that can scavenge superoxide and peroxyl radicals, hydrogen peroxide, hypochlorous acid, and oxidant air pollutants [207,208]. The antioxidant properties of vitamin C enable it to protect lung cells exposed to oxidants and oxidant-mediated damage caused by various pollutants, heavy metals, pesticides, and xenobiotics [204,209].

Tobacco smoke is an underestimated pollutant in many parts of the world. Both smokers and passive smokers have lower plasma and leukocyte vitamin C levels than non-smokers [10,210,211], partly due to increased oxidative stress and to both a lower intake and a higher metabolic turnover of vitamin C compared to non-smokers [10,211–213]. Mean serum concentrations of vitamin C in adults who smoke have been found to be one-third lower than those of non-smokers, and it has been recommended that smokers should consume an additional 35 mg/day of vitamin C to ensure there is sufficient ascorbic acid to repair oxidant damage [10,14]. Vitamin C levels are also lower in children and adolescents exposed to environmental tobacco smoke [214]. Research in vitamin C-deficient guinea pigs exposed to tobacco smoke has indicated that vitamin C can protect against protein damage and lipid peroxidation [213,215]. In passive smokers exposed to environmental tobacco smoke, vitamin C supplementation significantly reduced plasma F_2-isoprostane concentrations, a measure of oxidative stress [216]. Tobacco use increases susceptibility to bacterial and viral infections [217,218], in which vitamin C may play a role. For example, in a population-based study the risk of developing obstructive airways disease was significantly higher in those with the lowest plasma vitamin C concentrations (26 µmol/L) compared to never smokers, a risk that decreased with increasing vitamin C concentration [219].

Individuals with diabetes are at greater risk of common infections, including influenza, pneumonia, and foot infections, which are associated with increased morbidity and mortality [220,221]. Several immune-related changes are observed in obesity that contribute towards the development of type 2 diabetes. A major factor is persistent low-grade inflammation of adipose tissue in obese subjects, which plays a role in the progression to insulin resistance and type 2 diabetes, and which is not present in the adipose tissue of lean subjects [222,223]. The adipose tissue is infiltrated by pro-inflammatory macrophages and T-cells, leading to the accumulation of pro-inflammatory cytokines such as interleukins and TNF-α [224,225]. A decrease in plasma vitamin C levels has been observed in studies of type 2 diabetes [18,226], and a major cause of increased need for vitamin C in type 2 diabetes is thought to be the high level of oxidative stress caused by hyperglycemia [10,227,228]. Inverse correlations have been reported between plasma vitamin C concentrations and the risk of diabetes, hemoglobin A1c concentrations (an index of glucose tolerance), fasting and postprandial blood glucose, and oxidative stress [219,229–232]. Meta-analysis of interventional studies has indicted that supplementation with vitamin C can improve glycemic control in type 2 diabetes [233].

Elderly people are particularly susceptible to infections due to immunosenescence and decreased immune cell function [234]. For example, common viral infections such as respiratory illnesses, that are usually self-limiting in healthy young people, can lead to the development of complications such as pneumonia, resulting in increased morbidity and mortality in elderly people. A lower mean vitamin C status has been observed in free-living or institutionalized elderly people, indicated by lowered plasma and leukocyte concentrations [10,235,236], which is of concern because low vitamin C concentrations (<17 µmol/L) in older people (aged 75–82 years) are strongly predictive of all-cause mortality [237]. Acute and chronic diseases that are prevalent in this age group may also play an important part in the reduction of vitamin C reserves [238–240]. Institutionalization in particular is an aggravating factor in this age group, resulting in even lower plasma vitamin C levels than in non-institutionalized elderly people. It is noteworthy that elderly hospitalized patients with acute respiratory infections have been shown to fare significantly better with vitamin C supplementation than those not receiving the vitamin [241]. Decreased immunological surveillance in individuals older than 60 years also results in greater risk of cancer, and patients with cancer, particularly those undergoing cancer treatments, have compromised immune systems, decreased vitamin C status, and enhanced risk of developing sepsis [242,243]. Hospitalized patients, in general, have lower vitamin C status than the general population [244].

5. Vitamin C and Infection

A major symptom of the vitamin C deficiency disease scurvy is the marked susceptibility to infections, particularly of the respiratory tract, with pneumonia being one of the most frequent complications of scurvy and a major cause of death [7]. Patients with acute respiratory infections, such as pulmonary tuberculosis and pneumonia, have decreased plasma vitamin C concentrations relative to control subjects [245]. Administration of vitamin C to patients with acute respiratory infections returns their plasma vitamin C levels to normal and ameliorates the severity of the respiratory symptoms [246]. Cases of acute lung infections have shown rapid clearance of chest X-rays following administration of intravenous vitamin C [247,248]. This vitamin C-dependent clearance of neutrophils from infected lungs could conceivably be due to enhanced apoptosis and subsequent phagocytosis and clearance of the spent neutrophils by macrophages [73]. Pre-clinical studies of animals with sepsis-induced lung injury have indicated that vitamin C administration can increase alveolar fluid clearance, enhance bronchoalveolar epithelial barrier function, and attenuate sequestration of neutrophils [74], all essential factors for normal lung function.

Meta-analysis has indicated that vitamin C supplementation with doses of 200 mg or more daily is effective in ameliorating the severity and duration of the common cold, and the incidence of the common cold if also exposed to physical stress [249]. Supplementation of individuals who had an inadequate vitamin C status (i.e., <45 μmol/L) also decreased the incidence of the common cold [203]. Surprisingly, few studies have assessed vitamin C status during the common cold [250]. Significant decreases in both leukocyte vitamin C levels, and urinary excretion of the vitamin, have been reported to occur during common cold episodes, with levels returning to normal following the infection [251–254]. These changes indicate that vitamin C is utilized during the common cold infection. Administration of gram doses of vitamin C during the common cold episode ameliorated the decline in leukocyte vitamin C levels, suggesting that administration of vitamin C may be beneficial for the recovery process [251].

Beneficial effects of vitamin C on recovery have been noted in pneumonia. In elderly people hospitalized because of pneumonia, who were determined to have very low vitamin C levels, administration of vitamin C reduced the respiratory symptom score in the more severe patients [246]. In other pneumonia patients, low-dose vitamin C (0.25–0.8 g/day) reduced the hospital stay by 19% compared with no vitamin C supplementation, whereas the higher-dose group (0.5–1.6 g/day) reduced the duration by 36% [255]. There was also a positive effect on the normalization of chest X-ray, temperature, and erythrocyte sedimentation rate [255]. Since prophylactic vitamin C administration also appears to decrease the risk of developing more serious respiratory infections, such as pneumonia [256], it is likely that the low vitamin C levels observed during respiratory infections are both a cause and a consequence of the disease.

6. Conclusions

Overall, vitamin C appears to exert a multitude of beneficial effects on cellular functions of both the innate and adaptive immune system. Although vitamin C is a potent antioxidant protecting the body against endogenous and exogenous oxidative challenges, it is likely that its action as a cofactor for numerous biosynthetic and gene regulatory enzymes plays a key role in its immune-modulating effects. Vitamin C stimulates neutrophil migration to the site of infection, enhances phagocytosis and oxidant generation, and microbial killing. At the same time, it protects host tissue from excessive damage by enhancing neutrophil apoptosis and clearance by macrophages, and decreasing neutrophil necrosis and NETosis. Thus, it is apparent that vitamin C is necessary for the immune system to mount and sustain an adequate response against pathogens, whilst avoiding excessive damage to the host.

Vitamin C appears to be able to both prevent and treat respiratory and systemic infections by enhancing various immune cell functions. Prophylactic prevention of infection requires dietary vitamin C intakes that provide at least adequate, if not saturating plasma levels (i.e., 100–200 mg/day), which optimize cell and tissue levels. In contrast, treatment of established infections requires significantly higher (gram) doses of the vitamin to compensate for the increased metabolic demand.

Epidemiological studies indicate that hypovitaminosis C is still relatively common in Western populations, and vitamin C deficiency is the fourth leading nutrient deficiency in the United States. Reasons include reduced intake combined with limited body stores. Increased needs occur due to pollution and smoking, fighting infections, and diseases with oxidative and inflammatory components, e.g., type 2 diabetes, etc. Ensuring adequate intake of vitamin C through the diet or via supplementation, especially in groups such as the elderly or in individuals exposed to risk factors for vitamin C insufficiency, is required for proper immune function and resistance to infections.

Acknowledgments: Thanks are given to Mark Hampton for critically reviewing the manuscript and Deborah Nock (Medical WriteAway, Norwich, UK) for medical writing support and editorial assistance on behalf of Bayer Consumer Care Ltd. A.C.C. is the recipient of a Health Research Council of New Zealand Sir Charles Hercus Health Research Fellowship.

Author Contributions: A.C.C. and S.M. conceived and wrote the review, and A.C.C. had primary responsibility for the final content.

Conflicts of Interest: S.M. is employed by Bayer Consumer Care Ltd., a manufacturer of multivitamins, and wrote the section on 'Vitamin C insufficiency conditions'. A.C.C. has received funding, as a Key Opinion Leader, from Bayer Consumer Care Ltd.

References

1. Parkin, J.; Cohen, B. An overview of the immune system. *Lancet* **2001**, *357*, 1777–1789. [CrossRef]
2. Maggini, S.; Wintergerst, E.S.; Beveridge, S.; Hornig, D.H. Selected vitamins and trace elements support immune function by strengthening epithelial barriers and cellular and humoral immune responses. *Br. J. Nutr.* **2007**, *98*, S29–S35. [CrossRef] [PubMed]
3. Webb, A.L.; Villamor, E. Update: Effects of antioxidant and non-antioxidant vitamin supplementation on immune function. *Nutr. Rev.* **2007**, *65*, 181. [CrossRef] [PubMed]
4. Burns, J.J. Missing step in man, monkey and guinea pig required for the biosynthesis of L-ascorbic acid. *Nature* **1957**, *180*, 553. [CrossRef] [PubMed]
5. Nishikimi, M.; Fukuyama, R.; Minoshima, S.; Shimizu, N.; Yagi, K. Cloning and chromosomal mapping of the human nonfunctional gene for L-gulono-gamma-lactone oxidase, the enzyme for L-ascorbic acid biosynthesis missing in man. *J. Biol. Chem.* **1994**, *269*, 13685–13688. [PubMed]
6. Sauberlich, H.E. A history of scurvy and vitamin C. In *Vitamin C in Health and Disease*; Packer, L., Fuchs, J., Eds.; Marcel Dekker: New York, NY, USA, 1997; pp. 1–24.
7. Hemila, H. Vitamin C and Infections. *Nutrients* **2017**, *9*, 339. [CrossRef] [PubMed]
8. Carr, A.C.; McCall, C. The role of vitamin C in the treatment of pain: New insights. *J. Transl. Med.* **2017**, *15*, 77. [CrossRef] [PubMed]
9. Krebs, H.A. The Sheffield Experiment on the vitamin C requirement of human adults. *Proc. Nutr. Soc.* **1953**, *12*, 237–246. [CrossRef]
10. Institute of Medicine Panel on Dietary Antioxidants and Related Compounds. *Dietary Reference Intakes for Vitamin C, Vitamin E, Selenium, and Carotenoids*; National Academies Press: Washington, DC, USA, 2000.
11. Levine, M.; Dhariwal, K.R.; Welch, R.W.; Wang, Y.; Park, J.B. Determination of optimal vitamin C requirements in humans. *Am. J. Clin. Nutr.* **1995**, *62*, 1347S–1356S. [PubMed]
12. Carr, A.C.; Frei, B. Toward a new recommended dietary allowance for vitamin C based on antioxidant and health effects in humans. *Am. J. Clin. Nutr.* **1999**, *69*, 1086–1087. [PubMed]

13. Schleicher, R.L.; Carroll, M.D.; Ford, E.S.; Lacher, D.A. Serum vitamin C and the prevalence of vitamin C deficiency in the United States: 2003–2004 National Health and Nutrition Examination Survey (NHANES). *Am. J. Clin. Nutr.* **2009**, *90*, 1252–1263. [CrossRef] [PubMed]

14. US Centers for Disease Control and Prevention. *Second National Report on Biochemical Indicators of Diet and Nutrition in the US Population 2012*; National Center for Environmental Health: Atlanta, GA, USA, 2012.

15. Maggini, S.; Beveridge, S.; Sorbara, J.; Senatore, G. Feeding the immune system: The role of micronutrients in restoring resistance to infections. *CAB Rev.* **2008**, *3*, 1–21. [CrossRef]

16. Huskisson, E.; Maggini, S.; Ruf, M. The role of vitamins and minerals in energy metabolism and well-being. *J. Int. Med. Res.* **2007**, *35*, 277–289. [CrossRef] [PubMed]

17. Carr, A.; Frei, B. Does vitamin C act as a pro-oxidant under physiological conditions? *FASEB J.* **1999**, *13*, 1007–1024. [PubMed]

18. Mandl, J.; Szarka, A.; Banhegyi, G. Vitamin C: Update on physiology and pharmacology. *Br. J. Pharmacol.* **2009**, *157*, 1097–1110. [CrossRef] [PubMed]

19. England, S.; Seifter, S. The biochemical functions of ascorbic acid. *Annu. Rev. Nutr.* **1986**, *6*, 365–406. [CrossRef] [PubMed]

20. Carr, A.C.; Shaw, G.M.; Fowler, A.A.; Natarajan, R. Ascorbate-dependent vasopressor synthesis: A rationale for vitamin C administration in severe sepsis and septic shock? *Crit. Care* **2015**, *19*, e418. [CrossRef] [PubMed]

21. Kuiper, C.; Vissers, M.C. Ascorbate as a co-factor for Fe- and 2-oxoglutarate dependent dioxygenases: Physiological activity in tumor growth and progression. *Front. Oncol.* **2014**, *4*, 359. [CrossRef] [PubMed]

22. Young, J.I.; Zuchner, S.; Wang, G. Regulation of the epigenome by vitamin C. *Annu. Rev. Nutr.* **2015**, *35*, 545–564. [CrossRef] [PubMed]

23. Pullar, J.M.; Carr, A.C.; Vissers, M.C.M. The roles of vitamin C in skin health. *Nutrients* **2017**, *9*, 866. [CrossRef] [PubMed]

24. Rhie, G.; Shin, M.H.; Seo, J.Y.; Choi, W.W.; Cho, K.H.; Kim, K.H.; Park, K.C.; Eun, H.C.; Chung, J.H. Aging- and photoaging-dependent changes of enzymic and nonenzymic antioxidants in the epidermis and dermis of human skin in vivo. *J. Investig. Dermatol.* **2001**, *117*, 1212–1217. [CrossRef] [PubMed]

25. Shindo, Y.; Witt, E.; Han, D.; Epstein, W.; Packer, L. Enzymic and non-enzymic antioxidants in epidermis and dermis of human skin. *J. Investig. Dermatol.* **1994**, *102*, 122–124. [CrossRef] [PubMed]

26. McArdle, F.; Rhodes, L.E.; Parslew, R.; Jack, C.I.; Friedmann, P.S.; Jackson, M.J. UVR-induced oxidative stress in human skin in vivo: Effects of oral vitamin C supplementation. *Free Radic. Biol. Med.* **2002**, *33*, 1355–1362. [CrossRef]

27. Steiling, H.; Longet, K.; Moodycliffe, A.; Mansourian, R.; Bertschy, E.; Smola, H.; Mauch, C.; Williamson, G. Sodium-dependent vitamin C transporter isoforms in skin: Distribution, kinetics, and effect of UVB-induced oxidative stress. *Free Radic. Biol. Med.* **2007**, *43*, 752–762. [CrossRef] [PubMed]

28. Hodges, R.E.; Baker, E.M.; Hood, J.; Sauberlich, H.E.; March, S.C. Experimental scurvy in man. *Am. J. Clin. Nutr.* **1969**, *22*, 535–548. [PubMed]

29. Hodges, R.E.; Hood, J.; Canham, J.E.; Sauberlich, H.E.; Baker, E.M. Clinical manifestations of ascorbic acid deficiency in man. *Am. J. Clin. Nutr.* **1971**, *24*, 432–443. [PubMed]

30. Kivirikko, K.I.; Myllyla, R.; Pihlajaniemi, T. Protein hydroxylation: Prolyl 4-hydroxylase, an enzyme with four cosubstrates and a multifunctional subunit. *FASEB J.* **1989**, *3*, 1609–1617. [PubMed]

31. Geesin, J.C.; Darr, D.; Kaufman, R.; Murad, S.; Pinnell, S.R. Ascorbic acid specifically increases type I and type III procollagen messenger RNA levels in human skin fibroblast. *J. Investig. Dermatol.* **1988**, *90*, 420–424. [CrossRef] [PubMed]

32. Kishimoto, Y.; Saito, N.; Kurita, K.; Shimokado, K.; Maruyama, N.; Ishigami, A. Ascorbic acid enhances the expression of type 1 and type 4 collagen and SVCT2 in cultured human skin fibroblasts. *Biochem. Biophys. Res. Commun.* **2013**, *430*, 579–584. [CrossRef] [PubMed]

33. Nusgens, B.V.; Humbert, P.; Rougier, A.; Colige, A.C.; Haftek, M.; Lambert, C.A.; Richard, A.; Creidi, P.; Lapiere, C.M. Topically applied vitamin C enhances the mRNA level of collagens I and III, their processing enzymes and tissue inhibitor of matrix metalloproteinase 1 in the human dermis. *J. Investig. Dermatol.* **2001**, *116*, 853–859. [CrossRef] [PubMed]

34. Tajima, S.; Pinnell, S.R. Ascorbic acid preferentially enhances type I and III collagen gene transcription in human skin fibroblasts. *J. Dermatol. Sci.* **1996**, *11*, 250–253. [CrossRef]

35. Davidson, J.M.; LuValle, P.A.; Zoia, O.; Quaglino, D., Jr.; Giro, M. Ascorbate differentially regulates elastin and collagen biosynthesis in vascular smooth muscle cells and skin fibroblasts by pretranslational mechanisms. *J. Biol. Chem.* **1997**, *272*, 345–352. [CrossRef] [PubMed]

36. Fuchs, J.; Kern, H. Modulation of UV-light-induced skin inflammation by D-alpha-tocopherol and L-ascorbic acid: A clinical study using solar simulated radiation. *Free Radic. Biol. Med.* **1998**, *25*, 1006–1012. [CrossRef]

37. Lauer, A.C.; Groth, N.; Haag, S.F.; Darvin, M.E.; Lademann, J.; Meinke, M.C. Dose-dependent vitamin C uptake and radical scavenging activity in human skin measured with in vivo electron paramagnetic resonance spectroscopy. *Skin Pharmacol. Physiol.* **2013**, *26*, 147–154. [CrossRef] [PubMed]

38. Valacchi, G.; Sticozzi, C.; Belmonte, G.; Cervellati, F.; Demaude, J.; Chen, N.; Krol, Y.; Oresajo, C. Vitamin C compound mixtures prevent ozone-induced oxidative damage in human keratinocytes as initial assessment of pollution protection. *PLoS ONE* **2015**, *10*, e0131097. [CrossRef] [PubMed]

39. Valacchi, G.; Muresan, X.M.; Sticozzi, C.; Belmonte, G.; Pecorelli, A.; Cervellati, F.; Demaude, J.; Krol, Y.; Oresajo, C. Ozone-induced damage in 3D-skin model is prevented by topical vitamin C and vitamin E compound mixtures application. *J. Dermatol. Sci.* **2016**, *82*, 209–212. [CrossRef] [PubMed]

40. Lin, J.Y.; Selim, M.A.; Shea, C.R.; Grichnik, J.M.; Omar, M.M.; Monteiro-Riviere, N.A.; Pinnell, S.R. UV photoprotection by combination topical antioxidants vitamin C and vitamin E. *J. Am. Acad. Dermatol.* **2003**, *48*, 866–874. [CrossRef] [PubMed]

41. Pasonen-Seppanen, S.; Suhonen, T.M.; Kirjavainen, M.; Suihko, E.; Urtti, A.; Miettinen, M.; Hyttinen, M.; Tammi, M.; Tammi, R. Vitamin C enhances differentiation of a continuous keratinocyte cell line (REK) into epidermis with normal stratum corneum ultrastructure and functional permeability barrier. *Histochem. Cell Biol.* **2001**, *116*, 287–297. [CrossRef] [PubMed]

42. Savini, I.; Catani, M.V.; Rossi, A.; Duranti, G.; Melino, G.; Avigliano, L. Characterization of keratinocyte differentiation induced by ascorbic acid: Protein kinase C involvement and vitamin C homeostasis. *J. Investig. Dermatol.* **2002**, *118*, 372–379. [CrossRef] [PubMed]

43. Ponec, M.; Weerheim, A.; Kempenaar, J.; Mulder, A.; Gooris, G.S.; Bouwstra, J.; Mommaas, A.M. The formation of competent barrier lipids in reconstructed human epidermis requires the presence of vitamin C. *J. Investig. Dermatol.* **1997**, *109*, 348–355. [CrossRef] [PubMed]

44. Uchida, Y.; Behne, M.; Quiec, D.; Elias, P.M.; Holleran, W.M. Vitamin C stimulates sphingolipid production and markers of barrier formation in submerged human keratinocyte cultures. *J. Investig. Dermatol.* **2001**, *117*, 1307–1313. [CrossRef] [PubMed]

45. Kim, K.P.; Shin, K.O.; Park, K.; Yun, H.J.; Mann, S.; Lee, Y.M.; Cho, Y. Vitamin C stimulates epidermal ceramide production by regulating its metabolic enzymes. *Biomol. Ther.* **2015**, *23*, 525–530. [CrossRef] [PubMed]

46. Mohammed, B.M.; Fisher, B.J.; Kraskauskas, D.; Ward, S.; Wayne, J.S.; Brophy, D.F.; Fowler, A.A., III; Yager, D.R.; Natarajan, R. Vitamin C promotes wound healing through novel pleiotropic mechanisms. *Int. Wound J.* **2016**, *13*, 572–584. [CrossRef] [PubMed]

47. Duarte, T.L.; Cooke, M.S.; Jones, G.D. Gene expression profiling reveals new protective roles for vitamin C in human skin cells. *Free Radic. Biol. Med.* **2009**, *46*, 78–87. [CrossRef] [PubMed]

48. Desneves, K.J.; Todorovic, B.E.; Cassar, A.; Crowe, T.C. Treatment with supplementary arginine, vitamin C and zinc in patients with pressure ulcers: A randomised controlled trial. *Clin. Nutr.* **2005**, *24*, 979–987. [CrossRef] [PubMed]

49. Taylor, T.V.; Rimmer, S.; Day, B.; Butcher, J.; Dymock, I.W. Ascorbic acid supplementation in the treatment of pressure-sores. *Lancet* **1974**, *2*, 544–546. [CrossRef]

50. Stankova, L.; Gerhardt, N.B.; Nagel, L.; Bigley, R.H. Ascorbate and phagocyte function. *Infect. Immun.* **1975**, *12*, 252–256. [PubMed]

51. Winterbourn, C.C.; Vissers, M.C. Changes in ascorbate levels on stimulation of human neutrophils. *Biochim. Biophys. Acta* **1983**, *763*, 175–179. [CrossRef]

52. Parker, A.; Cuddihy, S.L.; Son, T.G.; Vissers, M.C.; Winterbourn, C.C. Roles of superoxide and myeloperoxidase in ascorbate oxidation in stimulated neutrophils and $H_{(2)}O_{(2)}$-treated HL60 cells. *Free Radic. Biol. Med.* **2011**, *51*, 1399–1405. [CrossRef] [PubMed]

53. Oberritter, H.; Glatthaar, B.; Moser, U.; Schmidt, K.H. Effect of functional stimulation on ascorbate content in phagocytes under physiological and pathological conditions. *Int. Arch. Allergy Appl. Immunol.* **1986**, *81*, 46–50. [CrossRef] [PubMed]

54. Goldschmidt, M.C. Reduced bactericidal activity in neutrophils from scorbutic animals and the effect of ascorbic acid on these target bacteria in vivo and in vitro. *Am. J. Clin. Nutr.* **1991**, *54*, 1214S–1220S. [PubMed]

55. Goldschmidt, M.C.; Masin, W.J.; Brown, L.R.; Wyde, P.R. The effect of ascorbic acid deficiency on leukocyte phagocytosis and killing of actinomyces viscosus. *Int. J. Vitam. Nutr. Res.* **1988**, *58*, 326–334. [PubMed]

56. Johnston, C.S.; Huang, S.N. Effect of ascorbic acid nutriture on blood histamine and neutrophil chemotaxis in guinea pigs. *J. Nutr.* **1991**, *121*, 126–130. [PubMed]

57. Rebora, A.; Dallegri, F.; Patrone, F. Neutrophil dysfunction and repeated infections: Influence of levamisole and ascorbic acid. *Br. J. Dermatol.* **1980**, *102*, 49–56. [CrossRef] [PubMed]

58. Patrone, F.; Dallegri, F.; Bonvini, E.; Minervini, F.; Sacchetti, C. Disorders of neutrophil function in children with recurrent pyogenic infections. *Med. Microbiol. Immunol.* **1982**, *171*, 113–122. [CrossRef] [PubMed]

59. Boura, P.; Tsapas, G.; Papadopoulou, A.; Magoula, I.; Kountouras, G. Monocyte locomotion in anergic chronic brucellosis patients: The in vivo effect of ascorbic acid. *Immunopharmacol. Immunotoxicol.* **1989**, *11*, 119–129. [CrossRef] [PubMed]

60. Anderson, R.; Theron, A. Effects of ascorbate on leucocytes: Part III. In vitro and in vivo stimulation of abnormal neutrophil motility by ascorbate. *S. Afr. Med. J.* **1979**, *56*, 429–433. [PubMed]

61. Johnston, C.S.; Martin, L.J.; Cai, X. Antihistamine effect of supplemental ascorbic acid and neutrophil chemotaxis. *J. Am. Coll. Nutr.* **1992**, *11*, 172–176. [PubMed]

62. Anderson, R.; Oosthuizen, R.; Maritz, R.; Theron, A.; Van Rensburg, A.J. The effects of increasing weekly doses of ascorbate on certain cellular and humoral immune functions in normal volunteers. *Am. J. Clin. Nutr.* **1980**, *33*, 71–76. [PubMed]

63. Anderson, R. Ascorbate-mediated stimulation of neutrophil motility and lymphocyte transformation by inhibition of the peroxidase/H_2O_2/halide system in vitro and in vivo. *Am. J. Clin. Nutr.* **1981**, *34*, 1906–1911. [PubMed]

64. Ganguly, R.; Durieux, M.F.; Waldman, R.H. Macrophage function in vitamin C-deficient guinea pigs. *Am. J. Clin. Nutr.* **1976**, *29*, 762–765. [PubMed]

65. Corberand, J.; Nguyen, F.; Fraysse, B.; Enjalbert, L. Malignant external otitis and polymorphonuclear leukocyte migration impairment. Improvement with ascorbic acid. *Arch. Otolaryngol.* **1982**, *108*, 122–124. [CrossRef] [PubMed]

66. Levy, R.; Schlaeffer, F. Successful treatment of a patient with recurrent furunculosis by vitamin C: Improvement of clinical course and of impaired neutrophil functions. *Int. J. Dermatol.* **1993**, *32*, 832–834. [CrossRef] [PubMed]

67. Levy, R.; Shriker, O.; Porath, A.; Riesenberg, K.; Schlaeffer, F. Vitamin C for the treatment of recurrent furunculosis in patients with imparied neutrophil functions. *J. Infect. Dis.* **1996**, *173*, 1502–1505. [CrossRef] [PubMed]

68. Nungester, W.J.; Ames, A.M. The relationship between ascorbic acid and phagocytic activity. *J. Infect. Dis.* **1948**, *83*, 50–54. [CrossRef] [PubMed]

69. Shilotri, P.G. Phagocytosis and leukocyte enzymes in ascorbic acid deficient guinea pigs. *J. Nutr.* **1977**, *107*, 1513–1516. [PubMed]

70. Shilotri, P.G. Glycolytic, hexose monophosphate shunt and bactericidal activities of leukocytes in ascorbic acid deficient guinea pigs. *J. Nutr.* **1977**, *107*, 1507–1512. [PubMed]

71. Sharma, P.; Raghavan, S.A.; Saini, R.; Dikshit, M. Ascorbate-mediated enhancement of reactive oxygen species generation from polymorphonuclear leukocytes: Modulatory effect of nitric oxide. *J. Leukoc. Biol.* **2004**, *75*, 1070–1078. [CrossRef] [PubMed]

72. Rebora, A.; Crovato, F.; Dallegri, F.; Patrone, F. Repeated staphylococcal pyoderma in two siblings with defective neutrophil bacterial killing. *Dermatologica* **1980**, *160*, 106–112. [CrossRef] [PubMed]

73. Vissers, M.C.; Wilkie, R.P. Ascorbate deficiency results in impaired neutrophil apoptosis and clearance and is associated with up-regulation of hypoxia-inducible factor 1alpha. *J. Leukoc. Biol.* **2007**, *81*, 1236–1244. [CrossRef] [PubMed]

74. Fisher, B.J.; Kraskauskas, D.; Martin, E.J.; Farkas, D.; Wegelin, J.A.; Brophy, D.; Ward, K.R.; Voelkel, N.F.; Fowler, A.A., III; Natarajan, R. Mechanisms of attenuation of abdominal sepsis induced acute lung injury by ascorbic acid. *Am. J. Physiol. Lung Cell. Mol. Physiol.* **2012**, *303*, L20–L32. [CrossRef] [PubMed]

75. Mohammed, B.M.; Fisher, B.J.; Kraskauskas, D.; Farkas, D.; Brophy, D.F.; Fowler, A.A.; Natarajan, R. Vitamin C: A novel regulator of neutrophil extracellular trap formation. *Nutrients* **2013**, *5*, 3131–3151. [CrossRef] [PubMed]

76. Huijskens, M.J.; Walczak, M.; Koller, N.; Briede, J.J.; Senden-Gijsbers, B.L.; Schnijderberg, M.C.; Bos, G.M.; Germeraad, W.T. Technical advance: Ascorbic acid induces development of double-positive T cells from human hematopoietic stem cells in the absence of stromal cells. *J. Leukoc. Biol.* **2014**, *96*, 1165–1175. [CrossRef] [PubMed]

77. Molina, N.; Morandi, A.C.; Bolin, A.P.; Otton, R. Comparative effect of fucoxanthin and vitamin C on oxidative and functional parameters of human lymphocytes. *Int. Immunopharmacol.* **2014**, *22*, 41–50. [CrossRef] [PubMed]

78. Tanaka, M.; Muto, N.; Gohda, E.; Yamamoto, I. Enhancement by ascorbic acid 2-glucoside or repeated additions of ascorbate of mitogen-induced IgM and IgG productions by human peripheral blood lymphocytes. *Jpn. J. Pharmacol.* **1994**, *66*, 451–456. [CrossRef] [PubMed]

79. Manning, J.; Mitchell, B.; Appadurai, D.A.; Shakya, A.; Pierce, L.J.; Wang, H.; Nganga, V.; Swanson, P.C.; May, J.M.; Tantin, D.; et al. Vitamin C promotes maturation of T-cells. *Antioxid. Redox Signal.* **2013**, *19*, 2054–2067. [CrossRef] [PubMed]

80. Kennes, B.; Dumont, I.; Brohee, D.; Hubert, C.; Neve, P. Effect of vitamin C supplements on cell-mediated immunity in old people. *Gerontology* **1983**, *29*, 305–310. [CrossRef] [PubMed]

81. Anderson, R.; Hay, I.; van Wyk, H.; Oosthuizen, R.; Theron, A. The effect of ascorbate on cellular humoral immunity in asthmatic children. *S. Afr. Med. J.* **1980**, *58*, 974–977. [PubMed]

82. Fraser, R.C.; Pavlovic, S.; Kurahara, C.G.; Murata, A.; Peterson, N.S.; Taylor, K.B.; Feigen, G.A. The effect of variations in vitamin C intake on the cellular immune response of guinea pigs. *Am. J. Clin. Nutr.* **1980**, *33*, 839–847. [PubMed]

83. Feigen, G.A.; Smith, B.H.; Dix, C.E.; Flynn, C.J.; Peterson, N.S.; Rosenberg, L.T.; Pavlovic, S.; Leibovitz, B. Enhancement of antibody production and protection against systemic anaphylaxis by large doses of vitamin C. *Res. Commun. Chem. Pathol. Pharmacol.* **1982**, *38*, 313–333. [CrossRef]

84. Prinz, W.; Bloch, J.; Gilich, G.; Mitchell, G. A systematic study of the effect of vitamin C supplementation on the humoral immune response in ascorbate-dependent mammals. I. The antibody response to sheep red blood cells (a T-dependent antigen) in guinea pigs. *Int. J. Vitam. Nutr. Res.* **1980**, *50*, 294–300. [PubMed]

85. Prinz, W.; Bortz, R.; Bregin, B.; Hersch, M. The effect of ascorbic acid supplementation on some parameters of the human immunological defence system. *Int. J. Vitam. Nutr. Res.* **1977**, *47*, 248–257. [PubMed]

86. Chen, Y.; Luo, G.; Yuan, J.; Wang, Y.; Yang, X.; Wang, X.; Li, G.; Liu, Z.; Zhong, N. Vitamin C mitigates oxidative stress and tumor necrosis factor-alpha in severe community-acquired pneumonia and LPS-induced macrophages. *Mediators Inflamm.* **2014**, *2014*, 426740. [CrossRef] [PubMed]

87. Jeng, K.C.; Yang, C.S.; Siu, W.Y.; Tsai, Y.S.; Liao, W.J.; Kuo, J.S. Supplementation with vitamins C and E enhances cytokine production by peripheral blood mononuclear cells in healthy adults. *Am. J. Clin. Nutr.* **1996**, *64*, 960–965. [PubMed]

88. Kim, Y.; Kim, H.; Bae, S.; Choi, J.; Lim, S.Y.; Lee, N.; Kong, J.M.; Hwang, Y.I.; Kang, J.S.; Lee, W.J. Vitamin C is an essential factor on the anti-viral immune responses through the production of interferon-a/b at the initial stage of influenza A virus (H_3N_2) infection. *Immune Netw.* **2013**, *13*, 70–74. [CrossRef] [PubMed]

89. Gao, Y.L.; Lu, B.; Zhai, J.H.; Liu, Y.C.; Qi, H.X.; Yao, Y.; Chai, Y.F.; Shou, S.T. The parenteral vitamin C improves sepsis and sepsis-induced multiple organ dysfunction syndrome via preventing cellular immunosuppression. *Mediat. Inflamm.* **2017**, *2017*, 4024672. [CrossRef] [PubMed]

90. Portugal, C.C.; Socodato, R.; Canedo, T.; Silva, C.M.; Martins, T.; Coreixas, V.S.; Loiola, E.C.; Gess, B.; Rohr, D.; Santiago, A.R.; et al. Caveolin-1-mediated internalization of the vitamin C transporter SVCT2 in microglia triggers an inflammatory phenotype. *Sci. Signal.* **2017**, *10*. [CrossRef] [PubMed]

91. Dahl, H.; Degre, M. The effect of ascorbic acid on production of human interferon and the antiviral activity in vitro. *Acta Pathol. Microbiol. Scand. B* **1976**, *84b*, 280–284. [CrossRef] [PubMed]

92. Karpinska, T.; Kawecki, Z.; Kandefer-Szerszen, M. The influence of ultraviolet irradiation, L-ascorbic acid and calcium chloride on the induction of interferon in human embryo fibroblasts. *Arch. Immunol. Ther. Exp.* **1982**, *30*, 33–37.

93. Siegel, B.V. Enhancement of interferon production by poly(rI)-poly(rC) in mouse cell cultures by ascorbic acid. *Nature* **1975**, *254*, 531–532. [CrossRef] [PubMed]

94. Canali, R.; Natarelli, L.; Leoni, G.; Azzini, E.; Comitato, R.; Sancak, O.; Barella, L.; Virgili, F. Vitamin C supplementation modulates gene expression in peripheral blood mononuclear cells specifically upon an inflammatory stimulus: A pilot study in healthy subjects. *Genes Nutr.* **2014**, *9*, 390. [CrossRef] [PubMed]

95. Dawson, W.; West, G.B. The influence of ascorbic acid on histamine metabolism in guinea-pigs. *Br. J. Pharmacol. Chemother.* **1965**, *24*, 725–734. [CrossRef] [PubMed]

96. Nandi, B.K.; Subramanian, N.; Majumder, A.K.; Chatterjee, I.B. Effect of ascorbic acid on detoxification of histamine under stress conditions. *Biochem. Pharmacol.* **1974**, *23*, 643–647. [CrossRef]

97. Subramanian, N.; Nandi, B.K.; Majumder, A.K.; Chatterjee, I.B. Role of L-ascorbic acid on detoxification of histamine. *Biochem. Pharmacol.* **1973**, *22*, 1671–1673. [CrossRef]

98. Chatterjee, I.B.; Gupta, S.D.; Majumder, A.K.; Nandi, B.K.; Subramanian, N. Effect of ascorbic acid on histamine metabolism in scorbutic guinea-pigs. *J. Physiol.* **1975**, *251*, 271–279. [CrossRef] [PubMed]

99. Clemetson, C.A. Histamine and ascorbic acid in human blood. *J. Nutr.* **1980**, *110*, 662–668. [PubMed]

100. Johnston, C.S.; Solomon, R.E.; Corte, C. Vitamin C depletion is associated with alterations in blood histamine and plasma free carnitine in adults. *J. Am. Coll. Nutr.* **1996**, *15*, 586–591. [CrossRef] [PubMed]

101. Hagel, A.F.; Layritz, C.M.; Hagel, W.H.; Hagel, H.J.; Hagel, E.; Dauth, W.; Kressel, J.; Regnet, T.; Rosenberg, A.; Neurath, M.F.; et al. Intravenous infusion of ascorbic acid decreases serum histamine concentrations in patients with allergic and non-allergic diseases. *Naunyn Schmiedebergs Arch. Pharmacol.* **2013**, *386*, 789–793. [CrossRef] [PubMed]

102. Bruno, R.S.; Leonard, S.W.; Atkinson, J.; Montine, T.J.; Ramakrishnan, R.; Bray, T.M.; Traber, M.G. Faster plasma vitamin E disappearance in smokers is normalized by vitamin C supplementation. *Free Radic. Biol. Med.* **2006**, *40*, 689–697. [CrossRef] [PubMed]

103. Parsons, K.K.; Maeda, N.; Yamauchi, M.; Banes, A.J.; Koller, B.H. Ascorbic acid-independent synthesis of collagen in mice. *Am. J. Physiol. Endocrinol. Metab.* **2006**, *290*, E1131–E1139. [CrossRef] [PubMed]

104. Ross, R.; Benditt, E.P. Wound healing and collagen formation. II. Fine structure in experimental scurvy. *J. Cell Biol.* **1962**, *12*, 533–551. [CrossRef] [PubMed]

105. Fukushima, R.; Yamazaki, E. Vitamin C requirement in surgical patients. *Curr. Opin. Clin. Nutr. Metab. Care* **2010**, *13*, 669–676. [CrossRef] [PubMed]

106. Blass, S.C.; Goost, H.; Tolba, R.H.; Stoffel-Wagner, B.; Kabir, K.; Burger, C.; Stehle, P.; Ellinger, S. Time to wound closure in trauma patients with disorders in wound healing is shortened by supplements containing antioxidant micronutrients and glutamine: A PRCT. *Clin. Nutr.* **2012**, *31*, 469–475. [CrossRef] [PubMed]

107. Cereda, E.; Gini, A.; Pedrolli, C.; Vanotti, A. Disease-specific, versus standard, nutritional support for the treatment of pressure ulcers in institutionalized older adults: A randomized controlled trial. *J. Am. Geriatr. Soc.* **2009**, *57*, 1395–1402. [CrossRef] [PubMed]

108. Martin, P.; Leibovich, S.J. Inflammatory cells during wound repair: The good, the bad and the ugly. *Trends Cell Biol.* **2005**, *15*, 599–607. [CrossRef] [PubMed]

109. Wilgus, T.A.; Roy, S.; McDaniel, J.C. Neutrophils and Wound Repair: Positive Actions and Negative Reactions. *Adv. Wound Care* **2013**, *2*, 379–388. [CrossRef] [PubMed]

110. Wong, S.L.; Demers, M.; Martinod, K.; Gallant, M.; Wang, Y.; Goldfine, A.B.; Kahn, C.R.; Wagner, D.D. Diabetes primes neutrophils to undergo NETosis, which impairs wound healing. *Nat. Med.* **2015**, *21*, 815–819. [CrossRef] [PubMed]

111. Washko, P.; Rotrosen, D.; Levine, M. Ascorbic acid transport and accumulation in human neutrophils. *J. Biol. Chem.* **1989**, *264*, 18996–19002. [PubMed]

112. Bergsten, P.; Amitai, G.; Kehrl, J.; Dhariwal, K.R.; Klein, H.G.; Levine, M. Millimolar concentrations of ascorbic acid in purified human mononuclear leukocytes. Depletion and reaccumulation. *J. Biol. Chem.* **1990**, *265*, 2584–2587. [PubMed]

113. Evans, R.M.; Currie, L.; Campbell, A. The distribution of ascorbic acid between various cellular components of blood, in normal individuals, and its relation to the plasma concentration. *Br. J. Nutr.* **1982**, *47*, 473–482. [CrossRef] [PubMed]

114. Levine, M.; Conry-Cantilena, C.; Wang, Y.; Welch, R.W.; Washko, P.W.; Dhariwal, K.R.; Park, J.B.; Lazarev, A.; Graumlich, J.F.; King, J.; et al. Vitamin C pharmacokinetics in healthy volunteers: Evidence for a recommended dietary allowance. *Proc. Natl. Acad. Sci. USA* **1996**, *93*, 3704–3709. [CrossRef] [PubMed]

115. Levine, M.; Wang, Y.; Padayatty, S.J.; Morrow, J. A new recommended dietary allowance of vitamin C for healthy young women. *Proc. Natl. Acad. Sci. USA* **2001**, *98*, 9842–9846. [CrossRef] [PubMed]

116. Carr, A.C.; Bozonet, S.M.; Pullar, J.M.; Simcock, J.W.; Vissers, M.C. Human skeletal muscle ascorbate is highly responsive to changes in vitamin C intake and plasma concentrations. *Am. J. Clin. Nutr.* **2013**, *97*, 800–807. [CrossRef] [PubMed]

117. Vissers, M.C.; Bozonet, S.M.; Pearson, J.F.; Braithwaite, L.J. Dietary ascorbate intake affects steady state tissue concentrations in vitamin C-deficient mice: Tissue deficiency after suboptimal intake and superior bioavailability from a food source (kiwifruit). *Am. J. Clin. Nutr.* **2011**, *93*, 292–301. [CrossRef] [PubMed]

118. Corpe, C.P.; Lee, J.H.; Kwon, O.; Eck, P.; Narayanan, J.; Kirk, K.L.; Levine, M. 6-Bromo-6-deoxy-l-ascorbic acid: An ascorbate analog specific for Na^+-dependent vitamin C transporter but not glucose transporter pathways. *J. Biol. Chem.* **2005**, *280*, 5211–5220. [CrossRef] [PubMed]

119. Washko, P.W.; Wang, Y.; Levine, M. Ascorbic acid recycling in human neutrophils. *J. Biol. Chem.* **1993**, *268*, 15531–15535. [PubMed]

120. Buettner, G.R. The pecking order of free radicals and antioxidants: Lipid peroxidation, alpha-tocopherol, and ascorbate. *Arch. Biochem. Biophys.* **1993**, *300*, 535–543. [CrossRef] [PubMed]

121. Sen, C.K.; Packer, L. Antioxidant and redox regulation of gene transcription. *FASEB J.* **1996**, *10*, 709–720. [PubMed]

122. Li, N.; Karin, M. Is NF-kappaB the sensor of oxidative stress? *Faseb J.* **1999**, *13*, 1137–1143. [PubMed]

123. Macdonald, J.; Galley, H.F.; Webster, N.R. Oxidative stress and gene expression in sepsis. *Br. J. Anaesth.* **2003**, *90*, 221–232. [CrossRef] [PubMed]

124. Tan, P.H.; Sagoo, P.; Chan, C.; Yates, J.B.; Campbell, J.; Beutelspacher, S.C.; Foxwell, B.M.; Lombardi, G.; George, A.J. Inhibition of NF-kappa B and oxidative pathways in human dendritic cells by antioxidative vitamins generates regulatory T cells. *J. Immunol.* **2005**, *174*, 7633–7644. [CrossRef] [PubMed]

125. Winterbourn, C.C.; Hampton, M.B. Thiol chemistry and specificity in redox signaling. *Free Radic. Biol. Med.* **2008**, *45*, 549–561. [CrossRef] [PubMed]

126. Griffiths, H.R.; Willetts, R.S.; Grant, M.M.; Mistry, N.; Lunec, J.; Bevan, R.J. In vivo vitamin C supplementation increases phosphoinositol transfer protein expression in peripheral blood mononuclear cells from healthy individuals. *Br. J. Nutr.* **2009**, *101*, 1432–1439. [CrossRef] [PubMed]

127. Grant, M.M.; Mistry, N.; Lunec, J.; Griffiths, H.R. Dose-dependent modulation of the T cell proteome by ascorbic acid. *Br. J. Nutr.* **2007**, *97*, 19–26. [CrossRef] [PubMed]

128. Lammermann, T. In the eye of the neutrophil swarm-navigation signals that bring neutrophils together in inflamed and infected tissues. *J. Leukoc. Biol.* **2016**, *100*, 55–63. [CrossRef] [PubMed]

129. Demaret, J.; Venet, F.; Friggeri, A.; Cazalis, M.A.; Plassais, J.; Jallades, L.; Malcus, C.; Poitevin-Later, F.; Textoris, J.; Lepape, A.; et al. Marked alterations of neutrophil functions during sepsis-induced immunosuppression. *J. Leukoc. Biol.* **2015**, *98*, 1081–1090. [CrossRef] [PubMed]

130. Arraes, S.M.; Freitas, M.S.; da Silva, S.V.; de Paula Neto, H.A.; Alves-Filho, J.C.; Auxiliadora Martins, M.; Basile-Filho, A.; Tavares-Murta, B.M.; Barja-Fidalgo, C.; Cunha, F.Q. Impaired neutrophil chemotaxis in sepsis associates with GRK expression and inhibition of actin assembly and tyrosine phosphorylation. *Blood* **2006**, *108*, 2906–2913. [CrossRef] [PubMed]

131. Chishti, A.D.; Shenton, B.K.; Kirby, J.A.; Baudouin, S.V. Neutrophil chemotaxis and receptor expression in clinical septic shock. *Intensive Care Med.* **2004**, *30*, 605–611. [CrossRef] [PubMed]

132. Tavares-Murta, B.M.; Zaparoli, M.; Ferreira, R.B.; Silva-Vergara, M.L.; Oliveira, C.H.; Murta, E.F.; Ferreira, S.H.; Cunha, F.Q. Failure of neutrophil chemotactic function in septic patients. *Crit. Care Med.* **2002**, *30*, 1056–1061. [CrossRef] [PubMed]

133. Hotchkiss, R.S.; Monneret, G.; Payen, D. Sepsis-induced immunosuppression: From cellular dysfunctions to immunotherapy. *Nat. Rev. Immunol.* **2013**, *13*, 862–874. [CrossRef] [PubMed]

134. Vohra, K.; Khan, A.J.; Telang, V.; Rosenfeld, W.; Evans, H.E. Improvement of neutrophil migration by systemic vitamin C in neonates. *J. Perinatol.* **1990**, *10*, 134–136. [PubMed]

135. Roos, D. Chronic granulomatous disease. *Br. Med. Bull.* **2016**, *118*, 50–63. [CrossRef] [PubMed]

136. Introne, W.; Boissy, R.E.; Gahl, W.A. Clinical, molecular, and cell biological aspects of Chediak-Higashi syndrome. *Mol. Genet. Metab.* **1999**, *68*, 283–303. [CrossRef] [PubMed]

137. Anderson, R.; Dittrich, O.C. Effects of ascorbate on leucocytes: Part IV. Increased neutrophil function and clinical improvement after oral ascorbate in 2 patients with chronic granulomatous disease. *S. Afr. Med. J.* **1979**, *56*, 476–480. [PubMed]

138. Anderson, R. Assessment of oral ascorbate in three children with chronic granulomatous disease and defective neutrophil motility over a 2-year period. *Clin. Exp. Immunol.* **1981**, *43*, 180–188. [PubMed]

139. Anderson, R. Effects of ascorbate on normal and abnormal leucocyte functions. *Int. J. Vitam. Nutr. Res. Suppl.* **1982**, *23*, 23–34. [PubMed]

140. Gallin, J.I.; Elin, R.J.; Hubert, R.T.; Fauci, A.S.; Kaliner, M.A.; Wolff, S.M. Efficacy of ascorbic acid in Chediak-Higashi syndrome (CHS): Studies in humans and mice. *Blood* **1979**, *53*, 226–234. [PubMed]

141. Boxer, L.A.; Watanabe, A.M.; Rister, M.; Besch, H.R., Jr.; Allen, J.; Baehner, R.L. Correction of leukocyte function in Chediak-Higashi syndrome by ascorbate. *N. Engl. J. Med.* **1976**, *295*, 1041–1045. [CrossRef] [PubMed]

142. Yegin, O.; Sanal, O.; Yeralan, O.; Gurgey, A.; Berkel, A.I. Defective lymphocyte locomotion in Chediak-Higashi syndrome. *Am. J. Dis. Child.* **1983**, *137*, 771–773. [PubMed]

143. Weening, R.S.; Schoorel, E.P.; Roos, D.; van Schaik, M.L.; Voetman, A.A.; Bot, A.A.; Batenburg-Plenter, A.M.; Willems, C.; Zeijlemaker, W.P.; Astaldi, A. Effect of ascorbate on abnormal neutrophil, platelet and lymphocytic function in a patient with the Chediak-Higashi syndrome. *Blood* **1981**, *57*, 856–865. [PubMed]

144. Boxer, L.A.; Vanderbilt, B.; Bonsib, S.; Jersild, R.; Yang, H.H.; Baehner, R.L. Enhancement of chemotactic response and microtubule assembly in human leukocytes by ascorbic acid. *J. Cell. Physiol.* **1979**, *100*, 119–126. [CrossRef] [PubMed]

145. Boxer, L.A.; Albertini, D.F.; Baehner, R.L.; Oliver, J.M. Impaired microtubule assembly and polymorphonuclear leucocyte function in the Chediak-Higashi syndrome correctable by ascorbic acid. *Br. J. Haematol.* **1979**, *43*, 207–213. [CrossRef] [PubMed]

146. Parker, W.H.; Rhea, E.M.; Qu, Z.C.; Hecker, M.R.; May, J.M. Intracellular ascorbate tightens the endothelial permeability barrier through Epac1 and the tubulin cytoskeleton. *Am. J. Physiol. Cell Physiol.* **2016**, *311*, C652–C662. [CrossRef] [PubMed]

147. Bozonet, S.M.; Carr, A.C.; Pullar, J.M.; Vissers, M.C.M. Enhanced human neutrophil vitamin C status, chemotaxis and oxidant generation following dietary supplementation with vitamin C-rich SunGold kiwifruit. *Nutrients* **2015**, *7*, 2574–2588. [CrossRef] [PubMed]

148. De la Fuente, M.; Ferrandez, M.D.; Burgos, M.S.; Soler, A.; Prieto, A.; Miquel, J. Immune function in aged women is improved by ingestion of vitamins C and E. *Can. J. Physiol. Pharmacol.* **1998**, *76*, 373–380. [CrossRef] [PubMed]

149. Winterbourn, C.C.; Kettle, A.J.; Hampton, M.B. Reactive oxygen species and neutrophil function. *Annu. Rev. Biochem.* **2016**, *85*, 765–792. [CrossRef] [PubMed]

150. Patrone, F.; Dallegri, F.; Bonvini, E.; Minervini, F.; Sacchetti, C. Effects of ascorbic acid on neutrophil function. Studies on normal and chronic granulomatous disease neutrophils. *Acta Vitaminol. Enzymol.* **1982**, *4*, 163–168. [PubMed]

151. Foroozanfar, N.; Lucas, C.F.; Joss, D.V.; Hugh-Jones, K.; Hobbs, J.R. Ascorbate (1 g/day) does not help the phagocyte killing defect of X-linked chronic granulomatous disease. *Clin. Exp. Immunol.* **1983**, *51*, 99–102. [PubMed]

152. Hampton, M.B.; Kettle, A.J.; Winterbourn, C.C. Inside the neutrophil phagosome: Oxidants, myeloperoxidase, and bacterial killing. *Blood* **1998**, *92*, 3007–3017. [PubMed]

153. Wenisch, C.; Graninger, W. Are soluble factors relevant for polymorphonuclear leukocyte dysregulation in septicemia? *Clin. Diagn. Lab. Immunol.* **1995**, *2*, 241–245. [PubMed]

154. Danikas, D.D.; Karakantza, M.; Theodorou, G.L.; Sakellaropoulos, G.C.; Gogos, C.A. Prognostic value of phagocytic activity of neutrophils and monocytes in sepsis. Correlation to CD64 and CD14 antigen expression. *Clin. Exp. Immunol.* **2008**, *154*, 87–97. [CrossRef] [PubMed]

155. Stephan, F.; Yang, K.; Tankovic, J.; Soussy, C.J.; Dhonneur, G.; Duvaldestin, P.; Brochard, L.; Brun-Buisson, C.; Harf, A.; Delclaux, C. Impairment of polymorphonuclear neutrophil functions precedes nosocomial infections in critically ill patients. *Crit. Care Med.* **2002**, *30*, 315–322. [CrossRef] [PubMed]

156. McGovern, N.N.; Cowburn, A.S.; Porter, L.; Walmsley, S.R.; Summers, C.; Thompson, A.A.; Anwar, S.; Willcocks, L.C.; Whyte, M.K.; Condliffe, A.M.; et al. Hypoxia selectively inhibits respiratory burst activity and killing of Staphylococcus aureus in human neutrophils. *J. Immunol.* **2011**, *186*, 453–463. [CrossRef] [PubMed]

157. Drifte, G.; Dunn-Siegrist, I.; Tissieres, P.; Pugin, J. Innate immune functions of immature neutrophils in patients with sepsis and severe systemic inflammatory response syndrome. *Crit. Care Med.* **2013**, *41*, 820–832. [CrossRef] [PubMed]

158. Bass, D.A.; Olbrantz, P.; Szejda, P.; Seeds, M.C.; McCall, C.E. Subpopulations of neutrophils with increased oxidative product formation in blood of patients with infection. *J. Immunol.* **1986**, *136*, 860–866. [PubMed]

159. Pillay, J.; Ramakers, B.P.; Kamp, V.M.; Loi, A.L.; Lam, S.W.; Hietbrink, F.; Leenen, L.P.; Tool, A.T.; Pickkers, P.; Koenderman, L. Functional heterogeneity and differential priming of circulating neutrophils in human experimental endotoxemia. *J. Leukoc. Biol.* **2010**, *88*, 211–220. [CrossRef] [PubMed]

160. Wenisch, C.; Fladerer, P.; Patruta, S.; Krause, R.; Horl, W. Assessment of neutrophil function in patients with septic shock: Comparison of methods. *Clin. Diagn. Lab. Immunol.* **2001**, *8*, 178–180. [CrossRef] [PubMed]

161. Fox, S.; Leitch, A.E.; Duffin, R.; Haslett, C.; Rossi, A.G. Neutrophil apoptosis: Relevance to the innate immune response and inflammatory disease. *J. Innate Immun.* **2010**, *2*, 216–227. [CrossRef] [PubMed]

162. Hampton, M.B.; Fadeel, B.; Orrenius, S. Redox regulation of the caspases during apoptosis. *Ann. N. Y. Acad. Sci.* **1998**, *854*, 328–335. [CrossRef] [PubMed]

163. Fadeel, B.; Ahlin, A.; Henter, J.I.; Orrenius, S.; Hampton, M.B. Involvement of caspases in neutrophil apoptosis: Regulation by reactive oxygen species. *Blood* **1998**, *92*, 4808–4818. [PubMed]

164. Wilkie, R.P.; Vissers, M.C.; Dragunow, M.; Hampton, M.B. A functional NADPH oxidase prevents caspase involvement in the clearance of phagocytic neutrophils. *Infect. Immun.* **2007**, *75*, 3256–3263. [CrossRef] [PubMed]

165. Keel, M.; Ungethum, U.; Steckholzer, U.; Niederer, E.; Hartung, T.; Trentz, O.; Ertel, W. Interleukin-10 counterregulates proinflammatory cytokine-induced inhibition of neutrophil apoptosis during severe sepsis. *Blood* **1997**, *90*, 3356–3363. [PubMed]

166. Jimenez, M.F.; Watson, R.W.; Parodo, J.; Evans, D.; Foster, D.; Steinberg, M.; Rotstein, O.D.; Marshall, J.C. Dysregulated expression of neutrophil apoptosis in the systemic inflammatory response syndrome. *Arch. Surg.* **1997**, *132*, 1263–1269. [CrossRef] [PubMed]

167. Harter, L.; Mica, L.; Stocker, R.; Trentz, O.; Keel, M. Mcl-1 correlates with reduced apoptosis in neutrophils from patients with sepsis. *J. Am. Coll. Surg.* **2003**, *197*, 964–973. [CrossRef] [PubMed]

168. Taneja, R.; Parodo, J.; Jia, S.H.; Kapus, A.; Rotstein, O.D.; Marshall, J.C. Delayed neutrophil apoptosis in sepsis is associated with maintenance of mitochondrial transmembrane potential and reduced caspase-9 activity. *Crit. Care Med.* **2004**, *32*, 1460–1469. [CrossRef] [PubMed]

169. Fotouhi-Ardakani, N.; Kebir, D.E.; Pierre-Charles, N.; Wang, L.; Ahern, S.P.; Filep, J.G.; Milot, E. Role for myeloid nuclear differentiation antigen in the regulation of neutrophil apoptosis during sepsis. *Am. J. Respir. Crit. Care Med.* **2010**, *182*, 341–350. [CrossRef] [PubMed]

170. Paunel-Gorgulu, A.; Flohe, S.; Scholz, M.; Windolf, J.; Logters, T. Increased serum soluble Fas after major trauma is associated with delayed neutrophil apoptosis and development of sepsis. *Crit. Care* **2011**, *15*, R20. [CrossRef] [PubMed]

171. Paunel-Gorgulu, A.; Kirichevska, T.; Logters, T.; Windolf, J.; Flohe, S. Molecular mechanisms underlying delayed apoptosis in neutrophils from multiple trauma patients with and without sepsis. *Mol. Med.* **2012**, *18*, 325–335. [CrossRef] [PubMed]

172. Tamayo, E.; Gomez, E.; Bustamante, J.; Gomez-Herreras, J.I.; Fonteriz, R.; Bobillo, F.; Bermejo-Martin, J.F.; Castrodeza, J.; Heredia, M.; Fierro, I.; et al. Evolution of neutrophil apoptosis in septic shock survivors and nonsurvivors. *J. Crit. Care* **2012**, *27*, 415. [CrossRef] [PubMed]

173. Fialkow, L.; Fochesatto Filho, L.; Bozzetti, M.C.; Milani, A.R.; Rodrigues Filho, E.M.; Ladniuk, R.M.; Pierozan, P.; de Moura, R.M.; Prolla, J.C.; Vachon, E.; et al. Neutrophil apoptosis: A marker of disease severity in sepsis and sepsis-induced acute respiratory distress syndrome. *Crit. Care* **2006**, *10*, R155. [CrossRef] [PubMed]

174. Ertel, W.; Keel, M.; Infanger, M.; Ungethum, U.; Steckholzer, U.; Trentz, O. Circulating mediators in serum of injured patients with septic complications inhibit neutrophil apoptosis through up-regulation of protein-tyrosine phosphorylation. *J. Trauma* **1998**, *44*, 767–775. [CrossRef] [PubMed]

175. Parlato, M.; Souza-Fonseca-Guimaraes, F.; Philippart, F.; Misset, B.; Adib-Conquy, M.; Cavaillon, J.M. CD24-triggered caspase-dependent apoptosis via mitochondrial membrane depolarization and reactive oxygen species production of human neutrophils is impaired in sepsis. *J. Immunol.* **2014**, *192*, 2449–2459. [CrossRef] [PubMed]

176. Colotta, F.; Re, F.; Polentarutti, N.; Sozzani, S.; Mantovani, A. Modulation of granulocyte survival and programmed cell death by cytokines and bacterial products. *Blood* **1992**, *80*, 2012–2020. [PubMed]

177. Mikirova, N.; Riordan, N.; Casciari, J. Modulation of Cytokines in Cancer Patients by Intravenous Ascorbate Therapy. *Med. Sci. Monit.* **2016**, *22*, 14–25. [CrossRef] [PubMed]

178. Ferron-Celma, I.; Mansilla, A.; Hassan, L.; Garcia-Navarro, A.; Comino, A.M.; Bueno, P.; Ferron, J.A. Effect of vitamin C administration on neutrophil apoptosis in septic patients after abdominal surgery. *J. Surg. Res.* **2009**, *153*, 224–230. [CrossRef] [PubMed]

179. Pechous, R.D. With Friends like These: The Complex Role of Neutrophils in the Progression of Severe Pneumonia. *Front. Cell. Infect. Microbiol.* **2017**, *7*, 160. [CrossRef] [PubMed]

180. Zawrotniak, M.; Rapala-Kozik, M. Neutrophil extracellular traps (NETs)—Formation and implications. *Acta Biochim. Pol.* **2013**, *60*, 277–284. [PubMed]

181. Fuchs, T.A.; Abed, U.; Goosmann, C.; Hurwitz, R.; Schulze, I.; Wahn, V.; Weinrauch, Y.; Brinkmann, V.; Zychlinsky, A. Novel cell death program leads to neutrophil extracellular traps. *J. Cell Biol.* **2007**, *176*, 231–241. [CrossRef] [PubMed]

182. Brinkmann, V.; Reichard, U.; Goosmann, C.; Fauler, B.; Uhlemann, Y.; Weiss, D.S.; Weinrauch, Y.; Zychlinsky, A. Neutrophil extracellular traps kill bacteria. *Science* **2004**, *303*, 1532–1535. [CrossRef] [PubMed]

183. Parker, H.; Albrett, A.M.; Kettle, A.J.; Winterbourn, C.C. Myeloperoxidase associated with neutrophil extracellular traps is active and mediates bacterial killing in the presence of hydrogen peroxide. *J. Leukoc. Biol.* **2012**, *91*, 369–376. [CrossRef] [PubMed]

184. Czaikoski, P.G.; Mota, J.M.; Nascimento, D.C.; Sonego, F.; Castanheira, F.V.; Melo, P.H.; Scortegagna, G.T.; Silva, R.L.; Barroso-Sousa, R.; Souto, F.O.; et al. Neutrophil extracellular traps induce organ damage during experimental and clinical sepsis. *PLoS ONE* **2016**, *11*, e0148142. [CrossRef] [PubMed]

185. Camicia, G.; Pozner, R.; de Larranaga, G. Neutrophil extracellular traps in sepsis. *Shock* **2014**, *42*, 286–294. [CrossRef] [PubMed]

186. Silk, E.; Zhao, H.; Weng, H.; Ma, D. The role of extracellular histone in organ injury. *Cell Death Dis.* **2017**, *8*, e2812. [CrossRef] [PubMed]

187. Margraf, S.; Logters, T.; Reipen, J.; Altrichter, J.; Scholz, M.; Windolf, J. Neutrophil-derived circulating free DNA (cf-DNA/NETs): A potential prognostic marker for posttraumatic development of inflammatory second hit and sepsis. *Shock* **2008**, *30*, 352–358. [CrossRef] [PubMed]

188. Natarajan, R.; Fisher, B.J.; Syed, A.A.; Fowler, A.A. Impact of intravenous ascorbic acid infusion on novel biomarkers in patients with severe sepsis. *J. Pulm. Respir. Med.* **2014**, *4*, 8. [CrossRef]

189. Elks, P.M.; van Eeden, F.J.; Dixon, G.; Wang, X.; Reyes-Aldasoro, C.C.; Ingham, P.W.; Whyte, M.K.; Walmsley, S.R.; Renshaw, S.A. Activation of hypoxia-inducible factor-1alpha (Hif-1alpha) delays inflammation resolution by reducing neutrophil apoptosis and reverse migration in a zebrafish inflammation model. *Blood* **2011**, *118*, 712–722. [CrossRef] [PubMed]

190. Hirota, K.; Semenza, G.L. Regulation of hypoxia-inducible factor 1 by prolyl and asparaginyl hydroxylases. *Biochem. Biophys. Res. Commun.* **2005**, *338*, 610–616. [CrossRef] [PubMed]

191. McInturff, A.M.; Cody, M.J.; Elliott, E.A.; Glenn, J.W.; Rowley, J.W.; Rondina, M.T.; Yost, C.C. Mammalian target of rapamycin regulates neutrophil extracellular trap formation via induction of hypoxia-inducible factor 1 alpha. *Blood* **2012**, *120*, 3118–3125. [CrossRef] [PubMed]

192. Hong, J.M.; Kim, J.H.; Kang, J.S.; Lee, W.J.; Hwang, Y.I. Vitamin C is taken up by human T cells via sodium-dependent vitamin C transporter 2 (SVCT2) and exerts inhibitory effects on the activation of these cells in vitro. *Anat. Cell Biol.* **2016**, *49*, 88–98. [CrossRef] [PubMed]

193. Bergsten, P.; Yu, R.; Kehrl, J.; Levine, M. Ascorbic acid transport and distribution in human B lymphocytes. *Arch. Biochem. Biophys.* **1995**, *317*, 208–214. [CrossRef] [PubMed]

194. Lenton, K.J.; Therriault, H.; Fulop, T.; Payette, H.; Wagner, J.R. Glutathione and ascorbate are negatively correlated with oxidative DNA damage in human lymphocytes. *Carcinogenesis* **1999**, *20*, 607–613. [CrossRef] [PubMed]

195. Campbell, J.D.; Cole, M.; Bunditrutavorn, B.; Vella, A.T. Ascorbic acid is a potent inhibitor of various forms of T cell apoptosis. *Cell. Immunol.* **1999**, *194*, 1–5. [CrossRef] [PubMed]

196. Huijskens, M.J.; Walczak, M.; Sarkar, S.; Atrafi, F.; Senden-Gijsbers, B.L.; Tilanus, M.G.; Bos, G.M.; Wieten, L.; Germeraad, W.T. Ascorbic acid promotes proliferation of natural killer cell populations in culture systems applicable for natural killer cell therapy. *Cytotherapy* **2015**, *17*, 613–620. [CrossRef] [PubMed]

197. Penn, N.D.; Purkins, L.; Kelleher, J.; Heatley, R.V.; Mascie-Taylor, B.H.; Belfield, P.W. The effect of dietary supplementation with vitamins A, C and E on cell-mediated immune function in elderly long-stay patients: A randomized controlled trial. *Age Ageing* **1991**, *20*, 169–174. [CrossRef] [PubMed]

198. Heuser, G.; Vojdani, A. Enhancement of natural killer cell activity and T and B cell function by buffered vitamin C in patients exposed to toxic chemicals: The role of protein kinase-C. *Immunopharmacol. Immunotoxicol.* **1997**, *19*, 291–312. [CrossRef] [PubMed]

199. Sasidharan Nair, V.; Song, M.H.; Oh, K.I. Vitamin C Facilitates Demethylation of the Foxp3 Enhancer in a Tet-Dependent Manner. *J. Immunol.* **2016**, *196*, 2119–2131. [CrossRef] [PubMed]

200. Nikolouli, E.; Hardtke-Wolenski, M.; Hapke, M.; Beckstette, M.; Geffers, R.; Floess, S.; Jaeckel, E.; Huehn, J. Alloantigen-Induced Regulatory T Cells Generated in Presence of Vitamin C Display Enhanced Stability of Foxp3 Expression and Promote Skin Allograft Acceptance. *Front. Immunol.* **2017**, *8*, 748. [CrossRef] [PubMed]

201. Monfort, A.; Wutz, A. Breathing-in epigenetic change with vitamin C. *EMBO Rep.* **2013**, *14*, 337–346. [CrossRef] [PubMed]

202. Song, C.X.; He, C. Potential functional roles of DNA demethylation intermediates. *Trends Biochem. Sci.* **2013**, *38*, 480–484. [CrossRef] [PubMed]

203. Johnston, C.S.; Barkyoumb, G.M.; Schumacher, S.S. Vitamin C supplementation slightly improves physical activity levels and reduces cold incidence in men with marginal vitamin C status: A randomized controlled trial. *Nutrients* **2014**, *6*, 2572–2583. [CrossRef] [PubMed]

204. Haryanto, B.; Suksmasari, T.; Wintergerst, E.; Maggini, S. Multivitamin supplementation supports immune function and ameliorates conditions triggered by reduced air quality. *Vitam. Miner.* **2015**, *4*, 1–15.

205. Romieu, I.; Castro-Giner, F.; Kunzli, N.; Sunyer, J. Air pollution, oxidative stress and dietary supplementation: A review. *Eur. Respir. J.* **2008**, *31*, 179–196. [CrossRef] [PubMed]

206. Kelly, F.; Dunster, C.; Mudway, I. Air pollution and the elderly: Oxidant/antioxidant issues worth consideration. *Eur. Respir. J.* **2003**, *21*, 70s–75s. [CrossRef]

207. Marmot, A.; Eley, J.; Stafford, M.; Stansfeld, S.; Warwick, E.; Marmot, M. Building health: An epidemiological study of "sick building syndrome" in the Whitehall II study. *Occup. Environ. Med.* **2006**, *63*, 283–289. [CrossRef] [PubMed]

208. Pozzer, A.; Zimmermann, P.; Doering, U.; van Aardenne, J.; Tost, H.; Dentener, F.; Janssens-Maenhout, G.; Lelieveld, J. Effects of business-as-usual anthropogenic emissions on air quality. *Atmos. Chem. Phys.* **2012**, *12*, 6915–6937. [CrossRef]

209. Sram, R.J.; Binkova, B.; Rossner, P., Jr. Vitamin C for DNA damage prevention. *Mutat. Res.* **2012**, *733*, 39–49. [CrossRef] [PubMed]

210. Tribble, D.; Giuliano, L.; Fortmann, S. Reduced plasma ascorbic acid concentrations in nonsmokers regularly exposed to environmental tobacco smoke. *Am. J. Clin. Nutr.* **1993**, *58*, 886–890. [PubMed]

211. Valkonen, M.; Kuusi, T. Passive smoking induces atherogenic changes in low-density lipoprotein. *Circulation* **1998**, *97*, 2012–2016. [CrossRef] [PubMed]

212. Schectman, G.; Byrd, J.C.; Hoffmann, R. Ascorbic acid requirements for smokers: Analysis of a population survey. *Am. J. Clin. Nutr.* **1991**, *53*, 1466–1470. [PubMed]

213. Preston, A.M.; Rodriguez, C.; Rivera, C.E.; Sahai, H. Influence of environmental tobacco smoke on vitamin C status in children. *Am. J. Clin. Nutr.* **2003**, *77*, 167–172. [PubMed]

214. Strauss, R. Environmental tobacco smoke and serum vitamin C levels in children. *Pediatrics* **2001**, *107*, 540–542. [CrossRef] [PubMed]

215. Panda, K.; Chattopadhyay, R.; Chattopadhyay, D.J.; Chatterjee, I.B. Vitamin C prevents cigarette smoke-induced oxidative damage in vivo. *Free Radic. Biol. Med.* **2000**, *29*, 115–124. [CrossRef]

216. Dietrich, M.; Block, G.; Benowitz, N.; Morrow, J.; Hudes, M.; Jacob, P., III; Norkus, E.; Packer, L. Vitamin C supplementation decreases oxidative stress biomarker f2-isoprostanes in plasma of nonsmokers exposed to environmental tobacco smoke. *Nutr. Cancer* **2003**, *45*, 176–184. [CrossRef] [PubMed]

217. Bagaitkar, J.; Demuth, D.; Scott, D. Tobacco use increases susceptibility to bacterial infection. *Tob. Induc. Dis.* **2008**, *4*, 12. [CrossRef] [PubMed]

218. Arcavi, L.; Benowitz, N.L. Cigarette smoking and infection. *Arch. Intern. Med.* **2004**, *164*, 2206–2216. [CrossRef] [PubMed]

219. Sargeant, L.; Jaeckel, A.; Wareham, N. Interaction of vitamin C with the relation between smoking and obstructive airways disease in EPIC Norfolk. European Prospective Investigation into Cancer and Nutrition. *Eur. Respir. J.* **2000**, *16*, 397–403. [CrossRef] [PubMed]

220. Peleg, A.Y.; Weerarathna, T.; McCarthy, J.S.; Davis, T.M. Common infections in diabetes: Pathogenesis, management and relationship to glycaemic control. *Diabetes Metab. Res. Rev.* **2007**, *23*, 3–13. [CrossRef] [PubMed]

221. Narayan, K.M.V.; Williams, D.; Gregg, E.W.; Cowie, C.C. (Eds.) *Diabetes Public Health: From Data to Policy*; Oxford University Press: Oxford, UK, 2011.

222. Pirola, L.; Ferraz, J. Role of pro- and anti-inflammatory phenomena in the physiopathology of type 2 diabetes and obesity. *World J. Biol. Chem.* **2017**, *8*, 120–128. [CrossRef] [PubMed]

223. Donath, M. Targeting inflammation in the treatment of type 2 diabetes: Time to start. *Nat. Rev. Drug Discov.* **2014**, *13*, 465–476. [CrossRef] [PubMed]

224. Ferrante, A.W., Jr. Macrophages, fat, and the emergence of immunometabolism. *J. Clin. Investig.* **2013**, *123*, 4992–4993. [CrossRef] [PubMed]

225. Osborn, O.; Olefsky, J.M. The cellular and signaling networks linking the immune system and metabolism in disease. *Nat. Med.* **2012**, *18*, 363–374. [CrossRef] [PubMed]

226. Wilson, R.; Willis, J.; Gearry, R.; Skidmore, P.; Fleming, E.; Frampton, C.; Carr, A. Inadequate vitamin C status in prediabetes and type 2 diabetes mellitus: Associations with glycaemic control, obesity, and smoking. *Nutrients* **2017**, *9*, 997. [CrossRef] [PubMed]

227. Maggini, S.; Wenzlaff, S.; Hornig, D. Essential role of vitamin C and zinc in child immunity and health. *J. Int. Med. Res.* **2010**, *38*, 386–414. [CrossRef] [PubMed]

228. Wintergerst, E.; Maggini, S.; Hornig, D. Immune-enhancing role of vitamin C and zinc and effect on clinical conditions. *Ann. Nutr. Metab.* **2006**, *50*, 85–94. [CrossRef] [PubMed]

229. Harding, A.H.; Wareham, N.J.; Bingham, S.A.; Khaw, K.; Luben, R.; Welch, A.; Forouhi, N.G. Plasma vitamin C level, fruit and vegetable consumption, and the risk of new-onset type 2 diabetes mellitus: The European prospective investigation of cancer—Norfolk prospective study. *Arch. Intern. Med.* **2008**, *168*, 1493–1499. [CrossRef] [PubMed]

230. Kositsawat, J.; Freeman, V.L. Vitamin C and A1c relationship in the National Health and Nutrition Examination Survey (NHANES) 2003–2006. *J. Am. Coll. Nutr.* **2011**, *30*, 477–483. [CrossRef] [PubMed]

231. Carter, P.; Gray, L.J.; Talbot, D.; Morris, D.H.; Khunti, K.; Davies, M.J. Fruit and vegetable intake and the association with glucose parameters: A cross-sectional analysis of the Let's Prevent Diabetes Study. *Eur. J. Clin. Nutr.* **2013**, *67*, 12–17. [CrossRef] [PubMed]

232. Mazloom, Z.; Hejazi, N.; Dabbaghmanesh, M.H.; Tabatabaei, H.R.; Ahmadi, A.; Ansar, H. Effect of vitamin C supplementation on postprandial oxidative stress and lipid profile in type 2 diabetic patients. *Pak. J. Biol. Sci.* **2011**, *14*, 900–904. [PubMed]

233. Ashor, A.W.; Werner, A.D.; Lara, J.; Willis, N.D.; Mathers, J.C.; Siervo, M. Effects of vitamin C supplementation on glycaemic control: A systematic review and meta-analysis of randomised controlled trials. *Eur. J. Clin. Nutr.* **2017**. [CrossRef] [PubMed]

234. Hajishengallis, G. Too old to fight? Aging and its toll on innate immunity. *Mol. Oral Microbiol.* **2010**, *25*, 25–37. [CrossRef] [PubMed]

235. Cheng, L.; Cohen, M.; Bhagavan, H. Vitamin C and the elderly. In *CRC Handbook of Nutrition in the Aged*; Watson, R., Ed.; CRC Press Inc.: Boca Raton, FL, USA, 1985; pp. 157–185.

236. Simon, J.; Hudes, E.; Tice, J. Relation of serum ascorbic acid to mortality among US adults. *J. Am. Coll. Nutr.* **2001**, *20*, 255–263. [CrossRef] [PubMed]

237. Fletcher, A.; Breeze, E.; Shetty, P. Antioxidant vitamins and mortality in older persons: Findings from the nutrition add-on study to the Medical Research Council Trial of Assessment and Management of Older People in the Community. *Am. J. Clin. Nutr.* **2003**, *78*, 999–1010. [PubMed]

238. Thurman, J.; Mooradian, A. Vitamin supplementation therapy in the elderly. *Drugs Aging* **1997**, *11*, 433–449. [CrossRef] [PubMed]

239. Hanck, A. Vitamin C in the elderly. *Int. J. Vitam. Nutr. Res. Suppl.* **1983**, *24*, 257–269. [PubMed]

240. Schorah, C.J. The level of vitamin C reserves required in man: Towards a solution to the controversy. *Proc. Nutr. Soc.* **1981**, *40*, 147–154. [CrossRef] [PubMed]

241. Hunt, C.; Chakravorty, N.; Annan, G. The clinical and biochemical effects of vitamin C supplementation in short-stay hospitalized geriatric patients. *Int. J. Vitam. Nutr. Res.* **1984**, *54*, 65–74. [PubMed]

242. Mayland, C.R.; Bennett, M.I.; Allan, K. Vitamin C deficiency in cancer patients. *Palliat. Med.* **2005**, *19*, 17–20. [CrossRef] [PubMed]

243. Danai, P.A.; Moss, M.; Mannino, D.M.; Martin, G.S. The epidemiology of sepsis in patients with malignancy. *Chest* **2006**, *129*, 1432–1440. [CrossRef] [PubMed]

244. Gan, R.; Eintracht, S.; Hoffer, L.J. Vitamin C deficiency in a university teaching hospital. *J. Am. Coll. Nutr.* **2008**, *27*, 428–433. [CrossRef] [PubMed]

245. Bakaev, V.V.; Duntau, A.P. Ascorbic acid in blood serum of patients with pulmonary tuberculosis and pneumonia. *Int. J. Tuberc. Lung Dis.* **2004**, *8*, 263–266. [PubMed]

246. Hunt, C.; Chakravorty, N.K.; Annan, G.; Habibzadeh, N.; Schorah, C.J. The clinical effects of vitamin C supplementation in elderly hospitalised patients with acute respiratory infections. *Int. J. Vitam. Nutr. Res.* **1994**, *64*, 212–219. [PubMed]

247. Bharara, A.; Grossman, C.; Grinnan, D.; Syed, A.A.; Fisher, B.J.; DeWilde, C.; Natarajan, R.; Fowler, A.A. Intravenous vitamin C administered as adjunctive therapy for recurrent acute respiratory distress syndrome. *Case Rep. Crit. Care* **2016**, *2016*, 8560871. [CrossRef] [PubMed]

248. Fowler, A.A.; Kim, C.; Lepler, L.; Malhotra, R.; Debesa, O.; Natarajan, R.; Fisher, B.J.; Syed, A.; DeWilde, C.; Priday, A.; et al. Intravenous vitamin C as adjunctive therapy for enterovirus/rhinovirus induced acute respiratory distress syndrome. *World J. Crit. Care Med.* **2017**, *6*, 85–90. [CrossRef] [PubMed]

249. Hemila, H.; Chalker, E. Vitamin C for preventing and treating the common cold. *Cochrane Database Syst. Rev.* **2013**, *1*, CD000980.

250. Hemila, H. Vitamin C and the common cold. *Br. J. Nutr.* **1992**, *67*, 3–16. [CrossRef] [PubMed]

251. Hume, R.; Weyers, E. Changes in leucocyte ascorbic acid during the common cold. *Scott. Med. J.* **1973**, *18*, 3–7. [CrossRef] [PubMed]

252. Wilson, C.W. Ascorbic acid function and metabolism during colds. *Ann. N. Y. Acad. Sci.* **1975**, *258*, 529–539. [CrossRef] [PubMed]

253. Schwartz, A.R.; Togo, Y.; Hornick, R.B.; Tominaga, S.; Gleckman, R.A. Evaluation of the efficacy of ascorbic acid in prophylaxis of induced rhinovirus 44 infection in man. *J. Infect. Dis.* **1973**, *128*, 500–505. [CrossRef] [PubMed]

254. Davies, J.E.; Hughes, R.E.; Jones, E.; Reed, S.E.; Craig, J.W.; Tyrrell, D.A. Metabolism of ascorbic acid (vitamin C) in subjects infected with common cold viruses. *Biochem. Med.* **1979**, *21*, 78–85. [CrossRef]

255. Mochalkin, N. Ascorbic acid in the complex therapy of acute pneumonia. *Voen. Med. Zhurnal* **1970**, *9*, 17–21. Available online: http://www.mv.helsinki.fi/home/hemila/T5.pdf (accessed on 5 December 2014).

256. Hemila, H.; Louhiala, P. Vitamin C for preventing and treating pneumonia. *Cochrane Database Syst. Rev.* **2013**, *8*, CD005532.

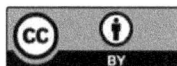

nutrients

MDPI

Article

Vitamin C Intake is Inversely Associated with Cardiovascular Mortality in a Cohort of Spanish Graduates: The SUN Project

Nerea Martín-Calvo [1,2,3] (iD) **and Miguel Ángel Martínez-González** [1,2,3,4,]*

1   Department of Preventive Medicine and Public Health, University of Navarra,
    31008 Pamplona, Navarra, Spain; nmartincalvo@unav.es
2   IdiSNA, Navarra Institute for Health Research, 31008 Pamplona, Navarra, Spain
3   CIBER Physiopathology of Obesity and Nutrition (CIBERobn), Carlos III Institute of Health,
    28029 Madrid, Spain
4   Department of Nutrition, Harvard T.H. Chan School of Public Health, Boston, MA 02115, USA
*   Correspondence: mamartinez@unav.es; Tel.: +34-948-254-600

Received: 14 July 2017; Accepted: 24 August 2017; Published: 29 August 2017

Abstract: Observational studies have found a protective effect of vitamin C on cardiovascular health. However, results are inconsistent, and residual confounding by fiber might be present. The aim of this study was to assess the association of vitamin C with the incidence of cardiovascular disease (CVD) and cardiovascular mortality (CVM) while accounting for fiber intake and adherence to the Mediterranean dietary pattern. We followed up 13,421 participants in the Seguimiento Universidad de Navarra (University of Navarra follow-up) (SUN) cohort for a mean time of 11 years. Information was collected at baseline and every two years through mailed questionnaires. Diet was assessed with a validated semi-quantitative food frequency questionnaire. Incident CVD was defined as incident fatal or non-fatal myocardial infarction, fatal or non-fatal stroke, or death due to any cardiovascular cause. CVM was defined as death due to cardiovascular causes. Events were confirmed by physicians in the study team after revision of medical records. Cox proportional hazard models were fitted to assess the associations of (a) energy-adjusted and (b) fiber-adjusted vitamin C intake with CVD and CVM. We found energy-adjusted vitamin C was inversely associated with CVD and CVM after adjusting for several confounding factors, including fiber from foods other than fruits and vegetables, and adherence to the Mediterranean dietary pattern. On the other hand, when vitamin C was adjusted for total fiber intake using the residuals method, we found a significant inverse association with CVM (HR (95% confidence interval (CI)) for the third tertile compared to the first tertile, 0.30 (0.12–0.72), but not with CVD in the fully adjusted model.

Keywords: vitamin C; cardiovascular disease; cardiovascular mortality; fiber

---

1. Introduction

Vitamin C, also known as L-ascorbic acid, is a water-soluble vitamin naturally present in some foods, added to others, and available as dietary supplement. Vitamin C is an essential dietary component, since humans, unlike most animals, are unable to synthetize it. Vitamin C is required for the synthesis of collagen, L-carnitine and some neurotransmitters. Based on vitamin C's antioxidant capacity, there is growing interest in assessing whether vitamin C intake might help prevent or delay some type of cancer, cardiovascular disease (CVD) or other diseases in which oxidative stress plays an important role.

Recommended dietary allowances (RDA) for vitamin C—75 mg/day for women and 90 mg/day for men [1]—are based on its known physiological and antioxidant functions in white blood cells and are higher than the amount required to prevent deficiency. Nevertheless, given that vitamin C may relate to cancer, CVD, or other diseases through different mechanisms, whether classical RDAs are optimal to obtain maximum benefits is unclear [2].

The belief that vitamin C relates to cardiovascular health stemmed from the benefits observed from fruit and vegetable consumption [3–5]. Observational studies have found an inverse association of dietary vitamin C [6] and ascorbic acid plasma levels [6–8] with cardiovascular risk factors, CVD, and cardiovascular mortality (CVM). Nevertheless, those studies showed some limitations, including suboptimal adjustment for potential confounders such as fiber intake.

Vitamin C from foods and supplements seemed to be equally bioavailable [9]. However, observational studies [6] and clinical trials [10–13] concluded that supplementation with vitamin C (500 to 1000 mg/day) had no effect on different cardiovascular endpoints. Moreover, higher CVM and total mortality has been reported among participants under vitamin C supplementation in both observational [14] and interventional studies [15]. On the other hand, two meta-analyses reported that high dose supplementation with vitamin C ((500 to 2000 mg/day) and (500 to 4000 mg/day) respectively) was associated to endothelial function improvements [16] and reduced blood pressure [17].

The aim of this study was to assess whether vitamin C intake was independently associated with lower CVD and CVM risk among participants in the Seguimiento Universidad de Navarra (University of Navarra follow-up) (SUN) cohort.

2. Materials and Methods

2.1. Study Population

The SUN project is an ongoing, prospective and multipurpose cohort of Spanish university graduates. As a dynamic cohort, enrolment is permanently open, and follow-up information is gathered by mailed questionnaires every two years. Regarding the obtention of informed consent of potential participants, we duly informed these potential candidates of their right to refuse to participate in the SUN study or to withdraw their consent to participate at any time without reprisal, according to the principles of the Declaration of Helsinki. Special attention was given to the specific information needs of individual potential candidates as well as to the methods used to deliver their information and the feedback that may receive in the future from the research team. After ensuring that the candidate had understood the information, we sought their potential freely-given informed consent, and their voluntary completion of the baseline questionnaire. These methods were accepted by our Institutional Review Board as to imply an appropriately-obtained informed consent. A more detailed description of the SUN methodology can be found elsewhere [18]. The study protocol was approved by the Institutional Review Board of the University of Navarra (approval code 010830).

We assessed 22,280 participants recruited before March 2014 to ensure they completed at least the two-year follow-up questionnaire. We excluded 308 participants due to prevalent cardiovascular disease, 7384 participants younger than 40 years old who were considered too young to present a cardiovascular event during the follow-up, 290 participants with energy intake out of the sex-specific limits (under p1 or above p99), and 284 participants with vitamin C intake out of the sex-specific limits (under p1 or above p99). Out of the rest of the participants, 593 were lost to follow-up (retention in the cohort: 96%), leading to a final sample of 13,421 participants (Figure 1).

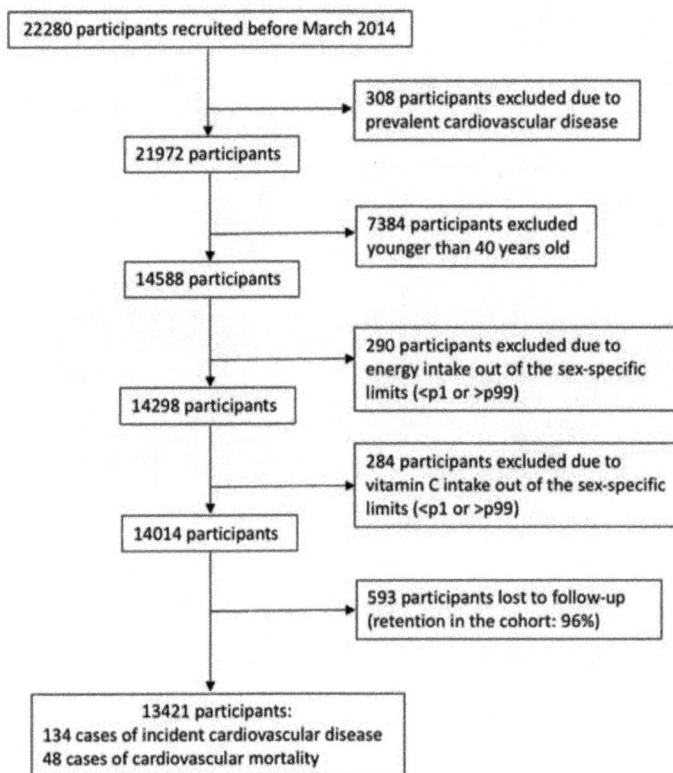

Figure 1. Flow chart of participants for the assessment of the association of cardiovascular disease and cardiovascular mortality with vitamin C intake in the Seguimiento Universidad de Navarra (University of Navarra follow-up) (SUN) cohort (follow-up 1999–2016).

2.2. Exposure Assessment

Participants were asked to complete a previously validated semi-quantitative food frequency questionnaire (FFQ) [19,20] and report how often on average they had consumed 136 foods and beverages during the past year. The FFQ had nine categories for intake frequency, from never to two or more servings per day. Multivitamin and supplements users were asked to specify the brand of multivitamin or supplement, the dose, and frequency of use. The nutritional content of each food was obtained from Spanish food composition guides [21,22] and supplemented with information from food and supplement manufacturers when needed. The nutrient contribution of each food item was calculated by multiplying the frequency of food consumption by the nutrient composition of the specified portion size. Dietary vitamin C intake was adjusted for energy intake using the residuals method, and categorized into tertiles. Total vitamin C intake was estimated by summing the vitamin C contribution of food items and supplements. In ancillary analyses, we assessed the independent effect of vitamin C from foods additionally adjusted for supplement intake (dichotomous variable).

In further analyses, to nullify the correlation between vitamin C and fiber, dietary vitamin C was alternatively adjusted for total fiber intake using the residuals method.

2.3. Outcome Assessment

Incident CVD was defined as either incident fatal or non-fatal myocardial infarction (with or without ST elevation), or fatal or non-fatal stroke and death due to other cardiovascular causes. CVM was defined as death due to cardiovascular causes.

Information about the events was initially gathered from follow-up questionnaires. When participants reported any of the previously mentioned events, they were asked for their medical reports, which were evaluated by physicians in the study team who were blinded to the nutritional information. Myocardial infarction was diagnosed using universal criteria. Non-fatal stroke was defined as sudden onset focal-neurological lack with a vascular mechanism that last more than 24 h. Confirmed events were classified according to the International Classification of Diseases (ICD-10). I21 and I63 codes were considered to define cardiovascular events [23]. The National Death Index is checked at least once a year to confirm the vital status of participants during follow-up. Deaths were reported by either participant's next of kin, work associates, or postal authorities.

Participants were followed-up from enrollment until December 2016, the diagnosis of the event, or death, whichever came first.

2.4. Covariates

Information about socio-demographic and anthropometric characteristics, lifestyle (physical activity, television watching, smoking status), classical cardiovascular risk factors (hypertension, hypercholesterolemia, hypertriglyceridemia and diabetes), prevalent diseases (cancer and cardiovascular related diseases), and family history of stroke and cardiovascular-related medication was collected at baseline.

Age was calculated as the difference between the date of recruitment and the date of birth. Body mass index (BMI) was calculated by dividing participants' weight (kg) by their squared height (m). A validation study in a subset of the SUN cohort showed that self-reported weight and height were highly reproducible and specific [24].

Dietary information was obtained from the baseline FFQ. Energy (kcal/day) and fiber (mg/day) intakes were calculated by multiplying the frequency of each food item consumed by the energy and fiber contribution of its specified portion size. Total energy and fiber intakes were calculated as the sum of energy and fiber provided by each food item. We also calculated the adherence to the Mediterranean dietary pattern based on the information from the FFQ using the classical Mediterranean Dietary Score (MDS) [25] without the fruit- and vegetable-related items (total seven items). We defined three categories of adherence to the MDS: Low (from 0 to 2 points), medium (from 3 to 4 points), and high (from 5 to 7 points).

Physical activity was collected at baseline with a previously validated questionnaire [26] that included 17 activities and 10 categories of response, from never to eleven or more hours per week. METs-h/week for each activity were calculated by multiplying the number of Metabolic Equivalent of Task (METs) of each activity [27] by the weekly participation in that activity, weighted according to the number of months dedicated to each activity. Total physical activity was quantified by summing the METs-h/week dedicated to all activities performed during leisure time. Time spent watching television was used as a proxy of sedentary behavior [28]. Hours per week of television watching were calculated as the mean of hours spent watching television during weekdays and hours spent watching television during weekends. Missing data were imputed based on the values of other covariates.

Cardiovascular-related diseases at baseline (coronary heart disease, tachycardia, atrial fibrillation, aortic aneurism, heart failure, venous thrombosis, and claudication) were grouped in a single quantitative variable (number of cardiovascular-related diseases) included in the multivariable adjustment. Validation studies in the SUN cohort showed self-reported information about cardiovascular risk factors was valid as to be used in epidemiological studies [29,30].

2.5. Statistical Analysis

Baseline characteristics of participants were presented by tertiles of total vitamin C intake as mean (standard deviation) for quantitative variables, and as proportions for qualitative variables. A *p* value for trend across tertiles was calculated using simple linear or logistic regressions.

We fitted Cox proportional hazard models to assess the association of energy-adjusted vitamin C intake with CVD and CVM. We estimated the hazard ratios (HR) and their 95% confidence intervals (CI) for second and third tertile of vitamin C intake compare to the lowest tertile (category of reference). Age was used as the underlying time variable in all the models. We fitted five multivariable adjusted models: (1) adjusted for age and sex; (2) additionally adjusted for body mass index (continuous), total energy intake (continuous), physical activity (continuous), television watching (continuous), smoking (never, current, or former), family history of stroke (dichotomus) and treatment with aspirin (dichotomus); (3) additionally adjusted for number of cardiovascular-related diseases at baseline (discrete), prevalent cancer (dichotomus), prevalent hypertension (dichotomus), prevalent diabetes (dichotomus), prevalent hypercholesterolemia (dichotomus) and prevalent hypertriglyceridemia (dichotomus); (4) additionally adjusted for dietary fiber (fiber from foods other than fruits and vegetables) (continuous); and (5) additionally adjusted for adherence to the MDS (without the fruit- and vegetable-related items (low, medium or high).

Interactions with vitamin C supplements intake, total fiber intake and age at the end of follow-up were assessed for both CVD and CVM by adding an interaction product term to the model and calculating the maximum likelihood ratio test.

In ancillary analyses, we evaluated the association of tertiles of dietary vitamin C with CVD and CVM fitting a model additionally adjusted for vitamin C supplements intake (dichotomus).

In further analyses, we re-ran the multivariable adjusted models for fiber-adjusted vitamin C intake categorized into tertiles.

Analyses were performed with STATA version 12.0 (StataCorp, College Station, TX, USA).

3. Results

We followed-up 13,421 participants for a mean time of 10.9 years (the standard deviation (SD) = 3.82). Baseline characteristics of participants by tertiles of vitamin C intake are described in Table 1. Participants in the highest tertile of vitamin C intake (from 320 to 1110 mg/day) were older, more likely to be women, and less likely to be current smokers. They were also more physically active and spent less time watching television. Moreover, they reported higher fiber intake and greater adherence to the Mediterranean dietary patter (MDP). We found total vitamin C intake showed a modest correlation with energy intake (*r* = 0.33), but it was highly correlated with total fiber intake (*r* = 0.72). Similar results were found for dietary vitamin C.

Aortic aneurism, heart failure, and hypertriglyceridemia at baseline were less prevalent among participants with higher vitamin C intake. However, cancer, venous thrombosis, diabetes, hypertension, and family history of stroke at baseline were more prevalent, probably due to the older age of participants with higher intake of vitamin C. Participants in the highest tertile of vitamin C intake were more likely to be under treatment with diuretics, antihypertensives, aspirin, and other cardiovascular treatment drugs.

Table 1. Baseline characteristics of participants over 40 years old in the SUN cohort by tertiles of total vitamin C intake. Numbers are means (SD) or percentages.

Baseline Characteristics	Tertiles of Vitamin C Intake			
	Q1	Q2	Q3	*p*
N	4474	4474	4473	
Vitamin C intake (mg/day)	148 (44.2)	257 (33.0)	445 (114)	<0.001
Fiber intake (g/day)	23.0 (10.0)	27.8 (9.8)	38.3 (14.1)	<0.001
Vittamin C range (mg/day)	0–205	206–319	320–1110	
Vitamin C from supplements (mg/day)	0.56 (4.2)	2.0 (10.0)	9.6 (33.4)	<0.001
Sex (female)	41.6	55.8	67.9	<0.001
Age (years)	41.2 (10.3)	42.8 (10.7)	43.7 (10.8)	<0.001
BMI (kg/m^2)	24.3 (3.6)	24.1 (3.5)	23.8 (3.5)	<0.001
Mediterranean Dietary Score [§]				<0.001
Low (0–2 points)	39.0	29.6	21.4	
Medium (3–4 points)	47.3	50.9	51.1	
High (5–7 points)	13.7	19.5	27.5	
Energy intake (kcal/day)	2548 (804)	2346 (710)	2530 (755)	0.26
Physical activity (MET-h/week)	23.4 (20.6)	25.8 (21.6)	29.2 (25.3)	<0.001
Television time (h/week)	1.63 (1.1)	1.57 (1.1)	1.51 (1.1)	<0.001
Family history of myocardial infarction	15.8	18.3	17.1	0.09
Smoking				0.03
Never	43	44	44	
Current	29	23	22	
Former	28	33	34	
Prevalent diseases				
Cancer	3.7	4.6	5.6	<0.001
Coronary heart disease	0.38	0.47	0.27	0.39
Tachycardia	1.9	1.6	2.3	0.12
Atrial fibrillation	0.65	0.72	0.69	0.80
Aortic aneurism	0.25	0.11	0.02	0.01
Heart failure	0.42	0.56	0.38	0.75
Pulmonary embolism	0.13	0.09	0.11	0.75
Venous thrombosis	0.51	0.92	0.92	0.03
Claudication	0.31	0.31	0.56	0.07
Diabetes	1.4	2.2	3.0	<0.001
Hypertension	9.7	11.3	10.9	0.07
Hypercholesterolemia	20.0	21.9	20.7	0.42
Hypertriglyceridemia	8.5	8.9	7.3	0.04
Drugs				
Digoxin	0.11	0.13	0.13	0.77
Diuretics	1.0	1.6	1.7	0.01
Beta blockers	1.7	2.3	1.9	0.40
Calcium antagonists	0.40	0.45	0.63	0.13
Nitrite	0.13	0.11	0.18	0.57
Antihypertensives	2.8	4.1	3.7	0.03
Aspirin	3.4	5.2	4.9	0.001
Other CV treatment drug	5.2	6.9	6.6	0.01

[§] Mediterranean Diet Score without the fruit- and vegetable-related items. *N* = 13,421.

Multivariable-adjusted associations of total vitamin C intake with both CVD and CVM are showed in Figure 2.

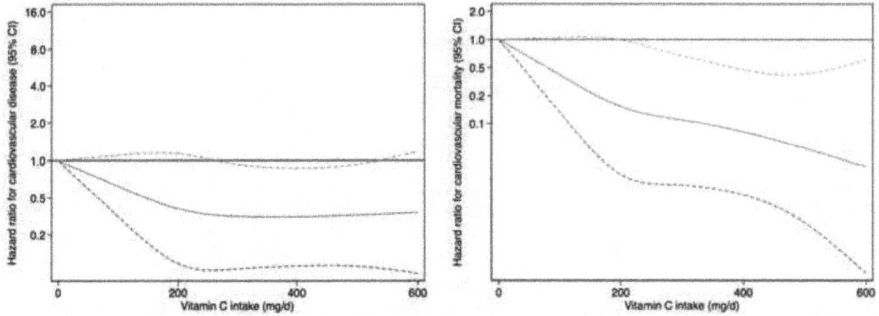

Figure 2. Restricted Cubic Splines for the Hazard Ratio (HR) and 95% Confidence Interval (CI) for cardiovascular disease and cardiovascular mortality associated with total vitamin C intake in the SUN cohort (follow-up 1999–2016). Age strata as underlying time variable. Multivariable model adjusted for sex, body mass index (continuous), total energy intake (continuous), physical activity (continuous), television watching (continuous), smoking (never, current or former), family history of stroke, treatment with aspirin, number of cardiovascular-related diseases at baseline, prevalent cancer, prevalent hypertension, prevalent diabetes, prevalent hypercholesterolemia, prevalent hypertriglyceridemia, fiber (from foods other than fruits and vegetables) (continuous), and Mediterranean Dietary Score (MDS) without fruit- and vegetable-related items (low, medium, high).

3.1. Cardiovascular Disease

A total of 134 cases of CVD were identified over 146,973 person-years at risk. The cumulative risk of a cardiovascular event was 0.07% in the highest tertile versus 0.12% in the lowest tertile of vitamin C intake.

We found that higher vitamin C intake was associated with a lower risk of CVD in the age-adjusted analysis (Table 2). Moreover, this association remained significant in the age and sex-adjusted model, in the model adjusted for demographic, metabolic, and lifestyle risk factors (multivariable adjusted model 1), and in the model additionally adjusted for prevalent diseases at baseline (multivariable adjusted model 2). Further adjustment for fiber intake (multivariable adjusted model 3) did not change the results. In the fully adjusted model (multivariable adjusted model 4), we found that, compared with participants in the first tertile of vitamin C intake, those in the second and third tertiles showed significant lower risk of CVD (HR (95% CI): 0.60 (0.40–0.91) and 0.62 (0.40–0.97), respectively).

High vitamin C intake showed no significant association with CVD when fiber from fruits and vegetables was also considered. HRs (95% CI) for the third tertile in models 3 and 4 were 0.66 (0.39–1.10) and 0.68 (0.40–1.13), respectively. Nevertheless, the association was still significant when the second and third tertiles were considered together (HR (95% CI): 0.63 (0.41–0.94) for model 3 and 0.64 (0.43–0.88) for model 4).

Neither age at the end of follow-up ($p = 0.79$) nor fiber intake ($p = 0.15$) resulted in effect modification. Marginally significant interaction was found between total vitamin C and vitamin C supplementation ($p = 0.05$).

Table 2. Hazard Ratio (HR) and 95% Confidence Interval (CI) for cardiovascular disease (CVD) associated with total vitamin C intake for participants over 40 years old in the SUN cohort (follow-up 1999–2016).

Main Analyses [§]	Tertiles of Vitamin C Intake		
	Q1 (*N* = 4474)	Q2 (*N* = 4474)	Q3 (*N* = 4473)
Incident CVD (person-years at risk)	61 (50,792)	38 (48,765)	35 (47,415)
Age-adjusted	1.00 (Ref.)	0.52 (0.35–0.78)	0.44 (0.29–0.67)
Sex- and age-adjusted	1.00 (Ref.)	0.59 (0.39–0.89)	0.56 (0.37–0.86)
Multivariable adjusted model 1	1.00 (Ref.)	0.59 (0.39–0.90)	0.60 (0.39–0.93)
T2 + T3 vs. T1	1.00 (Ref.)	0.60 (0.42–0.85)	
Multivariable adjusted model 2	1.00 (Ref.)	0.58 (0.38–0.88)	0.58 (0.37–0.90)
T2 + T3 vs. T1	1.00 (Ref.)	0.58 (0.41–0.83)	
Multivariable adjusted model 3	1.00 (Ref.)	0.58 (0.38–0.88)	0.58 (0.37–0.90)
T2 + T3 vs. T1	1.00 (Ref.)	0.58 (0.41–0.83)	
Multivariable adjusted model 4	1.00 (Ref.)	0.60 (0.40–0.91)	0.62 (0.40–0.97)
T2 + T3 vs. T1	1.00 (Ref.)	0.61 (0.43–0.88)	

[§] Age strata as underlying time variable in all the models; *N* = 13,421; Ref: reference category. Multivariable adjusted **model 1**: Additionally adjusted for sex, body mass index (continuous), total energy intake (continuous), physical activity (continuous), television watching (continuous), smoking (never, current or former), family history of stroke, and treatment with aspirin. Multivariable adjusted **model 2**: Additionally adjusted for the number of cardiovascular-related diseases at baseline, prevalent cancer, prevalent hypertension, prevalent diabetes, prevalent hypercholesterolemia and prevalent hypertrygliceridemia. Multivariable adjusted **model 3**: Additionally adjusted for dietary fiber (fiber from foods other than fruits and vegetables) (continuous). Multivariable adjusted **model 4**: Additionally adjusted for the MDS without fruit and vegetable intake related items (low, medium, or high).

3.2. Cardiovascular Mortality

A total of 48 cases of CVM occurred over 147,495 person-years at risk during the follow up. The cumulative risk was 0.02% in the third tertile versus 0.04% in the first tertile of vitamin C intake.

Compare to the category of reference, we found a significant inverse association for the highest tertile of vitamin C intake and CVM in the age-adjusted analysis (Table 3). Results were similar in the age and sex-adjusted model; the models adjusted for demographic, metabolic and lifestyle risk factors; (multivariable adjusted model 1); and in the model additionally adjusted for prevalent diseases at baseline (multivariable adjusted model 2). Additional adjustment for fiber from foods other than fruits and vegetables did not change the results, but they became non-significant when total fiber intake was considered (HR (95% CI): 0.48 (0.19–1.20)). No significant results were found in the fully-adjusted model that included the MDS.

Neither age at the end of follow-up ($p = 0.70$), fiber intake ($p = 0.42$), nor vitamin C supplements intake ($p = 0.12$) modified the association between total vitamin C intake and CVM.

Table 3. Hazard Ratios (HR) and 95% Confidence Intervals (CI) for cardiovascular mortality associated with total vitamin C intake for participants over 40 years old in the SUN cohort (follow-up 1999–2016).

Main Analyses [§]	Tertiles of Vitamin C Intake		
	Q1 (N = 4474)	Q2 (N = 4474)	Q3 (N = 4473)
Cardiovascular deaths (person-years at risk)	22 (51,016)	15 (48,901)	11 (47,577)
Age-adjusted	1.00 (Ref.)	0.55 (0.28–1.06)	0.34 (0.17–0.73)
Sex- and age-adjusted	1.00 (Ref.)	0.56 (0.29–1.10)	0.37 (0.17–0.79)
Multivariable adjusted model 1	1.00 (Ref.)	0.57 (0.29–1.12)	0.39 (0.18–0.86)
Multivariable adjusted model 2	1.00 (Ref.)	0.54 (0.27–1.08)	0.40 (0.18–0.89)
Multivariable adjusted model 3	1.00 (Ref.)	0.54 (0.27–1.09)	0.41 (0.19–0.92)
Multivariable adjusted model 4	1.00 (Ref.)	0.56 (0.28–1.12)	0.45 (0.20–1.01)

[§] Age strata as underlying time variable in all the models; *N* = 13,421; Ref: reference category. Multivariable adjusted **model 1**: Additionally adjusted for sex, body mass index (continuous), total energy intake (continuous), physical activity (continuous), television watching (continuous), smoking (never, current or former), family history of stroke, and treatment with aspirin. Multivariable adjusted **model 2**: Additionally adjusted for the number of cardiovascular-related diseases at baseline, prevalent cancer, prevalent hypertension, prevalent diabetes, prevalent hypercholesterolemia, and prevalent hypertrygliceridemia. Multivariable adjusted **model 3**: Additionally adjusted for dietary fiber (fiber from foods other than fruits and vegetables) (continuous). Multivariable adjusted **model 4**: Additionally adjusted for the MDS without fruit and vegetable intake related items (low, medium, or high).

3.3. Fiber-Adjusted Vitamin C Intake

In further analyses, dietary vitamin C was adjusted for total fiber intake using the residuals method to nullify the correlation between vitamin C and fiber (Table 4). We found a cumulative risk for CVD of 0.07% in the third versus 0.12% in the first tertile. However, no significant association was found for vitamin C intake and CVD.

On the other hand, the cumulative risk for CVM was 0.01% in the third tertile versus 0.05% in the first one. Compared with participants in the first tertile, those in the highest tertile of vitamin C intake showed significant lower risk of CVM in multivariable adjusted analyses (HR (95% CI): 0.30 (0.13–0.73)). Further adjustment for the MDS did not change the results.

Neither CVD nor CVM were significantly associated with dietary vitamin C, independently of vitamin C supplement intake (Figure S1).

Table 4. Hazard Ratio (HR) and 95% Confidence Interval (CI) for the association of total vitamin C intake, adjusted for fiber intake using the residuals method with both cardiovascular disease (CVD) and cardiovascular mortality (CVM) for participants over 40 years old in the SUN cohort (follow-up 1999–2016).

Main Analyses [§]	Tertiles of Vitamin C Intake		
	Q1 (N = 4474)	Q2 (N = 4474)	Q3 (N = 4473)
Incident CVD (person-time-1 at risk)	58 (49,706)	44 (49,080)	32 (48,186)
Multivariable adjusted [§‡]	1.00 (Ref.)	0.86 (0.57–1.29)	0.74 (0.47–1.15)
Additionally adjusted for MDS	1.00 (Ref.)	0.86 (0.57–1.29)	0.74 (0.47–1.15)
Cardiovascular deaths (person-years at risk)	27 (49,879)	14 (49,247)	7 (48,368)
Multivariable adjusted [§‡]	1.00 (Ref.)	0.52 (0.26–1.02)	0.30 (0.13–0.73)
Additionally adjusted for MDS	1.00 (Ref.)	0.52 (0.26–1.04)	0.30 (0.12–0.72)

MDS: Mediterranean Dietary Score without fruit and vegetable intake related items (low, medium, or high); [§] Age as underlying time variable in all the models; [‡] Adjusted for sex, body mass index (continuous), total energy intake (continuous), total fiber intake (continuous), physical activity (continuous), television watching (continuous), smoking (never, current or former), number of cardiovascular-related diseases at baseline, prevalent cancer, prevalent hypertension, prevalent diabetes, prevalent hypercholesterolemia, prevalent hypertriglyceridemia, family history of stroke, and treatment with aspirin. *N* = 13,421; Ref: reference category.

4. Discussion

In this large cohort of Spanish university graduates followed-up over a mean time of 11 years, we found that, compared with the lowest category, the third tertile of total vitamin C intake was associated with 70% (95% CI 18%–88%) lower risk of CVM, but not with CVD. This analysis was based on a multivariable adjusted model that thoroughly controlled potential confounding by fiber and accounted for the adherence to the Mediterranean dietary pattern.

The belief that vitamin C benefits cardiovascular health is based on its antioxidant capability. Vitamin C may prevent oxidative changes to low-density lipoprotein (LDL)-cholesterol [31] and reduce monocyte adhesion [32], which are key in reducing the risk of atherosclerosis. Moreover, vitamin C prevents vascular smooth muscle cells apoptosis, which keeps atheroma plaques stables [33]. In addition, vitamin C improves the nitric oxide production of the endothelium [34], which in turn contributes to reduced blood pressure. This evidence, when added to the results found in the analyses to account for confounding by fiber and dietary variables included in the MDS, suggests that the associations of vitamin C intake with CVM may not be due to confounding factors, but may instead represent a true biological effect.

Observational studies had reported inverse associations of vitamin C with cardiovascular outcomes, particularly on hypertension [6] and heart failure [7]. However, those studies did not account for fiber intake. Due to the high correlation between vitamin C and fiber intakes found in this study, it was difficult to assess the effect of vitamin C on cardiovascular health independently of fiber intake in a multivariable adjusted model. In order to nullify that correlation, dietary vitamin C was adjusted for total fiber intake using the residuals method. On the other hand, reduced CVM risk associated to vitamin C intake had been previously reported in observational studies [8]. However, this association has not been confirmed in randomized controlled trials [10,11].

We found that energy-adjusted total vitamin C intake was associated with a lower risk of CVD. We obtained similar estimates in the comparisons of the second and the third tertiles, which suggests a threshold effect or L-shaped association between total vitamin C and CVD. However, in further analyses, we found the association of fiber-adjusted vitamin C with CVD was not significant.

We also found that high energy-adjusted total vitamin C intake was associated with lower risk of CVM after multivariable adjustment for demographic, metabolic, and lifestyle risk factors, prevalent diseases at baseline, and fiber from foods other than fruits and vegetables. However, results became non-significant when the model was additionally adjusted for the MDS. Nevertheless, further analyses showed that, compared to the first tertile, the highest category of fiber-adjusted vitamin C intake was associated with lower CVM risk in the fully adjusted model (HR: 0.30, 95% CI (0.12–0.72)).

These results suggest that most of the confounding effect by fiber was due to fiber from fruits and vegetables. Since vitamin C and fiber were highly correlated ($r = 0.72$) it was difficult to assess the effect of one of them while keeping the other one constant (Tables 2 and 3). When vitamin C was adjusted for fiber using the residuals method (Table 4), the correlation was nullified ($r = 0$), which allowed for the assessment of the effect of vitamin C on cardiovascular health independently of fiber. Nevertheless, given that vitamin C is a single nutrient and may not represent the whole dietary pattern, these results must be taken with caution. Several reasons support the hypothesis that attributing all of the observed effect to a single nutrient or food may be too simplistic and that when assessing the association of dietary variables with non-communicable diseases, the whole dietary pattern should be considered [35].

None significant associations with either CVD or CVM were found when vitamin C from food was considered alone. Importantly, means (SD) (mg/day) of fiber-adjusted dietary vitamin C intake across successive tertiles were 184 (57), 266.7 (20.5), and 387.7 (75.6) respectively. Therefore, the absence of significant results might be explained by the low variability in the exposure.

Regarding vitamin C supplements, our results parallel previous intervention studies that reported no effect of vitamin C supplementation on cardiovascular health [10–13]. It must be acknowledged that some clinical trials permitted the control group to an intake of vitamin C and multivitamin supplements, which made it harder to find significant differences between groups. Vitamin C supplementation in our study ranged from 3.4 to 440 mg/day, which is much lower than the doses assessed in the available clinical trials. We found the effect of total vitamin C on CVD may depend on vitamin C supplementation (*p* for interaction 0.05). However, among the 1055 participants undertaking vitamin C supplementation (8%), we found two cases of CVD and one single case of CVM; thus, stratified analyses were not possible.

Some limitations of this study must be acknowledged. First, because information about exposure was self-reported, some degree of misclassification is possible. Nevertheless, information bias would more likely be non-differential with respect to the outcomes, resulting in an attenuation of the observed associations. Moreover, little variability observed in the exposure might have reduced the possibility of significant findings. Second, the SUN cohort is not a representative sample of the general population, and therefore generalization of these results must be based on biological mechanisms rather than on statistical representativeness. Third, given the observational design of the study, the possibility of residual confounding for factors that were not considered (such as vitamin E) must be taken into account. Thus, before causality is implied, these results must be confirmed in well-designed randomized controlled trials. Finally, because participants in the SUN cohort are relatively young and health conscious, few incident cases of CVM were observed during follow-up. Further studies are need to determine if the magnitude of the association we observed represents the upper bound of the association between vitamin C and CVM. Despite these limitations, our study has several strengths. The sample size is large, the follow-up period is long, and the retention rate is high. Dietary information was collected with a validated FFQ, and outcomes were confirmed by physicians checking participant's medical records. Finally, participants in the SUN cohort are highly educated, and more than half are health professionals themselves, which reduces potential confounding by educational level, leads to better quality in self-reported data, and increases the internal validity of the study.

5. Conclusions

Energy-adjusted analyses suggest a threshold effect in the association of vitamin C intake with CVD, but not with CVM. Nevertheless, the model fitted to thoroughly control potential confounding for fiber showed that compared with the category of reference, the highest tertile of total vitamin C intake was associated with a significantly lower risk of CVM, but not CVD, after adjusting for several confounding factors, including adherence to the Mediterranean dietary pattern. Further research is needed in order to fully understand the biological mechanisms explaining these associations. Moreover, these results must be reproduced in different populations before clinical implications can be assessed.

Supplementary Materials: The following are available online at www.mdpi.com/2072-6643/9/9/954/s1, Figure S1: Hazard Ratio (HR) and 95% Confidence Interval (CI), for cardiovascular disease and cardiovascular mortality associated with vitamin C intake by vitamin C source in the SUN cohort (follow-up 1999–2016).

Acknowledgments: The SUN project received funding from the Spanish Government-Instituto de Salud Carlos III and the European Regional Development Fund (FEDER) (RD 06/0045, CIBER-Obn Grants PI10/02658, PI10/02293, PI13/00615, PI14/01668, PI14/01798, PI14/01764 AND G03/140), the Navarra Regional Government (45/2011, 122/2014), and the University of Navarra. We also thank all the researchers in the SUN project, and all the participants for their collaboration.

Author Contributions: Miguel Ángel Martínez-González designed and started the SUN cohort. Miguel Ángel Martínez-González and Nerea Martín-Calvo designed the present study. Nerea Martín-Calvo conducted the statistical analyses and wrote the first version of the manuscript. Miguel Ángel Martínez Gonzalez helped in the interpretation of the results and critically review the manuscript. All the authors approved the final version of the paper.

Conflicts of Interest: The authors declare no conflict of interest.

Nutrients **2017**, *9*, 954

References

1. Chun, O.K.; Floegel, A.; Chung, S.J.; Chung, CE.; Song, W.O.; Koo, S.I. Estimation of Antioxidant Intakes from Diet and Supplements in U.S. Adults. *J. Nutr.* **2010**, *140*, 317–324. [CrossRef] [PubMed]
2. Moser, M.; Chun, O. Vitamin C and Heart Health: A Review Based on Findings from Epidemiologic Studies. *Int. J. Mol. Sci.* **2016**, *17*, 1328. [CrossRef] [PubMed]
3. Joshipura, K.J.; Hu, F.B.; Manson, J.E.; Stampfer, M.J.; Rimm, E.B.; Speizer, F.E.; Colditz, G.; Ascherio, A.; Rosner, B.; Spiegelman, D.; et al. The effect of fruit and vegetable intake on risk for coronary heart disease. *Ann. Intern. Med.* **2001**, *134*, 1106–1114. [CrossRef] [PubMed]
4. Holmberg, S.; Thelin, A.; Stiernström, E.L. Food Choices and Coronary Heart Disease: A Population Based Cohort Study of Rural Swedish Men with 12 Years of Follow-up. *Int. J. Environ. Res. Public Health* **2009**, *6*, 2626–2638. [CrossRef] [PubMed]
5. Martínez-González, M.A.; de la Fuente-Arrillaga, C.; López-Del-Burgo, C.; Vázquez-Ruiz, Z.; Benito, S.; Ruiz-Canela, M. Low consumption of fruit and vegetables and risk of chronic disease: A review of the epidemiological evidence and temporal trends among Spanish graduates. *Public Health Nutr.* **2011**, *14*, 2309–2315. [CrossRef] [PubMed]
6. Buijsse, B.; Jacobs, D.R.; Steffen, L.M.; Kromhout, D.; Gross, M.D.; Abbott, R. Plasma Ascorbic Acid, A Priori Diet Quality Score, and Incident Hypertension: A Prospective Cohort Study. *PLoS ONE* **2015**, *10*, e0144920. [CrossRef] [PubMed]
7. Pfister, R.; Sharp, S.J.; Luben, R.; Wareham, N.J.; Khaw, K.T. Plasma vitamin C predicts incident heart failure in men and women in European Prospective Investigation into Cancer and Nutrition-Norfolk prospective study. *Am. Heart J.* **2011**, *162*, 246–253. [CrossRef] [PubMed]
8. Khaw, K.T.; Bingham, S.; Welch, A.; Luben, R.; Wareham, N.; Oakes, S.; Day, N. Relation between plasma ascorbic acid and mortality in men and women in EPIC-Norfolk prospective study: A prospective population study. European Prospective Investigation into Cancer and Nutrition. *Lancet* **2001**, *357*, 657–663. [CrossRef]
9. Mangels, A.R.; Block, G.; Frey, C.M.; Patterson, B.H.; Taylor, P.R.; Norkus, E.P.; Levander, O.A. The bioavailability to humans of ascorbic acid from oranges, orange juice and cooked broccoli is similar to that of synthetic ascorbic acid. *J. Nutr.* **1993**, *123*, 1054–1061. [PubMed]
10. Sesso, H.D.; Buring, J.E.; Christen, W.G.; Kurth, T.; Belanger, C.; MacFadyen, J.; Bubes, V.; Manson, J.E.; Glynn, R.J.; Gaziano, J.M. Vitamins E and C in the Prevention of Cardiovascular Disease in Men. *JAMA* **2008**, *300*, 2123–2133. [CrossRef] [PubMed]
11. Cook, N.R.; Albert, C.M.; Gaziano, J.M.; Zaharris, E.; MacFadyen, J.; Danielson, E; Buring, J.E.; Manson, J.E. A Randomized Factorial Trial of Vitamins C and E and Beta Carotene in the Secondary Prevention of Cardiovascular Events in Women. *Arch. Intern. Med.* **2007**, *167*, 1610–1618. [CrossRef] [PubMed]
12. Ellulu, M.S.; Rahmat, A.; Ismail, P.; Khaza' ai, H.; Abed, Y. Effect of vitamin C on inflammation and metabolic markers in hypertensive and/or diabetic obese adults: A randomized controlled trial. *Drug Des. Devel. Ther.* **2015**, *9*, 3405–3412. [CrossRef] [PubMed]
13. Brown, B.G.; Zhao, X.Q.; Chait, A.; Fisher, L.D.; Cheung, M.C.; Morse, J.S.; Dowdy, A.A.; Marino, E.K.; Bolson, E.L.; Alaupovic, P. Simvastatin and Niacin, Antioxidant Vitamins, or the Combination for the Prevention of Coronary Disease. *N. Engl. J. Med.* **2001**, *345*, 1583–1592. [CrossRef] [PubMed]
14. Lee, D.H.; Folsom, A.R.; Harnack, L.; Halliwell, B.; Jacobs, D.R. Does supplemental vitamin C increase cardiovascular disease risk in women with diabetes? *Am. J. Clin. Nutr.* **2004**, *80*, 1194–1200. [PubMed]
15. Waters, D.D.; Alderman, E.L.; Hsia, J.; Howard, B.V.; Cobb, F.R.; Rogers, W.J.; Ouyang, P.; Thompsom, P.; Tardif, J.C.; Higginson, L. Effects of hormone replacement therapy and antioxidant vitamin supplements on coronary atherosclerosis in postmenopausal women: a randomized controlled trial. *JAMA* **2002**, *288*, 2432–2440. [CrossRef] [PubMed]
16. Ashor, A.W.; Lara, J.; Mathers, J.C.; Siervo, M. Effect of vitamin C on endothelial function in health and disease: A systematic review and meta-analysis of randomised controlled trials. *Atherosclerosis* **2014**, *235*, 9–20. [CrossRef] [PubMed]
17. Juraschek, S.P.; Guallar, E.; Appel, L.J.; Miller, E.R. Effects of vitamin C supplementation on blood pressure: A meta-analysis of randomized controlled trials. *Am. J. Clin. Nutr.* **2012**, *95*, 1079–1088. [CrossRef] [PubMed]

18. Seguí-Gómez, M.; de la Fuente, C.; Vázquez, Z.; de Irala, J.; Martínez-González, M.A. Cohort profile: The "Seguimiento Universidad de Navarra" (SUN) study. *Int. J. Epidemiol.* **2006**, *35*, 1417–1422. [CrossRef] [PubMed]

19. Martin-Moreno, J.M.; Boyle, P.; Gorgojo, L.; Maisonneuve, P.; Fernandez-Rodriguez, J.C.; Salvini, S.; Willett, W.C. Development and validation of a food frequency questionnaire in Spain. *Int. J. Epidemiol.* **1993**, *22*, 512–519. [CrossRef] [PubMed]

20. De la Fuente-Arrillaga, C.; Vázquez-Ruiz, Z.; Bes-Rastrollo, M.; Sampson, L.; Martínez-Gonzlez, M.A. Reproducibility of an FFQ validated in Spain. *Public Health Nutr.* **2010**, *13*, 1364–1372. [CrossRef] [PubMed]

21. Mataix-Verdu, J.; Manas, M.; Martinez-Victoria, E.; Sanchez, J.J.; Borregon, A. *Tabla de Composición de Alimentos Españoles (Spanish Food Composition Tables)*, 4th ed.; Universidad de Granada Press: Granada, Spain, 2003.

22. Moreiras, O.; Carbajal, A.; Cabrera, L. *Tablas de Composición de Alimentos (Food Composition Tables)*, 9th ed.; Pirámide: Madrid, Spain, 2005.

23. World Health Organization. *International Classification of Diseases*; 10th Revision (ICD-10); World Health Organization: Geneva, Switzerland, 2010.

24. Bes-Rastrollo, M.; Valdivieso, J.R.; Sánchez-Villegas, A.; Alonso, Á.; Martínez-González, M.A. Validación del peso e índice de masa corporal auto-declarados de los participantes de una cohorte de graduados universitarios. *Rev. Española. Obes.* **2005**, *3*, 183–189.

25. Trichopoulou, A.; Costacou, T.; Bamia, C.; Trichopoulos, D. Adherence to a Mediterranean Diet and Survival in a Greek Population. *N. Engl. J. Med.* **2003**, *348*, 2599–2608. [CrossRef] [PubMed]

26. Martínez-González, M.A.; López-Fontana, C.; Varo, J.J.; Sánchez-Villegas, A.; Martinez, J.A. Validation of the Spanish version of the physical activity questionnaire used in the Nurses' Health Study and the Health Professionals' Follow-up Study. *Public Health Nutr.* **2005**, *8*, 920–927. [CrossRef] [PubMed]

27. Ainsworth, B.E.; Haskell, W.L.; Whitt, M.C.; Irwin, M.L.; Swartz, A.M.; Strath, S.J.; O'brien, W.L.; Bassett, D.R.; Schmitz, K.H.; Emplaincourt, P.O. Compendium of physical activities: An update of activity codes and MET intensities. *Med. Sci. Sports Exerc.* **2000**, *32*, S498–S504. [CrossRef] [PubMed]

28. Javier Basterra-Gortari, F.; Bes-Rastrollo, M.; Gea, A.; Núñez-Córdoba, J.; Toledo, E.; Martínez-González, M.Á. Television Viewing, Computer Use, Time Driving and All-Cause Mortality: The SUN Cohort. *J. Am. Heart Assoc.* **2014**, *3*, e000864. [CrossRef] [PubMed]

29. Alonso, Á.; Beunza, J.J.; Delgado-Rodríguez, M.; Martínez-González, M.A. Validation of self reported diagnosis of hypertension in a cohort of university graduates in Spain. *BMC Public Health* **2005**, *5*, 94. [CrossRef] [PubMed]

30. Barrio-Lopez, M.T.; Bes-Rastrollo, M.; Beunza, J.J.; Fernández-Montero, A.; García-López, M.; Martínez-González, M.A. Validation of metabolic syndrome using medical records in the SUN cohort. *BMC Public Health* **2011**, *11*, 867. [CrossRef] [PubMed]

31. Salvayre, R.; Negre-Salvayre, A.; Camaré, C. Oxidative theory of atherosclerosis and antioxidants. *Biochimie* **2016**, *125*, 281–296. [CrossRef] [PubMed]

32. Weber, C.; Erl, W.; Weber, K.; Weber, P.C. Increased Adhesiveness of Isolated Monocytes to Endothelium Is Prevented by Vitamin C Intake in Smokers. *Circulation* **1996**, *93*, 1488–1492. [CrossRef] [PubMed]

33. Siow, R.C.M.; Richards, J.P.; Pedley, K.C.; Leake, D.S.; Mann, G.E. Vitamin C Protects Human Vascular Smooth Muscle Cells Against Apoptosis Induced by Moderately Oxidized LDL Containing High Levels of Lipid Hydroperoxides. *Arterioscler. Thromb. Vasc. Biol.* **1999**, *19*, 2387–2394. [CrossRef] [PubMed]

34. D'Uscio, L.V.; Milstien, S.; Richardson, D.; Smith, L.; Katusic, Z.S. Long-Term Vitamin C Treatment Increases Vascular Tetrahydrobiopterin Levels and Nitric Oxide Synthase Activity. *Circ. Res.* **2003**, *92*, 88–95. [CrossRef] [PubMed]

35. Hu, F.B. Dietary pattern analysis: A new direction in nutritional epidemiology. *Curr. Opin. Lipidol.* **2002**, *13*, 3–9. [CrossRef] [PubMed]

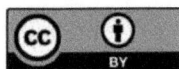

nutrients

MDPI

Article

Vitamin C Deficiency Reduces Muscarinic Receptor Coronary Artery Vasoconstriction and Plasma Tetrahydrobiopterin Concentration in Guinea Pigs

Gry Freja Skovsted *, Pernille Tveden-Nyborg, Maiken Marie Lindblad, Stine Normann Hansen and Jens Lykkesfeldt

Department of Veterinary and Animal Sciences, Faculty of Health and Medical Sciences,
University of Copenhagen, Ridebanevej 9, 1870 Frederiksberg C, Denmark; ptn@sund.ku.dk (P.T.-N.);
mali@sund.ku.dk (M.M.L.); snoha@sund.ku.dk (S.N.H.); jopl@sund.ku.dk (J.L.)
* Correspondence: gryfreja@sund.ku.dk; Tel.: +45-3533-7705

Received: 1 May 2017; Accepted: 29 June 2017; Published: 3 July 2017

Abstract: Vitamin C (vitC) deficiency is associated with increased cardiovascular disease risk, but its specific interplay with arteriolar function is unclear. This study investigates the effect of vitC deficiency in guinea pigs on plasma biopterin status and the vasomotor responses in coronary arteries exposed to vasoconstrictor/-dilator agents. Dunkin Hartley female guinea pigs ($n = 32$) were randomized to high (1500 mg/kg diet) or low (0 to 50 mg/kg diet) vitC for 10–12 weeks. At euthanasia, coronary artery segments were dissected and mounted in a wire-myograph. Vasomotor responses to potassium, carbachol, sodium nitroprusside (SNP), U46619, sarafotoxin 6c (S6c) and endothelin-1 (ET-1) were recorded. Plasma vitC and tetrahydrobiopterin were measured by HPLC. Plasma vitC status reflected the diets with deficient animals displaying reduced tetrahydrobiopterin. Vasoconstrictor responses to carbachol were significantly decreased in vitC deficient coronary arteries independent of their general vasoconstrictor/vasodilator capacity ($p < 0.001$). Moreover, in vitC deficient animals, carbachol-induced vasodilator responses correlated with coronary artery diameter ($p < 0.001$). Inhibition of cyclooxygenases with indomethacin increased carbachol-induced vasoconstriction, suggesting an augmented carbachol-induced release of vasodilator prostanoids. Atropine abolished carbachol-induced vasomotion, supporting a specific muscarinic receptor effect. Arterial responses to SNP, potassium, S6c, U46619 and ET-1 were unaffected by vitC status. The study shows that vitC deficiency decreases tetrahydrobiopterin concentrations and muscarinic receptor mediated contraction in coronary arteries. This attenuated vasoconstrictor response may be linked to altered production of vasoactive arachidonic acid metabolites and reduced muscarinic receptor expression/signaling.

Keywords: Vitamin C; ascorbic acid; vascular responses; biopterins

1. Introduction

The association between vitamin C (vitC) deficiency and an increased risk of cardiovascular disease (CVD) in humans is well-established [1–6], though a mechanistic link is yet to be elucidated. VitC is an essential nutrient for humans and an estimated 10–15% of adults in the Western populations suffer from hypovitaminosis C (plasma concentration <23 μM) [7]. Pathologies of vascular diseases are characterized by changed vasomotion as a consequence of an imbalance in vasodilation and vasoconstriction, leading to abnormal blood flow regulation and organ dysfunction. In the vasculature, vitC is a key component in maintaining collagen integrity of blood vessels; prolonged severe deficiency ultimately leads to the development of bleedings and haematoma hallmarking scurvy. However, little is known about how non-scorbutic vitC deficiency affects the function of the vascular cells and the vasomotion of arterioles proximal to the capillaries.

In human endothelial cells in vitro, vitC has been shown to act as specific redox modulator in the nitric oxide (NO) synthesis essential for vasodilation [8]. Furthermore, vitC provides reducing equivalents in the conversion of dihydrobiopterin (BH_2) to tetrahydrobiopterin (BH_4) [9,10], which in turn acts as co-factor for endothelial nitric oxide syntase (eNOS) to ensure the generation of NO [11]. Reduced BH_4 levels lead to eNOS uncoupling, and generation of superoxide rather than NO [12], likely to form the strong oxidant peroxynitrite and decreasing NO bioavailability [9]. We have previously shown that vitC deficiency in guinea pigs leads to decreased BH_4 plasma concentration in vivo [13], potentially weakening the vasodilator capacity.

Another important aspect of vitC is its antioxidant function, serving as a scavenger of reactive oxygen species (ROS) [14]. ROS play key roles in signal transduction related to both vasodilation and vasoconstiction [15] and can inhibit the two major endothelium-derived relaxing factors, NO and prostacyclin [15]. While eNOS uncoupling reduces NO bioavailability, peroxynitrite can inactivate prostacyclin synthase by tyrosin nitration of its active site [16,17]. Thus, as the primary vascular antioxidant, vitC protects the endothelium from oxidative stress [18].

A third mechanism of vitC-associated action could be on the cholinergic response of vascular smooth muscle cells (VSMCs). Increased oxidative stress has been found to reduce muscarinic receptor function in smooth muscle cells of the urinary bladder [19], and studies have shown an attenuated parasympathetic response [20] and muscarinic-cholinergic receptor density [21] in submandibular gland acinar cells in vitC deficient guinea pigs. As coronary arteries express muscarinic receptors in the endothelium and VSMCs, and an extensive network of cholinergic perivascular nerve fibres in the coronary artery tree is present in guinea pigs [22], the acetylcholine analogue carbachol was applied to study both vasodilator and vasoconstrictor responses.

In contrast to rats and mice, guinea pigs and humans share a requirement for dietary vitC. This makes the guinea pig an excellent in vivo model for studying effects of diet-imposed vitC deficiency. In this study, we examined a causal relationship between chronic vitC deficiency and plasma biopterin redox status, and putative consequences on the vasodilator and vasoconstrictor responses in isolated coronary arteries.

2. Materials and Methods

2.1. Animal Study

All experimental animal procedures were performed following protocols approved by the Danish Animal Experimental Inspectorate under the Ministry of Environment and Food of Denmark (No. 2012-15-2934-00205). Group sizes were determined by power analysis of sample size, applying a power of 80% and a 5% significance level. A difference of 30% was considered biologically relevant and variations of the chosen end-points were based on our previous experience with the model [23,24]. Animals were selected by randomization from a larger, extensive, study of diet imposed vitC deficiency in guinea pigs intended to investigate vitC transport to the brain (unpublished results). Thus, the current data-set depicts findings from a randomly defined subset of animals, representing high vitC intake (control) and low (deficient), thereby, reflecting the extremes of the imposed interventions of the main study.

Seven-day old, Dunkin Hartley female guinea pigs (Envigo, Horst, The Netherlands) were equipped with subcutaneous microchip implant for identification (Uno Pico Transponder, Zevenaar, The Netherlands) upon arrival to the facility. Animals were randomized into weight stratified groups and subjected to either high ($n = 16$; 1500 mg vitC/kg feed; Controls) or low vitC ($n = 16$, 0 mg vitC/kg feed for 3 weeks, followed by 50 mg vitC/kg feed until study termination; Deficient). All diets were chow based standard guinea pig diets for growing animals (Ssniff Spezialdiäten, Soesst, Germany), differing only in vitC levels as confirmed by post production analysis. Animals were group-housed in identical floor pens and allowed free access to feed, dried hay (devoid of vitC by analysis) and drinking water. Body-weight was monitored throughout the study period, and though vitC deficient animals experienced a brief period (1–3 days) of weight stagnation immediately prior to changing from 0 mg to 50 mg vitC/kg feed, clinical signs of vitC deficiency were absent and body weight was comparable between groups at the time of euthanasia, 10–12 weeks after study start.

2.2. Euthanasia

Guinea pigs were sedated with Torbugesic Vet (2 mL/kg) (Butorphanol 10 mg/mL; ScanVet Animal Health, Fredernsborg, Denmark) and anesthetized with 5% isofluorane (Isoba Vet 100%, Intervet International, Boxmeer, The Netherlands) in oxygen (Conoxia® 100%, AGA A/S, Copenhagen, Denmark) until cessation of voluntary reflexes. Blood was collected by cardiac puncture through the apex using a 18 G needle fitted onto a 1 mL syringe previously flushed with 15% tripotassium EDTA. Immediately hereafter, the guinea pig was euthanized by decapitation.

2.3. Wire Myography and Tissue Preparation

Immediately following euthanasia, the heart was isolated and placed into cold physiological buffer (in mM: 117.8 NaCl, 4.0 KCl, 2.0 CaCl$_2$, 0.9 MgCl$_2$, 1.25 NaH$_2$PO$_4$, 20 NaHCO$_3$, and 5.0 glucose). The left anterior descending (LAD) coronary artery was dissected from surrounding myocardial tissue, cut into 2 mm segments and directly mounted in a wire myograph (Danish Myo Technology, Aarhus, Denmark). The anatomical localization of the LAD coronary artery is illustrated in Supplemental Figure S1. Wire myography experiments were initiated by normalisation to an internal circumference corresponding to 0.9 of the circumference at 13.3 kPa. Following a 15 min equilibration period in physiological buffer the artery segments were contracted 2–3 times using 60 mM potassium (similar composition as the above physiological buffer, except that NaCl was exchanged with KCl on equimolar basis) to measure the vasoconstrictor reactivity of the arteries. Only segments with potassium induced contraction >0.5 mN/mm were included in the study. After washing to obtain baseline relaxation, the ETB receptor agonist, Sarafotoxin 6c (S6c) was added in a cumulative fashion (10^{-12} to 10^{-7} M). Carbachol induced vasodilation and vasoconstriction (10^{-12} to 3×10^{-4} M) was tested following pre-constriction with potassium (40 mM). In order to elucidate the carbachol vasomotor responses, carbachol concentration-response curves were acquired either in absence (controls) or in presence of the muscarinic receptor antagonist, atropine (10^{-5} M), the COX-inhibitor indomethacin (10^{-4} M) or the eNOS inhibitor L-NAME (10^{-5} M). Endothelium-independent vasodilation was tested by sodium nitroprusside (10^{-9} to 10^{-5} M) following pre-constriction with 40 mM potassium. U46619 (10^{-12} to 10^{-5} M) and endothelin-1 (ET-1)-induced (10^{-12} to 10^{-7} M) vasoconstriction were tested using cumulative additions.

2.4. Biochemical Analysis

EDTA-stabilized blood samples were centrifuged ($16,000 \times g$, 1 min, 4 °C). Plasma for ascorbate and dehydroascorbic acid (DHA) analysis was stabilized with meta-phosphoric acid prior to storage at -80 °C. Previous studies have shown that both ascorbate and DHA are stable under these conditions for at least five years [23]. Concentrations were measured by HPLC with colorimetric detection as previously described [25,26]. The remaining plasma aliquots were stored neat at -80 °C until further analysis, except for samples for BH$_2$ and BH$_4$ determination, where the blood was stabilized in 0.1% dithioerythritol prior to centrifugation ($2000 \times g$, 4 min, 4 °C), yielding a plasma fraction, which was analyzed by HPLC, as previously described [13].

2.5. Data and Statistical Analysis

Force data (mN) were transformed to tension (Nm^{-1}) by dividing by twice the artery segment length and subtracting the baseline tension values [24]. Active tension was calculated by subtracting the passive tension from the potassium-induced active tension. Agonist-induced tension was normalized to the potassium induced active tension. Carachol-induced relaxation was calculated by subtracting the active tensions from the potassium-induced (40 mM) active tension. All statistical analysis and graphs were performed in GraphPad Prism 7.00 (GraphPad Software, La Jolla, CA, USA). Differences between two groups were evaluated by a two-sided Student's *t*-test. For multiple comparisons (in functional myography data), two-way ANOVA repeated-measures with Sidak's multiple comparisons was applied. Correlations between specific outcomes were evaluated by Pearson correlation (r) coefficient with two-tailed *p*-values.

2.6. Materials

Endothelin-1, human, porcine (Catalogue No. SC324, PolyPeptide Group, Strassbourg, France), Sarafotoxin S6c (SC457, PolyPeptide Group, Strassbourg, France), 9,11-dideoxy-11α,9α-epoxy-methanoprostaglandin F2α (BML-PG023-0001, Enzo Life Sciences, Exeter, UK). Carbamoylcholine chloride (C4382-1G SIGMA, Sigma-Aldrich, St. Louis, MO, USA), indomethacin (I7378-5G SIGMA, Sigma-Aldrich, St. Louis, MO, USA), Nω-nitro-L-arginine methylester hydrochloride (N5751 Sigma, Sigma-Aldrich, St. Louis, MO, USA), atropine (A0132 SIGMA, Sigma-Aldrich, St. Louis, MO, USA), meta-phosphoric acid (239275, Sigma, Sigma-Aldrich, St. Louis, MO, USA), 1,4-dithioerythritol (D9680, Sigma, Sigma-Aldrich, St. Louis, MO, USA).

3. Results

3.1. Effects of Vitamin C Deficiency on Weight Gain of Animals, Plasma Ascorbate Concentration and Plasma BH_4 Concentration

Plasma vitC concentrations were measured at euthanasia, following 11 weeks on the experimental diets. The dietary regimen was reflected in plasma ascorbate and DHA concentrations, with marked ($p < 0.001$) reduction in plasma ascorbate concentration in the deficient group compared to the control group (Table 1). VitC deficiency also led to a significant reduction in plasma BH_4 concentration ($p < 0.0001$) (Figure 1).

Table 1. Animal weight and plasma analyses. Data are expressed as means ± SEM, N is number of animals, **** Different from controls, $p < 0.0001$, unpaired *t*-test.

	N	Controls	N	VitC Deficient
Weight (g)	16	625 ± 14	16	602 ± 16
Ascorbate concentration, (μM)	16	60.2 ± 5.1	16	2.3 ± 0.1 ****
Ascorbate total, (μM)	16	61.5 ± 5.3	16	2.3 ± 0.1 ****
% DHA	16	1.9 ± 0.5	16	2.2 ± 1.0

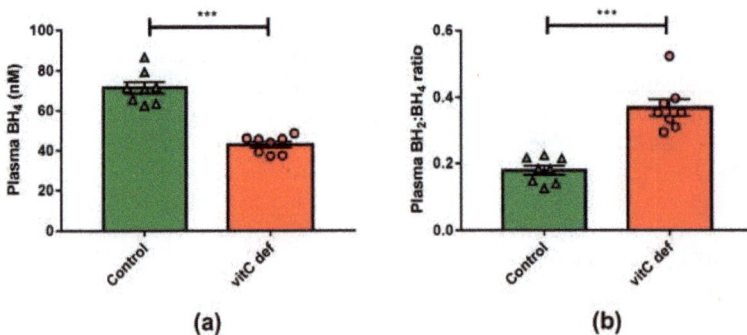

Figure 1. (a) Plasma concentrations of BH_4; (b) plasma BH_2:BH_4-ratio. Means ± SEM, *** $p < 0.0001$ (*n* = 8).

3.2. Contractile Reactivity

The potency and efficacy of ET-1 was significantly higher than that of U46619 ($p < 0.05$), and the selective ETB receptor agonist, S6c, induced only a negligible contraction in the coronary artery segments (Table 2). VitC status did not have a significant effect on the potassium, ET-1, U46619 or S6c vasoconstrictor responses (Figure 2a,b). In contrast to the other vasoconstrictors, potassium induced a long-lasting vasocontractile response persisting for at least 10 min and potassium was therefore used as a pre-constrictor in the studies of the relaxation-inducing agonists. Coronary arteries from vitC deficient guinea pigs were significantly smaller than the controls ($p < 0.05$, Table 2). Additionally, we found that for the vitC deficient group, the animal weight was positively correlated with the coronary artery diameter ($p < 0.002$, Table 3 and Figure 3a).

Table 2. Artery segment properties, diameter (μm), potassium tension (Nm^{-1}), agonist induced contraction (% of potassium contraction). Data are expressed as means $\pm$ SEM, N is number of animals, n is number of artery segments, NC = not calculated. * Different from controls, $p < 0.05$, unpaired t-test.

	N, n	Controls	N, n	VitC Deficient
Diameter	16, 35	366 $\pm$ 16	16, 35	312 $\pm$ 12 *
Potassium, tension	16, 35	3.2 $\pm$ 0.2	16, 35	3.1 $\pm$ 0.3
Endothelin-1	12, 17	Emax 116 $\pm$ 16 pEC$_{50}$ 8.2 $\pm$ 0.1	12, 17	Emax 108 $\pm$ 8 pEC$_{50}$ 8.3 $\pm$ 0.1
Sarafotoxin 6c	8, 20	Emax NC pEC$_{50}$ NC	8, 20	Emax 3 $\pm$ 1.6 pEC$_{50}$ 8.5 $\pm$ 0.7
U46619	16, 35	Emax 58 $\pm$ 9 pEC$_{50}$ 6.6 $\pm$ 0.1	16, 35	Emax 64 $\pm$ 13 pEC$_{50}$ 6.7 $\pm$ 0.2

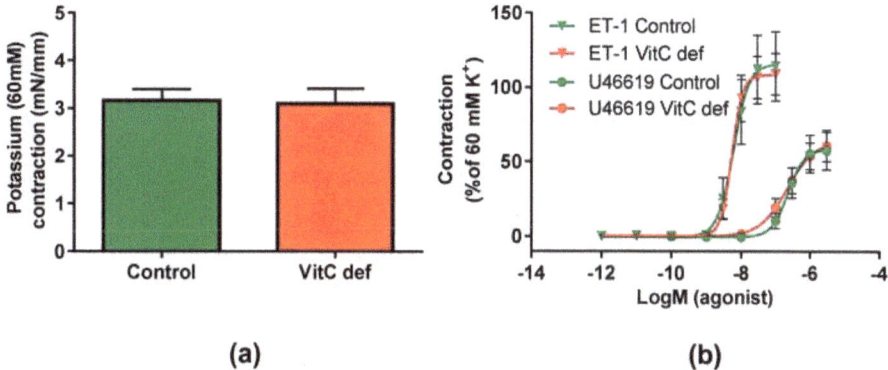

(a)

(b)

Figure 2. Contractile responses in coronary arteries. (**a**) Contractile responses to 60 mM extracellular potassium; (**b**) contractile responses to cumulative concentrations of ET-1 and U46610 in coronary arteries from control guinea pigs (green) and vitC deficient (red). Means $\pm$ SEM (K$^+$, $n = 16$; ET-1, $n = 12$; U46619, $n = 16$).

Table 3. Correlation analyses of specific outcomes in the control and vitC deficient groups. Pearson correlation analyses, N is number of animals, n is number of artery segments, r is Pearson correlation coefficient, ** p <0.002, *** p < 0.001.

	Controls			VitC Deficient		
	N, n	Pearson r	p Values	N, n	Pearson r	p Values
Diameter vs. weight	16, 35	0.182	0.500	16, 35	0.729	0.001 **
Diameter vs. carb induced dilatation	16, 35	0.010	0.954	16, 35	0.555	0.0005 ***
Diameter vs. carb induced contraction	16, 35	−0.174	0.518	16, 35	−0.286	0.284
BH₄ vs. carb induced dilatation	8, 15	0.403	0.105	8, 15	0.057	0.840
BH₄ vs. carb induced contraction	8, 15	−0.372	0.172	8, 15	0.232	0.406

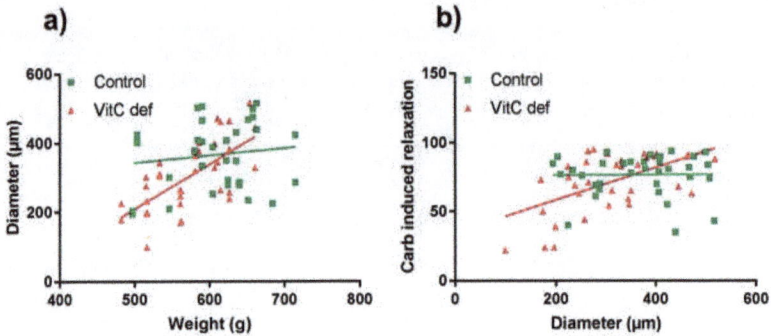

Figure 3. Scatter plots of coronary artery diameter vs. guinea pig body weight (**a**) and carbachol-induced vasorelaxation compared with coronary artery diameter (**b**). Control guinea pigs (green squares) and VitC deficient (red triangles).

3.3. Vascular Responses to Carbachol

Cumulative concentrations of carbachol in the range of 1 nM to 1 µM markedly relaxed coronary artery segments pre-contracted with 40 mM potassium (Figure 4a) and higher concentrations (1 µM to 0.3 mM) caused a rise in the isometric tension in a concentration-dependent fashion. Carbachol-induced relaxation and sensitivity was not significantly different in coronary arteries from vitC deficient guinea pigs compared to controls (Figure 3a); however, a significantly positive correlation between coronary artery diameter and carbachol-induced relaxation was found in coronary arteries from vitC deficient guinea pigs, but not in controls ($p < 0.001$), Table 3 and Figure 3b). The maximal carbachol-induced contraction response was significantly lower in segments from vitC deficient compared to controls ($p < 0.001$; Figure 4a) and in both vitC deficient and control animals the contractions were independent on coronary artery diameter ($p > 0.05$, Table 3). The muscarinic receptor antagonist, atropine (10 µM), blocked both the carbachol-induced vasodilation and vasoconstriction from both diet groups (Figure 2b). To evaluate the contribution of NO and prostanoids to carbachol-induced vasodilation and vasoconstriction, carbachol concentration- response curves were recorded during pre-contraction induced by potassium and in the presence of the COX inhibitor, indomethacin (10 µM), NOS inhibitor, L-NAME (100 µM) or in the presence of both indomethacin (10 µM) and L-NAME (100 µM). The presences of inhibitors alone or in combination revealed no differences in the vasodilator responses in control compared with vitC deficient animals, and the augmented vasoconstrictor responses in arteries from control animals compared to segments from vitC deficient animals were maintained in the presence of the inhibitors (Figure 4b–d).

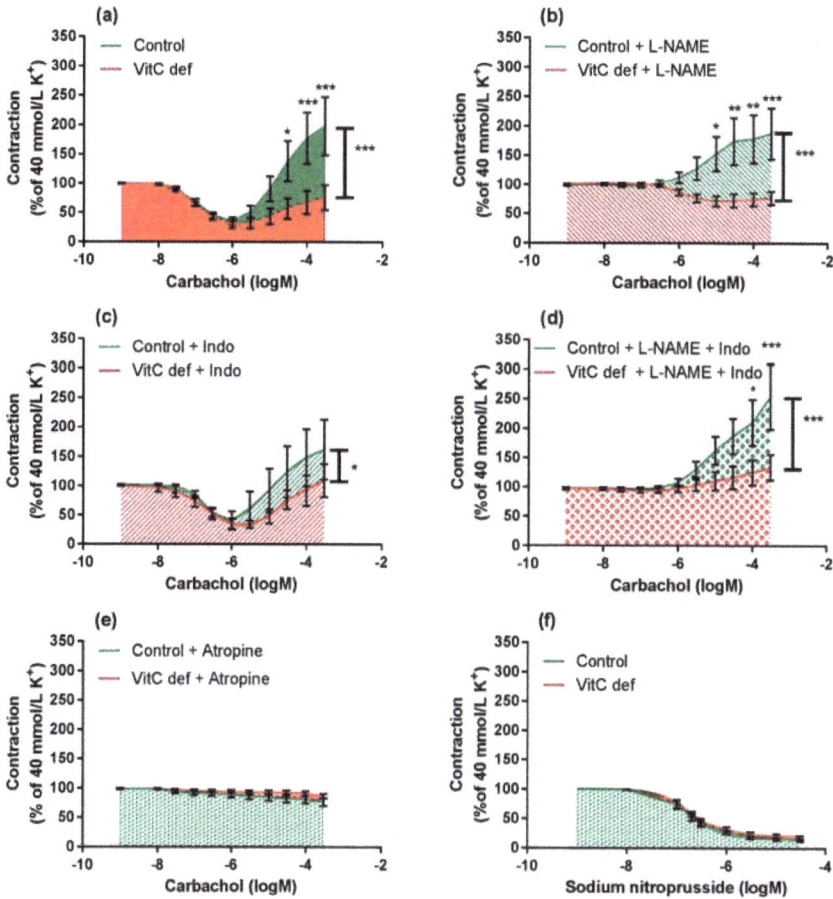

Figure 4. Log-concentration-response curves of coronary artery segments from vitC versus control guinea pigs. (**a**) Vasomotor responses to carbachol in coronary artery segments pre-constricted with 40 mM extracellular potassium; (**b**) in presence of L-NAME; (**c**) indomethacin; (**d**) both L-NAME and indomethacin; (**e**) atropine. (**f**) Vasodilator responses to sodium nitroprusside (SNP) in coronary arteries pre-constricted with 40 mM extracellular potassium. Control guinea pigs (green) and VitC deficient (red). Means ± SEM (n = 8–16), * $p < 0.05$, ** $p < 0.01$, *** $p < 0.001$.

L-NAME significantly inhibited the vasodilatory response to carbachol in segments from both control and vitC deficient guinea pigs ($p < 0.001$; Figure 5a,b); however L-NAME alone had no effect on the subsequent vasoconstrictor response compared to non-treated segments. In the presence of indomethacin alone, both carbachol-induced vasodilatation and vasoconstriction were restored (Figure 5c,d) in arteries from both groups compared to non-treated segments.

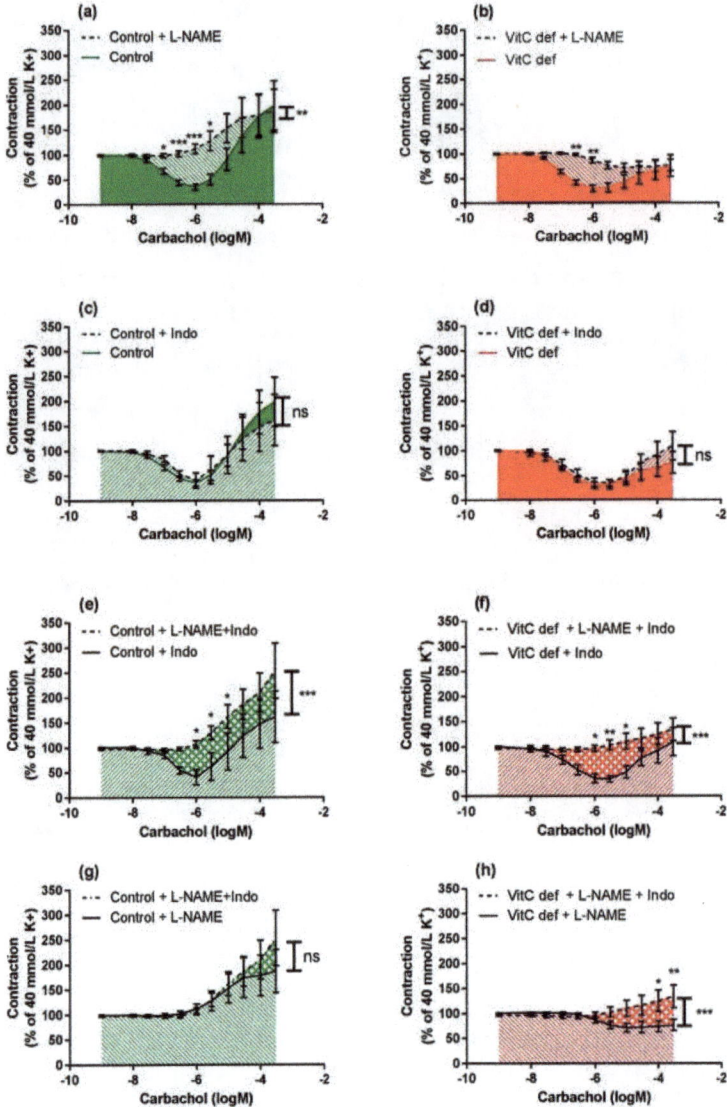

Figure 5. Log-concentration-response curves of coronary artery segments after treatment with L-NAME and/or indomethacin. The figures illustrate how the combination of inhibitors in artery segments from the same animal modulates the carbachol-induced vasodilator and constrictor responses. Vasomotor responses to carbachol in artery segments pre-constricted with 40 mM extracellular potassium: in absence versus presence of L-NAME in (**a**) control guinea pigs; (**b**) vitC deficient. In absence versus presence of indomethacin in (**c**) control; and (**d**) vitC deficient, in absence of L-NAME versus presence both L-NAME and indomethacin in (**e**) control guinea pigs; (**f**) VitC deficient, and in absence of indomethacin versus presence both L-NAME and indomethacin in (**g**) control guinea pigs; (**h**) VitC deficient. Means $\pm$ SEM ($n = 8$–16), * $p < 0.05$, ** $p < 0.01$, *** $p < 0.001$.

In the presence of L-NAME, indomethacin amplified the carbachol-induced vasoconstriction only in segments from vitC deficient guinea pigs, suggesting a potential effect arachidonic acid metabolites e.g., vasodilator prostanoids counteracting the vasoconstrictor effect of carbachol in coronary arteries from vitC deficient guinea pigs or increased production of vasoconstrictor leukotrienes, which is unmasked in the presence of indomethacine. This effect was not recorded for control animals.

In summary, we found that carbachol-induced vasodilator and constrictor responses were mediated by muscarinic receptors. In vitC deficient guinea pigs, the diameter of the coronary arteries were significantly and positively correlated with the weight of the animals and the endothelium-dependent vasorelaxation. These correlations were not present in the control group. In vitC deficient guinea pigs the muscarinic receptor-induced vasoconstrictor responses were significantly attenuated compared to controls and partly restored by COX-inhibition.

3.4. Relaxing Responses to SNP

To evaluate the endothelium-independent response to NO, relaxing response to the NO donor SNP (1 nM to 30 µM) was measured in potassium pre-contracted arteries. SNP induced a concentration dependent relaxation and the maximal relaxation and the sensitivity to SNP were not affected by the vitC status in the animals (Figure 4f).

4. Discussion

The present study shows that vasoconstrictor responses to carbachol are significantly decreased in arteries from vitC deficient guinea pigs as compared to arteries from control animals, proposing a link between vitC deficiency and compromised vascular function in vivo. Interestingly, contractions induced by other constrictors: potassium, S6c, U46619 and ET-1 were not affected by vitC status, suggesting that the contractile apparatus *per se* is not affected. Although vitC deficiency decreased plasma BH_4 levels, there was no significantly decreased vasodilator capacity compared to controls. However, vitC deficient guinea pigs had significantly smaller coronary artery diameters than controls, and in vitC deficient guinea pigs, the decreased diameter correlated with decreased carbachol-induced vasodilatation. Consequently, it appears that impaired vitC status affects the diameter of the coronary arteries and the endothelial function; furthermore vitC status induces a specific effect on the parasympathetic muscarinic receptor system, as measured by attenuated vasoconstrictor responses.

The parasympathetic neurotransmitter, acetylcholine and its analogue carbachol are widely used to study endothelial dependent/independent vasodilation and vasoconstriction, and the agonist is relevant since guinea pigs have an extensive network of cholinergic perivascular nerve fibres in the coronary artery tree [22]. In isolated coronary artery segments, carbachol induced a biphasic concentration-response pattern with an initial vasodilator response at low concentrations (from 10 nM to 1 µM) followed by a vasoconstrictor response at higher concentrations (from 1 µM to 0.3 mM). Carbachol-responses in the presence of atropine, indomethacin and/or L-NAME in the organ bath were assessed, revealing that atropine blocked both the carbachol-induced vasodilatation and vasoconstriction over the entire carbachol concentration interval. This suggests that carbachol elicits its effect via muscarinic receptors on guinea pig coronary arteries. This is consistent with previous studies showing that acetylcholine-induced vasodilator responses in bovine [25], simian [26] and mice [27] coronary arteries are mediated predominantly by endothelial muscarinic M_3 receptors, and that acetylcholine induced vasoconstrictor responses are mediated by vascular M_3 receptors in bovine [28,29] and porcine [30,31] coronary arteries.

In this study, we found that in vitC deficient guinea pigs, the endothelial-dependent vasodilation was significantly correlated with coronary artery diameter; a correlation that was not present in controls. Furthermore, we found coronary artery diameters were significantly smaller in vitC deficient guinea pigs as compared to control guinea pigs, despite sampling at uniform, anatomically defined, orientation. These results suggest that vitC deficiency potentially impair coronary artery growth and endothelial function of young guinea pigs. Hence, those guinea pigs that responded most sensitively to vitC restriction further developed more overall growth retardation with consequently impaired coronary artery growth and endothelial function. In the control group, in contrast, the variation in artery diameter did not reflect a pathophysiological response, but rather, a random variation in growth. Previously, degenerative changes in the capillary endothelium have been found in scorbutic guinea pigs whereas the larger arteries showed no abnormalities [32]. However, although we found this correlation between artery diameter and endothelial function in vitC deficient animals and not in controls; we found no overall effect of vitC deficiency when comparing the two groups. Treatment of the coronary artery segments with L-NAME abolished the initial carbachol-induced vasodilator response in both diet groups. In contrast, indomethacin did not significantly affect the vasodilator response between groups, suggesting that carbachol-induced vasodilator response was predominantly driven by endothelial-dependent NO release. Importantly, the vasodilator responses were investigated in arteries preconstricted with high extracellular concentration of potassium. High potassium concentrations depolarize VSMC and endothelial cells [33] which consequently hide a putative endothelium-derived hyperpolarizing factor (EDHF) mediated vasodilator effect [34]. Therefore, blocking the contribution of EDHF to vasodilation allowed the isolation of the effects of NO and prostaglandins on carbachol induced vasodilation.

Muscarinic receptors are widely expressed in smooth muscle cells in several organs, and diet-induced ascorbate deficiency in guinea pigs has previously been shown to reduce muscarinic-cholinergic receptor density [21]. Increased oxidative stress has been found to acutely reduce muscarinic receptor-mediated smooth muscle cell constriction in guinea pigs [19], and increased ROS production in ischemia/reperfusion reduce efficacy and sensitivity to cholinergic stimulation [35,36], linking redox imbalance to functional consequences mediated via muscarinic receptors.

Stimulating the arteries with the NO donor sodium nitroprussid revealed vasodilation with similar sensitivity and maximal effect in arteries from vitC deficient and control guinea pigs (Figure 4f). NO mediates a vasodilator effect by binding to soluble guanylyl cyclase (sGC) in VSMC. Guanylyl then catalyses the production of cGMP, which activates protein kinase G that via dephosphorylation of myosin light chain leads to vasorelaxation [37]. Oxidative stress has been showed to down-regulate soluble guanylyl cyclase expression and activity [38]. In present study, we found no effect of vitC deficiency on the NO-mediated vasodilation, indicating that the sGC activity was unaltered by the vitC status.

When coronary artery segments were treated with L-NAME and/or indomethacin, the carbachol-induced vasoconstrictor response remained reduced in arteries from vitC deficient compared to control animals. However, indomethacin increased the carbachol-induced vasoconstrictor response in eNOS blocked segments from vitC deficient animals, which was not present in arteries from control animals. This suggests that vitC deficiency promotes the release of vasodilator prostanoids in coronary arteries when stimulated with carbachol. Vasodilator prostanoids have previously been found to negate the effect of coronary vasoconstrictors after myocardial infarction [39], a condition known to induce oxidative stress [40] and be detrimental to cellular function and survival. In contrast, inhibition of prostanoid production has been found to have little effect in healthy humans [41] and dogs [42]. In this study, prostanoid-induced suppression of carbachol vasoconstrictor responses in coronary arteries were increased in vitC deficient guinea pigs, suggesting a compensatory role in the regulation of coronary vascular tone under vitC and BH$_4$ deficiency. The contractile responses induced by either extracellular potassium, U46619, S6c or ET-1 were not affected by vitC status, supporting the idea that the general vasoconstrictor capacity is not affected by vitC deficiency.

VitC deficiency (defined as plasma concentrations <23 μM) is surprisingly common, affecting ~15% of adults in the Western World with even higher prevalence among individuals who smoke, have high BMI, low socioeconomic status [7] as well as children with underlying medical conditions [43,44]. Epidemiological studies have shown an association between vitC deficiency and an increased risk of cardiovascular disease; however, the mechanistic link has not been elucidated [45,46]. Altered vasomotion and reactivity of coronary arteries plays an important role in pathophysiologic mechanisms involved in heart disease. The parasympathetic nervous system is known to provide a modulating influence on the response of coronary arteries to local metabolic requirements in the heart [47]. Moreover, muscarinic receptors are known to be expressed in human coronary arteries [48]. Patients with variant angina or coronary stenosis have been found to have altered coronary vasoconstriction after injection of acetylcholine, pointing toward a causal relationship with altered muscarinic receptor response and disease [49,50]. The observation that muscarinic receptor mediated contraction is impaired as a result of vitC deficiency is of potential importance, not only in regulation of coronary artery vasomotion, but also in other tissues that are highly dependent on parasympathetic-muscarinic receptor-mediated contraction (bladder, esophagus, intestines, pancreas, and salivary glands). For obvious ethical reasons, it is impossible to perform long-term controlled trials on humans to establish the consequence of vitC deficiency on vasculature and present knowledge is therefore restricted to indirect evidence. Applying the guinea pig as a unique and validated model of diet-induced vitC deficiency, this study shows that chronic vitC deficiency in vivo alters the response of the coronary arteries to parasympathetic stimuli. This provides a link between vitC deficiency and cardiovascular disease, proposing a yet undisclosed, specific, effect of vitC in the modulation of muscarinic receptor-modulated response within the vascular wall. Though requiring further investigation, the apparent association between vitC status and coronary artery contraction may prove relevant in the prevention and treatment of cardiovascular diseases in humans with poor vitC status.

The present study has several limitations. Based on existing literature, we expected that vitC deficiency reduced NO-mediated vasodilation as a consequence of the decreased BH_4 plasma concentration. The potential reason for the lack of correlation between the BH_4 plasma concentrations and endothelial function could be that we determined biopterines and vitC in the plasma, rather than in the arteries, which could potentially more adequately have reflected the vessel status. Interestingly, a correlation between animal weight, artery diameter and endothelial function in vitC deficient guinea pigs was found. Future studies are needed to elaborate on a causal relationship and putative functional consequences e.g., clarifying if vitC deficiency induces morphological changes of the heart muscle and vessels. Furthermore, measurements of intracellular calcium concentrations would be highly relevant to determine if vitC deficiency alters cytosolic calcium levels and handling, which can lead to increased tone and decreased vessel diameter. Here, the effect of vitC deficiency was evaluated in young guinea pigs—reproductive maturity is reached at around 10 weeks of age—with no other underlying pathophysiological condition. We found that the coronary arteries were highly resistant to mechanically endothelial denudation, suggesting that the animals, despite vitC deficiency, retained a high NO capacity and/or sensitivity in the coronary arteries. However, it could be speculated that in the presence of an additional vascular disease, such as atherosclerosis, left ventricular hypertension [51] or even age-related reductions in compensatory abilities, a decreased vitC concentration and consequently, a reduced capacity to recycle BH_4, may be crucial in preserving an adequate vasodilator capacity [52].

Our finding, that the muscarinic receptor system is highly sensitive to vitC deficiency, is a novel and so far unrecognized effect of in vivo vitC deficiency. Future studies are needed to elucidate the mechanisms underlying the impaired muscarinic receptor mediated contraction observed here and to study other tissues with highly dependent parasympathetic-muscarinic receptor-mediated contraction (e.g., bladder, esophagus, intestines, pancreas, and salivary glands).

5. Conclusions

The present study shows that chronic vitC deficiency impairs vasomotor function of coronary arteries. During vitC deficiency, the endothelial function is reduced, with decreasing vessel diameter and carbachol-induced vasoconstrictor responses being significantly impaired. The carbachol-induced effects are apparently mediated by altered muscarinic receptor activity. Although further studies are required to evaluate the underlying mechanisms and the potential clinical implications, these findings may provide a link between chronic vitC deficiency and increased risk of cardiovascular disease reported in numerous epidemiological studies.

Supplementary Materials: The following are available online at www.mdpi.com/2072-6643/9/7/691/s1; Figure S1: Localization of coronary artery segments used for myograph experiments.

Acknowledgments: We thank Joan Elisabeth Frandsen for her excellent technical expertise and assistance in the ascorbate measurements. This study was supported by the LIFEPHARM Centre for In Vivo Pharmacology.

Author Contributions: G.F.S., P.T.N. and J.L. conceived and designed the experiments; G.F.S. carried out the myography experiments and data analysis. P.T.N., M.M.L. and S.N.H. performed the animal study. G.F.S., P.T.N. and J.L. interpreted the data and wrote the manuscript. All authors read and commented on the final draft of the manuscript.

Conflicts of Interest: The authors declare no conflict of interest.

References

1. Myint, P.K.; Luben, R.N.; Wareham, N.J.; Khaw, K.-T. Association Between Plasma Vitamin C Concentrations and Blood Pressure in the European Prospective Investigation Into Cancer-Norfolk Population-Based Study. *Hypertension* **2011**, *58*, 372–379. [CrossRef] [PubMed]
2. Myint, P.K.; Luben, R.N.; Welch, A.A.; Bingham, S.A.; Wareham, N.J.; Khaw, K.T. Plasma vitamin C concentrations predict risk of incident stroke over 10 years in 20,649 participants of the European Prospective Investigation into Cancer Norfolk prospective population study. *Am. J. Clin. Nutr.* **2008**, *87*, 64–69. [PubMed]
3. NyyssÖnen, K.; Parviainen, M.T.; Salonen, R.; Tuomilehto, J.; Salonen, J.T. Vitamin C deficiency and risk of myocardial infarction: Prospective population study of men from eastern Finland. *BMJ* **1997**, *314*, 634–638. [CrossRef] [PubMed]
4. Pfister, R.; Michels, G.; Bragelmann, J.; Sharp, S.J.; Luben, R.; Wareham, N.J.; Khaw, K.T. Plasma vitamin C and risk of hospitalisation with diagnosis of atrial fibrillation in men and women in EPIC-Norfolk prospective study. *Int. J. Cardiol.* **2014**, *177*, 830–835. [CrossRef] [PubMed]
5. Pfister, R.; Sharp, S.J.; Luben, R.; Wareham, N.J.; Khaw, K.T. Plasma vitamin C predicts incident heart failure in men and women in European Prospective Investigation into Cancer and Nutrition-Norfolk prospective study. *Am. Heart J.* **2011**, *162*, 246–253. [CrossRef] [PubMed]
6. Wannamethee, S.G.; Bruckdorfer, K.R.; Shaper, A.G.; Papacosta, O.; Lennon, L.; Whincup, P.H. Plasma Vitamin C, but Not Vitamin E, Is Associated With Reduced Risk of Heart Failure in Older Men. *Circ. Heart Fail.* **2013**, *6*, 647–654. [CrossRef] [PubMed]
7. Schleicher, R.L.; Carroll, M.D.; Ford, E.S.; Lacher, D.A. Serum vitamin C and the prevalence of vitamin C deficiency in the United States: 2003–2004 National Health and Nutrition Examination Survey (NHANES). *Am. J. Clin. Nutr.* **2009**, *90*, 1252–1263. [CrossRef] [PubMed]
8. Heller, R.; Unbehaun, A.; Schellenberg, B.; Mayer, B.; Werner-Felmayer, G.; Werner, E.R. L-ascorbic acid potentiates endothelial nitric oxide synthesis via a chemical stabilization of tetrahydrobiopterin. *J. Biol. Chem.* **2001**, *276*, 40–47. [CrossRef] [PubMed]
9. Mortensen, A.; Lykkesfeldt, J. Does vitamin C enhance nitric oxide bioavailability in a tetrahydrobiopterin-dependent manner? In vitro, in vivo and clinical studies. *Nitric Oxide Biol. Chem. Off. J. Nitric Oxide Soc.* **2014**, *36*, 51–57. [CrossRef] [PubMed]
10. Baker, T.A.; Milstien, S.; Katusic, Z.S. Effect of vitamin C on the availability of tetrahydrobiopterin in human endothelial cells. *J. Cardiovasc. Pharmacol.* **2001**, *37*, 333–338. [CrossRef] [PubMed]
11. Tejero, J.; Stuehr, D. Tetrahydrobiopterin in nitric oxide synthase. *IUBMB Life* **2013**, *65*, 358–365. [CrossRef] [PubMed]
12. Vasquez-Vivar, J.; Martasek, P.; Whitsett, J.; Joseph, J.; Kalyanaraman, B. The ratio between tetrahydrobiopterin and oxidized tetrahydrobiopterin analogues controls superoxide release from endothelial nitric oxide synthase: An EPR spin trapping study. *Biochem. J.* **2002**, *362*, 733–739. [CrossRef] [PubMed]
13. Mortensen, A.; Hasselholt, S.; Tveden-Nyborg, P.; Lykkesfeldt, J. Guinea pig ascorbate status predicts tetrahydrobiopterin plasma concentration and oxidation ratio in vivo. *Nutr. Res.* **2013**, *33*, 859–867. [CrossRef] [PubMed]
14. Chen, X.; Touyz, R.M.; Park, J.B.; Schiffrin, E.L. Antioxidant effects of vitamins C and E are associated with altered activation of vascular NADPH oxidase and superoxide dismutase in stroke-prone SHR. *Hypertension* **2001**, *38*, 606–611. [CrossRef] [PubMed]

15. Lee, M.Y.; Griendling, K.K. Redox signaling, vascular function, and hypertension. *Antioxid. Redox Signal.* **2008**, *10*, 1045–1059. [CrossRef] [PubMed]

16. Zou, M.H. Peroxynitrite and protein tyrosine nitration of prostacyclin synthase. *Prostaglandins Lipid Mediat.* **2007**, *82*, 119–127. [CrossRef] [PubMed]

17. Zou, M.H.; Li, H.; He, C.; Lin, M.; Lyons, T.J.; Xie, Z. Tyrosine nitration of prostacyclin synthase is associated with enhanced retinal cell apoptosis in diabetes. *Am. J. Pathol.* **2011**, *179*, 2835–2844. [CrossRef] [PubMed]

18. Frei, B.; Stocker, R.; England, L.; Ames, B.N. Ascorbate: The most effective antioxidant in human blood plasma. *Adv. Exp. Med. Biol.* **1990**, *264*, 155–163. [PubMed]

19. De Jongh, R.; Haenen, G.R.; van Koeveringe, G.A.; Dambros, M.; De Mey, J.G.; van Kerrebroeck, P.E. Oxidative stress reduces the muscarinic receptor function in the urinary bladder. *Neurourol. Urodyn.* **2007**, *26*, 302–308. [CrossRef] [PubMed]

20. Sawiris, P.; Chanaud, N.; Enwonwu, C.O. Impaired inositol trisphosphate generation in carbachol-stimulated submandibular gland acinar cells from ascorbate deficient guinea pigs. *J. Nutr. Biochem.* **1995**, *6*, 557–563. [CrossRef]

21. Sawiris, P.G.; Enwonwu, C.O. Ascorbate deficiency impairs the muscarinic-cholinergic and ss-adrenergic receptor signaling systems in the guinea pig submandibular salivary gland. *J. Nutr.* **2000**, *130*, 2876–2882. [PubMed]

22. Gulbenkian, S.; Edvinsson, L.; Saetrum Opgaard, O.; Valenca, A.; Wharton, J.; Polak, J.M. Neuropeptide Y modulates the action of vasodilator agents in guinea-pig epicardial coronary arteries. *Regul. Pept.* **1992**, *40*, 351–362. [CrossRef]

23. Lykkesfeldt, J. Ascorbate and dehydroascorbic acid as reliable biomarkers of oxidative stress: Analytical reproducibility and long-term stability of plasma samples subjected to acidic deproteinization. *Cancer Epidemiol. Biomark. Prev.* **2007**, *16*, 2513–2516. [CrossRef] [PubMed]

24. DMT Normalization Guide. Available online: https://www.dmt.dk/uploads/6/5/6/8/65689239/dmt_normalization_guide.pdf (accessed on 22 June 2017).

25. Brunner, F.; Kuhberger, E.; Groschner, K.; Poch, G.; Kukovetz, W.R. Characterization of muscarinic receptors mediating endothelium-dependent relaxation of bovine coronary artery. *Eur. J. Pharmacol.* **1991**, *200*, 25–33. [CrossRef]

26. Ren, L.M.; Nakane, T.; Chiba, S. Muscarinic receptor subtypes mediating vasodilation and vasoconstriction in isolated, perfused simian coronary arteries. *J. Cardiovasc. Pharmacol.* **1993**, *22*, 841–846. [CrossRef] [PubMed]

27. Lamping, K.G.; Wess, J.; Cui, Y.; Nuno, D.W.; Faraci, F.M. Muscarinic (M) receptors in coronary circulation: Gene-targeted mice define the role of M_2 and M_3 receptors in response to acetylcholine. *Arterioscler. Thromb. Vasc. Biol.* **2004**, *24*, 1253–1258. [CrossRef] [PubMed]

28. Brunner, F.; Kuhberger, E.; Schloos, J.; Kukovetz, W.R. Characterization of muscarinic receptors of bovine coronary artery by functional and radioligand binding studies. *Eur. J. Pharmacol.* **1991**, *196*, 247–255. [CrossRef]

29. Duckles, S.P.; Garcia-Villalon, A.L. Characterization of vascular muscarinic receptors: Rabbit ear artery and bovine coronary artery. *J. Pharmacol. Exp. Ther.* **1990**, *253*, 608–613. [PubMed]

30. Entzeroth, M.; Doods, H.N.; Mayer, N. Characterization of porcine coronary muscarinic receptors. *Naunyn-Schmiedeberg's Arch. Pharmacol.* **1990**, *341*, 432–438. [CrossRef]

31. Van Charldorp, K.J.; van Zwieten, P.A. Comparison of the muscarinic receptors in the coronary artery, cerebral artery and atrium of the pig. *Naunyn-Schmiedeberg's Arch. Pharmacol.* **1989**, *339*, 403–408. [CrossRef]

32. Findlay, G.M. The Effects of an Unbalanced Diet in the Production of Guinea-pig Scurvy. *Biochem. J.* **1921**, *15*, 355–357. [CrossRef] [PubMed]

33. Karaki, H.; Urakawa, N.; Kutsky, P. Potassium-induced contraction in smooth muscle. *Nihon Heikatsukin Gakkai Zasshi* **1984**, *20*, 427–444. [CrossRef] [PubMed]

34. Mombouli, J.V.; Illiano, S.; Nagao, T.; Scott-Burden, T.; Vanhoutte, P.M. Potentiation of endothelium-dependent relaxations to bradykinin by angiotensin I converting enzyme inhibitors in canine coronary artery involves both endothelium-derived relaxing and hyperpolarizing factors. *Circ. Res.* **1992**, *71*, 137–144. [CrossRef] [PubMed]

35. Saito, M.; Wada, K.; Kamisaki, Y.; Miyagawa, I. Effect of ischemia-reperfusion on contractile function of rat urinary bladder: Possible role of nitric oxide. *Life Sci.* **1998**, *62*, PL149–PL156. [CrossRef]

36. Hisadome, Y.; Saito, M.; Kono, T.; Satoh, I.; Kinoshita, Y.; Satoh, K. Beneficial effect of preconditioning on ischemia-reperfusion injury in the rat bladder in vivo. *Life Sci.* **2007**, *81*, 347–352. [CrossRef] [PubMed]

37. Kots, A.Y.; Martin, E.; Sharina, I.G.; Murad, F. A short history of cGMP, guanylyl cyclases, and cGMP-dependent protein kinases. *Handb. Exp. Pharmacol.* **2009**, *191*, 1–14.

38. Priviero, F.B.; Zemse, S.M.; Teixeira, C.E.; Webb, R.C. Oxidative stress impairs vasorelaxation induced by the soluble guanylyl cyclase activator BAY 41-2272 in spontaneously hypertensive rats. *Am. J. Hypertens.* **2009**, *22*, 493–499. [CrossRef] [PubMed]

39. De Beer, V.J.; Taverne, Y.J.; Kuster, D.W.; Najafi, A.; Duncker, D.J.; Merkus, D. Prostanoids suppress the coronary vasoconstrictor influence of endothelin after myocardial infarction. *Am. J. Physiol. Heart Circ. Physiol.* **2011**, *301*, H1080–H1089. [CrossRef] [PubMed]

40. Hori, M.; Nishida, K. Oxidative stress and left ventricular remodelling after myocardial infarction. *Cardiovasc. Res.* **2009**, *81*, 457–464. [CrossRef] [PubMed]

41. Edlund, A.; Sollevi, A.; Wennmalm, A. The role of adenosine and prostacyclin in coronary flow regulation in healthy man. *Acta Physiol. Scand.* **1989**, *135*, 39–46. [CrossRef] [PubMed]

42. Dai, X.Z.; Bache, R.J. Effect of indomethacin on coronary blood flow during graded treadmill exercise in the dog. *Am. J. Physiol.* **1984**, *247*, H452–H458. [PubMed]

43. Lykkesfeldt, J.; Poulsen, H.E. Is vitamin C supplementation beneficial? Lessons learned from randomised controlled trials. *Br. J. Nutr.* **2010**, *103*, 1251–1259. [CrossRef] [PubMed]

44. Frei, B.; Birlouez-Aragon, I.; Lykkesfeldt, J. Authors' perspective: What is the optimum intake of vitamin C in humans? *Crit. Rev. Food Sci. Nutr.* **2012**, *52*, 815–829. [CrossRef] [PubMed]

45. Frikke-Schmidt, H.; Lykkesfeldt, J. Role of marginal vitamin C deficiency in atherogenesis: In vivo models and clinical studies. *Basic Clin. Pharmacol. Toxicol.* **2009**, *104*, 419–433. [CrossRef] [PubMed]

46. Tveden-Nyborg, P.; Lykkesfeldt, J. Does vitamin C deficiency increase lifestyle-associated vascular disease progression? Evidence based on experimental and clinical studies. *Antioxid. Redox Signal.* **2013**, *19*, 2084–2104. [CrossRef] [PubMed]

47. Dart, A.M.; Du, X.J.; Kingwell, B.A. Gender, sex hormones and autonomic nervous control of the cardiovascular system. *Cardiovasc. Res.* **2002**, *53*, 678–687. [CrossRef]

48. Niihashi, M.; Esumi, M.; Kusumi, Y.; Sato, Y.; Sakurai, I. Expression of muscarinic receptor genes in the human coronary artery. *Angiology* **2000**, *51*, 295–300. [PubMed]

49. Ludmer, P.L.; Selwyn, A.P.; Shook, T.L.; Wayne, R.R.; Mudge, G.H.; Alexander, R.W.; Ganz, P. Paradoxical vasoconstriction induced by acetylcholine in atherosclerotic coronary arteries. *N. Engl. J. Med.* **1986**, *315*, 1046–1051. [CrossRef] [PubMed]

50. Yasue, H.; Horio, Y.; Nakamura, N.; Fujii, H.; Imoto, N.; Sonoda, R.; Kugiyama, K.; Obata, K.; Morikami, Y.; Kimura, T. Induction of coronary artery spasm by acetylcholine in patients with variant angina: Possible role of the parasympathetic nervous system in the pathogenesis of coronary artery spasm. *Circulation* **1986**, *74*, 955–963. [CrossRef] [PubMed]

51. Bell, J.P.; Mosfer, S.I.; Lang, D.; Donaldson, F.; Lewis, M.J. Vitamin C and quinapril abrogate LVH and endothelial dysfunction in aortic-banded guinea pigs. *Am. J. Physiol. Heart Circ. Physiol.* **2001**, *281*, H1704–H1710. [PubMed]

52. LeBlanc, A.J.; Hoying, J.B. Adaptation of the Coronary Microcirculation in Aging. *Microcirculation* **2016**, *23*, 157–167. [CrossRef] [PubMed]

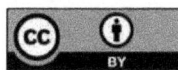

nutrients

MDPI

Review

Vitamin C, Aging and Alzheimer's Disease

Fiammetta Monacelli *, Erica Acquarone, Chiara Giannotti, Roberta Borghi and Alessio Nencioni

Section of Geriatrics, Department of Internal Medicine and Medical Specialties (DIMI), University of Genoa, Genoa 16132, Italy; erica88im@hotmail.com (E.A.); chiara.giannotti86@gmail.com (C.G.); robertaborghi@yahoo.it (R.B.); Alessio.Nencioni@unige.it (A.N.)

Received: 20 April 2017; Accepted: 13 June 2017; Published: 27 June 2017

Abstract: Accumulating evidence in mice models of accelerated senescence indicates a rescuing role of ascorbic acid in premature aging. Supplementation of ascorbic acid appeared to halt cell growth, oxidative stress, telomere attrition, disorganization of chromatin, and excessive secretion of inflammatory factors, and extend lifespan. Interestingly, ascorbic acid (AA) was also found to positively modulate inflamm-aging and immunosenescence, two hallmarks of biological aging. Moreover, ascorbic acid has been shown to epigenetically regulate genome integrity and stability, indicating a key role of targeted nutrition in healthy aging. Growing in vivo evidence supports the role of ascorbic acid in ameliorating factors linked to Alzheimer's disease (AD) pathogenesis, although evidence in humans yielded equivocal results. The neuroprotective role of ascorbic acid not only relies on the general free radical trapping, but also on the suppression of pro-inflammatory genes, mitigating neuroinflammation, on the chelation of iron, copper, and zinc, and on the suppression of amyloid-beta peptide (Aβ) fibrillogenesis. Epidemiological evidence linking diet, one of the most important modifiable lifestyle factors, and risk of Alzheimer's disease is rapidly increasing. Thus, dietary interventions, as a way to epigenetically modulate the human genome, may play a role in the prevention of AD. The present review is aimed at providing an up to date overview of the main biological mechanisms that are associated with ascorbic acid supplementation/bioavailability in the process of aging and Alzheimer's disease. In addition, we will address new fields of research and future directions.

Keywords: ascorbic acid; aging process; Alzheimer's disease

1. Ascorbic Acid and Its Relevance to the Aging Process

Due to the aging population and the increased life-expectancy [1] in developed and developing countries, a growing area of interest concerns the understanding of the mechanisms that regulate aging and that differentiate successful aging from pathological aging. Prolonged exposure to antigens throughout life produces a progressive modification of the individual homeostasis [2].

The free radical theory of aging allows an explanation of the molecular mechanisms underlying the aging process, at least partially, and the pathogenesis of age-related diseases, such as atherosclerosis, cardiovascular diseases, dementia, diabetes, and osteoporosis [3,4]. From a biological perspective, the process of aging is characterized by immunosenescence: this may be defined as the reduced ability to respond to foreign antigens and to tolerate self-antigens, leading to increased susceptibility to infections, cancer, and autoimmune diseases [5]. The most accredited molecular mechanisms for immunosenescence include redox-mediated and mitochondria-dependent oxidative pathways. High levels of free radicals and peroxidation products of lipid membranes, such as malondialdehyde (MDA), are able to modulate the activation of nuclear transcription factors, associated with cell aging and longevity, such as tumor protein p53, transcriptional protein AP-1 and nuclear factor kappa-light-chain-enhancer of activated B cells (NF-kB). In addition, these same mechanisms are responsible for altered T cell expression and the altered phenotype of immunological subpopulations [6].

Oxidative stress is increasingly considered to be the major epigenetic factor for aging and also plays an important role in inducing the low-grade inflammation, as the two processes are strictly intertwined. This pro-inflammatory phenotype, defined 'inflamm-aging', is characterized by an increased expression of genes related to inflammation and to the immune response. Indeed, it is known that the increased serum levels of C reactive protein (CRP) and pro-inflammatory cytokines, such as interleukin-6 (IL-6) and tumor necrosis factor alpha (TNF-α) induce the activation of NF-KB mediated superoxide production in mitochondria, promoting the release of oxygen reactive species (ROS) [2,6].

Inflamm-aging is also associated with decreased nitric oxide (NO) bioavailability in the endothelial layer, which induces endothelial dysfunction. Inflamm-aging may be considered a biological background for both the aging process and the pathophysiological process of frailty in humans [7].

The endogenous antioxidant enzymatic defense system superoxide dismutase (SOD), catalase and glutathione peroxidase (GSH) counteracts oxidative exogenous agents from diet and may undergo substantial decrease related to the aging process [8]. Accumulating evidence indicates that nutrition is a key relevant factor for inflamm-aging and an important modulator of the aging process as well [9–11].

Ascorbic acid (AA) is a powerful first-line antioxidant that mediates several beneficial effects on redox oxidative pathways and mitochondrial pathways on the immune system, on inflamm-aging, on endothelial integrity, and on lipoprotein metabolism [12,13]. AA, a lactone with six carbon atoms, is synthesized from glucose in the liver of many species of mammals. Humans have evolutionarily lost the gulonolactone oxidase enzyme, essential for the synthesis of 2-keto-L-gulonolactone, its direct precursor. As a result, people absorb AA exclusively from the diet. AA enters the cells through the sodium-dependent vitamin C transporters SVCT1 and SVCT2, a process favored by the electrochemical sodium gradient: due to its high capacity and low affinity, SVCT1 assures the intestinal and renal absorption and reabsorption [14].

All of the physiological and biochemical actions of AA are due to its ability to donate electrons (as a reducing agent). AA undergoes two consecutive and reversible oxidations: from the first electron loss, it generates an intermediate product, the ascorbate free radical (AFR), which is converted into dehydroascorbate (DHA) after the loss of the second electron. At physiological concentrations, AA is a powerful antioxidant and scavenger of free radicals in plasma and different tissues, including the central nervous system (CNS) [15,16].

AA is also implicated in the endothelial integrity associated with NO bioavailability [17]. The molecular mechanisms that induce endothelial dysfunction affect the enzyme NO synthase (eNOS) by impairing Gi- dependent signaling, decreasing mRNA stability for eNOS, and blocking eNOS translocation from the plasma membrane to the Golgi membranes. The reduced bioavailability of its substrate (L-arginine) or its co-factor (tetrahydrobiopterin BH4) was also observed [18]. Low levels of BH4 compromise eNOS function by promoting the transfer of electrons to oxygen molecules instead of L-arginine: in turn, eNOS produces a superoxide anion instead of generating NO [19].

2. Ascorbic Acid, Epigenetic Modulation and Nutrigenomics

In the last decades, the understanding of AA properties has undergone a major revolution, ranging from a simple antioxidant to a micronutrient, capable of epigenetic regulation [20,21].

Recent advances in epigenetics have identified a series of di-oxygenases Fe^{2+} and 2 oxoglutarate (2OG-dependent) enzymes that catalyze the epigenetic modifications of DNA and histones. Some of these enzymes require ascorbate to maintain their catalytic activity. Therefore, the availability of ascorbate might affect the epigenome, with a potential impact on health and age-related diseases. Methylation in the C5 position of cytosine (5-methylcytosine, 5mC) is the most important and well-studied epigenetic mark of mammalian DNA, which plays an essential role in the transcriptional and in the maintenance of genome stability.

DNA methyltransferase (DNMTs) is responsible for the transfer of a methyl group from the universal methyl donor, *S*-adenosyl-L-methionine (SAM), to the 5-position of cytosine residues in DNA. The presence of an unusual nucleotide, 5-hydroxymethylcytosine (5hmC) in mammalian DNA has been reported. Although 5hmC represents less than 1% of total nucleotides, high levels have been observed in the cerebellar Purkinje cells and in the granule neurons, suggesting a potential role for neuronal functions in epigenetic regulation. This nucleotide (5hmC) is formed by the activity of a group of enzymes, ten-eleven translocation methylcytosine dioxygenas (TET: TET1, TET2, TET3), that catalyze the ten-eleven translocation and oxidize 5mC to generate 5hmC. TET enzymes were shown to further oxidize 5hmC into 5-formylcytosine (5fC) and 5-carboxylcytosine (5caC). Ascorbic acid is known to increase 5hmC production in a TET-dependent way, probably by reactivating the catalytic site of TET enzyme, reducing Fe^{3+} to Fe^{2+}. Namely, AA induced a significant demethylation of 5-methylcytosine (5mC) to 5-hydroxymethyl cytosine (5hmC) [22,23].

Variation in ascorbate bioavailability can influence the demethylation of DNA and histones: in addition, ascorbate deficiency can present at different stages of aging and could be involved in the development of different age-related diseases. In particular, if additional ascorbate is not provided by supplementation or improved uptake, there would be progressive AA decline in the brain, which might be associated with neurodegeneration. So far, there is inconsistent data on epigenetic modifications in the human brain. Further studies could unravel the potential impact of age-related ascorbate decline on the epigenome and on neurodegeneration.

So far, AA seems to increasingly have beneficial effects on the aging processes and on the prevention of age-related diseases as atherosclerosis, cardiovascular diseases, cancer, and neurodegenerative diseases.

Nutrigenomics is a young area of research, but meaningful studies indicated a role for AA on gene expression. A previous study found that, although no diet-gene interactions were observed, genetic variation of SVCT1 can influence serum ascorbic acid concentrations. Moreover, both AA transporter genotypes modify the strength of the correlation between dietary AA and serum levels [24].

Recently, genetic variations of haptoglobin, polymorphisms in the transporters of AA, and deleted polymorphisms of glutathione-*S*-transferase have provided genetic information regarding possible relative AA levels [25–27].

Intriguingly, AA functions at the interface of different molecular pathways associated with aging, as illustrated by Figure 1.

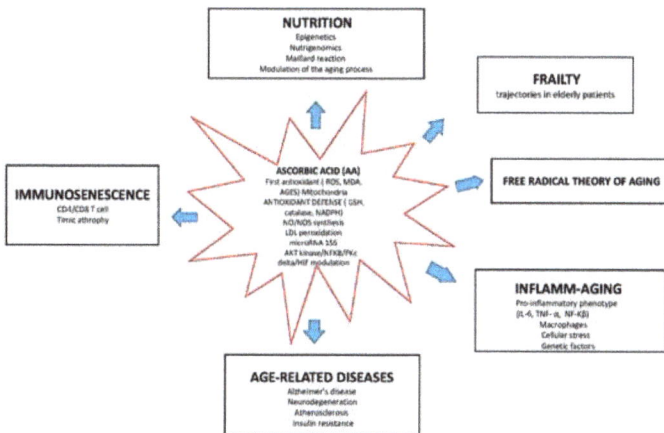

Figure 1. AA is at the crossroads of biological aging, intercepting immunosenescence, inflamm-aging, and oxidative stress (free radical theory of aging), with a potential role in the onset of age-related diseases and frailty trajectories.

3. Ascorbic Acid and the Aging Process: In Vitro Models

Several lines of research have increasingly accredited the role of AA in the aging process. The in vitro and in vivo evidence is reported herein and illustrated in Table 1.

Table 1. In vitro and in vivo evidence for a role of AA in the aging process.

Species	Model	Design and Methods	Conclusion	References
Human	ESCs	Methylation	Epigenetic regulation of Tet activity and DNA methylation	Blaschke, K. 2013 [28]
Mouse	Embryonic fibroblasts cultured	Expression of Tet genes, GSH antioxidant activity	Epigenetic modulation of genome activity and stability	Minor, E.A. [29]
Human	Umbilical cord vein endothelial cells (HUVEC)	Measurement of citrulline synthesis, determination of cGMP, eNOS activity, GTP Cyclohydrolase I	Anti-oxidative pathways (protection of tetrahydrobiopterin Endothelial integrity (cellular NO synthesis))	Heller, R. 2001 [18]
In Vitro	EA. hy926	Determination of BH4 levels, H_2O_2, expression of PP2Ac	Endothelial integrity (eNOS activity/eNOS phosphorylation)	Ladurner, A. 2012 [19]
Mouse	WrnΔhel/Δhel	Measurement ROS and oxidative DNA damage	Extended life span, improvement of inflammation, metabolic profile, lipid profile	Lebel, M. 2010 [30]
Mouse	Gulo−/−	Measurement cytokines and metabolites	Extended life span. Model of rejuvenation	Aumailley, L. 2016 [31]
Insect	Wrn-1(gk99) mutant	Gene expression and regulation	Extended mean life span of *C. elegans* (regulatory genes of lipid metabolism, ketones, organic acids, carboxylic acids. Locomotion and developmental anatomical structure)	Dallaire, A. 2014 [32]
In Vitro	WS MSC model	Oxidative stress levels, IL-6 anIL-8	Model of rejuvenation	Li, Y. 2016 [33]
Mouse	WrnΔhel/Δhel	Measurements of ROS and oxidative DNA damage, GSH, ATP, protein analysis, lactonase activity	Beneficial effects on oxidative pathways, genome stability	Massip, L. 2010 [34]
Human and Mouse	PBMCs and BMMC and BM from SOD1−/−	PBMC: IFN-γ ± NAC Human and mouse BM: BFA ± NAC	Beneficial effects on immunosenescence through inflamm-aging	Pangrazzi, L. 2016 [35]
Mouse and In Vitro	3T3-L1 cells, OP9 cells	Adipocytes differentiation	Adipocyte differentiation: implications for the aging process	Rahaman, F. 2014 [36]
Mouse	Embryonic stem cell line CGR8	Stem cells differentiation	AA-dependent differentiation (p38 MAPK/CREB pathway). Epigenetic regulation	Rahman, F. 2016 [37]
Human In Vitro	hBM-MSCs	Osteocyte and adipocyte differentiation	Beneficial effects on cells differentiation mediated by anti-oxidation	Jeong, S.G. 2015 [38]
Mouse	WrnΔhel/Δhel	Metabolite, cytokine and chemokine measurements	Potential predictive cardiometabolic biomarkers in patients with WS.	Aumailley, L. 2015 [39]
Mouse	SMP30KO	Immunosenescence and aging	Beneficial effect on the maintenance of immune cells (thymic atrophy)	Uchio, R. 2015 [40]
Mouse	SMP30/GNL KO	Model of senescence	Beneficial effects on liver protein oxidation in vivo	Sato, Y. 2014 [41]
In Vitro	Cortical precursor cells	Survival, proliferation, and differentiation of AA-treated CNS precursor cells	Brain development: the generation of neurons and glia	Lee, J.Y. 2003 [42]
Mouse	Hippocampal and cortical neurons from mice lacking one allele of the SVCT2	Combined treatment of AA and GSH	Beneficial effects on neuronal development, functional maturation, and antioxidant responses	Qiu, S. 2007 [43]

A mouse model of senescence showed that AA promotes proliferation of bone marrow mesenchymal cells derived from aging mice. The senescence-accelerated mouse prone 6 (SAMP6) mice and senescence-accelerated mouse resistant 1 (SAMR1) mice were used as the test group and the control group, respectively. Bone marrow mesenchymal stem cells (BMMSCs) derived from SAMP6 mice were treated with increasing concentrations of AA [44]. The treatment significantly improved the BMMSCs proliferation in a dose-dependent manner by increasing telomerase activity and TERT expression. The AA concentration of 100 μg/mL induced the strongest effect in promoting the proliferation of BMMSCs in SAMP6 mice, while at a concentration of 1.000 mg/mL, AA suppressed the cell growth. AA can promote the proliferation of BMMSCs from aging mice, possibly by increasing the cellular telomerase activity.

Interestingly, it is known that bone marrow (BM) plays a key role in immunological memory and surveillance, through inflamm-aging. Overexpression of IL-15 and IL-6 was stimulated by IFN-y and correlated with ROS. The plasma-cell survival factor a proliferation- inducing ligand (APRIL) was also reduced. AA was effective in counteracting inflammatory- and oxidative stress-related changes in the aging bone marrow, improving immunological memory in old age. This study is of key relevance in assessing the protective role for AA in immunosenescence [35].

The positive effects of AA on premature cellular events was confirmed by treatment with AA on Werner's syndrome protein (WRN-deficient) human mesenchymal stem cells (MSCs) [33]. In this model, the analysis of mRNA levels showed that AA altered gene expression was involved in chromatin condensation, the regulation of the cell cycle, and DNA replication and repair. AA promoted heterochromatin remodeling to a younger state (as demonstrated from the upregulation of heterochromatin Protein 1 (HP1α) markers and histone H3K9me3 by Western blotting). AA slowed down cellular senescence in mesenchymal WRN-deficient cells (as demonstrated by the SA-β-gal staining) restoring mesenchymal stem cells' vitality and proliferative potential. AA repressed telomere shortening, decreased the production of pro-inflammatory cytokines, such as IL-6 and IL-8, downregulated the expression of markers of aging, such as cyclin-dependent kinase inhibitor 2A, multiple tumor suppressor 1 p16Ink4a and zinc finger transcriptional GATA4, and repressed the SASP (elevated senescence-associated secretory phenotype). AA was effective at alleviating aging defects by reducing cell cycle regulation, telomere attrition, ROS burst, and nuclear laminin disorganization.

AA was also reported to stimulate/inhibit the differentiation of mesoderm-derived embryonic stem cells (ES) through the involvement of p38 mitogen activated protein kinase/cAMP response element binding (CREB) nuclear transcription factor activation (p38 MAPK/CREB pathway) and increased expression of the SVCT2 transporter. More precisely, AA was found to promote ES differentiation by regulating chromatin domain overlapping. These in vitro models have important implications for the aging process. The effect of AA in the context of body weight could be at least partially related to stem cell differentiation towards myogeneis and osteogenesis, inhibiting adipogenesis. Since aging is associated with sarcopenia and defects in body weight, the current observations suggest that AA-mediated stem cell effects could play a role in the aging process [36,37].

Furthermore, the same results were replicated in human bone marrow mesenchymal stromal cells (hBM-MSCs) undergoing replicative senescence to investigate the relationship between ROS levels and stem cell potential differentiation after AA treatment. Interestingly, AA supplementation eliminated ROS excess and restored the endogenous antioxidant enzymatic activity (catalase, SOD) by influencing phosphorylated fox head box O protein 1 (p-FOXO) and p53. Moreover, differentiation into adipocytes and osteocytes was significantly increased [38].

Thus, AA seems to be implicated in the regulation and differentiation of stem cells. Current knowledge on MSC cell surface biomarkers and molecular mechanisms of MSC differentiation emphasizes the role of Wnt/β-catenin signaling, the Notch signaling pathway, bone morphogenesis proteins, various growth factors, and oncogene and immunosuppressive activities of MSCs. Therefore, further investigations are needed to establish a role for AA in such targeting regulation of cell differentiation, which may have important clinical implications for the prevention of age-related disease [45].

Ascorbic Acid and the Aging Process: In Vivo Evidence

Murine models of Werner's syndrome (WS) (Wrn Δhel/Δhel mutants) exhibit many phenotypic characteristics similar to accelerated human aging. The supplementation with AA for nine months was found to reduce oxidative stress in hepatocytes and cardiomyocytes, and decrease hypertriglyceridemia and hyperglycemia. A significant improvement of the metabolic profile, including insulin resistance and the body fat in WrnΔhel/Δhel mutant mice was also observed.

Similarly, other Werner syndrome-like in vivo models have confirmed that AA supplementation rescued the shorter lifespan, reversing age-related abnormalities in adipose tissue, the liver, and genome integrity. In the metabolic profile, inflammatory status was improved and, at a molecular level, the normalization of the phosphorylation of AKT kinase, transcriptional levels of NF-kappa B, protein kinase delta (PKC delta), peroxisome proliferator-activated receptor alpha (PPAR-alpha) and hypoxia-inducible factor-1 alpha (HIF1-alpha), were observed [45].

A further study of WrnΔhel/Δhel mutant mouse models showed that the pro-oxidant and inflammatory state produced a premature defenestration of sinusoidal endothelium in liver tissue with consequent hepatic dysfunction and impaired hepatic lipoprotein metabolism. Long-term treatment with AA restored physiological levels of GSH and the fenestrated sinusoidal endothelium by quenching oxidative stress. It is noteworthy that in healthy mice, the beneficial effects of AA on health and lifespan were not significant and the supplementation significantly reduced the oxidative damage only in WrnΔhel/Δhel mouse liver [30,34].

AA had a positive impact on the cardiometabolic and inflammatory profiles of mice lacking the functional Werner syndrome protein helicase. AA reversed changes in the expression levels of plasminogen activator-1 (PAI-1) and improved, at a transcriptional level, fatty acid degradation. In addition, AA increased glutathione metabolism and reversed the oxidative stress. This study suggested that AA could be a potential cardiometabolic biomarker in patients with WS [39].

Caenorhabdilis elegans worm models, with a non-functional wrn-1 DNA helicase ortholog, exhibited a shorter lifespan. The supplementation with AA increased lifespan in the mutant strain, compared with the wild-type strain possibly by altering the expression of genes regulating the metabolism of lipids, ketones, organic acids, and carboxylic acids. AA modified the expression of genes involved in locomotion and development of the anatomical structure. Conversely, in the wild-type worms, AA only influenced the biological process of proteolysis [32].

Knockout (Gulo−/−) mice represent an interesting in vivo model that mimics human physiology, lacking the gulonolactone oxidase (Gulo) gene. Accumulating evidence from this in vivo model yielded additional information on the role of ascorbate in aging. Knockout (Gulo−/−) mice developed high oxidative stress, sensorimotor deficits, and behavior abnormalities. The lifespan of Gulo−/− mice appeared to inversely correlate with the phosphorylation levels of IRE1α and IF2α, in response to endoplasmic reticulum stress. In this model, AA supplementation reduced phosphorylated IRE1α, implicating its protective effect on endoplasmic reticulum stress and extended lifespan. In addition, in the same in vivo model, AA supplementation was shown to improve T cell-mediated acute response after liver injury, suggesting a modulation of the immune system [31].

Uchio et al. demonstrated the influence of long-term high-dose AA intake on the number and function of immune cells in SMP30KO mice. The total counts of leucocytes, lymphocytes, granulocytes, and monocytes in the peripheral blood, as well as the number of splenocytes and thymocytes, were all significantly higher in the treated group. In addition, the number of naive T cells in peripheral blood lymphocytes, the number of memory T-cell populations in splenocytes, and the number of clusters of differentiated CD4+ and CD8+ T cells in thymocytes were all remarkably elevated. High dietary AA intake was associated with the improvement of age-related thymic atrophy. The study indicated a role for AA in immunosenescence by targeting CD4+ and CD8+ cells. Further, AA was found to modulate immune cell surveillance in SMP30 knockout mice [40].

In line with these data, Sato and colleagues suggested that AA plays an important role in preventing protein oxidation in the liver of SM30/gluconolactonase knockout mice, with potential implications in overall health and aging [41].

4. Ascorbic Acid and the Aging Process: Oxidative Stress and Antioxidant Defense

Oxidative stress is considered noxious for lifespan and AA, and, as a first line antioxidant, has been thought to potentially increase longevity. These notions have recently been challenged by findings in model organisms that show beneficial effects on lifespan of increased ROS generation produced by mutations or pro-oxidant treatments [46,47]. Such a relationship would arise from a combination of beneficial effects from a moderate increase in ROS levels and their dose-dependent toxicity. Intriguingly, the small elevation of ROS levels that increase lifespan seems not to be stressful, nor do they induce an increased resistance to oxidative stress. In particular, in a *Caenorhabdilis elegans* model, [48] AA displayed an inverted U-shaped dose–response relationship between ROS levels and lifespan; both high and low levels of ROS were detrimental for longevity. This evidence further complicated the role of AA in aging. The fact that both antioxidant and pro-oxidant treatments reveal such a different behavior suggests that temporal administration of AA is of key relevance to obtain beneficial effects. Moreover, ROS levels still need to be optimized for lifespan in different cells, and the net balance between antioxidant and oxidant defense and their concentrations plays a relevant role in the aging process.

From a clinical perspective, AA functions at a true interface between aging, life span and age-related diseases. It is able to modulate telomeres activity, bioenergetics, DNA repair and oxidative stress, indicating a nutrigenomic role in the process of aging as well [49].

During aging, the antioxidant capacity of AA is finely regulated by the redox balance of DHA/ascorbate and the ability of the endogenous antioxidant enzymatic defense system (glutathione and nicotinamide adenine dinucleotide phosphate; NADPH) to recycle DHA back to AA. An increased ratio of DHA/AA becomes an indicator of a pro-oxidative ability of AA to mediate biological processes and may play a role in age-related diseases, intercepting different aging trajectories.

Similarly, cellular antioxidant enzymatic capacity declines during the aging process and oxidation of glutathione and NADPH may also explain different results in studies targeting aging and disease prevention. Recently, it has been shown that elderly people with lower peripheral antioxidant parameters, including AA and a decreased antioxidant capacity, are more prone to clinical vulnerability, disability, frailty and higher mortality over a 5-year follow up [50].

Conversely, two studies in healthy elderly subjects showed that daily intake of star fruit juice (Averrhoa Carambola, a fruit with high content of AA) acted as a scavenger of free radicals, and maintained low levels of lipoperoxidative stress (MDA), restoring GSH levels. The associated AA antioxidant capacity also mediated anti-inflammatory effects by the reduction of pro-inflammatory cytokine secretion, especially TNF-alpha and interleukin-23 (IL-23) excluding interleukin-2 (IL-2) [51,52].

Kim et al. investigated the effects of high-dose AA supplementation (1250 mg daily) in humans. After eight weeks, the analysis of serum lipoproteins showed a reduction of advanced glycation end products (AGEs). The anti-glycoxidative effect was significantly higher, especially in non-smoking men, and was associated with net improvement of plasma HDL levels. The quantitative analysis of the LDL fractions also showed an improvement of LDL lipid composition. Therefore, the supplementation with AA could exert protective effects against atherosclerosis and related systemic inflammation by reducing the oxidized LDL and macrophage phagocytosis, with reduced conversion to foam cells [42].

Interestingly, this study demonstrated that AA induced changes in gene expression of some microRNAs that negatively regulate target genes' post-transcriptional expression. After AA consumption, miR155 levels decreased by 90%, suggesting that high doses of AA may significantly modulate miRNA levels and the anti-inflammatory response [42]. Thus, AA may be considered an epigenetic key to personalized nutrition.

5. Evidence for Ascorbic Acid in Brain Aging

In the central nervous system, AA plays a complex role that is still only partially established. Cerebrospinal fluid (CSF) ascorbic acid concentrations (200–400 mM) are higher compared to those in cerebral parenchyma and in plasma (30–60 nM) [43].

AA is secreted into the CSF across the apical membrane of choroid plexus cells by an active and saturable transporter for AA, the sodium-dependent vitamin C transporter 2 (SVCT2). In turn, dehydroascorbate (DHA) can cross the blood-brain barrier (BBB) more efficiently through the GLUT1 transporter present in the BBB endothelial cells. SVCT2 mediates AA uptake through neurons or astrocytes in the brain while GLUT receptors (In particular GLUT1 and GLUT3) are primarily responsible for the DHA absorption from the central nervous system cells. Neurons likely use both mechanisms to maintain intracellular ascorbate, although SVCT2 transport mostly contributes to maintaining the ascorbate concentration gradient from CSF to neurons [43]. Moreover, AA recycling acts through a bystander effect by GLUT receptors mediated cellular uptake in pro-oxidative conditions. It favors the intracellular conversion from DHA to AA with increased intracellular accumulation. This bystander effect is responsible for AA recycling activity between neurons and astrocytes and plays a role in the fine balance between pro-oxidative and anti-oxidative status [53].

Recently, it has been shown that AA release mediated by neurons is linked to glutamate metabolism and kinetics in the brain. In particular, Wilson et al. [53] demonstrated that AA extracellular release is the direct consequence of astrocyte swelling mediated by glutamate receptors' increased sodium uptake. Heightened AA release in the brain and CSF is considered responsible for its antioxidant and neuroprotective mechanism against glutamate excitotoxicity [53].

Several in vivo studies documented that AA plays an antioxidative role, especially after an ischemic event or cerebral reperfusion. AA, at millimolar concentrations, was able to scavenge the superoxide anion, recycling the α-tocopherol within the lipid layers of the cellular membrane [54]. This, in turn, impeded the lipoperoxidation process. In addition, in the CNS, AA participated in several hydroxylation reactions that include the redox activity of Fe^{3+} and Cu^{2+} at dioxigenase sites. In vitro studies on cultured stem cells showed that AA is also implicated in neuronal developmental maturation and in neurotransmission. Lee et al. [55] further demonstrated that AA (at a 200 millimolar concentration) was effective in differentiating neuronal and astrocytes precursors, promoting synaptic maturation.

Using SVTC knockout mice as an in vivo model showed that AA, at lower doses, was able to mediate dendrite formation, increasing post-synaptic electrical potential [56].

AA is essential for the biosynthesis of catecholamines, peptide amination, myelin formation, synaptic function enhancement, along with the neuroprotective activity against glutamate toxicity [53,57]. In particular, AA plays an essential role in neurotransmission, because it is a co-factor of the dopamine beta–hydroxylase enzyme that catalyzes the conversion from dopamine to noradrenaline. AA is considered to modulate cerebral plasticity by orchestrating neurotransmitter balancing in the brain. The main AA-mediated mechanisms impacting neurotransmission could relate to redox modulating activity of the NMDA receptor, supporting a role for AA in counteracting glutamate excitotoxicity [57,58].

It is expected that better understanding of the physiological and molecular mechanisms associated with AA brain recycling and the differential expression of SVCT2 and GLUT receptors could contribute to disentangling the pathogenesis of complex neurodegenerative diseases, such as Alzheimer's disease and Huntington's disease.

6. Ascorbic Acid and Its Relevance to Alzheimer's Disease

Over the years, L-ascorbic acid (AA) has been increasingly found to promote several beneficial effects on neurodegeneration, with particular regard to Alzheimer's disease (AD) [59]. The increasing burden of this life-threatening condition [60] and the lack of disease-modifying drugs have guided the research towards preventive strategies, targeting AD modifiable risk factors [12]. Mounting evidence indicates a role for L-ascorbic acid in ameliorating specific factors linked to AD pathogenesis [61]. Namely, the main mechanisms associated with AA neuroprotection involve the scavenging activity against ROS, the modulation of neuroinflammation, the suppression of the fibrillation of amyloid-beta peptide (Aβ), and the chelation of iron, copper and zinc [62]. The amyloid cascade hypothesis is considered the primary event of AD pathogenesis [63]. The sequential cleavage by gamma and β secretase (BACE1) of the β-amyloid precursor protein (APP) results in the production of the β-amyloid species with neurotoxic oligomer accumulation. Brain accumulation of Aβ1-42 oligomers results in increased neuronal vulnerability to oxidative stress [64,65] neuroinflammation with impairment of synaptic plasticity [66], and neuronal death. Extracellular amyloid plaques are also responsible for the hyperphosphorylation of the cytoskeletal Tau protein [67]. In addition, Aβ oligomers interfere with mitochondrial dynamics [68,69].

Copper, zinc, and iron are present in Aβ plaques due to the presence of metal binding sites [70]. Metals can affect the morphology of Aβ, accelerating fibrillation and cytotoxicity of Aβ [71]. Therefore, redox active copper and iron linked to Aβ can generate hydroxyl radicals via the Fenton reaction, increasing protein and DNA oxidation and lipid peroxidation (MDA) in the AD brain. Metal redox activity also induces the production of AGEs, carbonyls, peroxynitrites, and increased levels of heme oxygenase-1 (HO-1), with decreased cytochrome c oxidase activity [61]. AGEs, through their interaction with receptors for advanced glycation end products (RAGEs), further activate pro-inflammatory pathways with the induction of pro-inflammatory cytokines, such as IL-6 [72]. In addition, lower concentrations of the fluorescent AGE pentosidine were observed in the CSF of AD patients, compared to healthy subjects, in support of a role for altered AGE metabolism in AD pathogenesis [73].

Oxidative stress is generally associated with chronological aging, while aging is the major epigenetic risk factor for AD. Recent evidence has found that oxidative stress plays an essential role in the pre-phase of AD, including mild cognitive impairment [74]. The brain is vulnerable to ROS damage due to neurons' post-mitotic state with higher oxygen consumption. With respect to lipid peroxidation products, oxidized proteins, and DNA damage, peroxynitrites have been increasingly detected in the AD temporal cortex, as well as oxidation of mitochondrial DNA and nuclear DNA in the parietal cortex [75]. In AD hippocampal neurons and astrocytes, a redox imbalance has been observed with an overexpression of heme oxygenase-1 and increased levels of Cu/Zn superoxide dismutase [76]. The conjugated aromatic ring of tyrosine residues is also a target for free-radical attack, and accumulation of dityrosine and 3-nitrotyrosine has also been reported in the AD brain [77]. Therefore, oxidative stress can directly activate glia with the priming of astrocytes and microglia at the injury site. In turn, the direct contact of activated glial cells with neurons may generate immune mediators (nitric oxide, ROS, pro-inflammatory cytokines, and chemokines) that are neurotoxins, spreading inflammation in the central nervous system [78,79]. Thus, extensive oxidative damage may act as a driver of brain aging, and early accumulation of oxidatively modified biomolecules may constitute the initial steps of AD neurodegeneration.

All of these findings could provide a mechanistic role for oxidative stress as a direct effect of aging and a consequence of the toxic effect of Aβ. Oxidative stress interacts with multiple features associated with AD pathogenesis, such as APP processing, mitochondrial dysfunction, and metal accumulation [80]. The main AA mediated neuroprotective effects on AD pathogenesis are reported and illustrated in Table 2.

Table 2. In vitro and in vivo evidence for a role of AA in Alzheimer's disease.

Species	Model	Design and Methods	Conclusion	References
Mouse	TASTPM	Evaluation of carbonyls, glutathione, Aβ, APP	Decreased oxidative stress markers, Nrf2, GSH, APP, soluble Aβ1-42. No increase of BACE 1, PS1and AB plaque	Choundhry, F. 2012 [58]
Mouse	Model with human APP695 and double mutation (K670N, M671L)	Evaluation of Aβ, BACE1, antioxidant system and IL-1β	Increased antioxidant system, reduced activity of BACE, IL-1β and NO levels, Aβ deposition	Apelt, J. 2004 [60]
Mouse	APP/PS1 transgenic	ROS scavengers and inhibitors effects on Aβ-induced impairments in LTP	Reversal of Aβ- deposition by mitochondria-targeted ROS scavenging	Ma, T. 2011 [62]
Mouse	HAPP/Sod1−/−	Anti-Aβ1-16 antibody	Inhibition of amyloid plaques (Aβ hexamers /BACE1 modulation)	Murakami, K. 2012 [65]
Mouse	Tg2576	Aβ levels brain deposition	Suppressed brain inflammatory and oxidative stress responses in mice, significant reduction of soluble and insoluble Aβ1-40 and Aβ1-42	Yao, Y. 2004 [57]
Mouse	APPS we/PSEN1ΔE9	MDA, Aβ levels, AChE activity. Learning and memory	Improvement of learning and memory Beneficial effects against MDA, and Beneficial effects on AChE function	Harrison, F.E. 2009 [50]
Mouse	APPSWE/PSEN1ΔE9 mice, SVCT2+/−	Behavioural test, GSH, MDA, isoprostanes	Decreased Aβ deposition (senile plaque formation and accumulation)	Dixit, S. 2015 [81]
Rat	F-344	Aβ deposition	Decreased-amyloid immunoreactive fibrils	Hauss-Wegrzyniak, B. 2002 [82]
Rat and Mouse	Charles-Foster, Swiss Albino mouse	Cognitive test, cytokines, ROS Cytotoxic Activity Assay	Enhancement of anti-oxidative pathway	Sil, S. 2016 [83]
Mouse	Gulo−/−5XFAD	Identification modification of cerebral capillaries	Reduction of Aβ accumulation	Kook, S.Y. 2014 [84]
In Vitro	neuroblastoma cell line SH-SY5Y	Apoptosis (phosphatidylserine, TUNEL assay, caspase-3 activity)	Prevention of toxicity induced by Aβ	Huang, J. 2006 [85]
Mouse	Tg2576, 3xTg-AD	Aβ staining, investigation APP and HS oligosaccharides	Modulation of Aβ fibrillogenesis	Cheng, F. 2011 [86]
Mouse	AD model	Fibrillogenesis: senile plaques	Modulation of synaptophysin and the phosphorylation of tau at Ser396	Murakami, K. 2011 [87]
Rat	Wistar	Lipoperoxidation, oxidation, Inflammation, nitrites	Reduction of pro-inflammatory cytokine Inhibition of Aβ deposition	Rosales-Corral, S. 2003 [88]
Human In Vitro	NT2 undifferentiated cells	Measurement levels of Aβx-40 and Aβx-42, HNE, expression of BACE-1. Evaluation apoptotic cell death induced by HNE	Increased anti-oxidative pathways against SAPK pathways and BACE-1 that regulate AβPP processing	Tamagno, E. 2005 [74]
Human In Vitro	Neuroblastoma cell line SH-SY5Y	Glutathione, superoxide dismutase, and catalase	Neuroprotection anti-oxidative pathways Improvement of antioxidant defense system	Ballaz, S. 2013 [80]
Rat	PND7	Induction of ROS, apoptotic markers. Quantification of Bax/Bcl-2 ratio, cytochrome c and caspases	Reduction of oxidation, neuroinflammation (both activated microglia and astrocytes). reduced ethanol-induced activation of PARP-1 and neurodegeneration	Ahmad, A. 2016 [89]
In Vitro	EA. hy926 cells	Measurement intracellular ascorbate and GSH	Endothelial integrity (NO: eNOS/guanylate cyclase pathway)	May, J.M. 2011 [90]

Table 2. *Cont.*

Nutrients 2017, 9, 670

Species	Model	Design and Methods	Conclusion	References
In Vitro	EA. hy926 cells	Quantification LDL-enriched lipoproteins, GSH, and lipid peroxidation	Endothelial integrity	May, J.M. 2010 [91]
Rat	Cortical neuron/glia co-cultures of neonatal	Measuring nitrites IL-6 and MIP-2, LDH. p38 and ERK MAPKs	Suppression of the LPS-stimulated production of inflammatory mediators	Huang, Y.N. 2014 [92]
Rat	Sprague–Dawley	Behavioural test BBB components	Modulation of cortical compression and/or BBB dysfunction	Lin, J.L. 2010 [12]
Rat	MCAO	Measurement of infarct and edema brain, measurement of serum MMP-9 levels, behavioural testing	decreased MMP-9 levels, Improvement of the vascular insult (BBB disruption and brain edema)	Allahtavakoli, M. 2015 [93]
Rat	Brains	Assessment the role of nanocapsulated ascorbic acid (NAA)	NAA exerted protection to brain mitochondria by preventing oxidative damage in ROS mediated CIR injury	Sarkar, S. 2016 [94]
Rat	Hippocampal neurons	Incubation with Aβ Os or 4-CMC ± NAC	NAC prevention of Aβ O-induced mitochondrial Fragmentation by anti-oxidative pathways	Sanmartin, C.D. 2012 [61]
Rat	Cortical neurons Neuroblastoma cells	Oxidative stress and DHA uptake, analysis of GLUTs	Improvement of anti-oxidative defense of neurons	García-Krauss, A. 2016 [75]
Rat	Primary neurons	Incubation with H_2O_2, ratio GSH/GSSG	Increased glutathione system of peroxide detoxification	Dringen, R. 1999 [78]
Rat	Astroglial cells	Treatment with H_2O_2 or hydro peroxide, NO release, Lipid Peroxidation, ROS	Reduction of neuroinflammation (microglial-astroglial cells)	Röhl, C. 2010 [79]
Rat	SD	Induction of transient focal cerebral ischemia, treatment with DHA	DHA reduced brain edema and vascular permeability formation following cerebral ischemia	Song, J. 2015 [95]
Human	Endothelial cell (HBMEC) and astrocyte co-colture	BBB after hyperglycaemic insult	Improvement of BBB permeability by reducing oxidative stress associated with glucose normalization	Allen, C.L. 2009 [96]

6.1. Ascorbic Acid and Oxidative Stress in Alzheimer's Disease

AA is suggested to play a major role in the pathogenesis of AD by direct neuroprotection against oxidative stress. Imbalance of AA homeostasis has been extensively demonstrated in neurodegeneration [58]. AA is a key antioxidant of the CNS, released from glial cells to the synaptic cleft, and taken up by neurons as an antioxidant defense to maintain neuronal metabolism and synaptic function. The astrocyte-neuron interaction was found to function as an essential mechanism for AA recycling, participating in the anti- oxidative defense of the brain [97].

It is well documented that AA is a first-line antioxidant defense to neutralize ROS reactivity, promoting the regeneration of endogenous antioxidants (GSH, catalase, vitamin E) [98].

Interestingly, it is also presumed that AA moderates the oxidative stress mediated by glutamate, protecting from excitotoxicity in the brain [56,88]. A previous study in APP/PSEN 1 transgenic mice showed that parenteral administration of AA possessed nootropic properties, without altering the AD-like features of plaque deposition, oxidative stress and acetylcholinesterase activity [85]. Therefore, several in vitro and in vivo studies underpin the therapeutic role of AA in AD, bolstering oxidative defense [99].

In rat hippocampal brains, oral administration of AA reduced oxidative stress and neuroinflammation mediated by Aβ fibrils [100]. Additionally, AA was shown to protect SH-SY5Y neuroblastoma cells from apoptosis mediated by Aβ [86], decreasing the rate of endogenous amyloid generation. Further, AA was reported to decrease acetylcholinesterase activity in mice [101] and to positively restore presynaptic acetylcholine release [102].

More recently, the NO-catalyzed release of anhydromannose in the presence of AA was detected [103] with an associated decreased formation of toxic Aβ oligomers. APP/PSEN 1 mice lacking the SVCT2 transporter and having AA mild deficiency showed accelerated amyloid pathogenesis, linked to oxidative stress pathways, compared to control mice with normal brain ascorbic acid [81]. Further, orally-administered AA reduced oxidative stress and pro-inflammatory cytokines induced by Aβ peptide injections in the CA1 area of the hippocampus in rat brains [99].

6.2. Metals, Oxidative Stress and Ascorbic Acid in Alzheimer's Disease: The AA Oxidative Balance in the Brain

The main features of enhanced oxidative stress in the AD brain are also related to the increased content of Cu and Fe, capable of stimulating free radical generation, lipid peroxidation, reactive nitrogen species (NRS) release, and stress-sensitive proteins [104]. In turn, the interaction of the redox-active copper ions with misfolded Aβ aggregates and oligomers may favor AD pathogenesis.

It is well known that at higher concentrations, AA acts as a pro-oxidant, either by generating reactive oxygen species or by inhibiting the antioxidant systems in the presence of iron, which, in turn, induces lipid peroxidation [105]. A pro-oxidant or antioxidant effect of AA mainly relies on the concentration gradient and redox state of a cell [106]. Evidence from a mouse model that selectively over-expressed the AA transporter SVCT2 in the eye [107] implicated AA in age-related damage to crystalline proteins in the lens. All of these experimental data contribute to heightening the debate on the potential pro-oxidant role of AA via the Fenton reaction.

A previous study undermined the protective role of AA in dementia, indicating that the interaction of AA with 'free' catalytically-active metal ions could contribute to oxidative damage through the production of hydroxyl and alkoxyl radicals [108]. Interestingly, some in vitro studies investigated the pro-oxidant properties of ascorbate [109], which were mainly attributed to the release of metal ions from damaged cells. It has been reported that neurotoxic forms of amyloid β, Aβ (1–42), Aβ (1–40), and also Aβ (25–35) induced copper-mediated oxidation of ascorbate, whereas non-toxic Aβ (40–1) did not [110,111]. It was concluded that toxic Aβ peptides mediated copper-oxidation of ascorbate with the generation of hydroxyl radicals, indicating a role for cupric-amyloid peptide's free radical generation in the pathogenesis of AD. In line with these last findings, Aβ was not found to silence the redox activity of $Cu^{2+/+}$ via chelation, but rather hydroxyl radicals were produced as a result of Fenton-Haber Weiss reactions of ascorbate and Cu^{2+}, rapidly quenching harmful radicals [112]. Moreover, reaction rates and mechanisms of AA oxidation resulted in greater biological relevance in the presence of Cu(II)-containing Aβ oligomers and fibrils, given the close proximity of ROS to cell membranes [104]. Further evidence indicated a pro-oxidative role for AA in the interaction of the redox-active copper ions with misfolded amyloid β and AD pathogenesis, with particular relevance to catalytic sites for Cu^+ present in full-length Aβ instead of in any particular Aβ conformation [82].

However, to complicate the issue, AA was observed to reduce in vivo oxidative damage in the presence of iron, despite its well-known in vitro pro-oxidant properties in buffer systems containing iron [83]. In addition, a recent report evaluated the in vitro effects of different food constituents on brain metal chelation, oxidative stress, and fibrillogenesis [89]. The results did not support the currently hypothesized AA neuroprotective mechanisms of action. Indeed, AA was found to be a good antioxidant with poor metal chelating activity. Strikingly, the study did not show any AA-mediated inhibiting effect on Aβ fibrillogenesis, compared to the multifunctional food abilities of epigallocatechin gallate (EGCG), gallic acid, and curcumin. Hence, due to good AA brain uptake, further investigation is needed to address the role of ascorbic acid in counteracting oxidative stress in an AD brain.

6.3. Ascorbic Acid and Neuroinflammation in Alzheimer's Disease

A previous study demonstrated that chronic administration of AA in the brain chronically infused with lipopolysaccharide and tiorphan was associated with increased deposition of Aβ amyloid plaques and increased Aβ neuronal immunoreactivity [92]. However, a body of evidence implicated AA in the suppression of glia-mediated inflammation. In particular, a colchicine-induced oxidative stress/neuroinflammation AD rat model [84] showed that administration of AA was effective in preventive memory impairment, and reducing inflammatory markers (TNF alpha, IL 1 beta), ROS, and nitrite levels in the hippocampus of AD rats. AA also significantly reduced amyloid plaque formation. Peripheral immune response (increased phagocytic activity of blood WBC and splenic PMN) was also recovered after AA administration and the observed changes were associated with the higher efflux of inflammatory mediators from the brain to peripheral circulation. The same results also addressed a pro-oxidant role of AA at higher doses (600 mg diet), supporting the dual role of AA in addressing the oxidative stress. In addition, a rat model of ethanol-induced oxidative stress showed that AA was effective in counteracting ethanol-induced oxidative stress, neuroinflammation, and apoptotic neuronal loss with beneficial effects against ethanol damage to brain development [87]. Even if the model is not a true AD model, the current findings add knowledge to the role of AA against oxidative stress and neuroinflammation in the brain. In particular, due to its free radical scavenging properties, AA treatment reduced the production of ROS and suppressed both activated microglia and astrocytes. AA also demonstrated mitigation of apoptosis and neurotoxicity by decreasing levels of the Bax/Bcl-2 ratio, cytochrome C, and different caspases, such as caspase-9 and caspase-3. Moreover, AA treatment reduced ethanol-induced activation of poly [ADP-ribose] polymerase 1 (PARP-1) and neurodegeneration. In line with these data, AA was also observed to suppress the lipopolysaccharide (LPS)-stimulated production of inflammatory mediators in neuron/glia co-cultures by inhibiting the MAPK and NF-κB signaling pathways [113].

6.4. Ascorbic Acid and Amyloid Plaque Accumulation in Alzheimer's Disease

Accumulating evidence indicates a role for AA on the toxic fibrillogenesis of Aβ. High doses of AA supplementation reduced the amyloid plaque burden in a 5 familial Alzheimer's disease mutation (5XFAD) AD mouse model. To better identify the pathogenetic importance of AA in an AD mouse model, the cross-breeding of 5XFAD mice with gulono-gamma-lactone oxidase (Gulo) knockout mice was performed (KO-Tg mice). The higher supplementation of AA in KO-Tg mice resulted in the amelioration of BBB disruption and mitochondrial alteration, with substantial reduction of amyloid plaque burden [114].

The APPSWE/PSEN1deltaE9 mouse model of AD, created by crossing APP/PSEN1(+) bigenic mice with SVCT2(+/−) heterozygous knockout mice, also showed interesting results [81]. By 14 months of age, increased oxidative stress was observed (malondialdehyde, protein carbonyls, F2-isoprostanes) with decreased total glutathione, compared to wild-type controls. In addition, increased amounts of both soluble and insoluble Aβ1-42, and a higher Aβ1-42/1-40 ratio with increased hippocampal and cortical amyloid-β plaque deposits were observed, compared to APP/PSEN1(+) mice with normal AA brains. These data suggested that AA deficiency plays an important role in accelerating amyloid accumulation, particularly during early stages of disease, and that these effects are likely modulated by oxidative stress pathways. Huang et al. showed that pre-loading cells with ascorbate substantially prevented apoptosis and death of SH-SY5Y cells, while also decreasing basal rates of endogenous beta-amyloid generation [86]. Cheng et al. demonstrated, in an in vitro model, that an inadequate supply of AA could contribute to the increased formation of toxic Aβ oligomers. In the absence of AA, the temporary interaction between the Aβ domain and small NO-catalyzed release of anhydromannose (anMan)-containing oligosaccharides is prevented, with the increased induction of neurotoxic fibrillogenesis [103]. Murakami et al. [91], in APP transgenic mice, showed that AA administration attenuated oligomerization, but not the total amyloid plaque volume. The authors concluded that the ability of mice to retain de novo synthesis of AA is possible, and a longer study duration is needed to appreciate the significant changes in amyloid plaque accumulation. These last findings are original and indicate the need to test the "sink hypothesis" through the systematic assessment of cerebrospinal fluid AA levels in order to support the role of AA in promoting healthy brain aging. Indeed, it is hypothesized that there is some form of equilibrium for the Aβ in the brain and the periphery such that Aβ can be transported across the blood-brain barrier. By modulating the peripheral Aβ levels, it is predicted that the brain Aβ levels will undergo concomitant changes, forming the basis of the "sink hypothesis" for Aβ lowering strategies.

6.5. Acid Ascorbic and Vascular Disease Associated with Alzheimer's Disease

Recently, a pathophysiological role of the vascular component in the pathogenesis of AD has been demonstrated [115]. Again, oxidative stress is considered a key relevant mediator, confirming the pathogenetic link between AD and vascular disease [116]. Oxidative stress may affect the neurovascular unit, by impairing the endothelial integrity with increased Aβ42 production. This series of pathological events resulted in automatically maintaining the cycle between ROS overproduction and new extracellular Aβ42 deposition. It was ascertained that AA mediates a series of protective effects on brain neurodegeneration by reducing intima-media thickness, lipid peroxidation, and endothelial dysfunction [90,116–119]. In keeping with this, it has been recently documented that the integrity of the endothelial lining in the blood-brain barrier is essential to prevent the onset of AD [120–122]. Each of these vascular risk factors may represent a biological target for AA and contribute to the preventative role of AA in the development of AD pathogenesis, associated with the vascular component.

Growing evidence indicates a role for AA in reducing cardiovascular related mortality and overall mortality, according to higher quartile plasma AA concentrations in humans [123]. Interestingly, it should be noted that the higher risk of carotid intima thickness >1.2 mm was exclusively associated with the lowest plasma AA tertile. This same increased risk was not observed with uric acid, vitamin A, or enzymatic antioxidant load (superoxide dismutase and glutathione oxidase activity). Similarly, dietetic interventions in elderly subjects showed that carotid intima thickness progression was reduced only in those subjects taking AA daily.

The risk of either AD or vascular dementia is higher in patients with elevated blood pressure, which suggests how arterial stiffness and atherosclerosis play important pathogenetic roles [123]. Endothelial dysfunction is associated with arterial stiffness which, in turn, is a strong predictor for cognitive decline [124]. All of these data support the role for AA in modifying vascular risk factors associated with Alzheimer's-type dementia.

Endothelial dysfunction is a crucial factor associated with AD pathogenesis. Aβ aggregates are cleared from the brain across the BBB, as the transport is finely regulated by RAGE receptors and LDL receptor-related protein (LRP-1). In patients with AD, brain endothelial LRP-1 expression throughout the BBB is reduced [125]. These data suggested an essential role of the endothelial cell integrity lining in the onset and progression of AD. The efficacy of AA against BBB breakdown due to cortical compression was reported [90]. A model of ischemic-reperfusion [126] and BBB breakdown with reduced NO bioavailability may be considered a prototypical model to understand the pleiotropic roles of AA on endothelial function. AA regulates endothelial integrity via oxidative pathways; superoxide generated by endothelial cells reacts with NO to form cytotoxic peroxynitrites and AA could decrease NO consumption by scavenging superoxide. In addition, AA was found to play a role in the function of endothelial nitric oxide synthase (eNOS) by recycling the eNOS co-factor, tetrahydrobiopterin, which is relevant for arterial elasticity and blood pressure regulation [18]. AA also favored the restoration of NO metabolism from *S*-nitrosothiols in plasma [127], reducing nitrite (NO2) to NO, which may preserve NO in tissues or plasma. AA was reported to reverse the generation and metabolism of NO [94], and to prevent endothelial dysfunction by inhibiting LDL oxidation. An oxidized endothelium is known to increase BBB permeability [117] and the AA-associated protective mechanism on lipid metabolism was found to improve BBB endothelial disruption. In addition, AA prevented the impaired response to the vasodilator acetylcholine (endothelium-dependent agonist) and reduced ROS (e.g., superoxide) produced by neutrophils [93]. Thus, a series of studies have suggested that AA may protect from AD onset, by protecting BBB integrity.

So far, scant investigations have explored the effects of anti-oxidative vitamins on dementia through the cerebrovascular axis [95]. The study of Kook et al. [87] recently reported that high-dose supplementation of AA reduced amyloidosis in AD mice (5XFAD) via the reduction of BBB disruption and mitochondrial alteration [96]. Additionally, AA was also reported to prevent the disruption of BBB by upregulating the expression of tight junction proteins, occludin and claudin-5.

In a model of stroke with substantial BBB disruption, AA significantly reduced BBB permeability [128]. Similarly, in a mouse model of cerebral ischemia, AA ameliorated BBB dysfunction by reversing tight junction claudin-5 and attenuated edema and neuronal loss [129]. Moreover, an in vitro study provided evidence that AA reversed hyperglycemia-mediated BBB disruption [130]. To date, AA seems to offer neuroprotection by restoring BBB integrity. However, further investigations should focus on simultaneously testing brain neuroprotective effects and BBB protective effects of antioxidants [95]. AA seems to possess both types of neuroprotection and could be further tested as a targeted dual agent for preventing cognitive decline.

Several cross-sectional studies have demonstrated a lower CSF-to-plasma AA ratio in AD patients compared to controls. In particular, recent findings [95] suggest that maintenance of a high CSF-to-plasma AA ratio is important in preventing cognitive decline in AD and that BBB impairment unfavorably affects this ratio. However, whether the AA transport carrier dysfunction (SVCT2) or the disturbed BBB integrity is responsible for it, is still a matter of debate.

Indeed, the loss of BBB integrity seen in elderly people with dementia may hamper the brain's ability to retain CNS AA regardless of the successful transport [131–133]. Genetic variations of the SVCT2 carrier at the choroid plexus and in neurons may also play a significant role. In line with these data, a recent review has concluded that CSF levels within the normal range for AA indicate the preservation of choroid plexus function and AA transport into the CSF [134], despite lower plasma levels.

7. From Bench to Bedside

Ascorbic acid levels in plasma are decreased in AD patients [135] and the association between cognitive impairment and low antioxidant status is accumulating. Indeed, it has been suggested that increased dietary intake may reduce the risk of developing AD. So far, whether oxidative stress associated with the disease is responsible for the reduction of antioxidants, or whether the low antioxidants contribute to the progression of the disease has not been ascertained.

However, plasma levels of AA were found to be lower both in patients with mild cognitive impairment and AD, compared to controls [136].

A further difference existed between undernourished patients with dementia and patients taking any antioxidant supplement.

From bench to bedside, eight large population studies [57] have investigated the association between AA intake and Alzheimer's-type dementia in both European countries and the US. However, the neuroprotection associated with AA has not yet been established. According to the CHAP study [137], none of the elderly dementia-free participants longitudinally developed dementia, due to AA supplementation. In contrast, a synergistic association between AA and vitamin E supplementation was shown in reducing the risk of AD [138]. Another large population study has shown a protective role for AA in vascular dementia and cognitively-intact subjects, but no protective role of AA was shown for Alzheimer's disease [139].

The Rotterdam study showed the most consistent association between higher AA intake and reduced relative risk for AD in the largest population study [140] with the higher magnitude of association in people most depleted of AA (e.g., smokers). The same study found an association for lower levels of vitamin E in AD patients at follow up an average of 9.6 years later, but not for AA intake.

Additionally, eleven studies have examined the relationship between plasma AA and cognitive decline, including AD, and four of them examined CSF AA and CSF-to-plasma AA ratios. An early study of Goodwin [29] assigned patients to AA plasmatic deficiency according to tertiles. The main findings suggested a significant association between AA deficiency below 20 μM, mild cognitive impairment, and AD patients compared to healthy controls, even after correction for co- morbidities, age, and fruit/vegetables intake.

The study of Quinn [141] showed that the mean CSF-to-plasma AA ratio was significantly lower in AD compared with controls. A further prospective analysis of CSF AA, rates of cognitive decline, and BBB did not draw final conclusions, but a higher CSF-to-plasma AA ratio was associated with a slower rate of decline [57].

Conversely, several clinical studies did not show any beneficial effect of AA on cognition in patients with AD. In a population study of North Carolina, 616 elders aged over 75 years and long-term supplement users of AA did not show any neuroprotection against developing AD [142]. However, no record was made of dietary intake, and the results outlined that less healthy behaviors and socioeconomic status were associated with the poorer cognitive outcomes. Vitamin E levels were significantly lower in the AD group than controls while AA levels did not differ significantly between groups.

A series of limitations may count for interpreting the clinical results. There is substantial inconsistency among the observational studies on AA intake, plasma levels, beneficial effects on aging and cognition.

It is noteworthy that a great deal of clinical studies usually excluded elderly people if they had polypharmacy or comorbidity. These exclusion criteria critically undermine the validity of results, leaving out the populations most at risk for AA deficiency.

Approximately 17% of the elderly population did not meet the RDA for AA intake, which critically suggests that large elderly population groups show depleted levels of AA; this determinant may count for the disparate conclusions of different clinical studies. In particular, as accurately summarized by Harrison F et al. [143], the classification of groups according to AA status differs greatly among studies. The deficiency levels of AA are lower than 11 μmol/L, with suboptimal concentrations between 11–38 μmol/L, adequate plasmatic concentrations of AA above 28 μmol/L and optimal concentrations between 50–60 μmol/L (μmol/L: conversion factor 56.78 from mg/dL concentrations of AA).

Moreover, the range of AA supplements greatly vary from 27 to 230–270 mg/day, introducing another element of variability.

Not least, the higher intakes of AA were associated with beneficial effects on cognition if not exceeding 500 mg/day; higher plasmatic values (1 g/day) of AA were associated with poorer cognitive performance.

The beneficial effects of AA need reliable plasmatic determinations with repeated points of measurement. The lack of accuracy in study designs and methodologies may also affect the reliability of the findings [57]. In addition, the lack of standardization between single nutrient consumption or multivitamins and the lack of systematic detection of plasmatic levels of AA also affect the accuracy of outcomes.

Moreover, the missing consideration of specific AA metabolism, the inaccurate daily estimate of AA consumption, and the erroneous intestine-to-bloodstream absorption due to saturable AA transporters being critical determinants for drawing appropriate conclusions [57]. The variability of the results may also be ascribed to difference of plasma AA concentrations according to polymorphisms of SVCT2 and SVCT1 despite equivalent AA intake. This difference indicates that SVCT1/2 genotype may play an important role in the association between AA intake and circulating AA levels. Furthermore, the difference between food intake and synthetic supplements and the mean of their bioavailability need to be clearly defined.

It should also be noted that the current intake of AA may not accurately reflect the subjects' lifetime habits; this, in turn, may substantially affect the biological trajectory of Alzheimer's disease with particular regard to early mid-life deposition of amyloid plaque. Thus, the stratification of different aging populations according to their clinical vulnerability, cognitive reserve, comorbidity and specific risk profile could add knowledge to this field [95]. Similarly, a greater understanding of the modulation between pro-oxidative AA status and antioxidative capacity during aging and age-related specific conditions, including dementia, is warranted.

Currently, the clinical data yield inconsistent results. AA supplementation showed beneficial effects when restoring a nutritional deficit or preventing vitamin deficiency; thus, it seems more plausible that avoiding AA deficiency is likely to be more beneficial than taking supplements on top of a normal healthy diet.

So far, the levels of AA needed to beneficially modify brain aging are largely unknown. A causal association between AA deficiency and cognitive decline, including dementia, is still debated and two main issues are unanswered. Namely, the co-causal role of AA deficiency versus its epiphenomenal role in AD neurodegeneration has not yet been established. However, AA's strong free radical scavenging properties, the well-characterized kinetics of transport, and the good bioavailability in the CNS provide a favorable background for further exploring its role in promoting brain function and healthy aging.

With testing by neuroimaging, recent research has demonstrated that it is possible to detect brain levels of AA by using a MEGA-PRESS mediated spectra (MEGA-PRESS, MEGA-point-resolved spectroscopy) [144]. The study indicated a relationship between brain and blood AA levels and provides a new conceptual framework for future studies, further exploring the role of AA in the brain.

8. Conclusions

In conclusion, randomized clinical trials have failed to demonstrate any association between AA-mediated antioxidant therapeutic activity and a delay in AD neurodegeneration.

However, the assessment of the "sink hypothesis" could substantiate a crucial role for AA in promoting healthy aging of the brain. The analysis of AA concentration in plasma, CSF, and the ratio of AA/glutamate, along with the role of AA-related carriers (SVCT2 SNPs) and barriers to its brain transport (BBB) could significantly spur this research field by directly analyzing the AA concentrations in the brain.

Neuroimaging measures also hold promise in offering deeper insights on the structural, metabolic, and connective role that AA plays in the brain [144], contributing to the larger picture.

Additionally, animal models need to be further investigated with a particular focus on gulonolactone oxidase knockout models that mimic human physiology, and may help identify novel AA mechanisms of action to promote healthy aging of the brain.

Another intriguing area of research could address the protective association between AA and glutamate transport/NMDA receptors to critically evaluate the AA role in neurodegeneration.

Finally, the field of epigenetics has recently answered the question as to why AA is disproportionally concentrated in CSF and brain parenchyma compared to plasma [28]. Nutrition represents one of the most powerful environmental modifications of the genome. Recent research has assessed a peculiar epigenetic role for AA. Namely, the oxidation of 5-mc (5-methylcytosine) to 5-hmc (5-hydroxymethylcytosine), as part of dynamic DNA demethylation, is catalyzed by TET (ten-eleven translocation) dioxygenase enzymes, for which AA is a critical co-factor [23,145]. Interestingly, no other antioxidant displayed such an epigenetic mechanism. Thus, AA can be considered vital for neuronal repair and offers new molecular mechanisms to understand the true neuroprotective role of AA in brain aging and neurodegeneration.

In addition, it has been recently documented that 75% of ascorbic acid degradation is due to Maillard degradation pathways (amide-AGEs) [146]. Knowledge of the mechanisms of Maillard model systems could help understand the changes occurring during storage and processing of AA-containing food, as well as in vivo modifications.

Thus, all of these lines of research could improve the understanding of the role of AA in brain aging and, hopefully, provide a new conceptual framework for AD in the near future.

Author Contributions: C.G., R.B. and E.A. revised the literature and significantly contributed to data acquisition; F.M. revised the literature, made the conception and design of the manuscript and drafted the manuscript; A.N. revised the manuscript critically and contributed to the manuscript drafting. All authors gave final approval of the version to be submitted and of any revised version.

Conflicts of Interest: The authors declare no conflict of interest.

References

1. Bloom, D.E. 7 billion and counting. *Science* **2011**, *333*, 562–569. [CrossRef] [PubMed]
2. Cannizzo, E.S.; Clement, C.C.; Sahu, R.; Follo, C.; Santambrogio, L. Oxidative stress, inflamm-aging and immunosenescence. *J. Proteom.* **2011**, *74*, 2313–2323. [CrossRef] [PubMed]
3. Franceschi, C.; Campisi, J. Chronic inflammation (inflammaging) and its potential contribution to age-associated diseases. *J. Gerontol. Ser. A Biol. Sci. Med. Sci.* **2014**, *69* (Suppl. 1), S4–S9. [CrossRef] [PubMed]
4. Vasto, S.; Candore, G.; Balistreri, C.R.; Caruso, M.; Colonna-Romano, G.; Grimaldi, M.P.; Listi, F.; Nuzzo, D.; Lio, D.; Caruso, C. Inflammatory networks in ageing, age-related diseases and longevity. *Mech. Ageing Dev.* **2007**, *128*, 83–91. [CrossRef] [PubMed]
5. Cevenini, E.; Monti, D.; Franceschi, C. Inflamm-ageing. *Curr. Opin. Clin. Nutr. Metab. Care* **2013**, *16*, 14–20. [CrossRef] [PubMed]
6. Michaud, M.; Balardy, L.; Moulis, G.; Gaudin, C.; Peyrot, C.; Vellas, B.; Cesari, M.; Nourhashemi, F. Proinflammatory cytokines, aging, and age-related diseases. *J. Am. Med. Dir. Assoc.* **2013**, *14*, 877–882. [CrossRef] [PubMed]
7. Franceschi, C.; Bonafe, M.; Valensin, S.; Olivieri, F.; De Luca, M.; Ottaviani, E.; De Benedictis, G. Inflamm-aging. An evolutionary perspective on immunosenescence. *Ann. N. Y. Acad. Sci.* **2000**, *908*, 244–254. [CrossRef] [PubMed]
8. Szarc vel Szic, K.; Declerck, K.; Vidakovic, M.; Vanden Berghe, W. From inflammaging to healthy aging by dietary lifestyle choices: Is epigenetics the key to personalized nutrition? *Clin. Epigenetics* **2015**, *7*, 33. [CrossRef] [PubMed]
9. Santoro, A.; Pini, E.; Scurti, M.; Palmas, G.; Berendsen, A.; Brzozowska, A.; Pietruszka, B.; Szczecinska, A.; Cano, N.; Meunier, N.; et al. Combating inflammaging through a Mediterranean whole diet approach: The nu-age project's conceptual framework and design. *Mech. Ageing Dev.* **2014**, *136*, 3–13. [CrossRef] [PubMed]

10. Berendsen, A.; Santoro, A.; Pini, E.; Cevenini, E.; Ostan, R.; Pietruszka, B.; Rolf, K.; Cano, N.; Caille, A.; Lyon-Belgy, N.; et al. Reprint of: A parallel randomized trial on the effect of a healthful diet on inflammageing and its consequences in European elderly people: Design of the nu-age dietary intervention study. *Mech. Ageing Dev.* **2014**, *136*, 14–21. [CrossRef] [PubMed]

11. Neufcourt, L.; Assmann, K.E.; Fezeu, L.K.; Touvier, M.; Graffouillere, L.; Shivappa, N.; Hebert, J.R.; Wirth, M.D.; Hercberg, S.; Galan, P.; et al. Prospective association between the dietary inflammatory index and metabolic syndrome: Findings from the su.Vi.Max study. *Nutr. Metab. Cardiovasc. Dis. NMCD* **2015**, *25*, 988–996. [CrossRef] [PubMed]

12. Padayatty, S.J.; Katz, A.; Wang, Y.; Eck, P.; Kwon, O.; Lee, J.H.; Chen, S.; Corpe, C.; Dutta, A.; Dutta, S.K.; et al. Vitamin C as an antioxidant: Evaluation of its role in disease prevention. *J. Am. Coll. Nutr.* **2003**, *22*, 18–35. [CrossRef] [PubMed]

13. Naidu, K.A. Vitamin C in human health and disease is still a mystery? An overview. *Nutr. J.* **2003**, *2*, 7. [CrossRef] [PubMed]

14. Michels, A.J.; Joisher, N.; Hagen, T.M. Age-related decline of sodium-dependent ascorbic acid transport in isolated rat hepatocytes. *Arch. Biochem. Biophys.* **2003**, *410*, 112–120. [CrossRef]

15. Grosso, G.; Bei, R.; Mistretta, A.; Marventano, S.; Calabrese, G.; Masuelli, L.; Giganti, M.G.; Modesti, A.; Galvano, F.; Gazzolo, D. Effects of vitamin c on health: A review of evidence. *Front. Biosci.* **2013**, *18*, 1017–1029.

16. Duarte, T.L.; Lunec, J. Review: When is an antioxidant not an antioxidant? A review of novel actions and reactions of vitamin C. *Free Radic. Res.* **2005**, *39*, 671–686. [CrossRef] [PubMed]

17. Regine, H.; Gabriele, W.-F.; Ernst, R.W. Antioxidants and endothelial nitric oxide synthesis. *Eur. J. Clin. Pharmacol.* **2006**, *62* (Suppl. 1), 21–28.

18. Heller, R.; Unbehaun, A.; Schellenberg, B.; Mayer, B.; Werner-Felmayer, G.; Werner, E.R. L-ascorbic acid potentiates endothelial nitric oxide synthesis via a chemical stabilization of tetrahydrobiopterin. *J. Biol. Chem.* **2001**, *276*, 40–47. [CrossRef] [PubMed]

19. Ladurner, A.; Schmitt, C.A.; Schachner, D.; Atanasov, A.G.; Werner, E.R.; Dirsch, V.M.; Heiss, E.H. Ascorbate stimulates endothelial nitric oxide synthase enzyme activity by rapid modulation of its phosphorylation status. *Free Radic. Biol. Med.* **2012**, *52*, 2082–2090. [CrossRef] [PubMed]

20. Halliwell, B. Vitamin C and genomic stability. *Mutat. Res.* **2001**, *475*, 29–35. [CrossRef]

21. Camarena, V.; Wang, G. The epigenetic role of vitamin C in health and disease. *Cell. Mol. Life Sci. CMLS* **2016**, *73*, 1645–1658. [CrossRef] [PubMed]

22. Young, J.I.; Zuchner, S.; Wang, G. Regulation of the epigenome by vitamin C. *Annu. Rev. Nutr.* **2015**, *35*, 545–564. [CrossRef] [PubMed]

23. Yin, R.; Mao, S.Q.; Zhao, B.; Chong, Z.; Yang, Y.; Zhao, C.; Zhang, D.; Huang, H.; Gao, J.; Li, Z.; et al. Ascorbic acid enhances Tet-mediated 5-methylcytosine oxidation and promotes DNA demethylation in mammals. *J. Am. Chem. Soc.* **2013**, *135*, 10396–10403. [CrossRef] [PubMed]

24. Cahill, L.E.; El-Sohemy, A. Vitamin c transporter gene polymorphisms, dietary vitamin C and serum ascorbic acid. *J. Nutr. Nutr.* **2009**, *2*, 292–301. [CrossRef] [PubMed]

25. Langlois, M.R.; Martin, M.E.; Boelaert, J.R.; Beaumont, C.; Taes, Y.E.; De Buyzere, M.L.; Bernard, D.R.; Neels, H.M.; Delanghe, J.R. The haptoglobin 2-2 phenotype affects serum markers of iron status in healthy males. *Clin. Chem.* **2000**, *46*, 1619–1625. [PubMed]

26. Horska, A.; Mislanova, C.; Bonassi, S.; Ceppi, M.; Volkovova, K.; Dusinska, M. Vitamin C levels in blood are influenced by polymorphisms in glutathione *S*-transferases. *Eur. J. Nutr.* **2011**, *50*, 437–446. [CrossRef] [PubMed]

27. Schwartz, B. New criteria for supplementation of selected micronutrients in the era of nutrigenetics and nutrigenomics. *Int. J. Food Sci. Nutr.* **2014**, *65*, 529–538. [CrossRef] [PubMed]

28. Blaschke, K.; Ebata, K.T.; Karimi, M.M.; Zepeda-Martinez, J.A.; Goyal, P.; Mahapatra, S.; Tam, A.; Laird, D.J.; Hirst, M.; Rao, A.; et al. Vitamin C induces Tet-dependent DNA demethylation and a blastocyst-like state in ES cells. *Nature* **2013**, *500*, 222–226. [CrossRef] [PubMed]

29. Goodwin, J.S.; Goodwin, J.M.; Garry, P.J. Association between nutritional status and cognitive functioning in a healthy elderly population. *JAMA* **1983**, *249*, 2917–2921. [CrossRef] [PubMed]

30. Lebel, M.; Massip, L.; Garand, C.; Thorin, E. Ascorbate improves metabolic abnormalities in *Wrn* mutant mice but not the free radical scavenger catechin. *Ann. N. Y. Acad. Sci.* **2010**, *1197*, 40–44. [CrossRef] [PubMed]

31. Aumailley, L.; Warren, A.; Garand, C.; Dubois, M.J.; Paquet, E.R.; Le Couteur, D.G.; Marette, A.; Cogger, V.C.; Lebel, M. Vitamin C modulates the metabolic and cytokine profiles, alleviates hepatic endoplasmic reticulum stress, and increases the life span of gulo−/− mice. *Aging* **2016**, *8*, 458–483. [CrossRef] [PubMed]

32. Dallaire, A.; Proulx, S.; Simard, M.J.; Lebel, M. Expression profile of *Caenorhabditis elegans* mutant for the Werner syndrome gene ortholog reveals the impact of vitamin C on development to increase life span. *BMC Genom.* **2014**, *15*, 940. [CrossRef] [PubMed]

33. Li, Y.; Zhang, W.; Chang, L.; Han, Y.; Sun, L.; Gong, X.; Tang, H.; Liu, Z.; Deng, H.; Ye, Y.; et al. Vitamin C alleviates aging defects in a stem cell model for Werner syndrome. *Protein Cell* **2016**, *7*, 478–488. [CrossRef] [PubMed]

34. Massip, L.; Garand, C.; Paquet, E.R.; Cogger, V.C.; O'Reilly, J.N.; Tworek, L.; Hatherell, A.; Taylor, C.G.; Thorin, E.; Zahradka, P.; et al. Vitamin C restores healthy aging in a mouse model for Werner syndrome. *FASEB J.* **2010**, *24*, 158–172. [CrossRef] [PubMed]

35. Pangrazzi, L.; Meryk, A.; Naismith, E.; Koziel, R.; Lair, J.; Krismer, M.; Trieb, K.; Grubeck-Loebenstein, B. "Inflamm-aging" influences immune cell survival factors in human bone marrow. *Eur. J. Immunol.* **2016**, *47*. [CrossRef] [PubMed]

36. Rahman, F.; Al Frouh, F.; Bordignon, B.; Fraterno, M.; Landrier, J.F.; Peiretti, F.; Fontes, M. Ascorbic acid is a dose-dependent inhibitor of adipocyte differentiation, probably by reducing camp pool. *Front. Cell Dev. Biol.* **2014**, *2*, 29. [CrossRef] [PubMed]

37. Rahman, F.; Bordignon, B.; Culerrier, R.; Peiretti, F.; Spicuglia, S.; Djabali, M.; Landrier, J.F.; Fontes, M. Ascorbic acid drives the differentiation of mesoderm-derived embryonic stem cells. Involvement of p38 MAPK/CREB and SVCT2 transporter. *Mol. Nutr. Food Res.* **2016**, *61*. [CrossRef] [PubMed]

38. Jeong, S.G.; Cho, G.W. Endogenous ROS levels are increased in replicative senescence in human bone marrow mesenchymal stromal cells. *Biochem. Biophys. Res. Commun.* **2015**, *460*, 971–976. [CrossRef] [PubMed]

39. Aumailley, L.; Dubois, M.J.; Garand, C.; Marette, A.; Lebel, M. Impact of vitamin C on the cardiometabolic and inflammatory profiles of mice lacking a functional Werner syndrome protein helicase. *Exp. Gerontol.* **2015**, *72*, 192–203. [CrossRef] [PubMed]

40. Uchio, R.; Hirose, Y.; Murosaki, S.; Yamamoto, Y.; Ishigami, A. High dietary intake of vitamin c suppresses age-related thymic atrophy and contributes to the maintenance of immune cells in vitamin C-deficient senescence marker protein-30 knockout mice. *Br. J. Nutr.* **2015**, *113*, 603–609. [CrossRef] [PubMed]

41. Sato, Y.; Amano, A.; Kishimoto, Y.; Takahashi, K.; Handa, S.; Maruyama, N.; Ishigami, A. Ascorbic acid prevents protein oxidation in livers of senescence marker protein-30/gluconolactonase knockout mice. *Geriatr. Gerontol. Int.* **2014**, *14*, 989–995. [CrossRef] [PubMed]

42. Kim, S.M.; Lim, S.M.; Yoo, J.A.; Woo, M.J.; Cho, K.H. Consumption of high-dose vitamin C (1250 mg per day) enhances functional and structural properties of serum lipoprotein to improve anti-oxidant, anti-atherosclerotic, and anti-aging effects via regulation of anti-inflammatory microrna. *Food Funct.* **2015**, *6*, 3604–3612. [CrossRef] [PubMed]

43. Harrison, F.E.; May, J.M. Vitamin c function in the brain: Vital role of the ascorbate transporter SVCT2. *Free Radic. Biol. Med.* **2009**, *46*, 719–730. [CrossRef] [PubMed]

44. Zheng, C.; Sui, B.; Hu, C.; Jin, Y. Vitamin c promotes in vitro proliferation of bone marrow mesenchymal stem cells derived from aging mice. *J. Sourn Med. Univ.* **2015**, *35*, 1689–1693.

45. Chen, B.Y.; Wang, X.; Chen, L.W.; Luo, Z.J. Molecular targeting regulation of proliferation and differentiation of the bone marrow-derived mesenchymal stem cells or mesenchymal stromal cells. *Curr. Drug Targets* **2012**, *13*, 561–571. [CrossRef] [PubMed]

46. Yang, W.; Hekimi, S. A mitochondrial superoxide signal triggers increased longevity in *Caenorhabditis elegans*. *PLoS Biol.* **2010**, *8*, e1000556. [CrossRef] [PubMed]

47. Van Raamsdonk, J.M.; Hekimi, S. Superoxide dismutase is dispensable for normal animal lifespan. *Proc. Natl. Acad. Sci. USA* **2012**, *109*, 5785–5790. [CrossRef] [PubMed]

48. Desjardins, D.; Cacho-Valadez, B.; Liu, J.L.; Wang, Y.; Yee, C.; Bernard, K.; Khaki, A.; Breton, L.; Hekimi, S. Antioxidants reveal an inverted U-shaped dose-response relationship between reactive oxygen species levels and the rate of aging in *Caenorhabditis elegans*. *Aging Cell* **2017**, *16*, 104–112. [CrossRef] [PubMed]

49. Riscuta, G. Nutrigenomics at the interface of aging, lifespan, and cancer prevention. *J. Nutr.* **2016**, *146*, 1931–1939. [CrossRef] [PubMed]

50. Soysal, P.; Isik, A.T.; Carvalho, A.F.; Fernandes, B.S.; Solmi, M.; Schofield, P.; Veronese, N.; Stubbs, B. Oxidative stress and frailty: A systematic review and synthesis of the best evidence. *Maturitas* **2017**, *99*, 66–72. [CrossRef] [PubMed]

51. Leelarungrayub, J.; Laskin, J.J.; Bloomer, R.J.; Pinkaew, D. Consumption of star fruit juice on pro-inflammatory markers and walking distance in the community dwelling elderly. *Arch. Gerontol. Geriatr.* **2016**, *64*, 6–12. [CrossRef] [PubMed]

52. Leelarungrayub, J.; Yankai, A.; Pinkaew, D.; Puntumetakul, R.; Laskin, J.J.; Bloomer, R.J. A preliminary study on the effects of star fruit consumption on antioxidant and lipid status in elderly Thai individuals. *Clin. Interv. Aging* **2016**, *11*, 1183–1192. [CrossRef] [PubMed]

53. Nualart, F.; Mack, L.; Garcia, A.; Cisternas, P.; Bongarzone, E.R.; Heitzer, M.; Jara, N.; Martinez, F.; Ferrada, L.; Espinoza, F.; et al. Vitamin C transporters, recycling and the bystander effect in the nervous system: SVCT2 versus gluts. *J. Stem Cell Res. Ther.* **2014**, *4*, 209. [CrossRef] [PubMed]

54. Rice, M.E. Ascorbate regulation and its neuroprotective role in the brain. *Trends Neurosci.* **2000**, *23*, 209–216. [CrossRef]

55. Lee, J.Y.; Chang, M.Y.; Park, C.H.; Kim, H.Y.; Kim, J.H.; Son, H.; Lee, Y.S.; Lee, S.H. Ascorbate-induced differentiation of embryonic cortical precursors into neurons and astrocytes. *J. Neurosci. Res.* **2003**, *73*, 156–165. [CrossRef] [PubMed]

56. Qiu, S.; Li, L.; Weeber, E.J.; May, J.M. Ascorbate transport by primary cultured neurons and its role in neuronal function and protection against excitotoxicity. *J. Neurosci. Res.* **2007**, *85*, 1046–1056. [CrossRef] [PubMed]

57. Harrison, F.E.; Bowman, G.L.; Polidori, M.C. Ascorbic acid and the brain: Rationale for the use against cognitive decline. *Nutrients* **2014**, *6*, 1752–1781. [CrossRef] [PubMed]

58. Covarrubias-Pinto, A.; Acuna, A.I.; Beltran, F.A.; Torres-Diaz, L.; Castro, M.A. Old things new view: Ascorbic acid protects the brain in neurodegenerative disorders. *Int. J. Mol. Sci.* **2015**, *16*, 28194–28217. [CrossRef] [PubMed]

59. Feng, Y.; Wang, X. Antioxidant therapies for Alzheimer's disease. *Oxid. Med. Cell. Longev.* **2012**, *2012*, 472932. [CrossRef] [PubMed]

60. Ientile, L.; De Pasquale, R.; Monacelli, F.; Odetti, P.; Traverso, N.; Cammarata, S.; Tabaton, M.; Dijk, B. Survival rate in patients affected by dementia followed by memory clinics (UVA) in Italy. *J. Alzheimers Dis.* **2013**, *36*, 303–309. [PubMed]

61. Yao, Y.; Chinnici, C.; Tang, H.; Trojanowski, J.Q.; Lee, V.M.; Pratico, D. Brain inflammation and oxidative stress in a transgenic mouse model of Alzheimer-like brain amyloidosis. *J. Neuroinflamm.* **2004**, *1*, 21. [CrossRef] [PubMed]

62. Choudhry, F.; Howlett, D.R.; Richardson, J.C.; Francis, P.T.; Williams, R.J. Pro-oxidant diet enhances beta/gamma secretase-mediated APP processing in APP/PS1 transgenic mice. *Neurobiol. Aging* **2012**, *33*, 960–968. [CrossRef] [PubMed]

63. McGeer, P.L.; McGeer, E.G. The amyloid cascade-inflammatory hypothesis of Alzheimer disease: Implications for therapy. *Acta Neuropathol.* **2013**, *126*, 479–497. [CrossRef] [PubMed]

64. Apelt, J.; Bigl, M.; Wunderlich, P.; Schliebs, R. Aging-related increase in oxidative stress correlates with developmental pattern of beta-secretase activity and beta-amyloid plaque formation in transgenic Tg2576 mice with Alzheimer-like pathology. *Int. J. Dev. Neurosci. Off. J. Int. Soc. Dev. Neurosci.* **2004**, *22*, 475–484. [CrossRef] [PubMed]

65. Sanmartin, C.D.; Adasme, T.; Hidalgo, C.; Paula-Lima, A.C. The antioxidant N-acetylcysteine prevents the mitochondrial fragmentation induced by soluble amyloid-beta peptide oligomers. *Neuro-Degener. Dis.* **2012**, *10*, 34–37. [CrossRef] [PubMed]

66. Ma, T.; Hoeffer, C.A.; Wong, H.; Massaad, C.A.; Zhou, P.; Iadecola, C.; Murphy, M.P.; Pautler, R.G.; Klann, E. Amyloid beta-induced impairments in hippocampal synaptic plasticity are rescued by decreasing mitochondrial superoxide. *J. Neurosci. Off. J. Soc. Neurosci.* **2011**, *31*, 5589–5595. [CrossRef] [PubMed]

67. Bloom, G.S. Amyloid-beta and tau: The trigger and bullet in Alzheimer disease pathogenesis. *JAMA Neurol.* **2014**, *71*, 505–508. [CrossRef] [PubMed]

68. Moreira, P.I.; Santos, M.S.; Oliveira, C.R. Alzheimer's disease: A lesson from mitochondrial dysfunction. *Antioxid. Redox Signal.* **2007**, *9*, 1621–1630. [CrossRef] [PubMed]

69. Murakami, K.; Shimizu, T. Cytoplasmic superoxide radical: A possible contributing factor to intracellular abeta oligomerization in Alzheimer disease. *Commun. Integr. Biol.* **2012**, *5*, 255–258. [CrossRef] [PubMed]

70. Bush, A.I.; Masters, C.L.; Tanzi, R.E. Copper, beta-amyloid, and Alzheimer's disease: Tapping a sensitive connection. *Proc. Natl. Acad. Sci. USA* **2003**, *100*, 11193–11194. [CrossRef] [PubMed]

71. Bush, A.I.; Curtain, C.C. Twenty years of metallo-neurobiology: Where to now? *Eur. Biophys. J. EBJ* **2008**, *37*, 241–245. [CrossRef] [PubMed]

72. Jomova, K.; Vondrakova, D.; Lawson, M.; Valko, M. Metals, oxidative stress and neurodegenerative disorders. *Mol. Cell. Biochem.* **2010**, *345*, 91–104. [CrossRef] [PubMed]

73. Monacelli, F.; Borghi, R.; Pacini, D.; Serrati, C.; Traverso, N.; Odetti, P. Pentosidine determination in CSF: A potential biomarker of Alzheimer's disease? *Clin. Chem. Lab. Med.* **2014**, *52*, 117–120. [CrossRef] [PubMed]

74. Butterfield, D.A.; Reed, T.; Newman, S.F.; Sultana, R. Roles of amyloid beta-peptide-associated oxidative stress and brain protein modifications in the pathogenesis of Alzheimer's disease and mild cognitive impairment. *Free Radic. Biol. Med.* **2007**, *43*, 658–677. [CrossRef] [PubMed]

75. Polidori, M.C.; Mecocci, P. Plasma susceptibility to free radical-induced antioxidant consumption and lipid peroxidation is increased in very old subjects with Alzheimer disease. *J. Alzheimers Dis.* **2002**, *4*, 517–522. [CrossRef] [PubMed]

76. Schipper, H.M.; Cisse, S.; Stopa, E.G. Expression of heme oxygenase-1 in the senescent and Alzheimer-diseased brain. *Ann. Neurol.* **1995**, *37*, 758–768. [CrossRef] [PubMed]

77. Ischiropoulos, H. Biological tyrosine nitration: A pathophysiological function of nitric oxide and reactive oxygen species. *Arch. Biochem. Biophys.* **1998**, *356*, 1–11. [CrossRef] [PubMed]

78. Garcia-Krauss, A.; Ferrada, L.; Astuya, A.; Salazar, K.; Cisternas, P.; Martinez, F.; Ramirez, E.; Nualart, F. Dehydroascorbic acid promotes cell death in neurons under oxidative stress: A protective role for astrocytes. *Mol. Neurobiol.* **2016**, *53*, 5847–5863. [CrossRef] [PubMed]

79. May, J.M. Vitamin c transport and its role in the central nervous system. *Sub-Cell. Biochem.* **2012**, *56*, 85–103.

80. Sultana, R.; Mecocci, P.; Mangialasche, F.; Cecchetti, R.; Baglioni, M.; Butterfield, D.A. Increased protein and lipid oxidative damage in mitochondria isolated from lymphocytes from patients with Alzheimer's disease: Insights into the role of oxidative stress in Alzheimer's disease and initial investigations into a potential biomarker for this dementing disorder. *J. Alzheimers Dis.* **2011**, *24*, 77–84. [PubMed]

81. Dixit, S.; Bernardo, A.; Walker, J.M.; Kennard, J.A.; Kim, G.Y.; Kessler, E.S.; Harrison, F.E. Vitamin C deficiency in the brain impairs cognition, increases amyloid accumulation and deposition, and oxidative stress in APP/PSEN1 and normally aging mice. *ACS Chem. Neurosci.* **2015**, *6*, 570–581. [CrossRef] [PubMed]

82. Parthasarathy, S.; Yoo, B.; McElheny, D.; Tay, W.; Ishii, Y. Capturing a reactive state of amyloid aggregates: Nmr-based characterization of copper-bound Alzheimer disease amyloid beta-fibrils in a redox cycle. *J. Biol. Chem.* **2014**, *289*, 9998–10010. [CrossRef] [PubMed]

83. Berger, T.M.; Polidori, M.C.; Dabbagh, A.; Evans, P.J.; Halliwell, B.; Morrow, J.D.; Roberts, L.J., II; Frei, B. Antioxidant activity of vitamin C in iron-overloaded human plasma. *J. Biol. Chem.* **1997**, *272*, 15656–15660. [CrossRef] [PubMed]

84. Sil, S.; Ghosh, T.; Gupta, P.; Ghosh, R.; Kabir, S.N.; Roy, A. Dual role of vitamin C on the neuroinflammation mediated neurodegeneration and memory impairments in colchicine induced rat model of Alzheimer disease. *J. Mol. Neurosci. MN* **2016**, *60*, 421–435. [CrossRef] [PubMed]

85. Harrison, F.E.; Hosseini, A.H.; McDonald, M.P.; May, J.M. Vitamin C reduces spatial learning deficits in middle-aged and very old APP/PSEN1 transgenic and wild-type mice. *Pharmacol. Biochem. Behav.* **2009**, *93*, 443–450. [CrossRef] [PubMed]

86. Huang, J.; May, J.M. Ascorbic acid protects SH-SY5Y neuroblastoma cells from apoptosis and death induced by beta-amyloid. *Brain Res.* **2006**, *1097*, 52–58. [CrossRef] [PubMed]

87. Ahmad, A.; Shah, S.A.; Badshah, H.; Kim, M.J.; Ali, T.; Yoon, G.H.; Kim, T.H.; Abid, N.B.; Rehman, S.U.; Khan, S.; et al. Neuroprotection by vitamin c against ethanol-induced neuroinflammation associated neurodegeneration in the developing rat brain. *CNS Neurol. Disord. Drug Targets* **2016**, *15*, 360–370. [CrossRef] [PubMed]

88. Ballaz, S.; Morales, I.; Rodriguez, M.; Obeso, J.A. Ascorbate prevents cell death from prolonged exposure to glutamate in an in vitro model of human dopaminergic neurons. *J. Neurosci. Res.* **2013**, *91*, 1609–1617. [CrossRef] [PubMed]

89. Chan, S.; Kantham, S.; Rao, V.M.; Palanivelu, M.K.; Pham, H.L.; Shaw, P.N.; McGeary, R.P.; Ross, B.P. Metal chelation, radical scavenging and inhibition of abeta(4)(2) fibrillation by food constituents in relation to Alzheimer's disease. *Food Chem.* **2016**, *199*, 185–194. [CrossRef] [PubMed]

90. Polidori, M.C.; Pientka, L.; Mecocci, P. A review of the major vascular risk factors related to Alzheimer's disease. *J. Alzheimers Dis.* **2012**, *32*, 521–530. [PubMed]

91. Murakami, K.; Murata, N.; Ozawa, Y.; Kinoshita, N.; Irie, K.; Shirasawa, T.; Shimizu, T. Vitamin c restores behavioral deficits and amyloid-beta oligomerization without affecting plaque formation in a mouse model of Alzheimer's disease. *J. Alzheimers Dis.* **2011**, *26*, 7–18. [PubMed]

92. Hauss-Wegrzyniak, B.; Wenk, G.L. Beta-amyloid deposition in the brains of rats chronically infused with thiorphan or lipopolysaccharide: The role of ascorbic acid in the vehicle. *Neurosci. Lett.* **2002**, *322*, 75–78. [CrossRef]

93. Deane, R.; Bell, R.D.; Sagare, A.; Zlokovic, B.V. Clearance of amyloid-beta peptide across the blood-brain barrier: Implication for therapies in Alzheimer's disease. *CNS Neurol. Disord. Drug Targets* **2009**, *8*, 16–30. [CrossRef] [PubMed]

94. Dede, D.S.; Yavuz, B.; Yavuz, B.B.; Cankurtaran, M.; Halil, M.; Ulger, Z.; Cankurtaran, E.S.; Aytemir, K.; Kabakci, G.; Ariogul, S. Assessment of endothelial function in Alzheimer's disease: Is Alzheimer's disease a vascular disease? *J. Am. Geriatr. Soc.* **2007**, *55*, 1613–1617. [CrossRef] [PubMed]

95. Lam, V.; Hackett, M.; Takechi, R. Antioxidants and dementia risk: Consideration through a cerebrovascular perspective. *Nutrients* **2016**, *8*, 828. [CrossRef] [PubMed]

96. Sarkar, S.; Mukherjee, A.; Swarnakar, S.; Das, N. Nanocapsulated ascorbic acid in combating cerebral ischemia reperfusion-induced oxidative injury in rat brain. *Curr. Alzheimer Res.* **2016**, *13*, 1363–1373. [CrossRef] [PubMed]

97. Dringen, R.; Kussmaul, L.; Gutterer, J.M.; Hirrlinger, J.; Hamprecht, B. The glutathione system of peroxide detoxification is less efficient in neurons than in astroglial cells. *J. Neurochem.* **1999**, *72*, 2523–2530. [CrossRef] [PubMed]

98. Rohl, C.; Armbrust, E.; Herbst, E.; Jess, A.; Gulden, M.; Maser, E.; Rimbach, G.; Bosch-Saadatmandi, C. Mechanisms involved in the modulation of astroglial resistance to oxidative stress induced by activated microglia: Antioxidative systems, peroxide elimination, radical generation, lipid peroxidation. *Neurotox. Res.* **2010**, *17*, 317–331. [CrossRef] [PubMed]

99. Heo, J.H.; Hyon, L.; Lee, K.M. The possible role of antioxidant vitamin C in Alzheimer's disease treatment and prevention. *Am. J. Alzheimers Dis. Other Dement.* **2013**, *28*, 120–125. [CrossRef] [PubMed]

100. Rosales-Corral, S.; Tan, D.X.; Reiter, R.J.; Valdivia-Velazquez, M.; Martinez-Barboza, G.; Acosta-Martinez, J.P.; Ortiz, G.G. Orally administered melatonin reduces oxidative stress and proinflammatory cytokines induced by amyloid-beta peptide in rat brain: A comparative, in vivo study versus vitamin C and E. *J. Pineal Res.* **2003**, *35*, 80–84. [CrossRef] [PubMed]

101. Dhingra, D.; Parle, M.; Kulkarni, S.K. Comparative brain cholinesterase-inhibiting activity of *Glycyrrhiza glabra*, *Myristica fragrans*, ascorbic acid, and metrifonate in mice. *J. Med. Food* **2006**, *9*, 281–283. [CrossRef] [PubMed]

102. Kuo, C.H.; Hata, F.; Yoshida, H.; Yamatodani, A.; Wada, H. Effect of ascorbic acid on release of acetylcholine from synaptic vesicles prepared from different species of animals and release of noradrenaline from synaptic vesicles of rat brain. *Life Sci.* **1979**, *24*, 911–915. [CrossRef]

103. Cheng, F.; Cappai, R.; Ciccotosto, G.D.; Svensson, G.; Multhaup, G.; Fransson, L.A.; Mani, K. Suppression of amyloid beta a11 antibody immunoreactivity by vitamin C: Possible role of heparan sulfate oligosaccharides derived from glypican-1 by ascorbate-induced, nitric oxide (no)-catalyzed degradation. *J. Biol. Chem.* **2011**, *286*, 27559–27572. [CrossRef] [PubMed]

104. Jiang, D.; Li, X.; Liu, L.; Yagnik, G.B.; Zhou, F. Reaction rates and mechanism of the ascorbic acid oxidation by molecular oxygen facilitated by cu(II)-containing amyloid-beta complexes and aggregates. *J. Phys. Chem. B* **2010**, *114*, 4896–4903. [CrossRef] [PubMed]

105. Chambial, S.; Dwivedi, S.; Shukla, K.K.; John, P.J.; Sharma, P. Vitamin c in disease prevention and cure: An overview. *Indian J. Clin. Biochem. IJCB* **2013**, *28*, 314–328. [CrossRef] [PubMed]

106. Rahal, A.; Kumar, A.; Singh, V.; Yadav, B.; Tiwari, R.; Chakraborty, S.; Dhama, K. Oxidative stress, prooxidants, and antioxidants: The interplay. *BioMed Res. Int.* **2014**, *2014*, 761264. [CrossRef] [PubMed]

107. Cheng, R.; Lin, B.; Lee, K.W.; Ortwerth, B.J. Similarity of the yellow chromophores isolated from human cataracts with those from ascorbic acid-modified calf lens proteins: Evidence for ascorbic acid glycation during cataract formation. *Biochim. Biophys. Acta* **2001**, *1537*, 14–26. [CrossRef]

108. Carr, A.; Frei, B. Does vitamin c act as a pro-oxidant under physiological conditions? *FASEB J. Off. Publ. Fed. Am. Soc. Exp. Biol.* **1999**, *13*, 1007–1024.

109. Valko, M.; Morris, H.; Cronin, M.T. Metals, toxicity and oxidative stress. *Curr. Med. Chem.* **2005**, *12*, 1161–1208. [CrossRef] [PubMed]

110. Dikalov, S.I.; Vitek, M.P.; Mason, R.P. Cupric-amyloid beta peptide complex stimulates oxidation of ascorbate and generation of hydroxyl radical. *Free Radic. Biol. Med.* **2004**, *36*, 340–347. [CrossRef] [PubMed]

111. Shearer, J.; Szalai, V.A. The amyloid-beta peptide of Alzheimer's disease binds Cu(I) in a linear Bis-His coordination environment: Insight into a possible neuroprotective mechanism for the amyloid-beta peptide. *J. Am. Chem. Soc.* **2008**, *130*, 17826–17835. [CrossRef] [PubMed]

112. Nadal, R.C.; Rigby, S.E.; Viles, J.H. Amyloid beta-Cu^{2+} complexes in both monomeric and fibrillar forms do not generate H_2O_2 catalytically but quench hydroxyl radicals. *Biochemistry* **2008**, *47*, 11653–11664. [CrossRef] [PubMed]

113. Huang, Y.N.; Lai, C.C.; Chiu, C.T.; Lin, J.J.; Wang, J.Y. L-ascorbate attenuates the endotoxin-induced production of inflammatory mediators by inhibiting MAPK activation and NF-kappaB translocation in cortical neurons/glia Cocultures. *PloS ONE* **2014**, *9*, e97276.

114. Kook, S.Y.; Lee, K.M.; Kim, Y.; Cha, M.Y.; Kang, S.; Baik, S.H.; Lee, H.; Park, R.; Mook-Jung, I. High-dose of vitamin c supplementation reduces amyloid plaque burden and ameliorates pathological changes in the brain of 5XFAD mice. *Cell Death Dis.* **2014**, *5*, e1083. [CrossRef] [PubMed]

115. Polidori, M.C.; Ruggiero, C.; Croce, M.F.; Raichi, T.; Mangialasche, F.; Cecchetti, R.; Pelini, L.; Paolacci, L.; Ercolani, S.; Mecocci, P. Association of increased carotid intima-media thickness and lower plasma levels of vitamin C and vitamin E in old age subjects: Implications for Alzheimer's disease. *J. Neural Transm.* **2015**, *122*, 523–530. [CrossRef] [PubMed]

116. Bomboi, G.; Castello, L.; Cosentino, F.; Giubilei, F.; Orzi, F.; Volpe, M. Alzheimer's disease and endothelial dysfunction. *Neurol. Sci. Off. J. Ital. Neurol. Soc. Ital. Soc. Clin. Neurophysiol.* **2010**, *31*, 1–8. [CrossRef] [PubMed]

117. May, J.M.; Qu, Z.C. Ascorbic acid prevents increased endothelial permeability caused by oxidized low density lipoprotein. *Free Radic. Res.* **2010**, *44*, 1359–1368. [CrossRef] [PubMed]

118. May, J.M.; Harrison, F.E. Role of vitamin C in the function of the vascular endothelium. *Antioxid. Redox Signal.* **2013**, *19*, 2068–2083. [CrossRef] [PubMed]

119. Polidori, M.C.; Pientka, L. Bridging the pathophysiology of Alzheimer's disease with vascular pathology: The feed-back, the feed-forward, and oxidative stress. *J. Alzheimers Dis.* **2012**, *28*, 1–9. [PubMed]

120. Miller, M.C.; Tavares, R.; Johanson, C.E.; Hovanesian, V.; Donahue, J.E.; Gonzalez, L.; Silverberg, G.D.; Stopa, E.G. Hippocampal rage immunoreactivity in early and advanced Alzheimer's disease. *Brain Res.* **2008**, *1230*, 273–280. [CrossRef] [PubMed]

121. Lin, J.L.; Huang, Y.H.; Shen, Y.C.; Huang, H.C.; Liu, P.H. Ascorbic acid prevents blood-brain barrier disruption and sensory deficit caused by sustained compression of primary somatosensory cortex. *J. Cereb. Blood Flow Metab. Off. J. Int. Soc. Cereb. Blood Flow Metab.* **2010**, *30*, 1121–1136. [CrossRef] [PubMed]

122. May, J.M.; Qu, Z.C. Nitric oxide mediates tightening of the endothelial barrier by ascorbic acid. *Biochem. Biophys. Res. Commun.* **2011**, *404*, 701–705. [CrossRef] [PubMed]

123. Scuteri, A.; Tesauro, M.; Appolloni, S.; Preziosi, F.; Brancati, A.M.; Volpe, M. Arterial stiffness as an independent predictor of longitudinal changes in cognitive function in the older individual. *J. Hypertens.* **2007**, *25*, 1035–1040. [CrossRef] [PubMed]

124. Ellingsen, I.; Seljeflot, I.; Arnesen, H.; Tonstad, S. Vitamin C consumption is associated with less progression in carotid intima media thickness in elderly men: A 3-year intervention study. *Nutr. Metab. Cardiovasc. Dis. NMCD* **2009**, *19*, 8–14. [CrossRef] [PubMed]

125. Donahue, J.E.; Flaherty, S.L.; Johanson, C.E.; Duncan, J.A., III; Silverberg, G.D.; Miller, M.C.; Tavares, R.; Yang, W.; Wu, Q.; Sabo, E.; et al. Rage, lrp-1, and amyloid-beta protein in Alzheimer's disease. *Acta Neuropathol.* **2006**, *112*, 405–415. [CrossRef] [PubMed]

126. Pleiner, J.; Schaller, G.; Mittermayer, F.; Marsik, C.; MacAllister, R.J.; Kapiotis, S.; Ziegler, S.; Ferlitsch, A.; Wolzt, M. Intra-arterial vitamin C prevents endothelial dysfunction caused by ischemia-reperfusion. *Atherosclerosis* **2008**, *197*, 383–391. [CrossRef] [PubMed]

127. Scorza, G.; Pietraforte, D.; Minetti, M. Role of ascorbate and protein thiols in the release of nitric oxide from S-nitroso-albumin and S-nitroso-glutathione in human plasma. *Free Radic. Biol. Med.* **1997**, *22*, 633–642. [CrossRef]

128. Allahtavakoli, M.; Amin, F.; Esmaeeli-Nadimi, A.; Shamsizadeh, A.; Kazemi-Arababadi, M.; Kennedy, D. Ascorbic acid reduces the adverse effects of delayed administration of tissue plasminogen activator in a rat stroke model. *Basic Clin. Pharmacol. Toxicol.* **2015**, *117*, 335–339. [CrossRef] [PubMed]

129. Song, J.; Park, J.; Kim, J.H.; Choi, J.Y.; Kim, J.Y.; Lee, K.M.; Lee, J.E. Dehydroascorbic acid attenuates ischemic brain edema and neurotoxicity in cerebral ischemia: An in vivo study. *Exp. Neurobiol.* **2015**, *24*, 41–54. [CrossRef] [PubMed]

130. Allen, C.L.; Bayraktutan, U. Antioxidants attenuate hyperglycaemia-mediated brain endothelial cell dysfunction and blood-brain barrier hyperpermeability. *Diabetes Obes. Metab.* **2009**, *11*, 480–490. [CrossRef] [PubMed]

131. Bowman, G.L. Ascorbic acid, cognitive function, and Alzheimer's disease: A current review and future direction. *BioFactors* **2012**, *38*, 114–122. [CrossRef] [PubMed]

132. Bowman, G.L.; Dodge, H.; Frei, B.; Calabrese, C.; Oken, B.S.; Kaye, J.A.; Quinn, J.F. Ascorbic acid and rates of cognitive decline in Alzheimer's disease. *J. Alzheimers Dis.* **2009**, *16*, 93–98. [CrossRef] [PubMed]

133. Bowman, G.L.; Kaye, J.A.; Moore, M.; Waichunas, D.; Carlson, N.E.; Quinn, J.F. Blood-brain barrier impairment in alzheimer disease: Stability and functional significance. *Neurology* **2007**, *68*, 1809–1814. [CrossRef] [PubMed]

134. Spector, R.; Johanson, C.E. Sustained choroid plexus function in human elderly and Alzheimer's disease patients. *Fluids Barriers CNS* **2013**, *10*, 28. [CrossRef] [PubMed]

135. Charlton, K.E.; Rabinowitz, T.L.; Geffen, L.N.; Dhansay, M.A. Lowered plasma vitamin C, but not vitamin E, concentrations in dementia patients. *J. Nutr. Health Aging* **2004**, *8*, 99–107. [PubMed]

136. Rinaldi, P.; Polidori, M.C.; Metastasio, A.; Mariani, E.; Mattioli, P.; Cherubini, A.; Catani, M.; Cecchetti, R.; Senin, U.; Mecocci, P. Plasma antioxidants are similarly depleted in mild cognitive impairment and in Alzheimer's disease. *Neurobiol. Aging* **2003**, *24*, 915–919. [CrossRef]

137. Morris, M.C.; Beckett, L.A.; Scherr, P.A.; Hebert, L.E.; Bennett, D.A.; Field, T.S.; Evans, D.A. Vitamin E and vitamin C supplement use and risk of incident Alzheimer disease. *Alzheimer Dis. Assoc. Disord.* **1998**, *12*, 121–126. [CrossRef] [PubMed]

138. Zandi, P.P.; Anthony, J.C.; Khachaturian, A.S.; Stone, S.V.; Gustafson, D.; Tschanz, J.T.; Norton, M.C.; Welsh-Bohmer, K.A.; Breitner, J.C.; Cache County Study, G. Reduced risk of Alzheimer disease in users of antioxidant vitamin supplements: The cache county study. *Arch. Neurol.* **2004**, *61*, 82–88. [CrossRef] [PubMed]

139. Devore, E.E.; Kang, J.H.; Stampfer, M.J.; Grodstein, F. The association of antioxidants and cognition in the nurses' health study. *Am. J. Epidemiol.* **2013**, *177*, 33–41. [CrossRef] [PubMed]

140. Engelhart, M.J.; Geerlings, M.I.; Ruitenberg, A.; van Swieten, J.C.; Hofman, A.; Witteman, J.C.; Breteler, M.M. Dietary intake of antioxidants and risk of Alzheimer disease. *JAMA* **2002**, *287*, 3223–3229. [CrossRef] [PubMed]

141. Quinn, J.; Suh, J.; Moore, M.M.; Kaye, J.; Frei, B. Antioxidants in Alzheimer's disease-vitamin c delivery to a demanding brain. *J. Alzheimers Dis.* **2003**, *5*, 309–313. [CrossRef] [PubMed]

142. Fillenbaum, G.G.; Kuchibhatla, M.N.; Hanlon, J.T.; Artz, M.B.; Pieper, C.F.; Schmader, K.E.; Dysken, M.W.; Gray, S.L. Dementia and Alzheimer's disease in community-dwelling elders taking vitamin C and/or vitamin E. *Ann. Pharmacother.* **2005**, *39*, 2009–2014. [CrossRef] [PubMed]

143. Harrison, F.E. A critical review of vitamin C for the prevention of age-related cognitive decline and Alzheimer's disease. *J. Alzheimers Dis.* **2012**, *29*, 711–726. [PubMed]

144. Emir, U.E.; Raatz, S.; McPherson, S.; Hodges, J.S.; Torkelson, C.; Tawfik, P.; White, T.; Terpstra, M. Noninvasive quantification of ascorbate and glutathione concentration in the elderly human brain. *NMR Biomed.* **2011**, *24*, 888–894. [CrossRef] [PubMed]

145. Minor, E.A.; Court, B.L.; Young, J.I.; Wang, G. Ascorbate induces ten-eleven translocation (Tet) methylcytosine dioxygenase-mediated generation of 5-hydroxymethylcytosine. *J. Biol. Chem.* **2013**, *288*, 13669–13674. [CrossRef] [PubMed]

146. Smuda, M.; Glomb, M.A. Maillard degradation pathways of vitamin C. *Angew. Chem.* **2013**, *52*, 4887–4891. [CrossRef] [PubMed]

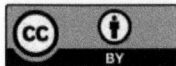

nutrients

MDPI

Review

Does Vitamin C Influence Neurodegenerative Diseases and Psychiatric Disorders?

Joanna Kocot * ⓘ, Dorota Luchowska-Kocot, Małgorzata Kiełczykowska, Irena Musik and Jacek Kurzepa

Chair and Department of Medical Chemistry, Medical University of Lublin, 4A Chodźki Street, 20-093 Lublin, Poland; dorota.luchowska-kocot@umlub.pl (D.L.-K.); malgorzata.kielczykowska@umlub.pl (M.K.); irena.musik@umlub.pl (I.M.); jacek.kurzepa@umlub.pl (J.K.)

Received: 15 May 2017; Accepted: 21 June 2017; Published: 27 June 2017

Abstract: Vitamin C (Vit C) is considered to be a vital antioxidant molecule in the brain. Intracellular Vit C helps maintain integrity and function of several processes in the central nervous system (CNS), including neuronal maturation and differentiation, myelin formation, synthesis of catecholamine, modulation of neurotransmission and antioxidant protection. The importance of Vit C for CNS function has been proven by the fact that targeted deletion of the sodium-vitamin C co-transporter in mice results in widespread cerebral hemorrhage and death on post-natal day one. Since neurological diseases are characterized by increased free radical generation and the highest concentrations of Vit C in the body are found in the brain and neuroendocrine tissues, it is suggested that Vit C may change the course of neurological diseases and display potential therapeutic roles. The aim of this review is to update the current state of knowledge of the role of vitamin C on neurodegenerative diseases including Alzheimer's disease, Parkinson's disease, Huntington's disease, multiple sclerosis and amyotrophic sclerosis, as well as psychiatric disorders including depression, anxiety and schizophrenia. The particular attention is attributed to understanding of the mechanisms underlying possible therapeutic properties of ascorbic acid in the presented disorders.

Keywords: vitamin C; Alzheimer's disease; Parkinson's disease; Huntington's disease; multiple sclerosis; amyotrophic sclerosis; depression; anxiety; schizophrenia

1. Introduction

Vitamin C (Vit C, ascorbic acid) belongs to a group of water-soluble vitamins. In organisms, Vit C can exist in two forms: reduced—the exact ascorbic acid (AA) which in physiological pH occurs in its anion form of an ascorbate—and oxidized one—dehydroascorbic acid (DHA), which is a product of two-electron oxidation of AA (Figure 1). In the course of metabolic processes an ascorbate free radical can be produced as a result of one-electron oxidation. This variety may subsequently undergo dismutation forming ascorbate and DHA [1].

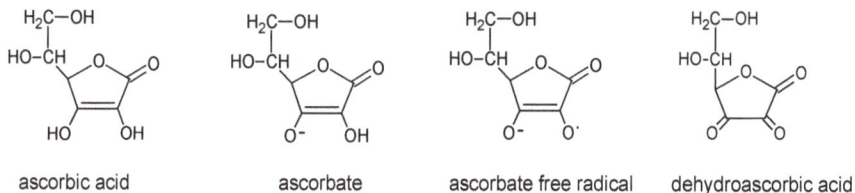

Figure 1. Forms of vitamin C occurring in organisms.

Mammalian organisms are generally capable of synthesizing Vit C themselves. However, some species like fruit bats, guinea pigs, other primates and humans are deprived of this ability due to the lack of L-gulono-1,4-lactone oxidase enzyme which is an element of the metabolic pathway responsible for synthesis of ascorbic acid from glucose [1,2]. Moreover, Vit C is not produced by intestinal microflora [3]. The above facts make these organisms strictly dependent on dietary intake. The recommended Vit C daily intake was established as 60 mg with the reservation that in smokers this value should be increased up to 140 mg [4]. According to the later recommendations, Vit C consumption should be 75 (women) and 90 (men) mg per day, whereas in smokers this value ought to be increased by 35 mg per day [3,5,6].

Vit C is a nutrient of greatest importance for proper functioning of nervous system and its main role in the brain is its participation in the antioxidant defense. Apart from this role, it is involved in numerous non-oxidant processes like biosynthesis of collagen, carnitine, tyrosine and peptide hormones as well as of myelin. It plays the crucial role in neurotransmission and neuronal maturation and functions [7]. For instance, its ability to alleviate seizure severity as well as reduction of seizure-induced damage have been proved [8,9]. On the other hand, disruption of vitamin C transport has been shown to contribute to brain damage in premature infants [10]. Furthermore, Vit C treatment has been reported to ameliorate neuropathological alterations as well as memory impairments and the neurodegenerative changes in rats exposed to neurotoxic substances like aluminum or colchicine [11,12].

Consequently, the growing interest in the issue of vitamin C deficiency, as well as vitamin C treatment in the nervous system diseases, was observed for many years. These facts made us decide to update the current state of knowledge of the role of Vit C in neurodegenerative diseases including Alzheimer's disease, Parkinson's disease, Huntington's disease, multiple sclerosis as well as amyotrophic sclerosis, as well as in psychiatric disorders including depression, anxiety disorders and schizophrenia.

2. Methods

To review the literature on brain Vit C transport/distribution and its function in central nervous system, PubMed and Scopus databases were searched using the following search terms: (vitamin C OR ascorbic acid) AND (central nervous system OR CNS) or (vitamin OR ascorbic acid) AND brain, separately.

To review the literature on the role of Vit C in neurodegenerative diseases and psychiatric disorders, PubMed and Scopus databases were searched using the following search terms: (vitamin C OR ascorbic acid) AND Alzheimer, (vitamin C OR ascorbic acid) AND Parkinson, (vitamin C OR ascorbic acid) AND Huntington, (vitamin C OR ascorbic acid) AND multiple sclerosis, (vitamin C OR ascorbic acid) AND amyotrophic sclerosis, (vitamin C OR ascorbic acid) AND depression, (vitamin C OR ascorbic acid) AND anxiety and (vitamin C OR ascorbic acid) AND schizophrenia, separately. The searching was limited to the last 10 years and human studies, but if none or a few human studies were found the criteria were expanded then to include in vitro or animal studies.

The final search was conducted in April 2017. The titles and abstracts of the articles identified through the initial search were reviewed, and the irrelevant articles were excluded. The full texts of the remaining articles were reviewed to detect studies that did were not suitable for this review.

3. Vitamin C Transport Systems and Distribution in the Brain

Two basic barriers limit the entry of Vit C (being a hydrophilic molecule) into the central nervous system: the blood-brain barrier and the blood-cerebrospinal fluid barrier (CSF) [13]. Considering the whole body, ascorbic acid uptake is mainly conditioned by two sodium-dependent transporters from the SLC23 family, the sodium-dependent Vit C transporter type 1 (SVCT1) and type 2 (SVCT2). These possess similar structure and amino acid sequence, but have different tissue distribution. SVCT1 is found predominantly in apical brush-border membranes of intestinal and renal tubular cells, whereas SVCT2 occurs in most tissue cells [14,15]. SVCT2 is especially important for the transport of Vit

C in the brain—it mediates the transport of ascorbate from plasma across choroid plexus to the cerebrospinal fluid and across the neuronal cell plasma membrane to neuronal cytosol [16]. Although dehydroascorbic acid (DHA) enters the central nervous system more rapidly than the ascorbate, the latter one readily penetrates CNS after oral administration. DHA is taken up by the omnipresent glucose transporters (GLUT), which have affinity to this form of Vit C [17,18]. GLUT1 and GLUT3 are mainly responsible for DHA uptake in the CNS [13]. Transport of DHA by GLUT transporter is bidirectional—each molecule of DHA formed inside the cells by oxidation of the ascorbate could be effluxed and lost. This phenomenon is prevented by efficient cellular mechanisms of DHA reduction and recycling in ascorbate [19]. Neurons can take up ascorbic acid using both described ways [20], whereas astrocytes acquire Vit C utilizing only GLUT transporters [21].

The brain has been found to belong to the organs of the highest ascorbate content, with neurons displaying the highest concentration of all the human organism and reaching 10 mmol/L [1,22]. Mefford et al. [23] and Milby et al. [24] showed high concentrations of Vit C in neuron-rich areas of hippocampus and neocortex in the human brain. Authors suggested that ascorbate content in above brain areas is as much as two-fold higher than in other regions. The difference in ascorbate content between neurons and glia appears to be significant [25]. It is postulated that in astrocytes and glial supported cells lacking the SVCT2, the uptake and reduction of DHA may be the only mechanism of ascorbate retention [26]. In addition to ascorbate motion in neurons and glial cells, it is also released from both types of cells. This release contributes to a certain extent to the homeostatic mechanism of extracellular ascorbate maintenance in the brain [15,19]. Moreover, the extracellular ascorbate concentration is regulated dynamically by glutamate release—increase in extracellular Vit C concentration causes heteroexchange with glutamate [27,28].

4. Vitamin C Function in Central Nervous System

It is well known that the main function of intracellular ascorbic acid in the brain is the antioxidant defense of the cells. However, vitamin C in the central nervous system (CNS) has also many non-antioxidant functions—it plays a role of an enzymatic co-factor participating in biosynthesis of such substances as collagen, carnitine, tyrosine and peptide hormones. It has also been indicated that myelin formation in Schwann cells could be stimulated by ascorbic acid [7,29].

The brain is an organ particularly exposed to oxidative stress and free radicals' activity, which is associated with high levels of unsaturated fatty acids and high cell metabolism rate [16]. Ascorbic acid, being an antioxidant, acts directly by scavenging reactive oxygen and nitrogen species produced during normal cell metabolism [30,31]. In vivo studies demonstrated that the ascorbate had the ability to inactivate superoxide radicals—the major byproduct of fast metabolism of mitochondrial neurons [32]. Moreover, the ascorbate is a key factor in the recycling of other antioxidants, e.g., alpha-tocopherol (Vitamin E). Alpha-tocopherol, found in all biological membranes, is involved in preventing lipid peroxidation by removing peroxyl radicals. During this process α-tocopherol is oxidized to the α-tocopheroxyl radical, which can result in a very harmful effect. The ascorbate could reduce the tocopheroxyl radical back to tocopherol and then its oxidized form is recycled by enzymatic systems with using NADH or NADPH [33]. Regarding these facts, vitamin C is considered to be an important neuroprotective agent.

One non-antioxidant function of vitamin C is its participation in CNS signal transduction through neurotransmitters [16]. Vit C is suggested to influence this process via modulating of binding of neurotransmitters to receptors as well as regulating their release [34–37]. In addition, ascorbic acid acts as a co-factor in the synthesis of neurotransmitters, particularly of catecholamines—dopamine and norepinephrine [26,38]. Seitz et al. [39] suggested that the modulating effect of the ascorbate could be divided into short- and long-term ones. The short-term effect refers to ascorbate role as a substrate for dopamine-β-hydroxylase. Vit C supplies electrons for this enzyme catalyzing the formation of norepinephrine from dopamine. Moreover, it may exert neuroprotective influence against ROS and quinones generated by dopamine metabolism [16]. On the other hand, the long-term effect could be connected with increased expression of the tyrosine hydroxylase gene, probably via a mechanism that entails the increase of intracellular cAMP [39]. It has been stated that the function of ascorbic acid as a neuromodulator of neural transmission may be also associated with amino acidic residues reduction [40] or scavenging of ROS generated in response to neurotransmitter receptor activation [34,41]. Moreover, some have studies showed that ascorbic acid modulates the activity of some receptors such as glutamate as well as γ-aminobutyric acid (GABA) ones [22,40,42–44]. Vit C has been shown to prevent excitotoxic damage caused by excessive extracellular glutamate leading to hyperpolarization of the *N*-methyl-D-aspartate (NMDA) receptor and therefore to neuronal damage [45]. Vit C inhibits the binding of glutamate to the NMDA receptor, thus demonstrating a direct effect in preventing excessive nerve stimulation exerted by the glutamate [26]. The effect of ascorbic acid on GABA receptors can be explained by a decrease in the energy barrier for GABA activation induced by this agent. Ascorbic acid could bind to or modify one or more sites capable of allosterically modulating single-channel properties. In addition, it is possible that ascorbic acid acts through supporting the conversion from the last GABA-bound closed state to the open state. Alternatively, ascorbic acid could induce the transition of channels towards additional open states in which the receptor adopts lower energy conformations with higher open probabilities [40,44].

There have also been reports concerning the effect of Vit C on cognitive processes such as learning, memory and locomotion, although the exact mechanism of this impact is still being investigated [26]. However, animal studies have shown a clear association between the ascorbate and the cholinergic and dopaminergic systems, they also suggested that the ascorbate can act as a dopamine receptor antagonist. This was also confirmed by Tolbert et al. [46], who showed that the ascorbate inhibits the binding of specific dopamine D1 and D2 receptor agonists.

Another non-antioxidant function of Vit C includes modulation of neuronal metabolism by changing the preference for lactate over glucose as an energy substrate to sustain synaptic activity. During ascorbic acid metabolic switch, this vitamin is released from glial cells and is taken up by neurons where it restraints glucose transport and its utilization. This allows lactate uptake and its usage as the primary energy source in neurons [47]. It was observed that intracellular ascorbic acid inhibited neuronal glucose usage via a mechanism involving GLUT3 [48].

Vit C is involved in collagen synthesis, which also occurs in the brain [26]. There is no doubt that collagen is needed for blood vessels and neural sheath formation. It is well recognized that vitamin C takes part in the final step of the formation of mature triple helix collagen. In this stage, ascorbic acid acts as an electron donor in the hydroxylation of procollagen propyl and lysyl residues [16]. The role of Vit C in collagen synthesis in the brain was confirmed by Sotiriou et al. [49]. According to these authors in mice deficient in SVCT2 ascorbate transporter, the concentration of ascorbate in the brain was below detection level. The animals died due to capillary hemorrhage in the penetrating vessels of the brain. Ascorbate-dependent collagen synthesis is also linked to the formation of the myelin sheath that surrounds many nerve fibers [26]. In vitro studies showed that ascorbate, added to a mixed culture of rat Schwann cells and dorsal root ganglion neurons, promoted myelin formation and differentiation of Schwann cells during formation of the basal lamina of the myelin sheath [7,29].

5. Role of Vitamin C in Neurodegenerative Diseases

Vit C is important for proper nervous system function and its abnormal concentration in nervous tissue is thought to be accompanied with neurological disorders. Studies have shown that disruption of vitamin C transport may cause brain damage in premature infants. Vit C was found to show alleviating effect on seizures severity as well as reducing influence on seizure-induced damage of hippocampus [8,9]. One of the recent studies also revealed that glutamate-induced negative changes in immature brain of rats were reduced by Vit C treatment [50]. Moreover, Vit C administration was shown to recover the colchicine-induced neuroinflammation-mediated neurodegeneration and memory impairments in rats [12] as well as ameliorate behavioral deficits and neuropathological alterations in rats exposed to aluminum chloride [11].

The fact that Vit C can neutralize superoxide radicals, which are generated in large amount during neurodegenerative processes, seems to support its role in neurodegeneration. Moreover, plasma and cellular Vit C levels decline steadily with age and neurodegenerative diseases are often associated with aging. An association of Vit C release with motor activity in central nervous system regions, glutamate-uptake-dependent release of Vit C, its possible role in modulation of N-methyl-D-aspartate receptor activity as well as ability to prevent peroxynitrite anion formation constitute further evidence pointing to the role of Vit C in neurodegenerative processes.

5.1. Alzheimer's Disease

Alzheimer's disease (AD) is the most common form of dementia, an incurable and progressive neurodegenerative disease, leading to far-reaching memory loss, cognitive decline and eventually death. There are two major forms of the AD disease: early onset (familial) and late onset (sporadic). Early-onset one is rare, accounting for less than 5% of all AD cases. Mutations in three genes, mainly amyloid precursor protein (21q21.3), presenilin-1 (14q24.3) and presenilin-2 (1q42.13), have been identified to be involved in the development of this form. Late-onset AD (LOAD) is common among individuals over 65 years of age. Although heritability of LOAD is high (79%), its etiology is considered to be polygenic and multifactorial. The apolipoprotein E ε4 allele (19q13.2) is the major known genetic risk factor for this form of AD. The E4/E4 genotype does not determine the occurrence of LOAD, but is a factor that increases susceptibility to this disease and lowers the age of disease onset. Moreover, a large number of genes have been suggested to be implicated in risk of late-onset Alzheimer's, e.g., clusterin (8p21), complement receptor 1 (1q32), phosphatidylinositol binding clathrin assembly protein (11q14.2), myc box-dependent-interacting protein 1 (2q14.3), ATP binding cassette transporter 7 (19p13.3), membrane-spanning 4-domains, subfamily A (11q12.2), ephrin type-A receptor 1 (7q34), CD33 antigen (19q13.3), CD2 associated protein (6p12.3), sortilin-related receptor 1 (11q24.1), GRB2 associated-binding protein 2 (11q13.4–13.5), insulin-degrading enzyme (10q24), death-associated protein kinase 1 (DAPK1) or gene encoding ubiquilin-1 (UBQLN1) [51,52]. The list of genes associated with AD is still growing. For instance, in the recent study, Lee et al. revealed that single-nucleotide polymorphisms in six genes, including 3-hydroxybutyrate dehydrogenase, type 1 (*BDH1*), ST6 beta-galactosamide alpha-2,6-sialyltranferase 1 (*ST6GAL1*), RAB20, member RAS oncogene family (*RAB20*), PDS5 cohesin associated factor B (*PDS5B*), adenosine deaminase, RNA-specific, B2 (*ADARB2*), and SplA/ryanodine receptor domain and SOCS box containing 1 (*SPSB1*), were directly or indirectly related to conversion of mild cognitive impairment to AD [53].

A neuropathological lesions characteristic of AD include neurofibrillary tangles (composed of hyperphosphorylated and aggregated tau protein) accumulated in the neuronal cytosol as well as the extracellular plaque deposits of the β-amyloid peptide (Aβ), with their frequency correlating with declining cognitive measures [54]. Proteolytic cleavage of amyloid precursor polypeptide chain by secretases (mainly β- and γ-secretase) produces Aβ40 and Aβ42 peptides, which consist of 40 and 42 amino acids, respectively. The latter one, due to its hydrophobicity, is characterized by a greater tendency to form fibrils and is believed to be the main factor responsible for the formation of amyloid deposits [55]. However, Nagababu et al. suggested that the enhanced toxic effect observed for Aβ42 could be attributed to a greater toxicity of the 1–42 aggregates than the 1–40 ones of a comparable size distribution and not to the formation of larger fibrils [56]. According to Ott et al. [54] pre-aggregated Aβ42 peptide induces hyperphosphorylation and pathological structural changes of tau protein and thereby directly links the "amyloid hypothesis" to tau pathology observed in AD [54]. Although the pathogenesis of AD has not been fully understood yet, many studies have demonstrated that ROS and oxidative stress are implicated in disease progression. Aβ peptide was found to enhance the neuronal vulnerability to oxidative stress and cause an impairment of electron transport chain, whereas oxidative stress was shown to induce accumulation of Aβ peptide which subsequently promotes ROS production [16,22,57]. Bartzokis et al. in turn [58] suggested that myelin breakdown in vulnerable late-myelinating regions released oligodendrocyte- and myelin-associated iron that promoted the development of the toxic amyloid oligomers and plaques. There is also the "amyloid cascade-inflammatory hypothesis" which assumes that AD probably results from the inflammatory response induced by extracellular β-amyloid protein deposits, which subsequently become enhanced by aggregates of tau protein [59]. Moreover, recent research has suggested that AD might be a prion-like disease [60,61].

The role of Vit C in AD disease was studied in APP/PSEN1 mice carrying human AD mutations in the amyloid precursor protein (APP) and presenilin (PSEN1) genes (transgenic mouse model of Alzheimer's disease) with partial ablation of vitamin C transport in the brain [9,62,63].

Warner et al. [9] demonstrated that decreased brain Vit C level in the 6-month-old SVCT2+/− APP/PSEN1 mice (obtained by crossing APP/PSEN1 bigenic mice with SVCT2+/− heterozygous knockout mice, which have the lower number of the sodium-dependent Vit C transporter) was associated with enhanced oxidative stress in brain, increased mortality, a shorter latency to seizure onset after kainic acid administration (10 mg/kg i.p.), and more ictal events following treatment with pentylenetetrazol (50 mg/kg i.p.). Furthermore, the authors reported that Vit C deficiency alone in SVCT2+/− mice increased the severity of kainic acid- and pentylenetetrazol-induced seizures [62]. According to another study even moderate intracellular Vit C deficiency displayed an important role in accelerating amyloid aggregation and brain oxidative stress formation, particularly during early stages of disease development. In 6-month-old SVCT2+/− APP/PSEN1 mice increased brain cortex oxidative stress (enhanced malondialdehyde, protein carbonyls, F2-isoprostanes) and decreased level of total glutathione as compared to wild-type controls were observed. Moreover, SVCT2+/− mice had elevated levels of both soluble and insoluble Aβ1-42 and a higher Aβ1-42/Aβ1-40 ratio. In 14-month old mice there were more amyloid-β plaque deposits in both hippocampus and cortex of SVCT2+/−APP/PSEN1+ mice as compared to APP/PSEN+ mice with normal brain Vit C level, whereas oxidative stress levels were similar between groups [62]. Ward et al. [63], in turn, showed that severe Vit C deficiency in Gulo−/− mice (lacking L-gulono-1,4-lactone oxidase (*Gulo*) responsible for the last step in Vit C synthesis) resulted in decreased blood glucose levels, oxidative damage to lipids and proteins in the cortex, and reduction in dopamine and serotonin metabolites in both the cortex and striatum. Moreover, Gulo−/− mice displayed a significant decrease in voluntary locomotor activity, reduced physical strength and elevated sucrose preference. All the above-mentioned behaviors were restored to control levels after treatment with Vit C (250 mg/kg, i.p.). The role of Vit C in preventing the brain against oxidative stress damage seems to be also proved by the recent study performed by Sarkar et al. [64]. The researchers share a view that cerebral ischemia-reperfusion-induced oxidative stress may initiate the pathogenic cascade leading eventually to neuronal loss, especially in hippocampus, with amyloid accumulation, tau protein pathology and irreversible Alzheimer's dementia. Being the prime source of ROS generation, neuronal mitochondria are the most susceptible to damage caused by oxidative stress. The study proved it that L-ascorbic acid loaded polylactide nanocapsules exerted a protective effect on brain mitochondria against cerebral ischemia-reperfusion-induced oxidative injury [64]. Kennard and Harrison, in turn, evaluated the effects of a single intravenous dose of Vit C on spatial memory (using the modified Y-maze test) in APP/PSEN1 mice. The study was performed on APP/PSEN1 and wild-type (WT) mice of three age spans (3, 9 or 20 months). It was shown that APP/PSEN1 mice displayed no behavioral impairment as compared to WT controls, but memory impairment along with aging was observed in both groups. Vit C treatment (125 mg/kg, i.v.) improved performance in 9-month old APP/PSEN1 and WT mice, but improvements in short-term spatial memory did not result from changes in the neuropathological features of AD or monoamine signaling, as acute Vit C administration did not alter monoamine levels in the nucleus accumbens [65]. Cognitive-enhancing effects of acute intraperitoneal (i.p.) Vit C treatment in APP/PSEN1 mice (12- and 24-month-old) were investigated by Harrison et al. Vit C treatment (125 mg/kg i.p.) improved Y-maze alternation rates and swim accuracy in the water maze in both APP/PSEN1 and wild-type mice; but like in the previous study had no significant effect on the age-associated increase in Aβ deposits and oxidative stress, and did not also affect acetylcholinesterase

(AChE) activity either, which was significantly reduced in APP/PSEN1 mice [66]. Murakami et al. [67] in turn reported that 6-month-treatment with Vit C resulted in reduced Aβ oligomer formation without affecting plaque formation, a significant decrease in brain oxidative damage and Aβ42/Aβ40 ratio as well as behavioral decline in an AD mouse model. Furthermore, this restored the declined synaptophysin and reduced the phosphorylation of tau protein at Ser396.

Besides the presented roles, Vit C has also been suggested to prevent neurodegenerative changes and cognitive decline by protecting blood–brain barrier (BBB) integrity [68].

Kook et al., in the study performed on KO-Tg mice (generating by crossing 5 familial Alzheimer's disease mutation (5XFAD) mice with mice lacking *Gulo*), found that oral Vit C supplementation (3.3 g/L of drinking water) reduced amyloid plaque burden in the cortex and hippocampus by ameliorating BBB disruption (via preventing tight junction structural changes) and morphological changes in the mitochondria [69]. This seems to be confirmed by other studies that proved that Vit C might affect levels of proteins responsible for the tightness of BBB, like tight junction-specific integral membrane proteins (occludin and claudin-5) as well as matrix metalloproteinase 9 (MMP-9). Allahtavakoli et al. demonstrated that in a rat stroke model Vit C administration (500 mg/kg; 5 h after stroke) significantly reduced BBB permeability by reducing serum levels of matrix metalloproteinase 9 [70]. Song et al. reported that Vit C (100 mg/kg i.p.) protected cerebral ischemia-induced BBB disruption by preserving the expression of claudin 5 [71], whereas Lin et al. observed that Vit C (500 mg/kg i.p.) prevented compression-induced BBB disruption and sensory deficit by upregulating the expression of both occludin and claudin-5 [72].

In the available literature, there were only few studies investigating the role of Vit C in AD disease in human and the existing ones have yielded equivocal results.

Some studies have shown significantly lower plasma/serum Vit C level in AD patients as compared to healthy individuals, whereas others have found no difference [73,74]. However, meta-analysis performed by Lopes da Silva et al. proved significantly lower plasma levels of Vit C in AD patients [75]. It seems that the above discrepancies may result from the fact that not plasma but rather intracellular Vit C may be associated with AD.

Generally, studies involving human participants are limited to assessing the effect of Vit C supplementation administered with other antioxidants on AD course.

Arlt et al. [76] found that 1-month and 1-year co-supplementation of Vit C (1000 mg/day) with vitamin E (400 IU/day) increased their concentrations not only in plasma but also in cerebrospinal fluid (which reflects the Vit C status of the brain), while cerebrospinal fluid lipid oxidation was significantly reduced only after 1 year. However, vitamins' supplementation did not have a significant effect on the course of AD [76]. These findings were aslo confirmed by the randomized clinical trial of Galasko et al. [77], which showed that treatment of AD patients for 16 weeks with vitamin E (800 IU/day) plus Vit C (500 mg/day) plus α-lipoic acid (900 mg/day) did not influence cerebrospinal fluid levels of Aβ42, tau and p181tau (widely accepted biomarkers related to amyloid or tau pathology), but decreased F2-isoprostane level (a validated biomarker of oxidative stress). Moreover, is should be emphasized that the above treatment increased risk of faster cognitive decline. This seems to be consistent with results of the recent study which revealed it that Vit C was a potent antioxidant within the AD brain, but it was not able to ameliorate other factors linked to AD pathogenesis as it was proved to be a poor metal chelator and did not inhibit Aβ42 fibrillation [78]. In the study considering an association between nutrient patterns and three brain AD-biomarkers, namely Aβ load, glucose metabolism and gray matter volumes (a marker of brain atrophy) in AD-vulnerable regions, it was found that the higher intake of carotenoids, vitamin A, vitamin C and dietary fibers was positively associated only with glucose metabolism [79].

On the other hand, a randomized control trial involving 276 elderly participants demonstrated that 16-week-co-supplementation of vitamin E and C with β-carotene significantly improved cognitive function (particularly with higher doses of β-carotene). Furthermore, the authors suggested that such a treatment markedly reduced plasma Aβ levels and elevated plasma estradiol levels [80]. Vit C and E co-supplementation for more than 3 years was also shown to be associated with a reduced prevalence and incidence of AD [81]. Moreover, an adequate Vit C plasma level seems to be associated with less progression in carotid intima-media thickness (C-IMT)—the greater C-IMT is suggested to be a risk factor in predicting cognitive decline in the general population, in the elderly population and in patients with Alzheimer's disease. Polidori et al. showed significant decrease (with a linear slope) in Vit C level among old individuals with no or very mild cognitive impairment from the first to the fourth C-IMT quartile [82].

5.2. Parkinson's Disease

Parkinson's disease (PD) is a common long-term neurodegenerative movement disorder characterized by the progressive loss of substantia nigra dopaminergic neurons and consequent depletion of dopamine in the striatum. Dementia, depression and behavioral deficiencies are common symptoms in the advanced stages of the disease [22]. PD is pathologically heterogeneous, but abnormal aggregation of α-synuclein (α-syn) within neuronal perikarya (Lewy bodies) and neurites (Lewy neurites) are neuropathological (but not pathognomonic) hallmarks of this disease [83]. The primary cause of the neurodegenerative process underlying PD is still unknown. Only about 10% of PD cases have shown to be hereditary, whereas the rest are sporadic and result from complex interactions between environmental and common genetic risk factors. Monogenic PD with autosomal-dominant inheritance is caused by mutation in α-synuclein gene (*SNCA*) or leucine-rich repeat kinase 2 gene (*LRRK2*), whereas the form with autosomal recessive inheritance by mutations in the genes encoding Parkin 2 (*PARK2*), PTEN-induced putative kinase 1 (*PINK1*), protein deglycase DJ-1 (*PARK7*), and protein ATP13A2 (*PARK9*). However, many diverse genetic defects in other loci have been suggested to be associated with PD. Candidate genes which have been reported to be associated with PD include e.g., β-glucocerebrosidase (*GBA*), diacylglycerol kinase θ, 110kD (*GAK-DGKQ*), *SNCA*, human leukocyte antigen (*HLA*), *RAD51B*, *DYRK1A*, *CHCHD2*, *VPS35*, *RAB39B* or *TMEM230* [84,85]. Different mechanisms, including genomic factors, epigenetic changes, toxic factors, mitochondrial dysfunction, oxidative stress, neuroimmune/neuroinflammatory reactions, hypoxic-ischemic conditions, metabolic deficiencies and ubiquitin–proteasome system dysfunction, seem to be involved in PD pathogenesis [84,86–92]. Mitochondrial dysfunction has been shown to be linked to mutations in *PINK1* and *DJ1* genes [87,88]. Moreover, it is known that dopamine metabolism produces oxidant species, whereas oxidative stress participates in protein aggregation in PD [22,90,93]. Glutamate-mediated excitotoxicity has been proposed to be a further PD factor. It is also suggested that, like in the case of AD, PD might be a prion-like disease [94–96]. Olanow et al. [94] proposed the hypothesis that α-synuclein is a prion-like protein that can adopt a self-propagating conformation and thereby cause neurodegeneration. Scheffold et al. [97], in turn, reported that telomere shortening (one of the hallmarks of ageing) led to an acceleration of synucleinopathy and impaired microglia response and thereby might contribute to PD pathology. It is likely that not the above factors per se, but rather their synergistic interactions result in the development of the nigrostriatal damage in PD.

Vit C is believed to play a role in dopaminergic neuron differentiation. He et al. [98] in in vitro study found that Vit C enhanced the differentiation of midbrain derived neural stem cell towards dopaminergic neurons by increasing 5-hydroxymethylcytosine (5hmC) and decreasing histone H3 lysine 27 tri-methylation (H3K27m3) generation in dopamine phenotype gene promoters, which are catalyzed by ten-eleven-translocation 1 methylcytosine dioxygenase 1 (Tet1) and histone H3K27 demethylase (Jmjd3), respectively [98,99]. It seems that Vit C acts through regulation of Tet1 and Jmjd3 activities (it acts as a co-factor), since Tet1 and Jmjd3 knockdown/inhibition resulted in no effect of Vit C on either 5hmC or H3K27m3 in the progenitor cells [98]. In another in vitro study, it was shown that mouse embryonic fibroblasts cultured in Vit C-free medium displayed extremely low content of 5hmC, whereas treatment with Vit C resulted in a dose- and time-dependent increase in 5-hmC generation, which was not associated with any change in *Tet* genes expression. Additionally, it was found that treatment with another reducing agent as glutathione did not affect 5-hmC, whereas blocking Vit C entry into cells or knocking down *Tet* expression significantly reduced the effect of Vit C on 5-hmC [100].

Vit C is also believed to play an indirect role in α-syn oligomerization. Posttranslational α-syn modifications caused by oxidative stress, including modification by 4-hydroxy-2-nonenal, nitration and oxidation, have been implicated to promote oligomerization of α-syn, whereas Vit C as an antioxidant prevents this effect [22,101]. Jinsmaa et al. [102] found that treatment with Vit C attenuated Cu^{2+}-mediated augmentation of 3,4-dihydroxyphenylacetaldehyde (DOPAL)-induced α-syn oligomerization in rat pheochromocytoma PC12 cells, but alone (without Cu^{2+}) did not exert such an effect. Khan et al. showed, in turn, that Vit C supplementation (227.1 μM, 454.2 μM or 681.3 μM in diet, 21 days) caused a significant dose-dependent delay in the loss of climbing ability of PD Drosophila model expressing normal human α-syn in the neurons [103].

Moreover, Vit C is thought to be involved in neuroprotection against glutamate-mediated excitotoxicity occurring in PD. Ballaz et al. [104] in in vitro study performed on dopaminergic neurons of human origin showed that Vit C prevented cell death following prolonged exposure to glutamate. Glutamate induced toxicity in a dose-dependent way via the stimulation of α-amino-3-hydroxy-5-methyl-4-isoxazole propionic acid (AMPA) and metabotropic receptors and to a lesser degree by *N*-methyl-D-aspartate (NMDA) and kainate receptors, whereas Vit C (25–300 μM) administration protected cells against glutamate excitotoxity. The authors emphasized the fact that such a neuroprotection effect was dependent on the inhibition of oxidative stress, as Vit C prevented the pro-oxidant action of quercetin occurred over the course of prolonged exposure [104]. Vit C neuroprotection effect against dose-dependent glutamate-induced neurodegeneration in the postnatal brain was also confirmed by Shah et al. [50].

The effect of Vit C on dopamine system has also been observed. Izumi et al. [105] showed that PC12 cells treated with paraquat (50 μM, 24 h) displayed increased levels of cytosolic and vesicular dopamine, whereas pretreatment with Vit C (0.3–10 μM, 24 h) suppressed the elevations of intracellular dopamine and almost completely prevented paraquat toxicity.

Human studies have shown that Vit C deficiency among PD patients is widespread [106,107]. However, similarly like in the case of AD, not plasma but rather intracellular Vit C seems to be associated with PD. This could to be confirmed by the study performed by Ide et al. [108] who investigated the association between both lymphocyte and plasma Vit C levels in various stages of PD. Lymphocyte Vit C levels in patients with severe PD was significantly lower compared to those at less severe stages, whereas plasma Vit C levels showed a decreasing tendency; however that effect was not significant [108].

Although in the newest literature data, there are only a few human studies considering the role of Vit C treatment in PD, the existing ones give some evidences that Vit C treatment may have beneficial effect in PD course. A cohort study involving 1036 PD patients showed that dietary Vit C intake was significantly associated with reduced PD risk. However, it was not significant in a 4-year lagged analysis [109]. Quiroga et al., in turn, reported a case of a 66-year-old man with PD, pleural effusion and bipolar disorder who was found to have low serum Vit C and zinc levels. Intravenous replacement of both Vit C and zinc resulted in resolution of the movement disorder in less than 24 h [107]. The other case report concerned 83-year-old men with dementia, diabetes mellitus, hypertension, benign prostatic hypertension, paroxysmal atrial fibrillation, congestive heart failure and suspected PD. The man was treated with Vit C (200 mg) and zinc (4 mg), which resulted in complete resolution of periungual and gingival bleeding as well as palatal petechiae. Moreover, the man's orientation and mental status were found to be markedly improved and no further delusions or agitations were observed [110].

Vit C was shown to increase L-dopa (3,4-dihydroxy-L-phenylalanine, one of the main drugs used in PD therapy) absorption in elderly PD patients. However, this effect was not observed in all patients but only in those with poor baseline L-dopa bioavailability [111]. Moreover, in vitro study performed by Mariam et al. revealed that Vit C is a strong inducer of L-dopa production from pre-grown mycelia of Aspergillus oryzae NRRL-1560 [112].

5.3. Huntington's Disease

Huntington's disease (HD) is a genetic, autosomal dominant disorder characterized by general neurodegeneration in brain with marked deterioration of medium-sized spiny neurons (MSNs) in the striatum [17,113]. HD is caused by a mutation (a CAG expansion) in the huntingtin gene (*HTT*), which results in an abnormal polyglutamine expansion in the huntingtin (HTT) protein and consequently HTT aggregation [113]. The mutant HTT alters intracellular Ca^{2+} homeostasis, induces mitochondrial dysfunction, disrupts intracellular trafficking and impairs gene transcription [114].

Clinically, HD is characterized by tripartite clinical features, namely progressive motor dysfunction (so-called choreic movements), neuropsychiatric symptoms and a variety of cognitive deficits [115,116]. Neuropathologically, HD is associated with a progressive, selective neuronal dysfunction and degeneration, especially in the both part of striatum (caudate and putamen) [117,118].

HD is known to be associated with a failure in energy metabolism, impaired mitochondrial ATP production and oxidative damage [113,119–121]. Other mechanisms, such as excitotoxicity, aberrant glutamatergic, dopaminergic and Ca^{2+} signaling mechanisms, metabolic damage, immune response, apoptosis as well as autophagy are also suggested to be involved in HD pathology [119,121–124].

Vit C flux from astrocytes to neurons during synaptic activity is regarded to be essential for protecting neurons against oxidative damage and modulation of neuronal metabolism, thus permitting optimal ATP production [119]. Under physiological conditions, Vit C is released from astrocytes to striatal extracellular fluid during increased synaptic activity. The enhancement of Vit C concentration in striatal extracellular fluid results in SVCT2 translocation to the plasma membrane and consequently Vit C uptake by neurons [119]. In neurons, Vit C is able to scavenge reactive oxygen species generated during synaptic activity and neuronal metabolism. As a result, Vit C is oxidized to dihydroascorbate, which is then released into the extracellular fluid and uptaken by neighboring astrocytes, where is subsequently turned back to a reduced form, which can be used again by neurons. Vit C can interact directly with reactive oxygen species but can also act as a co-factor in the reduction of other antioxidants as glutathione and α-tocopherol. Moreover, Vit C may function as a neuronal metabolic switch, which means that it is capable to inhibit glucose consumption and permit lactate uptake/use as a substrate to sustain synaptic activity. This function is not dependent on antioxidant activity of Vit C [47] and seems to be of great importance, taking into account that decreased expression of GLUT3 in both STHdhQ cells (striatal neurons derived from knock-in mice expressing mutant huntingtin; cell model of HD) and R6/2 mice (mouse model of HD) as well as impaired GLUT3 localization at the plasma membrane in HD cells were observed [125].

Unfortunately, the mechanism mentioned above does not work properly in HD. Abnormal Vit C flux from astrocytes to neurons was found both in R6/2 mice and STHdhQ cells. Acuña et al. proved that SVCT2 failed to reach the plasma membrane in cells expressing mutant Htt, which resulted in disturbed Vit C uptake by neurons [119]. Additionally, there is some evidence that altered glutamate transporter activity (GLT1—the protein primarily found on astrocytes and responsible for removing most extracellular glutamate), observed in HD, is related to deficient striatal Vit C release into extracellular fluid [126–128]. Miller et al. performed the study on R6/2 mice receiving ceftriaxone (200 mg/kg, once daily injection per 5 days)—a β-lactam antibiotic that selectively increases the expression of GLT1. To evaluate Vit C release in vivo voltammetry combined with corticostriatal afferent stimulation was used. R6/2 mice treated with saline displayed a marked decrease in striatal extracellular Vit C level compared to control group, whereas treatment with ceftriaxone restored striatal Vit C in R6/2 mice to control level and also improved the HD behavioral phenotype. It was also shown that intra-striatal infusion of GLT1 inhibitor (dihydrokainic acid or DL-*threo*-β-benzyloxyaspartate) blocked evoked striatal Vit C release [126]. Dorner et al., in turn, observed that cortical stimulation resulted in a rapid increase in Vit C release in both R6/2 and wild-type mice, but the response had a significantly shorter duration and smaller magnitude in R6/2 group. The researchers also measured striatal Vit C release in response to treatment with d-amphetamine (5 mg/kg)—a psychomotor stimulant known to release Vit C from corticostriatal terminals independently of dopamine. Both

Vit C release and behavioral activation were diminished in R6/2 mice compared to wild-type ones. The authors concluded that the corticostriatal pathway was directly involved in behavior-related Vit C release and that this system was dysfunctional in HD [127]. It is thought that Vit C is released into striatal extracellular fluid as glutamate is uptaken—glutamate/Vit C heteroexchange. Consequently, Vit C level decreases while glutamate level increases in extracellular fluid of HD striatum owing to a downregulation of GLT1 [127,128]. Elevated glutamate level in synaptic gaps leads to abnormal signal transmission.

In addition, it is also believed that long-term oxidative stress (one of the key players in HD progression) eliminates the ability of Vit C to modulate glucose utilization [125].

The effect of Vit C treatment on behavior-related neuronal activity was studied by Rebec et al. [129]. The authors showed that in the striatum of R6/2 mice impulse activity was consistently elevated compared to wild-type mice, whereas restoring extracellular Vit C to the wild-type level by Vit C treatment (300 mg/kg, 3 days) reversed this effect. This suggests Vit C involvement in normalization of neuronal function in HD striatum. In another study, the same researchers reported that regular injections of Vit C (300 mg/kg/day, 4 days/week) restored the behavior-related release of Vit C in striatum, which was associated with improved behavioral responding. Vit C treatment significantly attenuated the neurological motor signs of HD without altering overall motor activity [130].

Although studies performed on cell and animal models of HD appear to indicate the role of Vit C in HD course, to the best of our knowledge, in the newest literature there exists a lack of studies considering the role of Vit C or the effect of its supplementation in HD human subjects.

5.4. Multiple Sclerosis

Multiple sclerosis (MS) is a progressive demyelinating process considered as an autoimmune disease of unknown etiology. MS is characterized by infiltration of immune cells (in particular T cells and macrophages), demyelination (loss of myelin sheath that surrounds and protects nerve fibers allowing them to conduct electrical impulses) and axonal pathology resulting in multiple neurological deficits, which range from motor and sensory deficits to cognitive and psychological impairment [131,132]. The etiology of MS is still unknown, but it is suggested that genetic predisposition associated with environmental factors can lead to expression of the envelope protein of MS-associated retrovirus (MSRV) and thus trigger the disease [133]. Although pathogenesis of MS has not been fully clarified yet, either destruction by the immune system or a significant extent apoptosis, particularly apoptosis of oligodendroglia cells, are believed to be underlying mechanism. Oxidative/nitrosative stress and mitochondrial dysfunction are believed to contribute to the pathophysiology of MS [131,134–137].

Having regarded the presented facts, it seems to be justified that Vit C, being a very important brain antioxidant, may affect MS course. Vit C is known to affect numerous metabolic processes directly associated with immune system. Furthermore, Vit C-dependent collagen synthesis has also been linked to formation of the myelin sheath [7].

In the literature data, there are only a few studies considering association between MS and Vit C. However, the existing ones showed that MS patients displayed significantly lower Vit C level as compared to healthy individuals [135,136,138]. Besler et al. [138], in turn, observed an inverse correlation between the serum levels of Vit C and lipid peroxidation in MS patients. The authors concluded that decreased Vit C level, observed in MS patients during relapse of the disease, might be dependent on the elevated oxidative burden as reflected by increased lipid peroxidation. Hejazi et al. [139], in turn, found no significant difference between daily intake of Vit C (recorded from a 24-h dietary recall questionnaire for 3 days) in MS patients ($n = 37$) in comparison with healthy subjects. The intake of Vit C in both groups was below dietary reference intake (DRI), however in control group it was near the DRI value.

An efficiency of antioxidant therapy in relapsing-remitting multiple sclerosis patients ($n = 14$) treated with complex of antioxidants and neuroprotectors with various mechanisms of action (α-lipoic acid, nicotinamide, acetylcysteine, triovit beta-carotine, alpha-tocopheryl acetate, ascorbic acid, selenium, pentoxifylline, cerebrolysin, amantadine hydrochloride) during 1 month, 2 times a year was investigated by Odinak et al. [140]. The treatment resulted in significant reduction of relapse frequency, decrease of required corticosteroid courses and significantly reduced content of lipid peroxide products [140]. However, it should be underlined that Vit C was only one element of multicomponent treatment. However, in another study it was shown that intrahippocampal injection of Vit C (0.2, 1, 5 mg/kg, 7 days) improved memory acquisition of passive avoidance learning (PAL) in ethidium bromide-induced MS in rats. The injection of ethidium bromide caused significant deterioration of PAL, whereas treatment with Vit C at a dose of 5 mg/kg resulted in significant improvement in PAL [141].

Summing up, the possible role of Vit C in MS course remains to be explored.

5.5. Amyotrophic Lateral Sclerosis

Amyotrophic lateral sclerosis (ALS) is an incurable, chronic progressive neurodegenerative disease characterized by the degeneration of upper motor neurons in the motor cortex and lower motor neurons in the spinal cord and the brain stem [142]; the reason why only motor neurons are targeted remains unknown. ALS results in loss of power and function of skeletal muscles, which is reflected by difficulties in walking, using the arms, speaking and swallowing. ALS occurs in two forms: hereditary one, which is called familial (5–10% of ALS cases) and not hereditary one, called sporadic. Familial ALS is indistinguishable from the much more common sporadic form, but usually it begins at a slightly younger age. It is assumed that about 2% of all cases of ALS are caused by mutations in the gene encoding copper/zinc superoxide dismutase (SOD1) on chromosome 21, but the etiology of the remaining ALS cases is not fully understood. The course of ALS is variable, but usually relatively rapid. Most patients die, usually due to respiratory failure (respiratory muscles paralysis), within 3–5 years from the onset of symptoms [143].

Although the underlying causes of motor neuron degeneration remain still unknown, researchers have suggested a contribution of oxidative stress, mitochondrial dysfunction, glutamate-mediated excitotoxicity, cytoskeletal abnormalities, and protein aggregation [144]. Because of the above-presented facts and its activity-dependent release in the brain, it seems to be possible that Vit C may be involved in ALS pathogenesis. It appears to be confirmed by Blasco et al. who compared 1 H-NMR spectra of cerebrospinal fluid (CSF) samples collected from ALS patients ($n = 44$) and patients without a neurodegenerative disease. The authors found significantly higher Vit C level in the ALS group. Vit C, apart from being free radical scavenger, was suggested to modulate neuronal metabolism by reducing glucose consumption during episodes of glutamatergic synaptic activity and stimulating lactate uptake in neurons, which is consistent with lower lactate/pyruvate ratio seen in ALS patients [144].

However, in the available literature data, there are only a few studies evaluating an association between Vit C and ALS, and the existing ones have not proved its role in the course of this disease.

Nagano et al. [145] investigated the efficacy of Vit C treatment (0.8% *w/w* in the diet) in familiar ALS mice, administered before or after the onset of the disease. The mice treated with Vit C before disease onset survived significantly longer by 62% than the control. However, that treatment did not affect the mean age of onset appearance and administration after disease onset did not prolong survival. Netzahualcoyotzi and Tapia [146] found that the infusion of Vit C (20 mM), alone or in combination with glutathione ethylester, did not prevent the AMPA-induced motor alterations of the rear limbs and motor neuron degradation in rats. The pooled analysis of 5 large prospective studies of about 1100 ALS patients performed by Fitzgerald et al. showed that neither supplementation (even long-term) nor high dietary intake of Vit C affected risk of ALS [147]. Okamoto et al. [148] investigated the relationship between dietary intake of vegetables, fruit and antioxidants and the risk of ALS (153 ALS patients aged 18–81 years with disease duration of 3 years) in Japan. The study showed that a higher consumption of fruits and/or vegetables was associated with a significantly reduced risk of ALS. However, no significant dose-response relationship was observed between intake of beta-carotene,

Vit C and vitamin E and the risk of ALS. Spasojević et al. [149], in turn, suggested that the use of Vit C could have an unfavorable effect in ALS patients. The researchers examined the effect of Vit C on the production of hydroxyl radicals in CSF obtained from sporadic ALS patients. Using electron paramagnetic resonance spectroscopy, the authors detected ascorbyl radicals in CSF of ALS patients, whereas in control CSF they were undetectable. Moreover, the addition of hydrogen peroxide to the CSF of ALS patients provoked further formation of ascorbyl as well as hydroxyl radicals ex vivo. Thus, it seems that herein Vit C may paradoxically induce pro-oxidative effects. This may result from the fact that Vit C is an excellent one-electron reducing agent that can reduce ferric (Fe^{3+}) ion to ferrous (Fe^{2+}) one, while being oxidized to ascorbate radical. In a Fenton reaction, Fe^{2+} reacts with H_2O_2 generating Fe^{3+} and a very strong oxidizing agent—hydroxyl radical. The presence of Vit C allows the recycling of Fe^{3+} back to Fe^{2+}, which can subsequently catalyze the successive formation of hydroxyl radicals [1,150]. Moreover, it has also been shown that high concentrations of ascorbyl radical can reduce SOD activity.

6. Role of Vitamin C in Psychiatric Disorders

Vit C is also believed to be involved in anxiety, stress, depression, fatigue and mood state in humans. It has been hypothesized that oral Vit C supplementation can elevate mood as well as reduce distress and anxiety.

6.1. Depression

Depression (DP) is a mental disorder characterized by a number of basic symptoms like low mood, biological rhythm disorders, psychomotor slowdown, anxiety, somatic disorders as well other nonspecific symptoms [151]. It has a multifactorial etiology, with biological, psychological, social and lifestyle factors of important roles [152]. Several hypotheses have been proposed to explain the mechanisms underlying depression. Firstly, it is believed that depression is associated with disturbances of serotonin, norepinephrine and dopamine neurotransmission. Moreover, many observations have supported the involvement of GABAergic system in the pathomechanism of depression [153]. GABA level in plasma and CSF of patients suffering from depression was shown to be reduced [154,155] which points to its decreased synthesis in the brain. Recent data have suggested that chronic stress, via initiating changes in the hypothalamic-pituitary-adrenal axis and the immune system, acts as a trigger for the above-mentioned disturbance. For example, glucocorticoids and proinflammatory cytokines enhance the conversion of tryptophan to kynurenine thus leading to a decrease in the synthesis of brain serotonin (because less tryptophan is available for conversion to serotonin) and an increase in the formation of neurotoxic metabolites, e.g., glutamate antagonist quinolinic acid. The activity of the dopaminergic systems was also found to be reduced in response to inflammation [156]. Secondly, some genetic factors have been suggested to be implicated in depression etiology [157]. Thirdly, apoptosis of the brain cells seems to be involved in depression development, since a numerical and morphological alterations of astrocytes in patients with major depressive disorder were observed [158–161]. This may also be dependent, at least partially, on proinflammatory cytokine actions since quinolinic acid was shown to contribute to the increase in apoptosis of astrocytes or neurons [162,163].

Basing on several animal studies [153,155,164–166], there is preliminary evidence that Vit C exerts an antidepressant-like effect via:

1. modulation of monoaminergic systems [167] (e.g., Vit C was shown to activate the serotonin 1A (5-HT1A) receptor, this activation is a mechanism of action of many antidepressant, anxiolytic and antipsychotic drugs);
2. modulation of GABAergic systems (via activation of $GABA_A$ receptors and a possible inhibition of $GABA_B$ receptors) [155];

3. inhibition of *N*-methyl-D-aspartate (NMDA) receptors and L-arginine-nitric oxide (NO)-cyclic guanosine 3,5-monophosphate (cGMP) pathway—the blockade of NMDA receptor is associated with reduced levels of NO and cGMP, whereas reduction of NO levels within the hippocampus was shown to induce antidepressant-like effects [119];

4. blocking potassium (K$^+$) channels—Vit C administration was shown to produce an antidepressant-like effect in the tail suspension test via K$^+$ channel inhibition [119]; as K$^+$ channels were reported to belong to the physiological targets of NO and cGMP in the brain, their inhibition plays a significant role in the treatment of depression;

5. activation of phosphatidylinositol-3-kinase (PI3K) and inhibition of glycogen synthase kinase 3 beta (GSK-3β) activity [112,119];

6. induction of heme oxygenase 1 expression—it is a candidate depression biomarker which may be a link factor between inflammation, oxidative stress and the biological as well functional changes in brain activity in depression; its decreased expression is associated with depressive symptoms [166,168];

7. since depression is well known to be associated with altered anti- and prooxidant profiles, Vit C may play antidepressant function also by its antioxidant properties [118,119].

The available literature data indicate that Vit C deficiency is very common in patients with depressive disorders. Gariballa [169] in a randomized, double blind, placebo-controlled trial observed that low Vit C status was associated with increased depression symptoms following acute illness in older people. Parameters were measured at baseline as well as after 6 weeks and 6 months. Patients with Vit C depletion had significantly increased symptoms of depression as compared to those with its higher concentrations both at baseline and at 6 weeks. Significantly lower serum Vit C level in patients with depression vs. healthy controls was also shown by Bajpai et al. [170] and Gautam et al. [171]. Moreover, in the latter study dietary supplementation of Vit C (1000 mg/day) along with vitamins A and E for a period of 6 weeks resulted in a significant reduction in depression scores [171]. Furthermore, a case-control study carried out on 60 male university students showed that subjects diagnosed with depression had significantly lower intake of Vit C than the healthy ones [172]. Similarly, in another case-control study involving 116 girls identified as having depressive symptoms, depression was negatively associated with Vit C intake, even after adjusting for confounding variables [173]. Rubio-López et al. [174], in turn, examined the relationship between nutritional intake and depressive symptoms in 710 Valencian schoolchildren aged 6–9 years and also observed that nutrient intake of Vit C was significantly lower in children with depressive symptoms. Additionally, prevalence of Vit C inadequacy (below dietary recommended intakes) was significantly higher in subjects with depressive symptoms.

The efficacy of Vit C as an adjuvant agent in the treatment of pediatric major depressive disorder in a double-blind, placebo-controlled pilot trial was evaluated by Amr et al. [175]. Patients (*n* = 12) treated for six months with fluoxetine (10–20 mg/day) and Vit C (1000 mg/day) showed a significant decrease in depressive symptoms in comparison with the fluoxetine plus placebo group as measured by the Children's Depression Rating Scale and Children's Depression Inventory. No serious adverse effects were shown. Zhang et al. [176] in double-blind clinical trial investigated the effect of Vit C (500 mg twice daily) on mood in non-depressed acutely hospitalized patients. The applied therapy increased plasma and mononuclear leukocyte Vit C concentrations and was associated with a 34% reduction in mood disturbance (assessed with Profile of Mood States) [176]. Similarly, Wang et al. found that short-term Vit C (500 mg twice daily) treatment was associated with a 71% reduction in mood disturbance (assessed with Profile of Mood States) and a 51% reduction in psychological distress (assessed with Distress Thermometer) in acutely hospitalized patients with a high prevalence of hypovitaminosis C [177]. Khajehnasiri et al. [178] in a randomized, double-blind, placebo-controlled trial involving 136 depressed male shift workers observed, in turn, that Vit C administration (250 mg twice daily for 2 months) alone and in combination with omega-3 fatty acids significantly reduced the Beck Depression Inventory (BDI) score, however omega-3 fatty acid supplementation alone was more effective. Moreover, Vit C and omega-3 fatty acids supplementation alone (but not in combination) decreased significantly serum MDA levels. Fritz et al. [179] conducted a systematic review of human and observational studies assessing the efficiency of interventional Vit C as a contentious adjunctive cancer therapy and reported that it could improve quality of life, physical function, as well as prevent some side effects of chemotherapy, including fatigue, nausea, insomnia, constipation and depression.

6.2. Anxiety

Anxiety is an adaptive response to uncertain threat, but it becomes pathological when is disproportionate to the threat, persists beyond the presence of the stressor, or is triggered by innocuous stimuli or situations. Similarly like in the case of depression, neurotransmitter system disruptions (namely GABA, serotonin and noradrenalin) as well as an impaired regulation of the hypothalamic-pituitary-adrenal axis are involved in anxiety disorders [180]. Furthermore, several studies have suggested a positive correlation between oxidative stress and anxiety-like behavior.

The growing evidence, which has been recently emerged, suggests that anxiety is associated with Vit C deficit, whereas Vit C supplementation could help reduce feeling of anxiety. The underlying mechanism is not fully understood yet, but Vit C seems to play this role by: regulating neurotransmitters' activity, attenuating cortisol activity, preventing stress-induced oxidative damage and antioxidant defense in brain or some as yet undetermined effects on anxiety-related brain structures [181].

Kori et al. [182] observed that rats subjected to restrained stress (by placing in a wire mesh restrainer for 6 h per day for 21 days) displayed a significant increase in serum cortisol level with concomitant decrease in serum Vit C and E levels. Boufleur et al. [183], in turn, found decreased plasma Vit C levels in rats exposed to chronic mild stress. Interestingly, neonatal handling could prevent Vit C reduction in rats exposed to chronic mild stress in adulthood. Koizumi et al. [184] showed that Vit C status was critical for determining vulnerability to anxiety in a sex-specific manner. The study was performed on senescence marker protein–30/gluconolactones knockout mice (unable to synthesize Vit C) whose Vit C status was continuously shifted from adequate to depleted one (by providing a water with or without Vit C). It was observed that anxiety responses in the novelty-suppressed feeding paradigm were worse during Vit C depletion conditions, especially in females. Hughes et al. [181], in turn, reported that prolonged treatment with Vit C (approximately 80 mg/kg/day in drinking water, 83 days) markedly decreased anxiety-related behavior in the open field test in hooded rats. In another study, the same researchers examined the effect of Vit C treatment with three doses (61, 114 or 160 mg/kg/day in drinking water, 8 weeks) and observed that an anxiolytic effects of Vit C were displayed in higher frequencies of walking (with doses of 114 mg/kg/day and 160 mg/kg/day), higher frequencies of rearing (with dose of 61 mg/kg/day) and lower frequencies of grooming (with dose of 61 mg/kg/day) in the open-field as well as more frequent occupation of the open arms in the elevated plus-maze (with dose of 61 mg/kg/day). The authors concluded that anxiolytic effects of Vit C were more typical of the lowest dose and it was to some extent dependent on anxiety intensity [185]. The effect of Vit C on adrenal gland function (an element of the stress response system) was investigated by Choi et al. [186]. An adrenalectomized (ADX) and non-ADX rats were treated with Vit C (25 or 100 m/kg, 7 days) and subsequently subjected to both Vit C treatment and electroshock stress for next 5 days. Vit C supplementation reduced corticosterone level in non-ADX rats. Stress decreased the mean value of rearing frequency in both non-ADX and ADX rats, whereas Vit C partially attenuated this effect in non-ADX group. Moreover, Vit C treatment decreased adrenocorticotropic hormone in both groups and significantly reduced freezing time increased by stress. The authors suggested that the alleviating effect of Vit C on stress-related rearing behavior was exerted via modulation of corticosterone, whereas the effect on freezing behavior via modulation of corticotropin-releasing hormone or adrenocorticotropin-releasing hormone [186]. Puty et al. [187] in turn suggested that Vit C plays anxiolytic-like effect via affecting serotonergic system. The researchers evaluated the protective effect of Vit C against methylmercury (MeHg)-induced anxiogenic-like effect in zebrafish.

MeHg produced a marked anxiogenic effects in the light/dark box test, which was accompanied by a decrease in the extracellular levels of serotonin as well an increase in its oxidized metabolite tryptamine-4,5-dione, whereas pretreatment with Vit C (2 mg/g, i.p.) prevented such alterations. Furthermore, Angrini and Leslie [188] found that pretreatment with Vit C (100 mg or 200 mg/kg) could attenuate, especially the higher dose, behavioral and anxiogenic effects of prolonged exposure to noise (100 dB for 2 months, 5 days/week, 4 h daily) on male laboratory mice.

Although there are only a few studies considering the effects of vitamin C on anxiety and stress responses in humans, the existing ones seem to provide promising results.

De Oliveira et al. [189] examined the effects of short-term oral Vit C supplementation (500 mg/day, 14 days) in high school students (*n* = 42) in a randomized, double-blind, placebo-controlled trial. The treatment led to higher plasma Vit C concentration that was associated with reduced anxiety levels evaluated with BIA (Beck Anxiety Inventory). Moreover, the Vit C supplementation had positive effect on the heart rate. Gautam et al. [171] observed that patients with generalized anxiety disorder had significantly lower Vit C levels in comparison with healthy controls, whereas 6-week vitamins supplementation (vitamin C accompanied with A and E) led to a significant reduction in anxiety scores [171]. Mazloom et al. [190], in turn, showed that short-term supplementation of Vit C (1000 mg/day) reduced anxiety levels (evaluated basing on Depression Anxiety Stress Scales 21-item) in diabetic patients. This effect was exerted through alleviating oxidative damage. Furthermore, recently performed a systematic review also showed that high-dose Vit C supplementation was effective in reducing anxiety as well as stress-induced blood pressure increase [191].

6.3. Schizophrenia

Schizophrenia is a severe and complex neuropsychiatric disorder that affects 1% of the population worldwide [192–194]. Symptoms of schizophrenia are described as "positive" (also so-called productive) and "negative" ones: the first include hallucinations, paranoia and delusions, while negative examples are: limited motivation, impaired speech, weakening and social withdrawal. These symptoms usually appear in early adulthood and often persist in about three-fourths of patients despite optimum treatment [192]. Some authors have suggested that insufficient dopamine level due to the loss of dopamine producing cells may lead to schizophrenia [195]. On the other hand, it has been postulated that schizophrenia has been linked to hyperactivity of brain dopaminergic systems that may reflect an underlying dysfunction of NMDA receptor-mediated neurotransmission [194]. Furthermore, there is the increasing evidence that several physiological mechanisms such as oxidative stress, altered one carbon metabolism and atypical immune-mediated responses may be involved in schizophrenia pathomechanism [192,196].

Hoffer [197] summarized in the review study the evidence showing that among others Vit C deficiency could worsen the symptoms of schizophrenia and that large doses of this vitamin could improve the core metabolic abnormalities predisposing some people to development of this disease. According to the author, it is probable that the pathologic process responsible for schizophrenia could increase ascorbic acid utilization. Sarandol et al. [198] also noted lower levels of serum Vit C as compared to control group, but this was not regarded as a statistically significant difference. Moreover, a 6-week-long antipsychotic treatment did not modify the concentration of this vitamin. The authors explained that other factors, such as nutrition, physical activity, etc., might be the reason for the discrepancy between the results of their research and other studies. Similarly, Young et al. [199] observed only a slight decrease in Vit C levels in schizophrenic group vs. control one; but interestingly, a highly significant increase in Vit C level in the control female group as compared to both control as well as schizophrenic male group was observed. The authors pointed out that this information might be relevant particularly in the light of recent reports that the risk of schizophrenia is higher in men than women. The reduced supply of Vit C with the diet in patients with schizophrenia was noted by Konarzewska et al. [200].

The review of Magalhães et al. revealed that the implementation of Vit C as a low-molecular-weight antioxidant alleviated the effects of free radicals in the treatment of schizophrenia [201]. According to Bentsen et al. [202] membrane lipid metabolism and redox regulation may be disturbed in schizophrenia. These authors conducted a study aiming at examination of the clinical effect of adding vitamins E + C to antipsychotics (D_2 receptor antagonists). Patients with schizophrenia or related psychoses received Vit C (1000 mg/day) along with vitamin E (364 mg/day) for 16 weeks. Vitamins impaired the course of psychotic symptoms, especially of persecutory delusions. The authors pointed to the usefulness of supplementation of antioxidant vitamins as agents alleviating some side effects of antipsychotic drugs. This was also confirmed by the next study involving schizophrenia patients treated with haloperidol [203]. Classical antipsychotics like haloperidol are suggested to increase oxidative stress and oxidative cell injury in brain, which may influence the course as well as treatment effects of schizophrenia. In this study, chronic haloperidol treatment connected with supplementation of a combination of ω-3 fatty acids and vitamins E and C showed a significant beneficial effect on schizophrenia treatment as measured by SANS (Simpson Angus Scale) and BPRS (Brief Psychiatric Rating Scale) scales. BPRS total score and subscale scores as well as SANS scores were significantly improved starting from the 4th week of treatment. Moreover, in patients with schizophrenia after 16 weeks of treatment, serum Vit C levels were almost twice as high as at the beginning of the study. These results supported the hypothesis of a beneficial effect of the applied supplementation both on positive and negative symptoms of schizophrenia as well as the severity of side effects induced by haloperidol [203]. Heiser et al. [204] also stated that reactive oxygen species (ROS) were involved in the pathophysiology of psychiatric disorders such as schizophrenia. Their research demonstrated that antipsychotics induced ROS formation in the whole blood of rats, which could be reduced by the application of vitamin C. The aim of their study was to demonstrate the effects of clozapine, olanzapine and haloperidol at different doses (18, 90 and 180 μg/mL) on the formation of ROS in the whole blood by using electron spin resonance spectroscopy. To demonstrate the protective capacity of Vit C the blood samples were incubated the highest concentration of each drug with Vit C (1 mM) for 30 min. Olanzapine caused significantly greater ROS formation vs. control under all treatment conditions, while in the case of haloperidol and clozapine only two higher concentrations resulted in significantly increased ROS formation. Vitamin C reduced the ROS production of all tested drugs, but for olanzapine the attenuating effect did not reach a significant level.

A relatively novel approach as for the role of Vit C in etiology and treatment of schizophrenia was presented by Sershen et al. [193]. According to the researchers, deficits in N-methyl-D-aspartate receptor (NMDAR) function are linked to persistent negative symptoms and cognitive deficits in schizophrenia. This hypothesis is supported by the fact that the flavoprotein D-amino acid oxidase (DAO) was shown to degrade the gliotransmitter D-Ser, a potent activator of N-methyl-D-aspartate-type glutamate receptors, while a lot of evidence has suggested that DAO, together with its activator, G72 protein, may play a key role in the pathophysiology of schizophrenia. Furthermore, in a postmortem study the activity of DAO was found to be two-fold higher in schizophrenia subjects [205]. Sershen et al. [193] showed that acute ascorbic acid dose (300 mg/kg i.p.) inhibited PCP-induced and amphetamine-induced locomotor activity in mouse model, which was further attenuated in the presence of D-serine (600 mg/kg). The authors suggested that this effect could result from the Vit C-depended changes in dopamine carrier-membrane translocation and/or altered redox mechanisms that modulate NMDARs. However, this issue needs to be further investigated.

7. Conclusions

The crucial role of Vit C in neuronal maturation and functions, neurotransmitter action as well as responses to oxidative stress is well supported by the evidences presented in this review (Figure 2).

The aforementioned animal studies confirmed the usefulness of using of Vit C in the treatment of neurological diseases, both neurodegenerative and psychiatric ones. Only in the case of ALS, the possible unfavorable effects were suggested. However, studies on the role of Vit C in the course of neurological disorders in human are limited and the existing ones have aimed mostly at evaluating the effect of Vit C supplementation (often co-supplementation with other agents). Recently, a tendency toward using administration of large doses of Vit C as an adjuvant in curing of many diseases was observed. Unfortunately, in the available literature there is a lack of studies considering this issue in the context of neurological disorders.

NEURODEGENERATIVE DISEASES

Alzheimer's disease
- ↑ Oxidative stres
- ↑ Acceleration of amyloid aggregation
- ↑ Neuronal loss
- Influence on the blood-brain barrier integrity
- Influence on the phosphorylation of tau protein at Ser396

Parkinson's disease
- Oligomerization: ↑ posttranslational αSyn modifications
- ↓ Dopaminergic neuron differentiation
- ↓ Neuroprotection against glutamate-mediated excitotoxicity
- Effect on dopamine system

Huntington's disease
- ↑ Oxidative stres
- Disorders in glucose transport and metabolism
- Disorders in glutamine metabolism

Multiple sclerosis
- Disorders in collagen synthesis (demyelination)
- ↑ Oxidative stres

Amyotrophic lateral sclerosis
- ↑ Oxidative stres
- Disorders in glucose and lactate metabolism

PSYCHIATRIC DISORDERS

Depression
- Modulation of monoaminergic and GABAergic systems
- Inhibition of N-methyl-D-aspartatereceptors and L-arginine-nitric oxide-(NO)-cyclic guanosine 3,5-monophosphate (cGMP) pathway
- Blocking potassium (K^+) channels
- Activation of phosphatidylinositol-3-kinase (PI3K) and inhibition of glycogen synthase kinase 3 beta (GSK-3β) activity
- Induction of heme oxygenase 1 expression
- ↑ Oxidative stres

Anxiety
- ↑ Oxidative stres
- Disturbances in neurotransmitters' activities
- ↓ Cortisol activity

Vitamin C
deficiency in the brain

Schizophrenia
- Changes in dopamine carrier-membrane translocation
- Alteration of redox mechanisms modulating NMDARs
- ↑ Oxidative stres

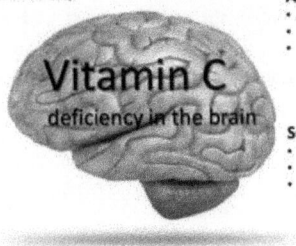

Figure 2. The main potential consequences of brain Vit C deficiency in the course and pathogenesis of neurological disorders.

In conclusion, the future studies concerning the question if Vit C could be a promising adjuvant in therapy of neurodegenerative and/or psychiatric disorders in humans, seem to be advisable.

Conflicts of Interest: The authors declare no conflict of interest.

References

1. Du, J.; Cullen, J.J.; Buettner, G.R. Ascorbic acid: Chemistry, biology and the treatment of cancer. *Biochim. Biophys. Acta* **2012**, *1826*, 443–457. [CrossRef] [PubMed]
2. Traber, M.G.; Stevens, J.F. Vitamins C and E: Beneficial effects from a mechanistic perspective. *Free Radic. Biol. Med.* **2011**, *51*, 1000–1013. [CrossRef] [PubMed]
3. Said, H.M. Intestinal absorption of water-soluble vitamins in health and disease. *Biochem. J.* **2011**, *437*, 357–372. [CrossRef] [PubMed]
4. Berger, M.M. Vitamin C requirements in parenteral nutrition. *Gastroenterology* **2009**, *137*, 70–78. [CrossRef] [PubMed]
5. Hart, A.; Cota, A.; Makhdom, A.; Harvey, E.J. The Role of Vitamin C in Orthopedic Trauma and Bone Health. *Am. J. Orthop.* **2015**, *44*, 306–311. [PubMed]
6. Waly, M.I.; Al-Attabi, Z.; Guizani, N. Low Nourishment of Vitamin C Induces Glutathione Depletion and Oxidative Stress in Healthy Young Adults. *Prev. Nutr. Food Sci.* **2015**, *20*, 198–203. [CrossRef] [PubMed]
7. Eldridge, C.F.; Bunge, M.B.; Bunge, R.P.; Wood, P.M. Differentiation of axon-related Schwann cells in vitro. I. Ascorbic acid regulates basal lamina assembly and myelin formation. *J. Cell. Biol.* **1987**, *105*, 1023–1034. [CrossRef] [PubMed]
8. Sawicka-Glazer, E.; Czuczwar, S.J. Vitamin C: A new auxiliary treatment of epilepsy? *Pharmacol. Rep.* **2014**, *66*, 529–533. [CrossRef] [PubMed]

Nutrients **2017**, *9*, 659

9. Warner, T.A.; Kang, J.Q.; Kennard, J.K.; Harrison, F.E. Low brain ascorbic acid increases susceptibility to seizures in mouse models of decreased brain ascorbic acid transport and Alzheimer's disease. *Epilepsy Res.* **2015**, *110*, 20–25. [CrossRef] [PubMed]

10. Tveden-Nyborg, P.; Vogt, L.; Schjoldager, J.G.; Jeannet, N.; Hasselholt, S.; Paidi, M.D.; Christen, S.; Lykkesfeldt, J. Maternal vitamin C deficiency during pregnancy persistently impairs hippocampal neurogenesis in offspring of guinea pigs. *PLoS ONE* **2012**, *7*, e48488. [CrossRef] [PubMed]

11. Olajide, O.J.; Yawson, E.O.; Gbadamosi, I.T.; Arogundade, T.T.; Lambe, E.; Obasi, K.; Lawal, I.T.; Ibrahim, A.; Ogunrinola, K.Y. Ascorbic acid ameliorates behavioural deficits and neuropathological alterations in rat model of Alzheimer's disease. *Environ. Toxicol. Pharmacol.* **2017**, *50*, 200–211. [CrossRef] [PubMed]

12. Sil, S.; Ghosh, T.; Gupta, P.; Ghosh, R.; Kabir, S.N.; Roy, A. Dual Role of Vitamin C on the Neuroinflammation Mediated Neurodegeneration and Memory Impairments in Colchicine Induced Rat Model of Alzheimer Disease. *J. Mol. Neurosci.* **2016**, *60*, 421–435. [CrossRef] [PubMed]

13. Nualart, F.; Mack, L.; García, A.; Cisternas, P.; Bongarzone, E.R.; Heitzer, M.; Jara, N.; Martínez, F.; Ferrada, L.; Espinoza, F.; et al. Vitamin C Transporters, Recycling and the Bystander Effect in the Nervous System: SVCT2 versus Gluts. *J. Stem Cell Res. Ther.* **2014**, *4*, 209. [CrossRef] [PubMed]

14. Corpe, C.P.; Tu, H.; Eck, P.; Wang, J.; Faulhaber-Walter, R.; Schnermann, J.; Margolis, S.; Padayatty, S.; Sun, H.; Wang, Y.; et al. Vitamin C transporter Slc23a1 links renal reabsorption, vitamin C tissue accumulation and perinatal survival in mice. *J. Clin. Investig.* **2010**, *120*, 1069–1083. [CrossRef] [PubMed]

15. Tsukaguchi, H.; Tokui, T.; Mackenzie, B.; Berger, U.V.; Chen, X.Z.; Wang, Y.; Brubaker, R.F.; Hediger, M.A. A family of mammalian Na1-dependent L-ascorbic acid transporters. *Nature* **1999**, *399*, 70–75. [CrossRef] [PubMed]

16. Hansen, S.N.; Tveden-Nyborg, P.; Lykkesfeldt, J. Does vitamin C deficiency affect cognitive development and function? *Nutrients* **2014**, *6*, 3818–3846. [CrossRef] [PubMed]

17. Hosoya, K.; Nakamura, G.; Akanuma, S.; Tomi, M.; Tachikawa, M. Dehydroascorbic acid uptake and intracellular ascorbic acid accumulation in cultured Müller glial cells (TR-MUL). *Neurochem. Int.* **2008**, *52*, 1351–1357. [CrossRef] [PubMed]

18. Parker, W.H.; Qu, Z.; May, J.M. Ascorbic Acid Transport in Brain Microvascular Pericytes. *Biochem. Biophys. Res. Commun.* **2015**, *458*, 262–267. [CrossRef] [PubMed]

19. May, J.M. Vitamin C transport and its role in the central nervous system. *Subcell. Biochem.* **2012**, *56*, 85–103. [CrossRef] [PubMed]

20. Castro, M.; Caprile, T.; Astuya, A.; Millán, C.; Reinicke, K.; Vera, J.C.; Vásquez, O.; Aguayo, L.G.; Nualart, F. High-affinity sodium-vitamin C co-transporters (SVCT) expression in embryonic mouse neurons. *J. Neurochem.* **2001**, *78*, 815–823. [CrossRef] [PubMed]

21. García-Krauss, A.; Ferrada, L.; Astuya, A.; Salazar, K.; Cisternas, P.; Martínez, F.; Ramírez, E.; Nualart, F. Dehydroascorbic Acid Promotes Cell Death in Neurons Under Oxidative Stress: A Protective Role for Astrocytes. *Mol. Neurobiol.* **2016**, *53*, 5847–5863. [CrossRef]

22. Covarrubias-Pinto, A.; Acuña, A.I.; Beltrán, F.A.; Torres-Díaz, L.; Castro, M.A. Old Things New View: Ascorbic Acid Protects the Brain in Neurodegenerative Disorders. *Int. J. Mol. Sci.* **2015**, *16*, 28194–28217.

23. Mefford, I.N.; Oke, A.F.; Adams, R.N. Regional distribution of ascorbate in human brain. *Brain Res.* **1981**, *212*, 223–226. [CrossRef]

24. Milby, K.; Oke, A.; Adams, R.N. Detailed mapping of ascorbate distribution in rat brain. *Neurosci. Lett.* **1982**, *28*, 169–174. [CrossRef]

25. Rice, M.E.; Russo-Menna, I. Differential compartmentalization of brain ascorbate and glutathione between neurons and glia. *Neuroscience* **1998**, *82*, 1213–1223. [CrossRef]

26. Harrison, F.E.; May, J.M. Vitamin C function in the brain: Vital role of the ascorbate transporter SVCT2. *Free Radic. Biol. Med.* **2009**, *46*, 719–730. [CrossRef] [PubMed]

27. Miele, M.; Boutelle, M.G.; Fillenz, M. The physiologically induced release of ascorbate in rat brain is dependent on impulse traffic, calcium influx and glutamate uptake. *Neuroscience* **1994**, *62*, 87–91. [CrossRef]

28. Rice, M.E. Ascorbate regulation and its neuroprotective role in the brain. *Trends Neurosci.* **2000**, *23*, 209–216. [CrossRef]

29. Olsen, C.L.; Bunge, R.P. Requisites for growth and myelination of urodele sensory neurons in tissue culture. *J. Exp. Zool.* **1986**, *238*, 373–384. [CrossRef] [PubMed]

30. May, J.M.; Qu, Z.C. Ascorbic acid prevents oxidant-induced increases in endothelial permeability. *Biofactors* **2011**, *37*, 46–50. [CrossRef] [PubMed]

31. Hu, T.M.; Chen, Y.J. Nitrosation-modulating effect of ascorbate in a model dynamic system of coexisting nitric oxide and superoxide. *Free Radic. Res.* **2010**, *44*, 552–562. [CrossRef] [PubMed]

32. Jackson, T.S.; Xu, A.; Vita, J.A.; Keaney, J.F., Jr. Ascorbate prevents the interaction of superoxide and nitric oxide only at very high physiological concentrations. *Circ. Res.* **1998**, *83*, 916–922. [CrossRef] [PubMed]

33. Mock, J.T.; Chaudhari, K.; Sidhu, A.; Sumien, N. The influence of vitamins E and C and exercise on brain aging. *Exp. Gerontol.* **2016**. [CrossRef] [PubMed]

34. Majewska, M.D.; Bell, J.A.; London, E.D. Regulation of the NMDA receptor by redox phenomena: Inhibitory role of ascorbate. *Brain Res.* **1990**, *537*, 328–332. [CrossRef]

35. Rebec, G.V.; Pierce, R.C. A vitamin as neuromodulator: Ascorbate release into the extracellular fluid of the brain regulates dopaminergic and glutamatergic transmission. *Prog. Neurobiol.* **1994**, *43*, 537–565. [CrossRef]

36. Serra, P.A.; Esposito, G.; Delogu, M.R.; Migheli, R.; Rocchitta, G.; Grella, G.; Miele, E.; Miele, M.; Desole, M.S. Analysis of 3-morpholinosydnonimine and sodium nitroprusside effects on dopamine release in the striatum of freely moving rats: Role of nitric oxide, iron and ascorbic acid. *Br. J. Pharmacol.* **2000**, *131*, 836–842. [CrossRef] [PubMed]

37. Todd, R.D.; Bauer, P.A. Ascorbate modulates 5-[3H]hydroxytryptamine binding to central 5-HT3 sites in bovine frontal cortex. *J. Neurochem.* **1988**, *50*, 1505–1512. [CrossRef] [PubMed]

38. Figueroa-Méndez, R.; Rivas-Arancibia, S. Vitamin C in Health and Disease: Its Role in the Metabolism of Cells and Redox State in the Brain. *Front. Physiol.* **2015**, *23*, 397. [CrossRef] [PubMed]

39. Seitz, G.; Gebhardt, S.; Beck, J.F.; Böhm, W.; Lode, H.N.; Niethammer, D.; Bruchelt, G. Ascorbic acid stimulates DOPA synthesis and tyrosine hydroxylase gene expression in the human neuroblastoma cell line SK-N-SH. *Neurosci. Lett.* **1998**, *244*, 33–36. [CrossRef]

40. Calero, C.I.; Vickers, E.; Cid, G.M.; Aguayo, L.G.; von Gersdorff, H.; Calvo, D.J. Allosteric modulation of retinal GABA receptors by ascorbic acid. *J. Neurosci.* **2011**, *31*, 9672–9682. [CrossRef] [PubMed]

41. Majewska, M.D.; Bell, J.A. Ascorbic acid protects neurons from injury induced by glutamate and NMDA. *Neuroreport* **1990**, *1*, 194–196. [CrossRef] [PubMed]

42. Fan, S.F.; Yazulla, S. Modulation of voltage-dependent k+ currents (Ik(v)) in retinal bipolar cells by ascorbate is mediated by dopamine d1 receptors. *Vis. Neurosci.* **1999**, *16*, 923–931. [CrossRef] [PubMed]

43. Nelson, M.T.; Joksovic, P.M.; Su, P.; Kang, H.W.; Van Deusen, A.; Baumgart, J.P.; David, L.S.; Snutch, T.P.; Barrett, P.Q.; Lee, J.H.; et al. Molecular mechanisms of subtype-specific inhibition of neuronal t-type calcium channels by ascorbate. *J. Neurosci.* **2007**, *27*, 12577–12583. [CrossRef] [PubMed]

44. Kara, Y.; Doguc, D.K.; Kulac, E.; Gultekin, F. Acetylsalicylic acid and ascorbic acid combination improves cognition; via antioxidant effect or increased expression of NMDARs and nAChRs? *Environ. Toxicol. Pharmacol.* **2014**, *37*, 916–927. [CrossRef] [PubMed]

45. Sandstrom, M.I.; Rebec, G.V. Extracellular ascorbate modulates glutamate dynamics: Role of behavioral activation. *BMC Neurosci.* **2007**, *8*, 32. [CrossRef] [PubMed]

46. Tolbert, L.C.; Morris, P.E., Jr.; Spollen, J.J.; Ashe, S.C. Stereospecific effects of ascorbic acid and analogues on D1 and D2 agonist binding. *Life Sci.* **1992**, *51*, 921–930. [CrossRef]

47. Castro, M.A.; Angulo, C.; Brauchi, S.; Nualart, F.; Concha, I.I. Ascorbic acid participates in a general mechanism for concerted glucose transport inhibition and lactate transport stimulation. *Pflugers Arch.* **2008**, *457*, 519–528. [CrossRef] [PubMed]

48. Beltrán, F.A.; Acuña, A.I.; Miro, M.P.; Anulo, C.; Concha, I.I.; Castro, M.A. Ascorbic acid-dependent GLUT3 inhibition is a critical step for switching neuronal metabolism. *J. Cell. Physiol.* **2011**, *226*, 3286–3294. [CrossRef] [PubMed]

49. Sotiriou, S.; Gispert, S.; Cheng, J.; Wang, Y.H.; Chen, A.; Hoogstraten-Miller, S.; Miller, G.F.; Kwon, O.; Levine, M.; Guttentag, S.H.; et al. Ascorbic-acid transporter Slc23a1 is essential for vitamin C transport into the brain and for perinatal survival. *Nat. Med.* **2002**, *8*, 514–517. [CrossRef] [PubMed]

50. Shah, S.A.; Yoon, G.H.; Kim, H.O.; Kim, M.O. Vitamin C neuroprotection against dose-dependent glutamate-induced neurodegeneration in the postnatal brain. *Neurochem. Res.* **2015**, *40*, 875–884. [CrossRef] [PubMed]

51. Bekris, L.M.; Yu, C.E.; Bird, T.D.; Tsuang, D.W. Genetics of Alzheimer Disease. *J. Geriatr. Psychiatry Neurol.* **2010**, *23*, 213–227. [CrossRef] [PubMed]

52. Barber, R.C. The Genetics of Alzheimer's Disease. *Scientifica (Cairo)* **2012**, *2012*, 46210. [CrossRef] [PubMed]
53. Lee, E.; Giovanello, K.S.; Saykin, A.J.; Xie, F.; Kong, D.; Wang, Y.; Yang, L.; Ibrahim, J.G.; Doraiswamy, P.M.; Zhu, H. Single-nucleotide polymorphisms are associated with cognitive decline at Alzheimer's disease conversion within mild cognitive impairment patients. *Alzheimers Dement.* **2017**, *8*, 86–95. [CrossRef] [PubMed]
54. Ott, S.; Henkel, A.W.; Henkel, M.K.; Redzic, Z.B.; Kornhuber, J.; Wiltfang, J. Pre-aggregated Aβ1 42 peptide increases tau aggregation and hyperphosphorylation after short-term application. *Mol. Cell. Biochem.* **2011**, *349*, 169–177. [CrossRef] [PubMed]
55. Marszałek, M. Alzheimer's disease against peptides products of enzymatic cleavage of APP protein. Forming and variety of fibrillating peptides—Some aspects. *Postepy Hig. Med. Dosw.* **2016**, *70*, 787–796. [CrossRef] [PubMed]
56. Nagababu, E.; UsatyuK, P.V.; Enika, D.; Natarajan, V.; Rifkind, J.M. Vascular Endothelial Barrier Dysfunction Mediated by Amyloid-β Proteins. *J. Alzheimers Dis.* **2009**, *17*, 845–854. [CrossRef] [PubMed]
57. Li, Q.; Cui, J.; Fang, C.; Liu, M.; Min, G.; Li, L. S-Adenosylmethionine Attenuates Oxidative Stress and Neuroinflammation Induced by Amyloid-β Through Modulation of Glutathione Metabolism. *J. Alzheimers Dis.* **2017**, *58*, 549–558. [CrossRef] [PubMed]
58. Bartzokis, G.; Lu, P.H.; Mintzd, J. Human brain myelination and amyloid beta deposition in Alzheimer's disease. *Alzheimers Dement.* **2007**, *3*, 122–125. [CrossRef] [PubMed]
59. McGeer, P.L.; McGeer, E.G. The amyloid cascade-inflammatory hypothesis of Alzheimer disease: Implications for therapy. *Acta Neuropathol.* **2013**, *126*, 479. [CrossRef] [PubMed]
60. Dinkins, M.B.; Dasgupta, S.; Wang, G.; Zhu, G.; Bieberich, E. Exosome reduction in vivo is associated with lower amyloid plaque load in the 5XFAD mouse model of Alzheimer's disease. *Neurobiol. Aging* **2014**, *35*, 1792–1800. [CrossRef] [PubMed]
61. Málaga-Trillo, E.; Ochs, K. Uncontrolled SFK-mediated protein trafficking in prion and Alzheimer's disease. *Prion* **2016**, *10*, 352–361. [CrossRef] [PubMed]
62. Dixit, S.; Bernardo, A.; Walker, J.M.; Kennard, J.A.; Kim, G.Y.; Kessler, E.S.; Harrison, F.E. Vitamin C deficiency in the brain impairs cognition, increases amyloid accumulation and deposition, and oxidative stress in APP/PSEN1 and normally aging mice. *ACS Chem. Neurosci.* **2015**, *6*, 570–581. [CrossRef] [PubMed]
63. Ward, M.S.; Lamb, J.; May, J.M.; Harrison, F.E. Behavioral and monoamine changes following severe vitamin C deficiency. *J. Neurochem.* **2013**, *124*, 363–375. [CrossRef] [PubMed]
64. Sarkar, S.; Mukherjee, A.; Swarnakar, S.; Das, N. Nanocapsulated Ascorbic Acid in Combating Cerebral Ischemia Reperfusion—Induced Oxidative Injury in Rat Brain. *Curr. Alzheimer. Res.* **2016**, *13*, 1363–1373. [CrossRef] [PubMed]
65. Kennard, J.A.; Harrison, F.E. Intravenous ascorbate improves spatial memory in middle-aged APP/PSEN1 and wild type mice. *Behav. Brain Res.* **2014**, *264*, 34–42. [CrossRef] [PubMed]
66. Harrison, F.E.; Hosseini, A.H.; McDonald, M.P.; May, J.M. Vitamin C reduces spatial learning deficits in middle-aged and very old APP/PSEN1 transgenic and wild-type mice. *Pharmacol. Biochem. Behav.* **2009**, *93*, 443–450. [CrossRef] [PubMed]
67. Murakami, K.; Murata, N.; Ozawa, Y.; Kinoshita, N.; Irie, K.; Shirasawa, T.; Shimizu, T. Vitamin C restores behavioral deficits and amyloid-β oligomerization without affecting plaque formation in a mouse model of Alzheimer's disease. *J. Alzheimers Dis.* **2011**, *26*, 7–18. [CrossRef] [PubMed]
68. Lam, V.; Hackett, M.; Takechi, R. Antioxidants and Dementia Risk: Consideration through a Cerebrovascular Perspective. *Nutrients* **2016**, *8*, 828. [CrossRef] [PubMed]
69. Kook, S.Y.; Lee, K.M.; Kim, Y.; Cha, M.Y.; Kang, S.; Baik, S.H.; Lee, H.; Park, R.; Mook-Jung, I. High-dose of vitamin C supplementation reduces amyloid plaque burden and ameliorates pathological changes in the brain of 5XFAD mice. *Cell Death Dis.* **2014**, *5*, 1083. [CrossRef] [PubMed]
70. Allahtavakoli, M.; Amin, F.; Esmaeeli-Nadimi, A.; Shamsizadeh, A.; Kazemi-Arababadi, M.; Kennedy, D. Ascorbic Acid Reduces the Adverse Effects of Delayed Administration of Tissue Plasminogen Activator in a Rat Stroke Model. *Basic Clin. Pharmacol. Toxicol.* **2015**, *117*, 335–339. [CrossRef] [PubMed]
71. Song, J.; Park, J.; Kim, J.H.; Choi, J.Y.; Kim, J.Y.; Lee, K.M.; Lee, J.E. Dehydroascorbic Acid Attenuates Ischemic Brain Edema and Neurotoxicity in Cerebral Ischemia: An in vivo Study. *Exp. Neurobiol.* **2015**, *24*, 41–54. [CrossRef] [PubMed]

72. Lin, J.L.; Huang, Y.H.; Shen, Y.C.; Huang, H.C.; Liu, pH. Ascorbic acid prevents blood-brain barrier disruption and sensory deficit caused by sustained compression of primary somatosensory cortex. *J. Cereb. Blood Flow. Metab.* **2010**, *30*, 1121–1136. [CrossRef] [PubMed]

73. Polidori, M.C.; Mattioli, P.; Aldred, S.; Cecchetti, R.; Stahl, W.; Griffiths, H.; Senin, U.; Sies, H.; Mecocci, P. Plasma antioxidant status, immunoglobulin g oxidation and lipid peroxidation in demented patients: Relevance to Alzheimer disease and vascular dementia. *Dement. Geriatr. Cogn. Disord.* **2004**, *18*, 265–270. [CrossRef] [PubMed]

74. Schippling, S.; Kontush, A.; Arlt, S.; Buhmann, C.; Sturenburg, H.J.; Mann, U.; Griffiths, H.; Senin, U.; Sies, H.; Mecocci, P. Increased lipoprotein oxidation in Alzheimer's disease. *Free Radic. Biol. Med.* **2000**, *28*, 351–360. [CrossRef]

75. Lopes da Silva, S.; Vellas, B.; Elemans, S.; Luchsinger, J.; Kamphuis, P.; Yaffe, K.; Sijben, J.; Groenendijk, M.; Stijnen, T. Plasma nutrient status of patients with Alzheimer's disease: Systematic review and meta-analysis. *Alzheimers Dement.* **2014**, *10*, 485–502. [CrossRef] [PubMed]

76. Arlt, S.; Müller-Thomsen, T.; Beisiegel, U.; Kontush, A. Effect of one-year vitamin C- and E-supplementation on cerebrospinal fluid oxidation parameters and clinical course in Alzheimer's disease. *Neurochem. Res.* **2012**, *37*, 2706–2714. [CrossRef] [PubMed]

77. Galasko, D.R.; Peskind, E.; Clark, C.M.; Quinn, J.F.; Ringman, J.M.; Jicha, G.A.; Cotman, C.; Cottrell, B.; Montine, T.J.; Thomas, R.G.; et al. Alzheimer's Disease Cooperative Study. Antioxidants for Alzheimer disease: A randomized clinical trial with cerebrospinal fluid biomarker measures. *Arch. Neurol.* **2012**, *69*, 836–841. [CrossRef] [PubMed]

78. Chan, S.; Kantham, S.; Rao, V.M.; Palanivelu, M.K.; Pham, H.L.; Shaw, P.N.; McGeary, R.P.; Ross, B.P. Metal chelation, radical scavenging and inhibition of $A\beta_{42}$ fibrillation by food constituents in relation to Alzheimer's disease. *Food Chem.* **2016**, *199*, 185–194. [CrossRef] [PubMed]

79. Berti, V.; Murray, J.; Davies, M.; Spector, N.; Tsui, W.H.; Li, Y.; Williams, S.; Pirraglia, E.; Vallabhajosula, S.; McHugh, P.; et al. Nutrient patterns and brain biomarkers of Alzheimer's disease in cognitively normal individuals. *J. Nutr. Health Aging* **2015**, *19*, 413–423. [CrossRef] [PubMed]

80. Li, Y.; Liu, S.; Man, Y.; Li, N.; Zhou, Y. Effects of vitamins E and C combined with β-carotene on cognitive function in the elderly. *Exp. Ther. Med.* **2015**, *9*, 1489–1493. [CrossRef] [PubMed]

81. Zandi, P.P.; Anthony, J.C.; Khachaturian, A.S.; Stone, S.V.; Gustafson, D.; Tschanz, J.T.; Norton, M.C.; Welsh-Bohmer, K.A.; Breitner, J.C. Cache County Study Group. Reduced risk of Alzheimer disease in users of antioxidant vitamin supplements: The Cache County Study. *Arch. Neurol.* **2004**, *61*, 82–88. [CrossRef] [PubMed]

82. Polidori, M.C.; Ruggiero, C.; Croce, M.F.; Raichi, T.; Mangialasche, F.; Cecchetti, R.; Pelini, L.; Paolacci, L.; Ercolani, S.; Mecocci, P. Association of increased carotid intima-media thickness and lower plasma levels of vitamin C and vitamin E in old age subjects: Implications for Alzheimer's disease. *J. Neural Transm.* **2015**, *122*, 523–530. [CrossRef] [PubMed]

83. Su, B.; Liu, H.; Wang, X.; Chen, S.G.; Siedlak, S.L.; Kondo, E.; Choi, R.; Takeda, A.; Castellani, R.J.; Perry, G.; et al. Ectopic localization of FOXO3a protein in Lewy bodies in Lewy body dementia and Parkinson's disease. *Mol. Neurodegener.* **2009**, *4*, 32. [CrossRef] [PubMed]

84. Cacabelos, R. Parkinson's Disease: From Pathogenesis to Pharmacogenomics. *Int. J. Mol. Sci.* **2017**, *18*, 551. [CrossRef] [PubMed]

85. Nalls, M.A.; Pankratz, N.; Lill, C.M.; Do, C.B.; Hernandez, D.G.; Saad, M.; DeStefano, A.L.; Kara, E.; Bras, J.; Sharma, M.; et al. Large-scale meta-analysis of genome-wide association data identifies six new risk loci for Parkinson's disease. *Nat. Genet.* **2014**, *46*, 989–993. [CrossRef] [PubMed]

86. Tanner, C.M.; Kamel, F.; Ross, G.W.; Hoppin, J.A.; Goldman, S.M.; Korell, M.; Marras, C.; Bhudhikanok, G.S.; Kasten, M.; Chade, A.R.; et al. Rotenone, paraquat, and Parkinson's disease. *Environ. Health. Perspect.* **2011**, *119*, 866–872. [CrossRef] [PubMed]

87. Hao, L.Y.; Giasson, B.L.; Bonini, N.M. DJ-1 is critical for mitochondrial function and rescues PINK1 loss of function. *Proc. Natl. Acad. Sci. USA* **2010**, *107*, 9747–9752. [CrossRef] [PubMed]

88. Gautier, C.A.; Kitada, T.; Shen, J. Loss of PINK1 causes mitochondrial functional defects and increased sensitivity to oxidative stress. *Proc. Natl. Acad. Sci. USA* **2008**, *105*, 11364–11369. [CrossRef] [PubMed]

89. Elkon, H.; Melamed, E.; Offen, D. Oxidative stress, induced by 6-hydroxydopamine, reduces proteasome activities in PC12 cells: Implications for the pathogenesis of Parkinson's disease. *J. Mol. Neurosci.* **2004**, *24*, 387–400. [CrossRef]

90. Belluzzi, E.; Bisaglia, M.; Lazzarini, E.; Tabares, L.C.; Beltramini, M.; Bubacco, L. Human SOD2 modification by dopamine quinones affects enzymatic activity by promoting its aggregation: Possible implications for Parkinson's disease. *PLoS ONE* **2012**, *7*, e38026. [CrossRef] [PubMed]

91. Rokad, D.; Ghaisas, S.; Harischandra, D.S.; Jin, H.; Anantharam, V.; Kanthasamy, A.; Kanthasamy, A.G. Role of neurotoxicants and traumatic brain injury in α-synuclein protein misfolding and aggregation. *Brain Res. Bull.* **2016**. [CrossRef] [PubMed]

92. Irwin, D.J.; Grossman, M.; Weintraub, D.; Hurtig, H.I.; Duda, J.E.; Xie, S.X.; Lee, E.B.; Van Deerlin, V.M.; Lopez, O.L.; Kofler, J.K.; et al. Neuropathological and genetic correlates of survival and dementia onset in synucleinopathies: A retrospective analysis. *Lancet. Neurol.* **2017**, *16*, 55–65. [CrossRef]

93. Rieder, C.R.; Williams, A.C.; Ramsden, D.B. Selegiline increases heme oxygenase-1 expression and the cytotoxicity produced by dopaminetreatment of neuroblastoma SK-N-SH cells. *Braz. J. Med. Biol. Res.* **2004**, *37*, 1055–1062. [CrossRef] [PubMed]

94. Olanow, C.W.; Brundin, P. Parkinson's disease and alpha synuclein: Is Parkinson's disease a prion-like disorder? *Mov. Disord.* **2013**, *28*, 31–40. [CrossRef] [PubMed]

95. Seidel, K.; Bouzrou, M.; Heidemann, N.; Krüger, R.; Schöls, L.; den Dunnen, W.F.A.; Korf, H.W.; Rüb, U. Involvement of the cerebellum in Parkinson disease and dementia with Lewy bodies. *Ann. Neurol.* **2017**. [CrossRef] [PubMed]

96. Armstrong, R.A. Evidence from spatial pattern analysis for the anatomical spread of α-synuclein pathology in Parkinson's disease dementia. *Folia Neuropathol.* **2017**, *55*, 23–30. [CrossRef] [PubMed]

97. Scheffold, A.; Holtman, I.R.; Dieni, S.; Brouwer, N.; Katz, S.F.; Jebaraj, B.M.; Kahle, P.J.; Hengerer, B.; Lechel, A.; Stilgenbauer, S.; et al. Telomere shortening leads to an acceleration of synucleinopathy and impaired microglia response in a genetic mouse model. *Acta Neuropathol. Commun.* **2016**, *4*, 87. [CrossRef] [PubMed]

98. He, X.B.; Kim, M.; Kim, S.Y.; Yi, S.H.; Rhee, Y.H.; Kim, T.; Lee, E.H.; Park, C.H.; Dixit, S.; Harrison, F.E.; et al. Vitamin C facilitates dopamine neuron differentiation in fetal midbrain through TET1- and JMJD3-dependent epigenetic control manner. *Stem Cells* **2015**, *33*, 1320–1332. [CrossRef] [PubMed]

99. Camarena, V.; Wang, G. The epigenetic role of vitamin C in health and disease. *Cell. Mol. Life Sci.* **2016**, *73*, 1645–1658. [CrossRef] [PubMed]

100. Minor, E.A.; Court, B.L.; Young, J.I.; Wang, G. Ascorbate Induces Ten-Eleven Translocation (Tet) Methylcytosine Dioxygenase-mediated Generation of 5-Hydroxymethylcytosine. *J. Biol. Chem.* **2013**, *288*, 13669–13674. [CrossRef] [PubMed]

101. Xiang, W.; Schlachetzki, J.C.; Helling, S.; Bussmann, J.C.; Berlinghof, M.; Schaffer, T.E.; Marcus, K.; Winkler, J.; Klucken, J.; Becker, C.M. Oxidative stress-induced posttranslational modifications of α-synuclein: Specific modification of α-synuclein by 4-hydroxy-2-nonenal increases dopaminergic toxicity. *Mol. Cell. Neurosci.* **2013**, *54*, 71–83. [CrossRef] [PubMed]

102. Jinsmaa, Y.; Sullivan, P.; Sharabi, Y.; Goldstein, D.S. DOPAL is transmissible to and oligomerizes alpha-synuclein in human glial cells. *Auton. Neurosci.* **2016**, *194*, 46–51. [CrossRef] [PubMed]

103. Khan, S.; Jyoti, S.; Naz, F.; Shakya, B.; Rahul, A.M.; Siddique, Y.H. Effect of L-ascorbic Acid on the climbing ability and protein levels in the brain of Drosophila model of Parkinson's disease. *J. Neurosci.* **2012**, *122*, 704–709. [CrossRef]

104. Ballaz, S.; Morales, I.; Rodríguez, M.; Obeso, J.A. Ascorbate prevents cell death from prolonged exposure to glutamate in an in vitro model of human dopaminergic neurons. *J. Neurosci. Res.* **2013**, *91*, 1609–1617. [CrossRef] [PubMed]

105. Izumi, Y.; Ezumi, M.; Takada-Takatori, Y.; Akaike, A.; Kume, T. Endogenous dopamine is involved in the herbicide paraquat-induced dopaminergic cell death. *Toxicol. Sci.* **2014**, *139*, 466–478. [CrossRef] [PubMed]

106. Medeiros, M.S.; Schumacher-Schuh, A.; Cardoso, A.M.; Bochi, G.V.; Baldissarelli, J.; Kegler, A.; Santana, D.; Chaves, C.M.; Schetinger, M.R.; Moresco, R.N.; et al. Iron and Oxidative Stress in Parkinson's Disease: An Observational Study of Injury Biomarkers. *PLoS ONE* **2016**, *11*, e0146129. [CrossRef] [PubMed]

107. Quiroga, M.J.; Carroll, D.W.; Brown, T.M. Ascorbate- and zinc-responsive parkinsonism. *Ann. Pharmacother.* **2014**, *48*, 1515–1520. [CrossRef] [PubMed]

108. Ide, K.; Yamada, H.; Umegaki, K.; Mizuno, K.; Kawakami, N.; Hagiwara, Y.; Matsumoto, M.; Yoshida, H.; Kim, K.; Shiosaki, E.; et al. Lymphocyte vitamin C levels as potential biomarker for progression of Parkinson's disease. *Nutrition* **2015**, *31*, 406–408. [CrossRef] [PubMed]

109. Hughes, K.C.; Gao, X.; Kim, I.Y.; Rimm, E.B.; Wang, M.; Weisskopf, M.G.; Schwarzschild, M.A.; Ascherio, A. Intake of antioxidant vitamins and risk of Parkinson's disease. *Mov. Disord.* **2016**, *31*. [CrossRef] [PubMed]

110. Noble, M.; Healey, C.S.; McDougal-Chukwumah, L.D.; Brown, T.M. Old disease, new look? A first report of parkinsonism due to scurvy, and of refeeding-induced worsening of scurvy. *Psychosomatics* **2013**, *54*, 277–283. [CrossRef] [PubMed]

111. Nagayama, H.; Hamamoto, M.; Ueda, M.; Nito, C.; Yamaguchi, H.; Katayama, Y. The effect of ascorbic acid on the pharmacokinetics of levodopa in elderly patients with Parkinson disease. *Clin. Neuropharmacol.* **2004**, *27*, 270–273. [CrossRef] [PubMed]

112. Mariam, I.; Ali, S.; Rehman, A. Ikram-Ul-Haq. L-Ascorbate, a strong inducer of L-dopa (3,4-dihydroxy-L-phenylalanine) production from pre-grown mycelia of Aspergillus oryzae NRRL-1560. *Biotechnol. Appl. Biochem.* **2010**, *55*, 131–137. [CrossRef] [PubMed]

113. Peña-Sánchez, M.; Riverón-Forment, G.; Zaldívar-Vaillant, T.; Soto-Lavastida, A.; Borrero-Sánchez, J.; Lara-Fernández, G.; Esteban-Hernández, E.M.; Hernández-Díaz, Z.; González-Quevedo, A.; Fernández-Almirall, I.; et al. Association of status redox with demographic, clinical and imaging parameters in patients with Huntington's disease. *Clin. Biochem.* **2015**, *48*, 1258–1263. [CrossRef] [PubMed]

114. Sari, Y. Huntington's Disease: From Mutant Huntingtin Protein to Neurotrophic Factor Therapy. *Int. J. Biomed. Sci.* **2011**, *7*, 89–100. [PubMed]

115. Paulsen, J.S. Cognitive Impairment in Huntington Disease: Diagnosis and Treatment. *Curr. Neurol. Neurosci. Rep.* **2011**, *11*, 474–483. [CrossRef] [PubMed]

116. Long, J.D.; Paulsen, J.S.; Marder, K.; Zhang, Y.; Kim, J.I.; Mills, J.A. Researchers of the PREDICT-HD Huntington's Study Group. Tracking motor impairments in the progression of Huntington's disease. *Mov. Disord.* **2014**, *29*, 311–319. [CrossRef] [PubMed]

117. Vonsattel, J.P.; Myers, R.H.; Stevens, T.J.; Ferrante, R.J.; Bird, E.D.; Richardson, E.P., Jr. Neuropathological classification of Huntington's disease. *J. Neuropathol. Exp. Neurol.* **1985**, *44*, 559–577. [CrossRef] [PubMed]

118. Postert, T.; Lack, B.; Kuhn, W.; Jergas, M.; Andrich, J.; Braun, B.; Przuntek, H.; Sprengelmeyer, R.; Agelink, M.; Büttner, T. Basal ganglia alterations and brain atrophy in Huntington's disease depicted by transcranial realtime sonography. *J. Neurol. Neurosurg. Psychiatry* **1999**, *67*, 457–462. [CrossRef] [PubMed]

119. Acuña, A.I.; Esparza, M.; Kramm, C.; Beltrán, F.A.; Parra, A.V.; Cepeda, C.; Toro, C.A.; Vidal, R.L.; Hetz, C.; Concha, I.I.; et al. A failure in energy metabolism and antioxidant uptake precede symptoms of Huntington's disease in mice. *Nat. Commun.* **2013**, *4*, 2917. [CrossRef] [PubMed]

120. Weydt, P.; Pineda, V.V.; Torrence, A.E.; Libby, R.T.; Satterfield, T.F.; Lazarowski, E.R.; Gilbert, M.L.; Morton, G.J.; Bammler, T.K.; Strand, A.D.; et al. Thermoregulatory and metabolic defects in Huntington's disease transgenic mice implicate PGC-1alpha in Huntington's disease neurodegeneration. *Cell. Metab.* **2006**, *4*, 349–362. [CrossRef] [PubMed]

121. Tereshchenko, A.; McHugh, M.; Lee, J.K.; Gonzalez-Alegre, P.; Crane, K.; Dawson, J.; Nopoulos, P. Abnormal Weight and Body Mass Index in Children with Juvenile Huntington's Disease. *J. Huntingtons. Dis.* **2015**, *4*, 231–238. [CrossRef] [PubMed]

122. Ross, C.A.; Tabrizi, S.J. Huntington's disease: From molecular pathogenesis to clinical treatment. *Lancet Neurol.* **2011**, *10*, 83–98. [CrossRef]

123. Labbadia, J.; Morimoto, R.I. Huntington's disease: Underlying molecular mechanisms and emerging concepts. *Trends Biochem. Sci.* **2013**, *38*, 378–385. [CrossRef] [PubMed]

124. Tang, T.S.; Chen, X.; Liu, J.; Bezprozvanny, I. Dopaminergic Signaling and Striatal Neurodegeneration in Huntington's Disease. *J. Neurosci.* **2007**, *27*, 7899–7910. [CrossRef] [PubMed]

125. Covarrubias-Pinto, A.; Moll, P.; Solís-Maldonado, M.; Acuña, A.I.; Riveros, A.; Miró, M.P.; Papic, E.; Beltrán, F.A.; Cepeda, C.; Concha, I.I.; et al. Beyond the redox imbalance: Oxidative stress contributes to an impaired GLUT3 modulation in Huntington's disease. *Free Radic. Biol. Med.* **2015**, *89*, 1085–1096. [CrossRef] [PubMed]

126. Miller, B.R.; Dorner, J.L.; Bunner, K.D.; Gaither, T.W.; Klein, E.L.; Barton, S.J.; Rebec, G.V. Up-regulation of GLT1 reverses the deficit in cortically evoked striatal ascorbate efflux in the R6/2 mouse model of Huntington's disease. *J. Neurochem.* **2012**, *121*, 629–638. [CrossRef] [PubMed]

127. Dorner, J.L.; Miller, B.R.; Klein, E.L.; Murphy-Nakhnikian, A.; Andrews, R.L.; Barton, S.J.; Rebec, G.V. Corticostriatal dysfunction underlies diminished striatal ascorbate release in the R6/2 mouse model of Huntington's disease. *Brain Res.* **2009**, *1290*, 111–120. [CrossRef] [PubMed]

128. Rebec, G.V. Dysregulation of corticostriatal ascorbate release and glutamate uptake in transgenic models of Huntington's disease. *Antioxid. Redox Signal.* **2013**, *19*, 2115–2128. [CrossRef] [PubMed]

129. Rebec, G.V.; Conroy, S.K.; Barton, S.J. Hyperactive striatal neurons in symptomatic Huntington R6/2 mice: Variations with behavioral state and repeated ascorbate treatment. *Neuroscience* **2006**, *137*, 327–336. [CrossRef] [PubMed]

130. Rebec, G.V.; Barton, S.J.; Marseilles, A.M.; Collins, K. Ascorbate treatment attenuates the Huntington behavioral phenotype in mice. *Neuroreport* **2003**, *14*, 1263–1265. [CrossRef] [PubMed]

131. Hadžović-Džuvo, A.; Lepara, O.; Valjevac, A.; Avdagić, N.; Hasić, S.; Kiseljaković, E.; Ibragić, S.; Alajbegović, A. Serum total antioxidant capacity in patients with multiple sclerosis. *Bosn. J. Basic Med. Sci.* **2011**, *11*, 33–36. [PubMed]

132. Rottlaender, A.; Kuerten, S. Stepchild or Prodigy? Neuroprotection in Multiple Sclerosis (MS) Research. *Int. J. Mol. Sci.* **2015**, *16*, 14850–14865. [CrossRef] [PubMed]

133. Morandi, E.; Tarlinton, R.E.; Gran, B. Multiple Sclerosis between Genetics and Infections: Human Endogenous Retroviruses in Monocytes and Macrophages. *Front. Immunol.* **2015**, *6*, 647. [CrossRef] [PubMed]

134. Pagano, G.; Talamanca, A.A.; Castello, G.; Cordero, M.D.; d'Ischia, M.; Gadaleta, M.N.; Pallardó, F.V.; Petrović, S.; Tiano, L.; Zatterale, A. Oxidative stress and mitochondrial dysfunction across broad-ranging pathologies: Toward mitochondria-targeted clinical strategies. *Oxid. Med. Cell. Longev.* **2014**, *2014*, 541230. [CrossRef] [PubMed]

135. Polachini, C.R.; Spanevello, R.M.; Zanini, D.; Baldissarelli, J.; Pereira, L.B.; Schetinger, M.R.; da Cruz, I.B.; Assmann, C.E.; Bagatini, M.D.; Morsch, V.M. Evaluation of Delta Aminolevulinic Dehydratase Activity, Oxidative Stress Biomarkers, and Vitamin D Levels in Patients with Multiple Sclerosis. *Neurotox. Res.* **2016**, *29*, 230–242. [CrossRef] [PubMed]

136. Tavazzi, B.; Batocchi, A.P.; Amorini, A.M.; Nociti, V.; D'Urso, S.; Longo, S.; Gullotta, S.; Picardi, M.; Lazzarino, G. Serum metabolic profile in multiple sclerosis patients. *Epub Mult. Scler. Int.* **2011**, *2011*, 167156. [CrossRef] [PubMed]

137. Patel, J.; Balabanov, R. Molecular mechanisms of oligodendrocyte injury in multiple sclerosis and experimental autoimmune encephalomyelitis. *Int. J. Mol. Sci.* **2012**, *13*, 10647–10659. [CrossRef] [PubMed]

138. Besler, H.T.; Comoğlu, S.; Okçu, Z. Serum levels of antioxidant vitamins and lipid peroxidation in multiple sclerosis. *Nutr. Neurosci.* **2002**, *5*, 215–220. [CrossRef] [PubMed]

139. Hejazi, E.; Amani, R.; SharafodinZadeh, N.; Cheraghian, B. Comparison of Antioxidant Status and Vitamin D Levels between Multiple Sclerosis Patients and Healthy Matched Subjects. *Mult. Scler. Int.* **2014**, *2014*, 539854. [CrossRef] [PubMed]

140. Odinak, M.M.; Bisaga, G.N.; Zarubina, I.V. New Approaches to Antioxidant Therapy in Multiple Sclerosis. Available online: http://www.ncbi.nlm.nih.gov/pubmed/12418396 (accessed on 26 June 2017).

141. Babri, S.; Mehrvash, F.; Mohaddes, G.; Hatami, H.; Mirzaie, F. Effect of intrahippocampal administration of vitamin C and progesterone on learning in a model of multiple sclerosis in rats. *Adv. Pharm. Bull.* **2015**, *5*, 83–87. [CrossRef] [PubMed]

142. Matic, I.; Strobbe, D.; Frison, M.; Campanella, M. Controlled and Impaired Mitochondrial Quality in Neurons: Molecular Physiology and Prospective Pharmacology. *Pharmacol. Res.* **2015**, *99*, 410–424. [CrossRef] [PubMed]

143. Orrell, R.W.; Lane, R.J.; Ross, M. A systematic review of antioxidant treatment for amyotrophic lateral sclerosis/motor neuron disease. *Amyotroph. Lateral Scler.* **2008**, *9*, 195–211. [CrossRef] [PubMed]

144. Blasco, H.; Corcia, P.; Moreau, C.; Veau, S.; Fournier, C.; Vourc'h, P.; Emond, P.; Gordon, P.; Pradat, P.F.; Praline, J.; et al. 1H-NMR-based metabolomic profiling of CSF in early amyotrophic lateral sclerosis. *PLoS ONE* **2010**, *5*, e13223. [CrossRef]

145. Nagano, S.; Fujii, Y.; Yamamoto, T.; Taniyama, M.; Fukada, K.; Yanagihara, T.; Sakoda, S. The efficacy of trientine or ascorbate alone compared to that of the combined treatment with these two agents in familial amyotrophic lateral sclerosis model mice. *Exp. Neurol.* **2003**, *179*, 176–180. [CrossRef]

146. Netzahualcoyotzi, C.; Tapia, R. Degeneration of spinal motor neurons by chronic AMPA-induced excitotoxicity in vivo and protection by energy substrates. *Acta Neuropathol. Commun.* **2015**, *3*, 27. [CrossRef] [PubMed]

147. Fitzgerald, K.C.; O'Reilly, É.J.; Fondell, E.; Falcone, G.J.; McCullough, M.L.; Park, Y.; Kolonel, L.N.; Ascherio, A. Intakes of vitamin C and carotenoids and risk of amyotrophic lateral sclerosis: Pooled results from 5 cohort studies. *Ann. Neurol.* **2013**, *73*, 236–245. [CrossRef] [PubMed]

148. Okamoto, K.; Kihira, T.; Kobashi, G.; Washio, M.; Sasaki, S.; Yokoyama, T.; Miyake, Y.; Sakamoto, N.; Inaba, Y.; Nagai, M. Fruit and vegetable intake and risk of amyotrophic lateral sclerosis in Japan. *Neuroepidemiology* **2009**, *32*, 251–256. [CrossRef] [PubMed]

149. Spasojević, I.; Stević, Z.; Nikolić-Kokić, A.; Jones, D.R.; Blagojević, D.; Spasić, M.B. Different roles of radical scavengers—Ascorbate and urate in the cerebrospinal fluid of amyotrophic lateral sclerosis patients. *Redox Rep.* **2010**, *15*, 81–86. [CrossRef] [PubMed]

150. Liu, Y.; Hu, N. Electrochemical detection of natural DNA damage induced by ferritin/ascorbic acid/H2O2 system and amplification of DNA damage by endonuclease Fpg. *Biosens. Bioelectron.* **2009**, *25*, 185–190. [CrossRef] [PubMed]

151. Bembnowska, M.; Jośko, J. Depressive behaviours among adolescents as a Public Health problem. *Zdr. Publ.* **2011**, *121*, 4260430.

152. Lopresti, A.L. A review of nutrient treatments for paediatric depression. *J. Affect. Disord.* **2015**, *181*, 24–32. [CrossRef] [PubMed]

153. Moretti, M.; Budni, J.; Ribeiro, C.M.; Rieger, D.; Leal, R.B.; Rodrigues, A.L. Subchronic administration of ascorbic acid elicits antidepressant-like effect and modulates cell survival signaling pathways in mice. *J. Nutr. Biochem.* **2016**, *38*, 50–56. [CrossRef] [PubMed]

154. Luscher, B.; Shen, Q.; Sahir, N. The GABAergic Deficit Hypothesis of Major Depressive Disorder. *Mol. Psychiatry* **2011**, *16*, 383–406. [CrossRef] [PubMed]

155. Rosa, P.B.; Neis, V.B.; Ribeiro, C.M.; Moretti, M.; Rodrigues, A.L.S. Antidepressant-like effects of ascorbic acid and ketamine involve modulation of GABAA and GABAB receptors. *Pharmacol. Rep.* **2016**, *68*, 996–1001. [CrossRef]

156. Capuron, L.; Pagnoni, G.; Drake, D.F.; Woolwine, B.J.; Spivey, J.R.; Crowe, R.J.; Votaw, J.R.; Goodman, M.M.; Miller, A.H. Dopaminergic mechanisms of reduced basal ganglia responses to hedonic reward during interferon alfa administration. *Arch. Gen. Psychiatry* **2012**, *69*, 1044–1053. [CrossRef] [PubMed]

157. Bigdeli, T.B.; Ripke, S.; Peterson, R.E.; Trzaskowski, M.; Bacanu, S.A.; Abdellaoui, A.; Andlauer, T.F.; Beekman, A.T.; Berger, K.; Blackwood, D.H.; et al. Genetic effects influencing risk for major depressive disorder in China and Europe. *Transl. Psychiatry* **2017**, *7*, e1074. [CrossRef] [PubMed]

158. Altshuler, L.L.; Abulseoud, O.A.; Foland-Ross, L.; Bartzokis, G.; Chang, S.; Mintz, J.; Hellemann, G.; Vinters, H.V. Amygdala astrocyte reduction in subjects with major depressive disorder but not bipolar disorder. *Bipolar Disord.* **2010**, *12*, 541–549. [CrossRef] [PubMed]

159. Cobb, J.A.; O'Neill, K.; Milner, J.; Mahajan, G.J.; Lawrence, T.J.; May, W.T.; Miguel-Hidalgo, J.; Rajkowska, G.; Stockmeiera, C.A. Density of GFAP-immunoreactive astrocytes is decreased in left hippocampi in major depressive disorder. *Neuroscience* **2016**, *316*, 209–220. [CrossRef] [PubMed]

160. Rajkowska, G.; Hughes, J.; Stockmeier, C.A.; Javier Miguel-Hidalgo, J.; Maciag, D. Coverage of blood vessels by astrocytic endfeet is reduced in major depressive disorder. *Biol. Psychiatry* **2013**, *73*, 613–621. [CrossRef] [PubMed]

161. Rubinow, M.J.; Mahajan, G.; May, W.; Overholser, J.C.; Jurjus, G.J.; Dieter, L.; Herbst, N.; Steffens, D.C.; Miguel-Hidalgo, J.J.; Rajkowska, G.; et al. Basolateral amygdala volume and cell numbers in major depressive disorder: A postmortem stereological study. *Brain Struct. Funct.* **2016**, *21*, 171–184. [CrossRef] [PubMed]

162. Guillemin, G.J.; Wang, L.; Brew, B.J. Quinolinic acid selectively induces apoptosis of human astrocytes: Potential role in AIDS dementia complex. *J. Neuroinflammation* **2005**, *2*, 16. [CrossRef] [PubMed]

163. Braidy, N.; Grant, R.; Adams, S.; Brew, B.J.; Guillemin, G.J. Mechanism for quinolinic acid cytotoxicity in human astrocytes and neurons. *Neurotox. Res.* **2009**, *16*, 77–86. [CrossRef] [PubMed]

164. Moretti, M.; Budni, J.; Ribeiro, C.M.; Rodrigues, A.L. Involvement of different types of potassium channels in the antidepressant-like effect of ascorbic acid in the mouse tail suspension test. *Eur. J. Pharmacol.* **2012**, *687*, 21–27. [CrossRef] [PubMed]

165. Moretti, M.; Budni, J.; Freitas, A.E.; Neis, V.B.; Ribeiro, C.M.; de Oliveira Balen, G.; Rieger, D.K.; Leal, R.B.; Rodrigues, A.L. TNF-α-induced depressive-like phenotype and p38(MAPK) activation are abolished by ascorbic acid treatment. *Eur. Neuropsychopharmacol.* **2015**, *25*, 902–912. [CrossRef] [PubMed]

166. Zhao, B.; Fei, J.; Chen, Y.; Ying, Y.L.; Ma, L.; Song, X.Q.; Wang, L.; Chen, E.Z.; Mao, E.Q. Pharmacological preconditioning with vitamin C attenuates intestinal injury via the induction of heme oxygenase-1 after hemorrhagic shock in rats. *PLoS ONE* **2014**, *9*, 99134. [CrossRef]

167. Binfaré, R.W.; Rosa, A.O.; Lobato, K.R.; Santos, A.R.; Rodrigues, A.L.S. Ascorbic acid administration produces an antidepressant-like effect: Evidence for the involvement of monoaminergic neurotransmission. *Prog. Neuropsychopharmacol. Biol. Psychiatry* **2009**, *33*, 530–540. [CrossRef] [PubMed]

168. Robaczewska, J.; Kędziora-Kornatowska, K.; Kucharski, R.; Nowak, M.; Muszalik, M.; Kornatowski, M.; Kędziora, J. Decreased expression of heme oxygenase is associated with depressive symptoms and may contribute to depressive and hypertensive comorbidity. *Redox Rep.* **2016**, *21*, 209–218. [CrossRef] [PubMed]

169. Gariballa, S. Poor vitamin C status is associated with increased depression symptoms following acute illness in older people. *Int. J. Vitam. Nutr. Res.* **2014**, *84*, 12–17. [CrossRef] [PubMed]

170. Bajpai, A.; Verma, A.K.; Srivastava, M.; Srivastava, R. Oxidative stress and major depression. *J. Clin. Diagn. Res.* **2014**, *8*, 4–7. [CrossRef] [PubMed]

171. Gautam, M.; Agrawal, M.; Gautam, M.; Sharma, P.; Gautam, A.S.; Gautam, S. Role of antioxidants in generalised anxiety disorder and depression. *Indian J. Psychiatry* **2012**, *54*, 244–247. [CrossRef] [PubMed]

172. Prohan, M.; Amani, R.; Nematpour, S.; Jomehzadeh, N.; Haghighizadeh, M.H. Total antioxidant capacity of diet and serum, dietary antioxidant vitamins intake, and serum hs-CRP levels in relation to depression scales in university male students. *Redox Rep.* **2014**, *19*, 133–139. [CrossRef] [PubMed]

173. Kim, T.H.; Choi, J.Y.; Lee, H.H.; Park, Y. Associations between Dietary Pattern and Depression in Korean Adolescent Girls. *J. Pediatr. Adolesc. Gynecol.* **2015**, *28*, 533–537. [CrossRef] [PubMed]

174. Rubio-López, N.; Morales-Suárez-Varela, M.; Pico, Y.; Livianos-Aldana, L.; Llopis-González, A. Nutrient Intake and Depression Symptoms in Spanish Children: The ANIVA Study. *Int. J. Environ. Res. Public Health* **2016**, *13*, 352. [CrossRef] [PubMed]

175. Amr, M.; El-Mogy, A.; Shams, T.; Vieira, K.; Lakhan, S.E. Efficacy of vitamin C as an adjunct to fluoxetine therapy in pediatric major depressive disorder: A randomized, double-blind, placebo-controlled pilot study. *Nutr. J.* **2013**, *12*, 31. [CrossRef] [PubMed]

176. Zhang, M.; Robitaille, L.; Eintracht, S.; Hoffer, L.J. Vitamin C provision improves mood in acutely hospitalized patients. *Nutrition* **2011**, *27*, 530–533. [CrossRef] [PubMed]

177. Wang, Y.; Liu, X.J.; Robitaille, L.; Eintracht, S.; MacNamara, E.; Hoffer, L.J. Effects of vitamin C and vitamin D administration on mood and distress in acutely hospitalizedpatients. *Am. J. Clin. Nutr.* **2013**, *98*, 705–711. [CrossRef] [PubMed]

178. Khajehnasiri, F.; Akhondzadeh, S.; Mortazavi, S.B.; Allameh, A.; Sotoudeh, G.; Khavanin, A.; Zamanian, Z. Are Supplementation of Omega-3 and Ascorbic Acid Effective in Reducing Oxidative Stress and Depression among Depressed Shift Workers? *Int. J. Vitam. Nutr. Res.* **2016**, *10*, 1–12. [CrossRef] [PubMed]

179. Fritz, H.; Flower, G.; Weeks, L.; Cooley, K.; Callachan, M.; McGowan, J.; Skidmore, B.; Kirchner, L.; Seely, D. Intravenous Vitamin C and Cancer: A Systematic Review. *Integr. Cancer Ther.* **2014**, *13*, 280–300. [CrossRef] [PubMed]

180. Grillon, C.H. Models and mechanisms of anxiety: Evidence from startle studies. *Psychopharmacology* **2008**, *199*, 421–437. [CrossRef] [PubMed]

181. Hughes, R.N.; Lowther, C.L.; van Nobelen, M. Prolonged treatment with vitamins C and E separately and together decreases anxiety-related open-field behavior and acoustic startle in hooded rats. *Pharmacol. Biochem. Behav.* **2011**, *97*, 494–499. [CrossRef] [PubMed]

182. Kori, R.S.; Aladakatti, R.H.; Desai, S.D.; Das, K.K. Effect of Drug Alprazolam on Restrained Stress Induced Alteration of Serum Cortisol and Antioxidant Vitamins (Vitamin C and E) in Male Albino Rats. *J. Clin. Diagn. Res.* **2016**, *10*, AF07–AF09. [CrossRef] [PubMed]

183. Boufleur, N.; Antoniazzi, C.T.; Pase, C.S.; Benvegnú, D.M.; Dias, V.T.; Segat, H.J.; Roversi, K.; Roversi, K.; Nora, M.D.; Koakoskia, G.; et al. Neonatal handling prevents anxiety-like symptoms in rats exposed to chronic mild stress: Behavioral and oxidative parameters. *Stress* **2013**, *16*, 321–330. [CrossRef] [PubMed]

184. Koizumi, M.; Kondob, Y.; Isakaa, A.; Ishigamib, A.; Suzukia, E. Vitamin C impacts anxiety-like behavior and stress-induced anorexia relative to social environment in SMP30/GNL knockout mice. *Nutr. Res.* **2016**, *36*, 1379–1391. [CrossRef] [PubMed]

185. Hughes, N.R.; Hancock, J.N.; Thompson, R.M. Anxiolysis and recognition memory enhancement with long-term supplemental ascorbic acid (vitamin C) in normal rats: Possible dose dependency and sex differences. *Ann. Neurosci. Psychol.* **2015**, *2*, 2. Available online: http://www.vipoa.org/neuropsychol (accessed on 26 June 2017).

186. Choi, J.Y.; dela Peña, I.C.; Yoon, S.Y.; Woo, T.E.; Choi, Y.J.; Shin, C.Y.; Ryu, J.H.; Lee, Y.S.; Yu, G.Y.; Cheong, J.H. Is the anti-stress effect of vitamin C related to adrenal gland function in rat? *Food Sci. Biotechnol.* **2011**, *20*, 429–435. [CrossRef]

187. Puty, B.; Maximino, C.; Brasil, A.; da Silva, W.L.; Gouveia, A., Jr.; Oliveira, K.R.; Batista Ede, J.; Crespo-Lopez, M.E.; Rocha, F.A.; Herculano, A.M. Ascorbic acid protects against anxiogenic-like effect induced by methylmercury in zebrafish: Action on the serotonergic system. *Zebrafish* **2014**, *11*, 365–370. [CrossRef] [PubMed]

188. Angrini, M.A.; Leslie, J.C. Vitamin C attenuates the physiological and behavioural changes induced by long-term exposure to noise. *Behav. Pharmacol.* **2012**, *23*, 119–125. [CrossRef] [PubMed]

189. De Oliveira, I.J.; de Souza, V.V.; Motta, V.; Da-Silva, S.L. Effects of Oral Vitamin C Supplementation on Anxiety in Students: A Double-Blind, Randomized, Placebo-Controlled Trial. *Pak. J. Biol. Sci.* **2015**, *18*, 11–18. [CrossRef] [PubMed]

190. Mazloom, Z.; Ekramzadeh, M.; Hejazi, N. Efficacy of supplementary vitamins C and E on anxiety, depression and stress in type 2 diabetic patients: A randomized, single-blind, placebo-controlled trial. *Pak. J. Biol. Sci.* **2013**, *16*, 1597–1600. [PubMed]

191. McCabe, D.; Lisy, K.; Lockwood, C.; Colbeck, M. The impact of essential fatty acid, B vitamins, vitamin C, magnesium and zinc supplementation on stress levels in women: A systematic review. *JBI Database Syst. Rev. Implement. Rep.* **2017**, *15*, 402–453. [CrossRef]

192. Arroll, M.A.; Wilder, L.; Neil, J. Nutritional interventions for the adjunctive treatment of schizophrenia: A brief review. *Nutr. J.* **2014**, *13*, 91. [CrossRef] [PubMed]

193. Sershen, H.; Hashim, A.; Dunlop, D.S.; Suckow, R.F.; Cooper, T.B.; Javitt, D.C. Modulating NMDA Receptor Function with D-Amino Acid Oxidase Inhibitors: Understanding Functional Activity in PCP-Treated Mouse Model. *Neurochem. Res.* **2016**, *41*, 398–408. [CrossRef] [PubMed]

194. Javitt, D.C. Twenty-five years of glutamate in schizophrenia: Are we there yet? *Schizophr. Bull.* **2012**, *38*, 911–913. [CrossRef] [PubMed]

195. Wabaidur, S.M.; Alothman, Z.A.; Naushad, M. Determination of dopamine in pharmaceutical formulation using enhanced luminescence from europium complex. *Spectrochim. Acta A Mol. Biomol. Spectrosc.* **2012**, *93*, 331–334. [CrossRef] [PubMed]

196. Morera-Fumero, A.L.; Díaz-Mesa, E.; Abreu-Gonzalez, P.; Fernandez-Lopez, L.; Cejas-Mendez, M.D. Low levels of serum total antioxidant capacity and presence at admission and absence at discharge of a day/night change as a marker of acute paranoid schizophrenia relapse. *Psychiatry Res.* **2017**, *249*, 200–205. [CrossRef] [PubMed]

197. Hoffer, L.J. Vitamin Therapy in Schizophrenia. *Isr. J. Psychiatry Relat. Sci.* **2008**, *45*, 3–10. [PubMed]

198. Sarandol, A.; Kirli, S.; Akkaya, C.; Altin, A.; Demirci, M.; Sarandol, E. Oxidative-antioxidative systems and their relation with serum S100 B levels in patients with schizophrenia: Effects of short term antipsychotic treatment. *Prog. Neuropsychopharmacol. Biol. Psychiatry* **2007**, *31*, 1164–1169. [CrossRef] [PubMed]

199. Young, J.; McKinney, S.B.; Ross, B.M.; Wahle, K.W.; Boyle, S.P. Biomarkers of oxidative stress in schizophrenic and control subjects. *Prostaglandins Leukot. Essent. Fatty Acids* **2007**, *76*, 73–85. [CrossRef] [PubMed]

200. Konarzewska, B.; Stefańska, E.; Wendołowicz, A.; Cwalina, U.; Golonko, A.; Małus, A.; Kowzan, U.; Szulc, A.; Rudzki, L.; Ostrowska, L. Visceral obesity in normal-weight patients suffering from chronic schizophrenia. *BMC Psychiatry* **2014**, *14*, 35. [CrossRef] [PubMed]

201. Magalhães, P.V.; Dean, O.; Andreazza, A.C.; Berk, M.; Kapczinski, F. Antioxidant treatments for schizophrenia. *Cochrane Database Syst. Rev.* **2016**, *2*, CD008919. [CrossRef] [PubMed]

202. Bentsen, H.; Osnes, K.; Refsum, H.; Solberg, D.K.; Bøhmer, T. A randomized placebo-controlled trial of an omega-3 fatty acid and vitamins E + C in schizophrenia. *Transl. Psychiatry* **2013**, *3*, e335. [CrossRef] [PubMed]

203. Sivrioglu, E.Y.; Kirli, S.; Sipahioglu, D.; Gursoy, B.; Sarandöl, E. The impact of omega-3 fatty acids, vitamins E and C supplementation on treatment outcome and side effects in schizophrenia patients treated with haloperidol: An open-label pilot study. *Prog. Neuropsychopharmacol. Biol. Psychiatry* **2007**, *31*, 1493–1499. [CrossRef] [PubMed]

204. Heiser, P.; Sommer, O.; Schmidt, A.J.; Clement, H.W.; Hoinkes, A.; Hopt, U.T.; Schulz, E.; Krieg, J.C.; Dobschütz, E. Effects of antipsychotics and vitamin C on the formation of reactive oxygen species. *J. Psychopharmacol.* **2010**, *24*, 1499–1504. [CrossRef] [PubMed]

205. Kawazoe, T.; Park, H.K.; Iwana, S.; Tsuge, H.; Fukui, K. Human D-amino acid oxidase: An update and review. *Chem. Rec.* **2007**, *7*, 305–315. [CrossRef] [PubMed]

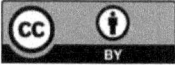

nutrients

MDPI

Review

Vitamin C Status and Cognitive Function: A Systematic Review

Nikolaj Travica [1,*], Karin Ried [2], Avni Sali [2], Andrew Scholey [1] (ID), Irene Hudson [1] and Andrew Pipingas [1]

1   Centre for Human Psychopharmacology, Swinburne University of Technology, John St, Hawthorn, Melbourne 3122, Australia; andrew@scholeylab.com (A.Sc.); Ihudson@swin.edu.au (I.H.); apipingas@swin.edu.au (A.P.)
2   The National Institute of Integrative Medicine, 21 Burwood Rd, Hawthorn, Melbourne 3122, Australia; karinried@niim.com.au (K.R.); asali@niim.com.au (A.Sa.)

Received: 28 July 2017; Accepted: 28 August 2017; Published: 30 August 2017

Abstract: Vitamin C plays a role in neuronal differentiation, maturation, myelin formation and modulation of the cholinergic, catecholinergic, and glutaminergic systems. This review evaluates the link between vitamin C status and cognitive performance, in both cognitively intact and impaired individuals. We searched the PUBMED, SCOPUS, SciSearch and the Cochrane Library from 1980 to January 2017, finding 50 studies, with randomised controlled trials (RCTs, $n = 5$), prospective ($n = 24$), cross-sectional ($n = 17$) and case-control ($n = 4$) studies. Of these, 36 studies were conducted in healthy participants and 14 on cognitively impaired individuals (including Alzheimer's and dementia). Vitamin C status was measured using food frequency questionnaires or plasma vitamin C. Cognition was assessed using a variety of tests, mostly the Mini-Mental-State-Examination (MMSE). In summary, studies demonstrated higher mean vitamin C concentrations in the cognitively intact groups of participants compared to cognitively impaired groups. No correlation between vitamin C concentrations and MMSE cognitive function was apparent in the cognitively impaired individuals. The MMSE was not suitable to detect a variance in cognition in the healthy group. Analysis of the studies that used a variety of cognitive assessments in the cognitively intact was beyond the scope of this review; however, qualitative assessment revealed a potential association between plasma vitamin C concentrations and cognition. Due to a number of limitations in these studies, further research is needed, utilizing plasma vitamin C concentrations and sensitive cognitive assessments that are suitable for cognitively intact adults.

Keywords: vitamin C; ascorbic acid; central nervous system; cognition; Alzheimer's; dementia; MMSE

1. Introduction

The biological benefits of the water soluble molecule vitamin C (L-ascorbic acid or ascorbate) have been well documented [1–5]. Based on its unique chemistry, the biological role of ascorbate is to act as a reducing agent, donating electrons in various enzymatic and non-enzymatic reactions [6]. It is a cofactor for at least eight enzymatic reactions involved in key bodily processes including the production of collagen, preventing harmful genetic mutations, protecting white blood cells [7] and the production of carnitine, vital for energy [8]. Ascorbate is reversibly oxidized with the loss of two electrons to form dehydroascorbic acid (DHAA).

Despite the extensive research into its enzymatic roles and antioxidant properties, the biological roles of vitamin C on the brain have only recently been described in detail. Animal studies have explored this biological link. In particular, research has focused on guinea pigs, due to their inability to biosynthesize vitamin C from glucose, similar to humans [9]. As a result of this biological limitation, the human brain relies on dietary sources of vitamin C. Animal studies have shown that vitamin C plays a vital role in neurodevelopment by influencing neuronal differentiation and the general development of neurons and myelin formation [9]. Additional, specific neurotransmitter functions include modulation of the cholinergic, catecholinergic, and glutaminergic systems of the brain. Ascorbic acid affects synaptic neurotransmission by preventing neurotransmitter binding to receptors [10], by modulating their release and reuptake [11], and also acting as a cofactor in neurotransmitter synthesis [12]. Another neuromodulatory role of Vitamin C appears to be its involvement in presynaptic re-uptake of glutamate [13], exhibiting a direct effect in the prevention of neuronal over-stimulation by glutamate [14].

Less research has been conducted on ascorbate in collagen synthesis in brain than in other organs, but minimal amounts are essential for blood vessel formation (angiogenesis). Vitamin C is essential for the formation of procollagen which then acts as an intracellular "glue" that gives support, shape and bulk to blood vessels [15]. Studies indicate that vitamin C deficiency in the brain is associated with a reduction in angiogenesis and vascular dysfunction [16,17] and the production of nitric oxide, responsible for vasodilation.

Neurons are especially sensitive to ascorbate deficiency, possibly due to 10-fold higher rates of oxidative metabolism than supporting glia [18]. Ascorbate at the concentrations present in CSF and neurons in vivo has been shown to effectively scavenge superoxide [19]. Once a superoxide radical is formed in the mitochondria of neurons, ascorbate catalyses its conversion to H_2O_2 and is oxidised in the process to an ascorbate free radical and DHAA. Ascorbate also supports the regeneration of other antioxidants, such as vitamin E and glutathione [19].

Indicative of its vital role in the brain is its recycling, homeostatic mechanism [20] which maintains vitamin C concentrations in the brain and neuronal tissues relative to other bodily organs and tissues. In the healthy brain, the content of vitamin C in cerebrospinal fluid (CSF) is highly concentrated compared to plasma (2–4 times more, 150–400 µmol/L) [21]. In whole brain, 1 to 2 mM of ascorbic acid has been detected, while intracellular neuronal concentrations are much higher, reaching up to 10 mM [22]. These high concentrations are the result of DHAA being recycled into ascorbate within astrocytes, which consist of glutathione [23]. The most saturated vitamin C brain regions include the cerebral cortex, hippocampus and amygdala [24,25].

Although higher plasma ascorbic acid concentrations generally result in higher CSF concentrations, these concentrations start to reach a steady state. As plasma concentrations decline, relatively more ascorbate is pumped into the CSF in order to maintain homeostasis [26]. Studies have demonstrated a higher CSF: plasma ratio in those with lower plasma vitamin C [26,27]. This could be a reflection of the increased "consumption" of ascorbate by the oxidative stressed brain, leading to lower plasma concentrations [26].

Thus, not only is it difficult to deplete brain ascorbate, it is also difficult to increase levels above those set by uptake and recycling mechanisms. In neuronal cells, the apparent Michaelis–Menten transport kinetics (K_m) for ascorbate appears to be somewhat high (113 µmol/L); this affinity corresponds well to plasma ascorbate concentrations of 30–60 µmol/L [28]. Thus, plasma vitamin C can only relate to brain vitamin C status in a narrow window, likely levels below 30 µmol/L.

Duration of deficiency has shown to influence brain ascorbate concentrations to a higher degree than the amount of depletion. This is exemplified by observations in acute scurvy where brain concentrations of ascorbate are relatively maintained through depletion of peripheral tissues [29], whereas marginal deficiency for longer periods of time resulted in greater brain ascorbate depletions [30].

Given the various biological roles on the central nervous system, a number of studies have been conducted with the intention of exploring whether vitamin C status is associated with cognitive performance in cognitively intact participants as well as those diagnosed with a neurodegenerative condition. This systematic review is the first to explore the effects of blood vitamin C status and cognitive performance in both cognitively impaired and intact groups of participants. This systematic review summarises current knowledge and provides recommendations for future studies.

2. Methods

2.1. Search Strategy

We searched the PUBMED, SCOPUS, SciSearch and the Cochrane Library for publications from 1980 to January 2017. Keywords used were vitamin C, ascorbic acid, antioxidant, cognition, memory, Alzheimer's and dementia. Additional published reports were obtained by checking references of screened articles. Studies only examining cognitive function and vitamin C status were included.

2.2. Selection of Trials

Study designs included randomised controlled trials, prospective cohort, cross-sectional, and case-control, restricted to those in the English language. This selection included adult participants who were either cognitively intact or diagnosed with a neurodegenerative condition such as Alzheimer's or dementia. Studies that administered some form of vitamin C measure and quantitative cognitive assessment were accepted.

2.3. Quality Assessment

Quality of studies was independently assessed by two investigators (NT and KR). Appraisal was determined using established guidelines for randomised, controlled trials (RCT), and observational studies (prospective and cohort) established from the Cochrane collaboration [31]. Quality was assessed on selection bias, allocation bias, attrition bias, methods to control confounding factors, and conflict of interest. Compliance was further assessed in RCTs. Higher-quality trials (score ≥ 4 of 8 points for RCT, ≥ 3 of 4 points for prospective and ≥ 2 of 3 for cross-sectional and case control) were compared with lower-quality studies.

2.4. Analysis of Trials Using Comparable Methods

An initial survey of the literature revealed that many studies used comparable cognitive and vitamin C measures—The Mini Mental State Examination (MMSE) and blood plasma vitamin C concentrations. Given this consistency in measurement we decided to further explore these trends across studies. A brief summary of these inclusions and methods is presented below. We contacted authors for mean values and standard deviations of studies which did not report numerical mean vitamin C concentrations or MMSE scores (0–30) but instead placed the means into categories (e.g., MMSE score of over/under 27, vitamin C concentrations into deficient/adequate ranges).

2.5. Blood Plasma Vitamin C

Given the practicality and accuracy of measuring absorbed vitamin C status through blood plasma, plasma vitamin C has been considered the ideal measure of vitamin C status [32]. A number of investigated studies have used this measure to determine vitamin C status. vitamin C blood concentrations, based on population studies, indicate that a plasma concentration of <11 µmol/L is considered to be deficient, 11–28 µmol/L is depleted or marginally deficient, 28–40 µmol/L is adequate, and >40 µmol/L is optimal [33]. Other studies measured CSF vitamin C concentrations or incorporated a variety of FFQs and supplementation questionnaires, measuring daily intake in milligrams. A recommended daily intake of 200 mg/day has been suggested, as this corresponds with optimal vitamin C blood concentrations [34].

2.6. Measure of Cognition

The MMSE is a simple validated and reliable paper and pen questionnaire designed to estimate the severity and progression of cognitive impairment and used to follow the course of cognitive changes in an individual over time [35]. Any score greater than or equal to 24 points (out of 30) indicates normal cognition. Below this, scores can indicate severe ($\leq$9 points), moderate (10–18 points) or mild (19–23 points) cognitive impairment [36]. The cognitive domains measured include attention and calculation, recall, language, ability to follow simple commands and orientation. Descriptive analyses were conducted for all included studies, which assessed vitamin C concentrations (means and standard deviations in μmol/L for blood tests and mg/day for FFQs), and mean MMSE scores.

2.7. Z Statistical Analysis-Correlation Between Blood Vitamin C and MMSE Score

Using IBM SPSS (version 23, Chicago, IL, USA) *t*-tests were conducted, comparing the baseline blood vitamin C concentrations and baseline MMSE scores between cognitively intact and impaired participants. Due to the ordinal nature of MMSE scores and ratio scales for blood test concentrations, a Spearman's correlation coefficient analysis (*r* values) was conducted. R-squared values, assessing goodness of fit and test of normality were conducted to establish the correlation between mean vitamin C concentrations and MMSE scores.

Only studies which measured blood vitamin C concentrations and cognition through the MMSE were compared. Comparable mean vitamin C blood concentrations and MMSE scores were extracted as separate data points from each of the studies and plotted graphically. A number of studies assessing cognitively impaired individuals also used healthy controls. The mean MMSE and vitamin C concentrations from these controls was added to the mean scores of other cognitively intact samples for comparison.

FFQ-based vitamin C levels were also converted to predicted blood concentrations, where every 1.97 mg of consumed vitamin C equates to 1 μmol/L of ascorbate plasma. A constant plateau in ascorbic acid concentration (60–80 μmol/L) is reached at 150 mg of consumed vitamin C [34]. Given the non-linear link between vitamin C consumption and absorption, the converted FFQ blood concentrations were added to the scatterplot for comparison, but were not included in the analysis. Additionally, ascorbate CSF concentrations were not included in the analysis due to a non-linear relationship with plasma vitamin C.

Additionally, qualitative analyses were conducted on the studies that utilized a range of other cognitive assessments and direct plasma vitamin C measures. These studies were reported qualitatively due to a large diversity in cognitive assessments and statistical reporting of results (odds ratios, confidence intervals, etc.). The overall trend of results and quality of these trials was taken into account for the qualitative analysis.

3. Results

The search captured exactly 500 articles, of which 50 studies were included in the systematic review (Figure 1). Of these, 14 studies involved cognitively impaired participants, e.g., dementia including Alzheimer's disease and 36 studies were conducted on cognitively intact participants. The cognitively impaired subgroup included 3 RCTS [37–39], 4 prospective [26,40,41], 4 cross-sectional [42–45] and 4 case-control [46–49] studies (Table 1). The cognitively intact subgroup included 2 RCTS [50,51], 21 prospective [52–72], 13 cross-sectional [73–85], and no case-control studies (Table 2). Table 3 summarises the trials that were excluded from the review, and the reason for their exclusion.

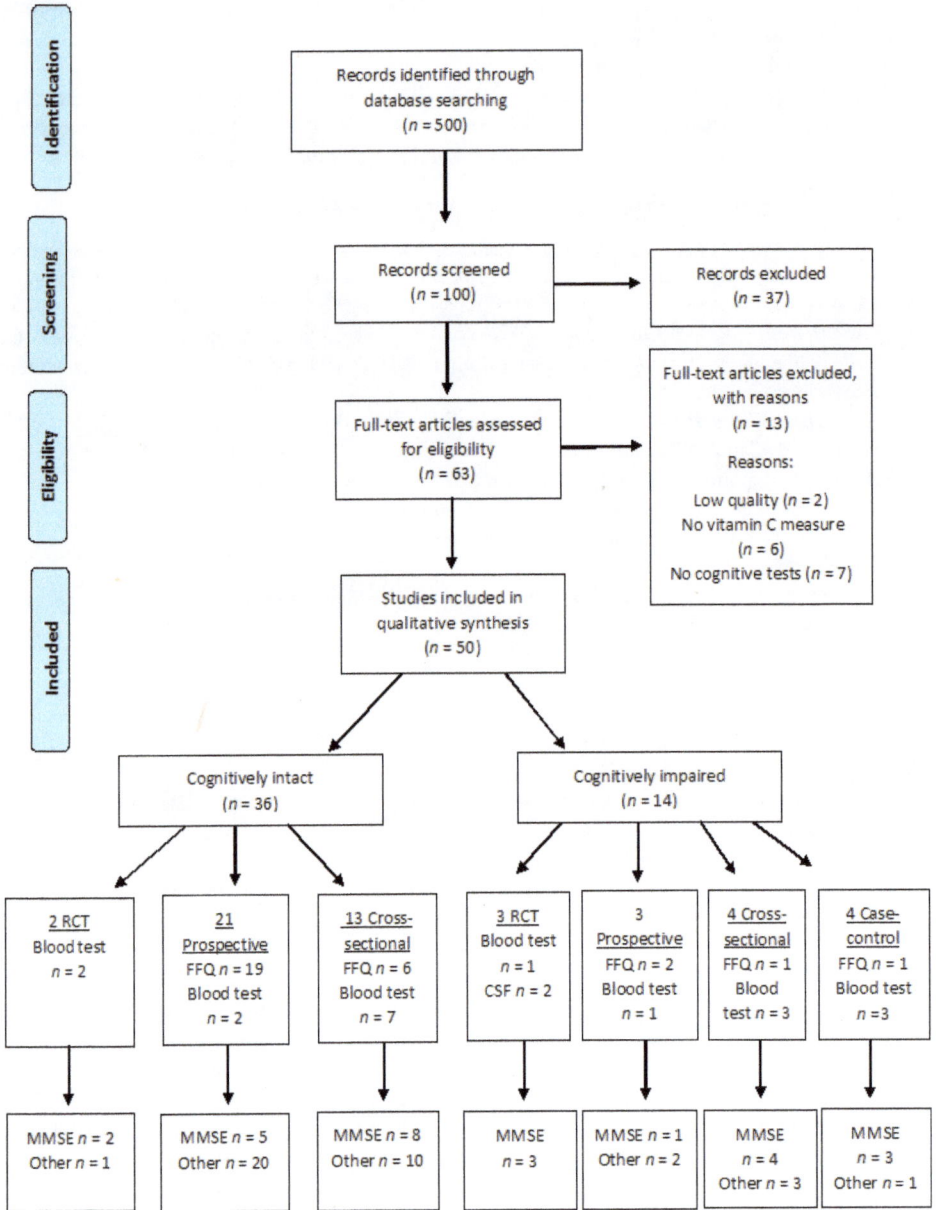

Figure 1. Flow chart of steps in systematic review.

Table 1. Characteristics and outcomes of studies using cognitively impaired samples.

Paper	Study Design	N	Age (years)	Condition	Quality Rating	Cognitive Measure	Vitamin C Measure	Outcome
Arlt, 2012 [37]	RCT	23	60–80	AD	6	MMSE, Word fluency, Immediate/delayed verbal recall, Trail-making task	CSF	1000 mg/day of vit C and E (400 mg/day) increased CSF concentrations after 1 year, but decreased MMSE score and no effect on other measures
Galasko, 2012 [47]	RCT	78	50–85	AD	4.5	MMSE	CSF	Decline in MMSE score occurred in E/C/ALA group. (500 mg/day vit C, vit E, alpha lipoic acid) did not influence CSF biomarkers related to amyloid
Burns, 1989 [39]	RCT	81	≥65	Senile Dementia, Community dementia	4.5	MMSE	Blood tests	200 mg Vit C, vits B1, B2, B3 No correlation between vit C intake and cognitive impairment
Bowman, 2009 [26]	Pros	32	71	AD	5	MMSE	CSF, plasma ascorbate	Neither Plasma nor CSF AA predictive of AD across 1 year
Zandi, 2004 [40]	Pros	4740 (4540 healthy)	≥65	AD	3.5	3MS, Dementia Questionnaire (DQ)	Supplement, Interview	vit E (>400 IU) and C (500 mg) supplements reduced the AD prevalence and incidence. Supplements alone had no protective affect across 2 years
Deijen, 2003 [41]	Pros	90	>65	Psychiatry nursing home	4.5	Dutch geriatric nursing scale, Zorg Index geriatrie (ZIG)	Food record	Higher vitamin intakes were associated with a worse daily functioning across 6 months
Rinaldi, 2003 [42]	Cross	141	>70	MCI, AD	3	Clinical dementia rating scale, MMSE, clock drawing test, Babcock story recall, auditory verbal learning test, Corsi block tapping test, Token test, category naming test, Oral word association test, visual search test, digit forward and backward test, Raven's progressive colored matrices	Plasma ascorbate	Lower vit C concentrations in patients with AD and MCI. MCI sig lower then controls
Polidori, 2004 [43]	Cross	141	≥65	AD, VaD	2	MMSE	Plasma ascorbate	Plasma AA lower in AD and VD
Richardson, 2002 [44]	Cross	37	65–97	In-patient ward	2	MMSE	Plasma ascorbate	75% with dementia had low concentrations of vitamin C
Lu, 2016 [45]	Cross	2892 (768 MCI)	58	MCI	2.5	Montreal cognitive assessment	FFQ	Carotenoids, vit C, and vitamin B6 exhibited the highest protective factor loadings
Charlton, 2004 [46]	CC	93	≥65	Dementia	4	MMSE	Plasma Ascorbate/FFQ	Plasma AA lower in dementia, not explained by diet
Glaso, 2004 [47]	CC	38	75–85	AD	4	MMSE	Serum ascorbate/CSF	Both plasma vitamin C and CSF lower in AD. CSF: plasma AA ratio higher in AD
Riviere, 1999 [48]	CC	69	>75	Severe AD, Moderate AD, Hospitalised AD	3.5	MMSE	Plasma ascorbate, FFQ	Nutritional intake lower in Severe AD, plasma vit C lower in more severe AD, not explained by vit C intake
Masaki, 2000 [49]	CC	3735 men	71–93	Dementia	3	Hasegawa scale, MMSE	Self-report supplementation	After controlling for factors such as age, education, stroke, there was an association with cognitive performance

Key: MCI = Mild cognitive impairment, AD = Alzheimer's, VaD = vascular dementia RCT = Randomized control trial, Pros = prospective, Cross = cross-sectional, CC = case-control, Vit = vitamin, FFQ = food frequency questionnaire, CSF = cerebrospinal fluid, MMSE = Mini mental state examination, 3MS = Modified Mini Mental State Examination, ALA = alpha lipoic acid.

Table 2. Characteristics and outcomes of studies using cognitively intact samples.

Paper	Study Design	N	Age (years)	Quality Assessment	Cognitive Measure	Vitamin C Measure	Outcome
Chandra, 2001 [50]	RCT	86	≥65	5.5	Wechsler memory test, Halstead-Reitan categories test, Buschke consistent long-term retrieval, digit span forward, salthouse listening span test, long-term memory recall, MMSE	Plasma spectrophotometry	80 mg of vitamin C in a multivitamin improved cognitive performance, not Long-term memory across 1 year
Dror, 1996 [51]	RCT	21	>80	3.5	MMSE	Plasma Assay	No changes in MMSE scores following 42-day supplementation with 45mg/day of vitamin C with other vitamins (Vit D, E B12, B6)
Gale, 1996 [52]	Pros	921	≥65	2.5	Hodkinson mental test (Dementia assessment)	Dietary intake/Ascorbate plasma	Cognitive function was poorest in those with the lowest vitamin C over 1 year
La Rue, 1997 [53]	Pros	137	66–90	5	Abstract performance, visuospatial performance, memory assessment	Plasma Ascorbate, Nutritional status	Visuospatial performance was higher with higher ascorbate concentrations after 6 years
Paleologos, 1998 [54]	Pros	117	69–91	4	MMSE, Reid brief neuropsychological Screen, the animals test of category fluency, the F, A, S test of verbal fluency	Semi-quantitative food frequency	After adjusting for age, sex, smoking, education, energy, vit C supplement linked to less severe cognitive decline, not verbal/category fluency across 4 years
Devore, 2002 [55]	Pros	16,010	>70 Women	5	MMSE, Telephone interview for cognitive status (TICS). East Boston memory test (immediate/delayed) category fluency, Delayed TICS, Digit span backwards	Semi-quantitative food frequency	Dietary vitamin C intake not associated with cognitive decline. Supplemental vit C associated with worse decline over 6 years
Engelhart, 2002 [56]	Pros	5395	>55	3.5	DSM-III-R criteria, MMSE	Semi-quantitative food frequency (SFFQ)	Higher dietary vit C intake associated with less AD after a mean of 6.5 years, controlling for supplements
Kalmijn, 1997 [57]	Pros	342 Men	69–89	3	MMSE	Dietary history FFQ	Higher vit C intake not correlated with cognitive decline or impairment after 3 years
Laurin, 2003 [58]	Pros	2549 Men	45–68	4	Hasegawa dementia screening instrument, MMSE, 3MS	24-h dietary recall	Vit C was not associated with the risk of dementia or its subtypes across an 8-year period
Basambombo, 2016 [59]	Pros	5269	≥65	2.5	Diagnostic and Statistical Manual of Mental Disorders (DSM-III-R)	Self-reported supplementation	The use of vitamin C supplements associated with a reduced risk of cognitive decline during 3, 5 year intervals
Nooyens, 2015 [60]	Pros	2613	43–70	5	15 Words Learning Test, the Stroop Test, Word Fluency test, Letter Digit Substitution Test	178-item semi-quantitative FFQ	No associations between intakes of vit C and cognitive decline across 5 years
Peneau, 2011 [61]	Pros	2533	45–60	4.5	RI-48 cued recall, semantic, and phonemic fluency tests, trail-making and forward and backward digit span tests	24-h dietary record	vit C–rich FVs (P-trend = 0.03), vitamin C (P-trend = 0.005) positively associated with verbal memory across 13 years
Fotuhi, 2008 [62]	Pros	3376	≥65	2.5	3MS	Self-report	Combined vit C, E, and anti-inflammatory resulted in a lower decline on the 3MS across 8 years. Vit C alone had no affect
Gray, 2008 [63]	Pros	2969	≥65	3.5	Cognitive abilities screening instrument	Self-report	No association between vitamin C and AD incidence, or vit C and E together after 2.8–8.7 years

Table 2. *Cont.*

Paper	Study Design	N	Age (years)	Quality Assessment	Cognitive Measure	Vitamin C Measure	Outcome
Wengreen, 2007 [64]	Pros	3831	≥65	3.5	3MS	Food frequency	Higher quartiles of vit C intake had a greater 3MS score and lower vit C intake had a greater rate of decline during 7 years
Fillenbaum, 2005 [65]	Pros	616	65–105	3.5	Short portable mental status questionnaire	In home interview	Vitamin C did not reduce AD or dementia incidence over either 3 or 14-year interval
Maxwell, 2005 [66]	Pros	894	≥65	3.5	3MS	Self-report	Subjects reporting supplementation of vit C were less likely to have cognitive decline or to be diagnosed with VCI after 5 years
Grodstein, 2003 [67]	Pros	14,968	70–79 women	4.5	Telephone Interview of Cognitive Status, Delayed recall of 10 word lists, Immediate and delayed recall of paragraph, Verbal fluency, Digit span backwards	Supplementation questionnaire	Vit C and E had higher mean global scores than non-supplemented. Vit C alone did not affect global score after 5 years
Luchsinger, 2003 [68]	Pros	980	≥65	4.5	Neuropsychological test battery	Semi quantitative food frequency	Neither dietary, supplemental nor total intake of vit C across 4 years was linked to AD Incidence
Morris, 2002 [69]	Pros	815	>65	3	Consortium Established for Research on AD	FFQ	Intake of vitamin C was not significantly associated with risk of AD across 3.9 years
Peacock, 2000 [70]	Pros	12,187	48–67	4.5	Delayed word recall test, Wechsler adult intelligence scale, Revised digit symbol subtest, word fluency test	Food frequency questionnaire	No consistent association between dietary and supplemental vit C and cognition across 8 years
Morris, 1998 [71]	Pros	633	≥65	3.5	Criteria for clinical diagnosis	Supplementation questionnaire	None of the vitamin C users were diagnosed after a mean of 4.3 years
Mendelsohn, 1996 [72]	Pros	1059	≥65	2.5	Neuropsychological battery (15 items)	297 vitamin C self-report supplementation	After adjustment for age, race, income, education, vit C supplementation did not relate to cognitive scores during 2 years
Berti, 2015 [73]	Cross	52 Women	54–66	1.5	Clinical dementia rating, Global deterioration score, MMSE	Harvard/Willet FFQ	Antioxidant consumption positively associated with METglc ($p < 0.001$)
Beydoun, 2015 [74]	Cross	1274	30–60	2	MMSE, CLVT-list A, CVLT-DFR, digit span forward/backwards, Benton visual retention test, Animal fluency test, Brief test of attention, trail making test, Clock drawing test, card rotations, identical pictures	Two 24-h recalls	Vitamin C not associated with cognition on either cognitive task, MMSE error count ($p = 0.17$)
Chaudhari, 2015 [75]	Cross	582	40–96	2	Repeatable battery for the assessment of neurological status, The executive interview	Ascorbate supplementation (self-report)	Vit C led to better immediate memory ($p = 0.04$), visuospatial skills ($p = 0.0002$), language ($p = 0.01$), global cognition ($p = 0.006$)
Goodwin, 1983 [76]	Cross	260	>60	2	Halstead-Reitan Categories, (Non-verbal abstract thinking), Wechsler Memory Test	Dietary intake/Ascorbate plasma	Performance worse on both tasks in those with low vit C (5–10% lowest levels)
Jama, 1996 [77]	Cross	5182	55–95	2.5	MMSE	Semi-quantitative food frequency questionnaire	No association between cognitive function and intake of vitamin C intake (<70mg/day (odd ratio) = 1.14, 130–160 mg/day (od) = 1.21

Table 2. *Cont.*

Paper	Study Design	N	Age (years)	Quality Assessment	Cognitive Measure	Vitamin C Measure	Outcome
Lindemann, 2000 [78]	Cross	195	≥65	3	MMSE, WAIS-R Digits Forward, Fuld Object Memory Evaluation, Clock drawing, Two Color Trail Making Tests	Serum ascorbate	Lower vit C not associated with cognition. There was a trend. Low vit C linked with a history of depression
Perrig, 1997 [79]	Cross	442	≥65	3	Computerised cognitive test (assessed working, implicit and explicit memory), WAIS-R vocabulary test	Plasma Ascorbate	Free recall, recognition, and vocabulary (not priming or working memory) correlated with ascorbic acid concentrations (semantic memory $p = 0.034$, vocabulary test $p \leq 0.021$)
Schmidt, 1998 [80]	Cross	1769	50–75	2	Mattis Dementia Rating Scale	Plasma (chromatograph)	No association between cognitive scores and plasma concentrations (odds ratio = 1, $p = 0.87$)
Sato, 2006 [81]	Cross	544	≥65	2.5	Digit symbol substitution task (DSST), MMSE	Ascorbate plasma, Block's FFQ	Highest fifth of plasma ascorbate associated with better DSST, marginally with MMSE
Whalley, 2003 [82]	Cross	176	77	2.5	MMSE, Raven's Progressive Matrices	Ascorbate plasma, FFQ (MONICA)	No difference between those taking vitamin C supplements and controls, after controlling for childhood IQ, education, socioeconomic status and cardiovascular health
Perkins, 1998 [83]	Cross	4809	>60	2	Delayed word recall, Delayed story recall	Serum ascorbate	After adjusting for socioeconomic factors and other trace elements, vitamin C concentrations were not associated with poor memory performance
Ortega, 1997 [84]	Cross	260	65–90	1.5	MMSE, Pfeiffer's mental status questionnaire	Food frequency for 7 days	Higher cognition correlated with great vitamin C intake across 7 days
Requejo, 2003 [85]	Cross	168	65–90	0.5	MMSE	Food record	Those with a greater intake of vitamin C were more likely to display adequate cognitive ability

Key: MCI = Mild cognitive impairment, AD = Alzheimer's, VaD = vascular dementia RCT = Randomized control trial, Pros = prospective, Cross = cross-sectional, CC = case-control, Vit = vitamin, FFQ = food frequency questionnaire, CSF = cerebrospinal fluid, MMSE = Mini mental state examination, 3MS = Modified Mini Mental State Examination.

Table 3. List of studies with reasons for exclusion.

Study	Study Design	Reason for Exclusion
Kennedy (2011) [86]	RCT	Mood/fatigue primary measures, vitamin C status not assessed
Smith (1999) [87]	RCT	Self-reported cognitive failures (subjective cognitive assessment)
Kumar (2008) [88]	RCT	Vitamin C status not assessed
Yaffe (2004) [89]	RCT	Cognition not assessed at baseline, vitamin C status not assessed
Kang (2009) [90]	RCT	Cognition not assessed at baseline, only 3.5 years after intervention
Chui (2008) [91]	RCT	Vitamin C status not assessed, no placebo/blinding
Day (1988) [92]	RCT	Vitamin C status not assessed, assessed only confusion
Paraskevas (1997) [93]/Quinn (2004) [27]/Woo (1989) [94]/Polidori (2002) [95]/Foy (1998) [96]	CS	No cognitive tests administered
Talley [97]	Pre-test post-test	Simple orientation/consciousness assessment

Legend: RCT = Randomised control trial, CS = case-control.

In the cognitively impaired samples, eight out of 14 studies used blood tests to measure vitamin C [26,39,42–44,46–48], two used CSF [37,38] and four used FFQs alone [40,41,45,49]. A series of cognitive tests were conducted in these studies. Eleven studies [26,37–39,42–44,47–49] used the MMSE and six [37,40–42,45,49] used alternate forms of cognitive assessment. In the cognitively intact samples, 11 out of 36 used blood tests to measure vitamin C status [50–53,76,78–83], and 25 studies conducted FFQs [54–75,77,84,85]. A series of cognitive tests were conducted in these studies. Fifteen studies [50,51,54–58,73,74,77,78,81,82,84,85] used the MMSE and 31 studies [50,52–56,58–67,69–76,78–84,98] used other forms of cognitive assessment.

Mean MMSE scores and measured or derived blood vitamin C concentrations are plotted in Figure 2 and presented in Tables 4 and 5. In the cognitively impaired group, these means were extracted from seven studies (sample sizes ranged from 12–88 participants, with a total of 391 participants). Independent samples t-tests revealed that mean vitamin C concentrations in the cognitively intact subgroup were significantly higher than in the cognitively impaired (t (15) = 4.5, $p < 0.01$) and mean MMSE scores were also significantly higher in this subgroup (t (10.3) = 5.7, $p < 0.01$).

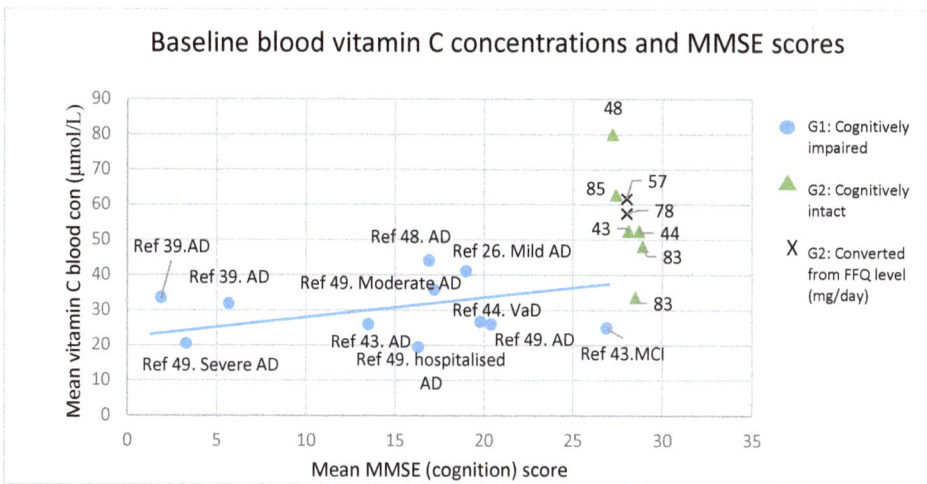

Figure 2. Scatterplot of baseline mean MMSE scores against blood vitamin C concentrations. Blue circles represent cognitively impaired groups of participants, and green triangles and crosses represent cognitively intact groups (triangles: direct plasma vit C measure, cross: converted from FFQ). No correlation analyses were conducted on the cognitively intact data points. The blue line represents the correlation slope amongst the studies of cognitively impaired groups of participants (r_s (11) = 0.009, $p = 0.98$). Key: Ref = study reference, * Not included in the analysis, AD = Alzheimer's disease, CSF = Cerebral Spinal Fluid, FFQ = Food Frequency Questionnaire; MCI = mild cognitive impairment, mg/day = milligram per day, VaD = Vascular dementia, Con = concentration, MMSE = Mini Mental State Examination.

Table 4. Cognitively impaired participants (Mean blood vitamin C/MMSE scores).

Paper	Study Design	N	Mean Vitamin C Level in μmol/L (SD)	Mean MMSE Score (SD)
Burns (1989) [39]	RCT	81	Intervention baseline-33.5 (28)	1.9 (3.3)
			Placebo baseline-31.8 (31)	5.7 (9.1)
			Placebo final-25 (28) [#]	5.7 (10.6) [#]
Bowman (2009) [26]	Pros	32	41 (30)	19 (5)
Rinaldi (2003) [42]	CS	25	MCI-24.9 (2.4)	26.9 (2)
		63	AD-25.9 (8.9)	13.5 (6.5)
Polidori (2004) [43]	CS	63	AD-25.9 (8.9)	20.4 (3)
		23	Vascular AD-26.6 (11.3)	19.8 (3)
Glaso (2004) [47]	CC	20	AD-44 (25)	16.9
Rivierie (1999) [48]	CC	24	Moderate AD-35.7	17.2 (4.9)
		9	Hospitalized AD-19.3	16.3 (6.1)
		20	Severe AD-20.4	3.3 (3.1)

Legend: SD, standard deviation; RCT = randomised controlled trial, Pros = prospective, CS = cross-sectional, CC = case-control, # not a baseline value therefore not included in analysis, blue circles representing cognitively impaired blood values.

Table 5. Cognitively intact participants (Mean blood vitamin C/MMSE scores).

Paper	Study Design	N	Vitamin C Level in μmol/L (SD)	MMSE Score (SD)
Engelhart (2002) [56] *	Pros	5395	61.7 (27)	28
Jama (1996) [77] *	CS	5182	57.5	28
Ortega (1997) [84]	CS	260	62.7 (33.5)	27.4 (4.8)
Whalley (2003) [82]	CS	79	Non-supplement user-33.7 (26.2)	28.5 (1.4)
		31	Supplement user-48.2 (25.7)	28.9 (1.4)
Glaso (2004) [47]	CC	18	Control group-80 (28)	27.2
Polidori (2004) [43]	CS	55	Control group-52.4 (16.4)	28.7 (1)
Rinaldi (2003) [42]	CS	53	Control group-52.4 (16.5)	28.1 (1.4)
Chandra (2001) [50] [#]	RCT	86	Adequate	28 (6.3)
			Deficient	17 (4)
Lindemann (2003) [78] [#]	CC	195	>57	27.2 (2.4)
			<57	26.4 (2.9)
Sato (2006) [81] [#]	CC	544	Median = 74.9 (interquartile range = 57.8–90.7)	<27
			Median = 78.9 (interquartile range = 64.1–99.2)	>27
Richardson (2002) [44] [#]	CC	37	<11	23 (12.3)
			11–40	25 (6.0)
			40–100	27 (5.1)

Legend: RCT = randomised controlled trial, Pros = prospective, CS = cross-sectional, CC = case-control, * converted FFQ to blood vitamin C (μmol/L) represented by crosses on Figure 2 (not included in analysis), green circles representing cognitively intact blood values (Figure 2), # Not included in analysis.

In the cognitively impaired subgroup, there was a wide distribution of both MMSE scores (mean score range = 1.9–26.9) and vitamin C concentrations (19–44 μmol/L) (Figure 2). Mean vitamin C concentration (Mean score ± standard deviation (SD) = 29.91 ± 8 μmol/L) corresponded with a borderline vitamin C depletion (<28 μmol/L) [33]. Mean MMSE scores (Mean score = 14.63 ± 7.8) corresponded to a severe cognitive impairment (scores >17) [99].

In the cognitively intact subgroup, mean vitamin C and MMSE scores were extracted from 5 studies (sample sizes ranged 18–260 participants, with a total of 496 participants). In this group, mean vitamin C concentrations (Mean score ± SD = 54.9 ± 16) μmol/L) were widely spread (33.7–80 μmol/L) but mean MMSE scores (Mean score = 28.1 ± 0.7) were not (27.2–28.9). The lack of variance in MMSE scores precluded correlational analysis in this subgroup.

In the cognitively impaired subgroup the scatterplot (Figure 2/Table 4) and a Pearson r^2 value of 0.0016 revealed low variance and a spread in means around the fitted regression line. The Spearman's correlation also revealed no significant correlation between MMSE scores and vitamin C concentrations (r_s (11) = 0.009, $p = 0.98$).

A number of studies [44,50,78,81] (Table 5) did not report numerical mean vitamin C concentrations or MMSE scores (0–30) but instead placed the means into categories (e.g., MMSE score of over/under 27, Vitamin C concentrations into deficient/adequate ranges). The results from these studies followed our observed trend where participants whose vitamin C concentrations were categorized into adequate ranges produced higher mean MMSE scores and those who were categorized into scoring under 27 on the MMSE had lower mean vitamin C concentrations.

Additional studies using cognitively intact groups of participants (Table 2) assessed cognition using a number of different cognitive measures and plasma vitamin C. Examples of these cognitive measures included the digit span backwards/forwards, the East Boston memory test, Wechsler memory test, clock drawing, delayed word recall, etc. (Table 2). A majority of these studies [50,52,78,79,81] revealed an association between vitamin C blood concentrations and cognitive performance on various cognitive tasks. Some of the cognitive domains included short-term memory, information processing, abstract thinking and working memory. A number of studies [80,82,83] did fail to demonstrate a link between vitamin C and cognition. However, the quality assessment revealed lower ratings for these studies than for those demonstrating a link. Additionally, one study [42] using cognitively impaired groups of participants (Table 1) assessed cognition with alternative assessments to the MMSE and demonstrated superior performance in those with higher vitamin C concentrations.

The predicted blood vitamin C concentrations generated from FFQs in the cognitively intact participants when plotted (Figure 2), were relatively similar to the blood concentrations generated by studies primarily using blood tests. These converted values were not used in correlation analyses.

4. Discussion

This review evaluated 50 studies exploring the link between vitamin C and cognitive function. Extrapolated mean vitamin C concentrations and MMSE scores from a number of these studies indicated that the cognitively intact groups of participants had higher mean vitamin C concentrations and MMSE scores than the cognitively impaired groups. However, there was no significant correlation between mean vitamin C concentrations and mean MMSE scores in the cognitively impaired studies ($n = 7$, $n = 391$ participants). In contrast, correlation analysis between blood vitamin C concentrations and MMSE scores in the cognitively intact studies was not feasible due to the low variance in MMSE scores, demonstrating the unsuitability of the MMSE in the cognitively healthy participants. Quantitative assessment of those studies in the cognitively intact groups revealed a potential association between plasma vitamin C concentrations and cognition. Our findings are consistent with a number of studies [42,48,95] that showed a significantly lower vitamin C blood concentrations between cognitively impaired compared to healthy individuals.

This may be explained by a reduction in dietary intake amongst the elderly in general [100], and those living alone or in aged care/hospital facilities [101] who are often unable to prepare their own meals, may have chewing problems, and may make poor food choices such as not including fruits and vegetables in their diet.

Subjects with AD may be nutrient deficient, particularly in the later phase of the disease. However, case-control studies have also demonstrated lower plasma vitamin C concentrations in the early AD stages in well-nourished subjects [48].

A more recent, second hypothesis for the depleted blood vitamin C concentrations in the cognitively impaired is the increased oxidation of vitamin C in response to elevated free radical production in the brain. Vitamin C has been reported to be the first barrier to free radicals produced in biological fluids [102]. In the cognitively impaired, studies have demonstrated an increased sensitivity to free radicals in the cerebral cortex [103]. The mechanisms of free radical production hypothesized for AD include: activated microglia surrounding senile plaques [104], neuronal mitochondrial dysfunction [105], intraneuronal amyloid accumulation [106] and presence of redox active metals [107]. Thirdly, disturbances in iron metabolism found in the vicinity of the senile plaques [108], could catalyse the production of free radicals. Noradrenergic and serotoninergic deficiencies have also been reported in AD [109], requiring the utilisation of vitamin C to restore these deficiencies.

The lack of linearity in vitamin C concentrations and MMSE scores in the cognitively impaired group could be explained by the non-linear relationship between plasma vitamin C and ascorbate CSF absorption. Due to a homeostatic mechanism [26], the amount of ascorbate CSF and vitamin C reaching the brain could show little variability at varying plasma concentrations, even with deficient plasma concentrations (<28 μmol/L). This could result in similar cognitive scores at varying plasma vitamin C concentrations.

4.1. Limitations

The results from the current review do need to be interpreted cautiously due to a number of limitations:

While blood samples are a more reliable measure of vitamin C status than FFQ-based Vitamin C determination, a number of further methodical issues may exist. Many factors can contribute to the instability of ascorbic acid in biological samples due to the oxidation of vitamin C in plasma is accelerated by heat, light, and elevated pH (acidity). These issues arise as a result of a lack of full appreciation of the redox chemistry and biology of ascorbic acid [110]. A number of handling techniques should be incorporated in order to ensure quality measures.

A majority of studies included in this review failed to thoroughly explain blood sample handling and biochemical analysis. Ideal handling conditions of samples intended for ascorbate analysis include immediate coverage from light, immediate plasma isolation, rapid acidification, and freezing below −20 °C to avoid misinterpretations compounded by the use of poorly preserved samples [110]. In order for plasma to be transported, it needs to be covered from light and transported on dry ice (−70 °C) before thawing and analysis.

Underestimation of vitamin C concentrations could occur if samples were not handled properly. Frequent freeze-thaw cycles or exposure to any metals (such as iron in the haemolysis of red blood cells) could both lead to rapid degradation of vitamin C in the sample [111]. It has been shown that there is a significant loss of ascorbate plasma in EDTA tubes [112], with lithium heparin tubes being ideal.

Several limitations can arise from the use of FFQs in determining nutrient level [32]. Plasma vitamin C concentrations are dependent on recent dietary intake, due to the vitamin's water soluble properties and excretion, therefore blood plasma measures would be most reflective of foods consumed recently (1–2 weeks). Incorporating food questionnaires relating to most recent food consumption, would be most indicative of blood concentrations. Given the overreliance on FFQs in the reviewed studies, especially in those incorporating prospective designs, instead of blood samples interpretation of findings is limited. A direct comparison between FFQ and blood samples could validate the effective of the questionnaire. A recent meta-analysis demonstrated that FFQ and food diaries have a moderate relationship with plasma vitamin C, with multiple factors affecting this relationship [32].

While converted FFQ-based vitamin C levels were of a similar range to blood concentrations, this conversion needs to be interpreted with caution. The conversion ratio of 1.95 mg to 1 μmol/L in plasma was based on a study that used 8 healthy participants [34]. However, this ratio may not be applicable for all individuals as individual factors could affect vitamin C absorption and distribution (i.e., oxidative stress, infection, etc.).

Plasma vitamin C differs according to polymorphisms of sodium dependent active transporters (SVCT2 and SVCT1) despite equivalent vitamin C intake indicating that SVCT1 and 2 genotype may determine the strength of the association between vitamin C intake and circulating vitamin C concentrations [113]. Some people may require greater than the recommended daily allowance to maintain optimal vitamin C concentrations. These differences could render food diary information even less accurate as perceived intake may not be equivalent to absorption [111].

In addition, dietary assessment has reliability and validity issues in relation to even mild cognitive deficits, which are frequent in older populations [114]. These include recall errors but even when food types and amounts are recalled correctly, differences in storage and cooking can decrease the vitamin C level in the food [115]. It is close to impossible to determine the concentrations retained in foods following manipulations such as cooking [116]. Furthermore, high levels of vitamin C gained from dietary sources will often be accompanied by higher levels of a number of other beneficial compounds (vitamins, phytochemicals) also found from the same sources [111].

Moreover, the reviewed randomised controlled studies have failed to assess the effects of a vitamin C intervention on its own, by using multivitamins. A large portion of the included studies have made efforts to statistically control for potential confounders. Although our review did demonstrate lower plasma vitamin C concentrations in the cognitively impaired, other studies using impaired samples have shown depletions in a number of other vitamin and minerals including: vitamin B12 [117], vitamin E [118], vitamin D [119], vitamin K [120], folate [117], and elevated homocysteine [117]. Additionally, it is important to note that when antioxidant function is involved, vitamins can work synergistically with other vitamins, e.g., vitamin C recycles α-tocopherol radical (vitamin E) [111]. The consumption and supplementation of these vitamins should be considered as potential confounders and should be monitored, especially in cognitive impaired participants.

Moreover, it can be speculated that a consistently high Vitamin C status acts in a preventive manner, while vitamin C supplementation per se is not a treatment for clinical AD [48]. Thus, infrequent supplement users may not achieve the same benefits as individuals with consistent intake of adequate vitamin C. Controlling for vitamin C supplementation use, or taking it into account, is crucial.

Intake at the time of measurement may not reflect lifetime dietary habits and given data that suggest that amyloid plaque burden begins to form well before middle age [121], intakes during younger adulthood may be equally as important as supplements taken by older adults, perhaps contributing to a biological buffer against disease pathogenesis. Measuring and controlling for a history of consumption and supplementation is crucial, especially in longer prospective studies where the development of neurodegeneration is being investigated.

In addition to the limitations on vitamin C levels, there were limitations regarding the type of cognitive measures. A number of long term prospective studies incorporated cognitive tests suitable for screening and assessing the incidence of Alzheimer's, such as the MMSE. Given the simplicity of such tests, and the scales used to measure performance, it becomes difficult to establish cognitive changes unless the cognitive decline is extremely severe. These MMSE scales have been effective in measuring cognition in those clinically diagnosed with a neurodegenerative condition [48,96], and were useful in the cognitively impaired subgroup in this review.

The sensitivity of the MMSE to detect differences in cognitively intact samples has been questioned [122,123]. This can lead to a lack of variance in MMSE scores. In our review, the mean MMSE score ranged 27.2–28.9 in this group (<24 = mild cognitive impairment). In this review, a number of studies conducted on the cognitively intact group did use a range of other, more suitable cognitive tests, including the digit span forwards/backwards, delayed word recall, letter digit substitution test, etc., with mixed results. A number of these studies [55,67,70,74,83] failed to demonstrate a link between vitamin C status and cognition whereas a number of studies [50,61,76,79,81] demonstrated the effects of vitamin C on a number of cognitive domains such as free recall, short-term memory, abstract thinking, visuospatial performance and recognition. However, comparison of different cognitive tests was beyond the scope of this review.

A further limitation to be considered is the often self-selection of healthier, more cognitively-able population in population studies. As a consequence of high baseline performance in cognitively intact participants, ceiling effects with narrow ranges in results can occur [124]. This effectively minimizes several confounding factors, but narrows the chance of detecting cognitive effects.

In cognitively intact samples, cognitive tests sensitive to age-associated cognitive decline should be employed to maximize the observation of any potential effects. Programs such as The Cambridge Neuropsychological Test Automated Battery [125] and The National Institute of Health (NIH) Toolbox [126] are available that tap into a wide range of cognitive domains sensitive to change from mid adulthood such as fluid intelligence would be ideal for establishing its association with nutrition or intervention [127]. In the present review, one study [79] using cognitively intact participants incorporated a computerized test battery assessing a number of cognitive domains. This study demonstrated a significant link between vitamin C status and free recall, recognition and vocabulary.

4.2. Future Directions

Future studies should incorporate a number of recommendations. Firstly, the most reliable and practical measure of vitamin C is the measurement of biological blood samples. Moreover, the incorporation of FFQs would allow a measure of possible confounding variables (vitamin B12, vitamin E, etc.). Age-sensitive cognitive tests assessing response time and accuracy should be administered [127], particularly in the case of cognitively intact individuals. A number of potential confounding factors such as supplementation, and the long term intake of other vitamins and minerals associated with cognition need to be take into account.

5. Conclusions

In summary, studies included in this systematic review demonstrated higher mean vitamin C concentrations in the cognitively intact groups of participants compared to the impaired groups. No correlation was found between vitamin C concentrations and MMSE scores in the cognitively impaired groups of participants. Analysis of the studies that used a variety of cognitive assessments was beyond the scope of this review, however, qualitative assessment in the cognitively intact groups revealed a potential association between plasma vitamin C concentrations and cognition. Due to a number of limitations, further research, assessing plasma vitamin C concentrations, taking confounding factors such as vitamin B12 and vitamin E into account, and the use of more sensitive cognitive assessment methodology for cognitively intact participants are needed to provide more insights into the relationship between vitamin C and cognition.

Author Contributions: A.S. and N.T. conceptualised the study in discussion with K.R. and A.P. I.H. provided statistical knowledge advice. N.T. undertook data analysis and interpreted findings in discussion with K.R. and I.H. N.T. and K.R. prepared the manuscript with contributions from co-authors A.P., A.Sa., and A.Sc. All authors approved the final version.

Conflicts of Interest: A.Sc. and A.P. have received research funding, consultancy, travel support and speaking fees from the nutrition and supplement industry. N.T., K.R., A.S. and I.H. declare no conflict of interest.

References

1. Trout, D.L. Vitamin c and cardiovascular risk factors. *Am. J. Clin. Nutr.* **1991**, *53*, 322S–325S. [PubMed]
2. Vojdani, A.; Ghoneum, M. In vivo effect of ascorbic acid on enhancement of human natural killer cell activity. *Nutr. Res.* **1993**, *13*, 753–764. [CrossRef]
3. Jacques, P.F.; Chylack, L.T. Epidemiologic evidence of a role for the antioxidant vitamins and carotenoids in cataract prevention. *Am. J. Clin. Nutr.* **1991**, *53*, 352S–355S. [PubMed]
4. Hatch, G.E. Asthma, inhaled oxidants, and dietary antioxidants. *Am. J. Clin. Nutr.* **1995**, *61*, 625S–630S. [PubMed]
5. Hemilä, H. Does vitamin c alleviate the symptoms of the common cold?—A review of current evidence. *Scand. J. Infect. Dis.* **1994**, *26*, 1–6. [CrossRef] [PubMed]
6. Gund, P. Three-dimensional pharmacophoric pattern searching. In *Progress in Molecular and Subcellular Biology*; Springer: Berlin/Heidelberg, Germany, 1977; pp. 117–143.
7. Gaby, S.K.; Bendich, A.; Singh, V.; Machlin, L.J. *Vitamin Intake and Health: A Scientific Review*; CRC Press: Boca Raton, FL, USA, 1991; pp. 71–103.
8. Levine, M.; Asher, A.; Pollard, H.; Zinder, O. Ascorbic acid and catecholamine secretion from cultured chromaffin cells. *J. Biol. Chem.* **1983**, *258*, 13111–13115. [PubMed]
9. Hansen, S.N.; Tveden-Nyborg, P.; Lykkesfeldt, J. Does vitamin c deficiency affect cognitive development and function? *Nutrients* **2014**, *6*, 3818–3846. [CrossRef] [PubMed]
10. Majewska, M.D.; Bell, J.A. Ascorbic acid protects neurons from injury induced by glutamate and nmda. *Neuroreport* **1990**, *1*, 194–196. [CrossRef] [PubMed]

11. Levine, M.; Morita, K.; Heldman, E.; Pollard, H.B. Ascorbic acid regulation of norepinephrine biosynthesis in isolated chromaffin granules from bovine adrenal medulla. *J. Biol. Chem.* **1985**, *260*, 15598–15603. [PubMed]
12. Levine, M.; Morita, K.; Pollard, H. Enhancement of norepinephrine biosynthesis by ascorbic acid in cultured bovine chromaffin cells. *J. Biol. Chem.* **1985**, *260*, 12942–12947. [PubMed]
13. Sandstrom, M.I.; Rebec, G.V. Extracellular ascorbate modulates glutamate dynamics: Role of behavioral activation. *BMC Neurosci.* **2007**, *8*, 1. [CrossRef] [PubMed]
14. Majewska, M.D.; Bell, J.A.; London, E.D. Regulation of the nmda receptor by redox phenomena: Inhibitory role of ascorbate. *Brain Res.* **1990**, *537*, 328–332. [CrossRef]
15. Liu, X.; Wu, H.; Byrne, M.; Krane, S.; Jaenisch, R. Type iii collagen is crucial for collagen i fibrillogenesis and for normal cardiovascular development. *Proc. Natl. Acad. Sci. USA* **1997**, *94*, 1852–1856. [CrossRef] [PubMed]
16. Huang, J.; Agus, D.B.; Winfree, C.J.; Kiss, S.; Mack, W.J.; McTaggart, R.A.; Choudhri, T.F.; Kim, L.J.; Mocco, J.; Pinsky, D.J. Dehydroascorbic acid, a blood-brain barrier transportable form of vitamin c, mediates potent cerebroprotection in experimental stroke. *Proc. Natl. Acad. Sci. USA* **2001**, *98*, 11720–11724. [CrossRef] [PubMed]
17. Iyer, N.V.; Kotch, L.E.; Agani, F.; Leung, S.W.; Laughner, E.; Wenger, R.H.; Gassmann, M.; Gearhart, J.D.; Lawler, A.M.; Aimee, Y.Y. Cellular and developmental control of o2 homeostasis by hypoxia-inducible factor 1α. *Genes Dev.* **1998**, *12*, 149–162. [CrossRef] [PubMed]
18. Hediger, M.A. New view at c. *Nat. Med.* **2002**, *8*, 445–446. [CrossRef] [PubMed]
19. Jackson, T.S.; Xu, A.; Vita, J.A.; Keaney, J.F. Ascorbate prevents the interaction of superoxide and nitric oxide only at very high physiological concentrations. *Circ. Res.* **1998**, *83*, 916–922. [CrossRef] [PubMed]
20. Spector, R.; Johanson, C.E. Sustained choroid plexus function in human elderly and alzheimer's disease patients. *Fluids Barriers CNS* **2013**, *10*, 1. [CrossRef] [PubMed]
21. Harrison, F.; Allard, J.; Bixler, R.; Usoh, C.; Li, L.; May, J.; McDonald, M. Antioxidants and cognitive training interact to affect oxidative stress and memory in app/psen1 mice. *Nutr. Neurosci.* **2009**, *12*, 203–218. [CrossRef] [PubMed]
22. Harrison, F.E.; Green, R.J.; Dawes, S.M.; May, J.M. Vitamin c distribution and retention in the mouse brain. *Brain Res.* **2010**, *1348*, 181–186. [CrossRef] [PubMed]
23. May, J.M. Vitamin c transport and its role in the central nervous system. In *Water Soluble Vitamins*; Springer: Dordrecht, The Netherlands, 2012; pp. 85–103.
24. Mefford, I.N.; Oke, A.F.; Adams, R.N. Regional distribution of ascorbate in human brain. *Brain Res.* **1981**, *212*, 223–226. [CrossRef]
25. Oke, A.F.; May, L.; Adams, R.N. Ascorbic acid distribution patterns in human brain. *Ann. N. Y. Acad. Sci.* **1987**, *498*, 1–12. [CrossRef] [PubMed]
26. Bowman, G.L.; Dodge, H.; Frei, B.; Calabrese, C.; Oken, B.S.; Kaye, J.A.; Quinn, J.F. Ascorbic acid and rates of cognitive decline in alzheimer's disease. *J. Alzheimers Dis.* **2009**, *16*, 93–98. [CrossRef] [PubMed]
27. Quinn, J.; Suh, J.; Moore, M.M.; Kaye, J.; Frei, B. Antioxidants in alzheimer's disease-vitamin c delivery to a demanding brain. *J. Alzheimers Dis.* **2003**, *5*, 309–313. [CrossRef] [PubMed]
28. May, J.M.; Li, L.; Hayslett, K.; Qu, Z.-C. Ascorbate transport and recycling by sh-sy5y neuroblastoma cells: Response to glutamate toxicity. *Neurochem. Res.* **2006**, *31*, 785–794. [CrossRef] [PubMed]
29. Spector, R. Vitamin homeostasis in the central nervous system. *N. Engl. J. Med.* **1977**, *296*, 1393–1398. [PubMed]
30. Hornig, D. Distribution of ascorbic acid, metabolites and analogues in man and animals. *Ann. N. Y. Acad. Sci.* **1975**, *258*, 103–118. [CrossRef] [PubMed]
31. Higgins, J.P.; Green, S. *Cochrane Handbook for Systematic Reviews of Interventions*; John Wiley & Sons: Hoboken, NJ, USA, 2011; Volume 4.
32. Dehghan, M.; Akhtar-Danesh, N.; McMillan, C.R.; Thabane, L. Is plasma vitamin c an appropriate biomarker of vitamin c intake? A systematic review and meta-analysis. *Nutr. J.* **2007**, *6*, 41. [CrossRef] [PubMed]
33. Hampl, J.S.; Taylor, C.A.; Johnston, C.S. Vitamin c deficiency and depletion in the united states: The third national health and nutrition examination survey, 1988 to 1994. *Am. J. Public Health* **2004**, *94*, 870–875. [CrossRef] [PubMed]

34. Levine, M.; Conry-Cantilena, C.; Wang, Y.; Welch, R.W.; Washko, P.W.; Dhariwal, K.R.; Park, J.B.; Lazarev, A.; Graumlich, J.F.; King, J. Vitamin c pharmacokinetics in healthy volunteers: Evidence for a recommended dietary allowance. *Proc. Natl. Acad. Sci. USA* **1996**, *93*, 3704–3709. [CrossRef] [PubMed]

35. Tombaugh, T.N.; McIntyre, N.J. The mini-mental state examination: A comprehensive review. *J. Am. Geriatr. Soc.* **1992**, *40*, 922–935. [CrossRef] [PubMed]

36. Mungas, D. Iii-office mental status testing: A practical guide. *Geriatrics* **1991**, *46*, 54–67. [PubMed]

37. Arlt, S.; Müller-Thomsen, T.; Beisiegel, U.; Kontush, A. Effect of one-year vitamin c-and e-supplementation on cerebrospinal fluid oxidation parameters and clinical course in alzheimer's disease. *Neurochem. Res.* **2012**, *37*, 2706–2714. [CrossRef] [PubMed]

38. Galasko, D.R.; Peskind, E.; Clark, C.M.; Quinn, J.F.; Ringman, J.M.; Jicha, G.A.; Cotman, C.; Cottrell, B.; Montine, T.J.; Thomas, R.G. Antioxidants for alzheimer disease: A randomized clinical trial with cerebrospinal fluid biomarker measures. *Arch. Neurol.* **2012**, *69*, 836–841. [CrossRef] [PubMed]

39. Burns, A.; Marsh, A.; Bender, D.A. A trial of vitamin supplementation in senile dementia. *Int. J. Geriatr. Psychiatry* **1989**, *4*, 333–338. [CrossRef]

40. Zandi, P.P.; Anthony, J.C.; Khachaturian, A.S.; Stone, S.V.; Gustafson, D.; Tschanz, J.T.; Norton, M.C.; Welsh-Bohmer, K.A.; Breitner, J.C. Reduced risk of alzheimer disease in users of antioxidant vitamin supplements: The cache county study. *Arch. Neurol.* **2004**, *61*, 82–88. [CrossRef] [PubMed]

41. Deijen, J.; Slump, E.; Wouters-Wesseling, W.; De Groot, C.; Galle, E.; Pas, H. Nutritional intake and daily functioning of psychogeriatric nursing home residents. *J. Nutr. Health Aging* **2002**, *7*, 242–246.

42. Rinaldi, P.; Polidori, M.C.; Metastasio, A.; Mariani, E.; Mattioli, P.; Cherubini, A.; Catani, M.; Cecchetti, R.; Senin, U.; Mecocci, P. Plasma antioxidants are similarly depleted in mild cognitive impairment and in alzheimer's disease. *Neurobiol. Aging* **2003**, *24*, 915–919. [CrossRef]

43. Polidori, M.C.; Mattioli, P.; Aldred, S.; Cecchetti, R.; Stahl, W.; Griffiths, H.; Senin, U.; Sies, H.; Mecocci, P. Plasma antioxidant status, immunoglobulin g oxidation and lipid peroxidation in demented patients: Relevance to alzheimer disease and vascular dementia. *Dement. Geriatr. Cogn. Disord.* **2004**, *18*, 265–270. [CrossRef] [PubMed]

44. Richardson, T.; Ball, L.; Rosenfeld, T. Will an orange a day keep the doctor away? *Postgrad. Med. J.* **2002**, *78*, 292–294. [CrossRef] [PubMed]

45. Lu, Y.; An, Y.; Guo, J.; Zhang, X.; Wang, H.; Rong, H.; Xiao, R. Dietary intake of nutrients and lifestyle affect the risk of mild cognitive impairment in the chinese elderly population: A cross-sectional study. *Front. Behav. Neurosci.* **2016**, *10*, 229. [CrossRef] [PubMed]

46. Charlton, K.E.; Rabinowitz, T.L.; Geffen, L.; Dhansay, M. Lowered plasma vitamin c, but not vitamin e, concentrations in dementia patients. *J. Nutr. Health Aging* **2004**, *8*, 99–108. [PubMed]

47. Glasø, M.; Nordbø, G.; Diep, L.; Bøhmer, T. Reduced concentrations of several vitamins in normal weight patients with late-onset dementia of the alzheimer type without vascular disease. *J. Nutr. Health Aging* **2003**, *8*, 407–413.

48. Rivière, S.; Birlouez-Aragon, I.; Nourhashémi, F.; Vellas, B. Low plasma vitamin c in alzheimer patients despite an adequate diet. *Int. J. Geriatr. Psychiatry* **1998**, *13*, 749–754. [CrossRef]

49. Masaki, K.; Losonczy, K.; Izmirlian, G.; Foley, D.; Ross, G.; Petrovitch, H.; Havlik, R.; White, L. Association of vitamin e and c supplement use with cognitive function and dementia in elderly men. *Neurology* **2000**, *54*, 1265–1272. [CrossRef] [PubMed]

50. Chandra, R.K. Retracted: Effect of vitamin and trace-element supplementation on cognitive function in elderly subjects. *Nutrition* **2001**, *17*, 709–712. [CrossRef]

51. Dror, Y.; Stern, F.; Nemesh, L.; Hart, J.; Grinblat, J. Estimation of vitamin needs—Riboflavin, vitamin b6 and ascorbic acid-according to blood parameters and functional-cognitive and emotional indices in a selected well-established group of elderly in a home for the aged in israel. *J. Am. Coll. Nutr.* **1996**, *15*, 481–488. [CrossRef] [PubMed]

52. Gale, C.R.; Martyn, C.N.; Cooper, C. Cognitive impairment and mortality in a cohort of elderly people. *BMJ* **1996**, *312*, 608–611. [CrossRef] [PubMed]

53. La Rue, A.; Koehler, K.M.; Wayne, S.J.; Chiulli, S.J.; Haaland, K.Y.; Garry, P.J. Nutritional status and cognitive functioning in a normally aging sample: A 6-y reassessment. *Am. J. Clin. Nutr.* **1997**, *65*, 20–29. [PubMed]

54. Paleologos, M.; Cumming, R.G.; Lazarus, R. Cohort study of vitamin c intake and cognitive impairment. *Am. J. Epidemiol.* **1998**, *148*, 45–50. [CrossRef] [PubMed]

55. Devore, E.E.; Kang, J.H.; Stampfer, M.J.; Grodstein, F. The association of antioxidants and cognition in the nurses' health study. *Am. J. Epidemiol.* **2013**, *177*, 33–41. [CrossRef] [PubMed]

56. Engelhart, M.J.; Geerlings, M.I.; Ruitenberg, A.; van Swieten, J.C.; Hofman, A.; Witteman, J.C.; Breteler, M.M. Dietary intake of antioxidants and risk of alzheimer disease. *JAMA* **2002**, *287*, 3223–3229. [CrossRef] [PubMed]

57. Kalmijn, S.; Feskens, E.; Launer, L.J.; Kromhout, D. Polyunsaturated fatty acids, antioxidants, and cognitive function in very old men. *Am. J. Epidemiol.* **1997**, *145*, 33–41. [CrossRef] [PubMed]

58. Laurin, D.; Masaki, K.H.; Foley, D.J.; White, L.R.; Launer, L.J. Midlife dietary intake of antioxidants and risk of late-life incident dementia the honolulu-asia aging study. *Am. J. Epidemiol.* **2004**, *159*, 959–967. [CrossRef] [PubMed]

59. Basambombo, L.L.; Carmichael, P.-H.; Côté, S.; Laurin, D. Use of vitamin e and c supplements for the prevention of cognitive decline. *Ann. Pharmacother.* **2016**, *51*, 118–124. [CrossRef] [PubMed]

60. Nooyens, A.C.; Milder, I.E.; Van Gelder, B.M.; Bueno-de-Mesquita, H.B.; Van Boxtel, M.P.; Verschuren, W.M. Diet and cognitive decline at middle age: The role of antioxidants. *Br. J. Nutr.* **2015**, *113*, 1410–1417. [CrossRef] [PubMed]

61. Péneau, S.; Galan, P.; Jeandel, C.; Ferry, M.; Andreeva, V.; Hercberg, S.; Kesse-Guyot, E.; Group, S.V.M.R. Fruit and vegetable intake and cognitive function in the su. Vi. Max 2 prospective study. *Am. J. Clin. Nutr.* **2011**, *94*, 1295–1303. [CrossRef] [PubMed]

62. Fotuhi, M.; Zandi, P.P.; Hayden, K.M.; Khachaturian, A.S.; Szekely, C.A.; Wengreen, H.; Munger, R.G.; Norton, M.C.; Tschanz, J.T.; Lyketsos, C.G. Better cognitive performance in elderly taking antioxidant vitamins e and c supplements in combination with nonsteroidal anti-inflammatory drugs: The cache county study. *Alzheimers Dement.* **2008**, *4*, 223–227. [CrossRef] [PubMed]

63. Gray, S.L.; Anderson, M.L.; Crane, P.K.; Breitner, J.; McCormick, W.; Bowen, J.D.; Teri, L.; Larson, E. Antioxidant vitamin supplement use and risk of dementia or alzheimer's disease in older adults. *J. Am. Geriatr. Soc.* **2008**, *56*, 291–295. [CrossRef] [PubMed]

64. Wengreen, H.; Munger, R.; Corcoran, C.; Zandi, P. Antioxidant intake and cognitive function of elderly men and women: The cache county study. *J. Nutr. Health Aging* **2007**, *11*, 230. [PubMed]

65. Fillenbaum, G.G.; Kuchibhatla, M.N.; Hanlon, J.T.; Artz, M.B.; Pieper, C.F.; Schmader, K.E.; Dysken, M.W.; Gray, S.L. Dementia and alzheimer's disease in community-dwelling elders taking vitamin c and/or vitamin e. *Ann. Pharmacother.* **2005**, *39*, 2009–2014. [CrossRef] [PubMed]

66. Maxwell, C.J.; Hicks, M.S.; Hogan, D.B.; Basran, J.; Ebly, E.M. Supplemental use of antioxidant vitamins and subsequent risk of cognitive decline and dementia. *Dement. Geriatr. Cogn. Disord.* **2005**, *20*, 45–51. [CrossRef] [PubMed]

67. Grodstein, F.; Chen, J.; Willett, W.C. High-dose antioxidant supplements and cognitive function in community-dwelling elderly women. *Am. J. Clin. Nutr.* **2003**, *77*, 975–984. [PubMed]

68. Luchsinger, J.A.; Tang, M.-X.; Shea, S.; Mayeux, R. Antioxidant vitamin intake and risk of alzheimer disease. *Arch. Neurol.* **2003**, *60*, 203–208. [CrossRef] [PubMed]

69. Morris, M.C.; Evans, D.A.; Bienias, J.L.; Tangney, C.C.; Bennett, D.A.; Aggarwal, N.; Wilson, R.S.; Scherr, P.A. Dietary intake of antioxidant nutrients and the risk of incident alzheimer disease in a biracial community study. *JAMA* **2002**, *287*, 3230–3237. [CrossRef] [PubMed]

70. Peacock, J.M.; Folsom, A.R.; Knopman, D.S.; Mosley, T.H.; Goff, D.C.; Szklo, M. Dietary antioxidant intake and cognitive performance in middle-aged adults. *Public Health Nutr.* **2000**, *3*, 337–343. [CrossRef] [PubMed]

71. Morris, M.C.; Beckett, L.A.; Scherr, P.A.; Hebert, L.E.; Bennett, D.A.; Field, T.S.; Evans, D.A. Vitamin e and vitamin c supplement use and risk of incident alzheimer disease. *Alzheimer Dis. Assoc. Disord.* **1998**, *12*, 121–126. [CrossRef] [PubMed]

72. Mendelsohn, A.B.; Belle, S.H.; Stoehr, G.P.; Ganguli, M. Use of antioxidant supplements and its association with cognitive function in a rural elderly cohort the movies project. *Am. J. Epidemiol.* **1998**, *148*, 38–44. [CrossRef] [PubMed]

73. Berti, V.; Murray, J.; Davies, M.; Spector, N.; Tsui, W.; Li, Y.; Williams, S.; Pirraglia, E.; Vallabhajosula, S.; McHugh, P. Nutrient patterns and brain biomarkers of alzheimer's disease in cognitively normal individuals. *J. Nutr. Health Aging* **2015**, *19*, 413–423. [CrossRef] [PubMed]

74. Beydoun, M.A.; Kuczmarski, M.F.; Kitner-Triolo, M.H.; Beydoun, H.A.; Kaufman, J.S.; Mason, M.A.; Evans, M.K.; Zonderman, A.B. Dietary antioxidant intake and its association with cognitive function in an ethnically diverse sample of us adults. *Psychosom. Med.* **2015**, *77*, 68. [CrossRef] [PubMed]

75. Chaudhari, K.; Sumien, N.; Johnson, L.; D'Agostino, D.; Edwards, M.; Paxton, R.; Hall, J.; O'Bryant, S.E. Vitamin c supplementation, apoe4 genotype and cognitive functioning in a rural-dwelling cohort. *J. Nutr. Health Aging* **2016**, *20*, 841–844. [CrossRef] [PubMed]

76. Goodwin, J.S.; Goodwin, J.M.; Garry, P.J. Association between nutritional status and cognitive functioning in a healthy elderly population. *JAMA* **1983**, *249*, 2917–2921. [CrossRef] [PubMed]

77. Jama, J.W.; Launer, L.J.; Witteman, J.; Den Breeijen, J.; Breteler, M.; Grobbee, D.; Hofman, A. Dietary antioxidants and cognitive function in a population-based sample of older persons the rotterdam study. *Am. J. Epidemiol.* **1996**, *144*, 275–280. [CrossRef] [PubMed]

78. Lindeman, R.D.; Romero, L.J.; Koehler, K.M.; Liang, H.C.; LaRue, A.; Baumgartner, R.N.; Garry, P.J. Serum vitamin b12, c and folate concentrations in the new mexico elder health survey: Correlations with cognitive and affective functions. *J. Am. Coll. Nutr.* **2000**, *19*, 68–76. [CrossRef] [PubMed]

79. Perrig, W.J.; Perrig, P.; Stähelin, H. The relation between antioxidants and memory performance in the old and very old. *J. Am. Geriatr. Soc.* **1997**, *45*, 718–724. [CrossRef] [PubMed]

80. Schmidt, R.; Hayn, M.; Reinhart, B.; Roob, G.; Schmidt, H.; Schumacher, M.; Watzinger, N.; Launer, L. Plasma antioxidants and cognitive performance in middle-aged and older adults: Results of the austrian stroke prevention study. *J. Am. Geriatr. Soc.* **1998**, *46*, 1407–1410. [CrossRef] [PubMed]

81. Sato, R.; Helzlsouer, K.; Comstock, G.; Hoffman, S. A cross-sectional study of vitamin c and cognitive function in older adults: The differential effects of gender. *J. Nutr. Health Aging* **2006**, *10*, 37. [PubMed]

82. Whalley, L.; Fox, H.; Lemmon, H.; Duthie, S.; Collins, A.; Peace, H.; Starr, J.; Deary, I. Dietary supplement use in old age: Associations with childhood iq, current cognition and health. *Int. J. Geriatr. Psychiatry* **2003**, *18*, 769–776. [CrossRef] [PubMed]

83. Perkins, A.J.; Hendrie, H.C.; Callahan, C.M.; Gao, S.; Unverzagt, F.W.; Xu, Y.; Hall, K.S.; Hui, S.L. Association of antioxidants with memory in a multiethnic elderly sample using the third national health and nutrition examination survey. *Am. J. Epidemiol.* **1999**, *150*, 37–44. [CrossRef] [PubMed]

84. Ortega, R.M.; Requejo, A.M.; Andrés, P.; López-Sobaler, A.M.; Quintas, M.E.; Redondo, M.R.; Navia, B.; Rivas, T. Dietary intake and cognitive function in a group of elderly people. *Am. J. Clin. Nutr.* **1997**, *66*, 803–809. [PubMed]

85. Requejo, A.; Ortega, R.; Robles, F.; Navia, B.; Faci, M.; Aparicio, A. Influence of nutrition on cognitive function in a group of elderly, independently living people. *Eur. J. Clin. Nutr.* **2003**, *57*, S54–S57. [CrossRef] [PubMed]

86. Kennedy, D.O.; Veasey, R.C.; Watson, A.W.; Dodd, F.L.; Jones, E.K.; Tiplady, B.; Haskell, C.F. Vitamins and psychological functioning: A mobile phone assessment of the effects of a b vitamin complex, vitamin c and minerals on cognitive performance and subjective mood and energy. *Hum. Psychopharmacol.* **2011**, *26*, 338–347. [CrossRef] [PubMed]

87. Smith, A.P.; Clark, R.; Nutt, D.; Haller, J.; Hayward, S.; Perry, K. Vitamin c, mood and cognitive functioning in the elderly. *Nutr. Neurosci.* **1999**, *2*, 249–256. [CrossRef] [PubMed]

88. Kumar, M.V.; Rajagopalan, S. Trial using multiple micronutrient food supplement and its effect on cognition. *Indian J. Pediatr.* **2008**, *75*, 671–678. [CrossRef] [PubMed]

89. Yaffe, K.; Clemons, T.; McBee, W.; Lindblad, A. Impact of antioxidants, zinc, and copper on cognition in the elderly: A randomized, controlled trial. *Neurology* **2004**, *63*, 1705–1707. [PubMed]

90. Kang, J.H.; Cook, N.R.; Manson, J.E.; Buring, J.E.; Albert, C.M.; Grodstein, F. Vitamin e, vitamin c, beta carotene, and cognitive function among women with or at risk of cardiovascular disease. *Circulation* **2009**, *119*, 2772–2780. [CrossRef] [PubMed]

91. Chui, M.H.; Greenwood, C.E. Antioxidant vitamins reduce acute meal-induced memory deficits in adults with type 2 diabetes. *Nutr. Res.* **2008**, *28*, 423–429. [CrossRef] [PubMed]

92. Day, J.; Bayer, A.; McMahon, M.; Pathy, M.; Spragg, B.; Rowlands, D. Thiamine status, vitamin supplements and postoperative confusion. *Age Ageing* **1988**, *17*, 29–34. [CrossRef] [PubMed]

93. Paraskevas, G.; Kapaki, E.; Libitaki, G.; Zournas, C.; Segditsa, I.; Papageorgiou, C. Ascorbate in healthy subjects, amyotrophic lateral sclerosis and alzheimer's disease. *Acta Neurol. Scand.* **1997**, *96*, 88–90. [CrossRef] [PubMed]

94. Woo, J.; Ho, S.; Mak, Y.; MacDonald, D.; Swaminathan, R. Vitamin nutritional status in elderly chinese subjects living in chronic care institutions. *Nutr. Res.* **1989**, *9*, 1071–1080. [CrossRef]

95. Polidori, M.C.; Mecocci, P. Plasma susceptibility to free radical-induced antioxidant consumption and lipid peroxidation is increased in very old subjects with alzheimer disease. *J. Alzheimers Dis.* **2002**, *4*, 517–522. [CrossRef] [PubMed]

96. Foy, C.; Passmore, A.; Vahidassr, M.; Young, I.; Lawson, J. Plasma chain-breaking antioxidants in alzheimer's disease, vascular dementia and parkinson's disease. *QJM* **1999**, *92*, 39–45. [CrossRef] [PubMed]

97. Talley V, H.C.; Wicks, M.N.; Carter, M.; Roper, B. Ascorbic acid does not influence consciousness recovery after anesthesia. *Biol. Res. Nurs.* **2009**, *10*, 292–298. [CrossRef] [PubMed]

98. Luchsinger, J.A.; Mayeux, R. Dietary factors and alzheimer's disease. *Lancet Neurol.* **2004**, *3*, 579–587. [CrossRef]

99. Folstein, M.F.; Folstein, S.E.; McHugh, P.R. "Mini-mental state": A practical method for grading the cognitive state of patients for the clinician. *J. Psychiatr. Res.* **1975**, *12*, 189–198. [CrossRef]

100. Mowe, M.; Bøhmer, T.; Kindt, E. Reduced nutritional status in an elderly population (>70 years) is probable before disease and possibly contributes to the development of disease. *Am. J. Clin. Nutr.* **1994**, *59*, 317–324. [PubMed]

101. Monget, A.; Galan, P.; Preziosi, P.; Keller, H.; Bourgeois, C.; Arnaud, J.; Favier, A.; Hercberg, S. Micronutrient status in elderly people. Geriatrie/min. Vit. Aux network. *Int. J. Vitam. Nutr. Res.* **1996**, *66*, 71–76. [PubMed]

102. Frei, B.; Stocker, R.; Ames, B.N. Antioxidant defenses and lipid peroxidation in human blood plasma. *Proc. Natl. Acad. Sci. USA* **1988**, *85*, 9748–9752. [CrossRef] [PubMed]

103. Richardson, J.S. Free radicals in the genesis of alzheimer's disease. *Ann. N. Y. Acad. Sci.* **1993**, *695*, 73–76. [CrossRef] [PubMed]

104. Markesbery, W.R.; Carney, J.M. Oxidative alterations in alzheimer's disease. *Brain Pathol.* **1999**, *9*, 133–146. [CrossRef] [PubMed]

105. Beal, M.F. Aging, energy, and oxidative stress in neurodegenerative diseases. *Ann. Neurol.* **1995**, *38*, 357–366. [CrossRef] [PubMed]

106. Gouras, G.K.; Tsai, J.; Naslund, J.; Vincent, B.; Edgar, M.; Checler, F.; Greenfield, J.P.; Haroutunian, V.; Buxbaum, J.D.; Xu, H. Intraneuronal aβ42 accumulation in human brain. *Am. J. Pathol.* **2000**, *156*, 15–20. [CrossRef]

107. Sayre, L.; Perry, G.; Atwood, C.; Smith, M. The role of metals in neurodegenerative diseases. *Cell. Mol. Biol.* **2000**, *46*, 731–741. [PubMed]

108. Connor, J.; Menzies, S.; St Martin, S.; Mufson, E. A histochemical study of iron, transferrin, and ferritin in alzheimer's diseased brains. *J. Neurosci. Res.* **1992**, *31*, 75–83. [CrossRef] [PubMed]

109. Thomas, T.; Thomas, G.; McLendon, C.; Sutton, T.; Mullan, M. Beta-amyloid-mediated vasoactivity and vascular endothelial damage. *Nature* **1996**, *380*, 168. [CrossRef] [PubMed]

110. Michels, A.J.; Frei, B. Myths, artifacts, and fatal flaws: Identifying limitations and opportunities in vitamin c research. *Nutrients* **2013**, *5*, 5161–5192. [CrossRef] [PubMed]

111. Harrison, F.E. A critical review of vitamin c for the prevention of age-related cognitive decline and alzheimer's disease. *J. Alzheimers Dis.* **2012**, *29*, 711–726. [PubMed]

112. Benzie, I.; Strain, J. Simultaneous automated measurement of total'antioxidant'(reducing) capacity and ascorbic acid concentration. *Redox Rep.* **1997**, *3*, 233–238. [CrossRef] [PubMed]

113. Cahill, L.E.; El-Sohemy, A. Vitamin c transporter gene polymorphisms, dietary vitamin c and serum ascorbic acid. *J. Nutrigenet. Nutrigenomics* **2010**, *2*, 292–301. [CrossRef] [PubMed]

114. Bowman, G.L.; Shannon, J.; Ho, E.; Traber, M.G.; Frei, B.; Oken, B.S.; Kaye, J.A.; Quinn, J.F. Reliability and validity of food frequency questionnaire and nutrient biomarkers in elders with and without mild cognitive impairment. *Alzheimer Dis. Assoc. Disord.* **2011**, *25*, 49. [CrossRef] [PubMed]

115. Weinstein, M.; Babyn, P.; Zlotkin, S. An orange a day keeps the doctor away: Scurvy in the year 2000. *Pediatrics* **2001**, *108*, e55. [CrossRef] [PubMed]

116. Vizuete, A.A.; Robles, F.; Rodríguez-Rodríguez, E.; López-Sobaler, A.M.; Ortega, R.M. Association between food and nutrient intakes and cognitive capacity in a group of institutionalized elderly people. *Eur. J. Nutr.* **2010**, *49*, 293–300. [CrossRef] [PubMed]

117. Clarke, R.; Smith, A.D.; Jobst, K.A.; Refsum, H.; Sutton, L.; Ueland, P.M. Folate, vitamin b12, and serum total homocysteine levels in confirmed alzheimer disease. *Arch. Neurol.* **1998**, *55*, 1449–1455. [CrossRef] [PubMed]

118. Grundman, M. Vitamin e and alzheimer disease: The basis for additional clinical trials. *Am. J. Clin. Nutr.* **2000**, *71*, 630S–636S. [PubMed]

119. Evatt, M.L.; DeLong, M.R.; Khazai, N.; Rosen, A.; Triche, S.; Tangpricha, V. Prevalence of vitamin d insufficiency in patients with parkinson disease and alzheimer disease. *Arch. Neurol.* **2008**, *65*, 1348–1352. [CrossRef] [PubMed]

120. Presse, N.; Shatenstein, B.; Kergoat, M.-J.; Ferland, G. Low vitamin k intakes in community-dwelling elders at an early stage of alzheimer's disease. *J. Am. Diet. Assoc.* **2008**, *108*, 2095–2099. [CrossRef] [PubMed]

121. Rodrigue, K.; Kennedy, K.; Devous, M.; Rieck, J.; Hebrank, A.; Diaz-Arrastia, R.; Mathews, D.; Park, D. B-amyloid burden in healthy aging regional distribution and cognitive consequences. *Neurology* **2012**, *78*, 387–395. [CrossRef] [PubMed]

122. WIND, A.W.; Schellevis, F.G.; Van Staveren, G.; Scholten, R.J.; Jonker, C.; Van Eijk, J.T.M. Limitations of the mini-mental state examination in diagnosing dementia in general practice. *Int. J. Geriatr. Psychiatry* **1997**, *12*, 101–108. [CrossRef]

123. Crum, R.M.; Anthony, J.C.; Bassett, S.S.; Folstein, M.F. Population-based norms for the mini-mental state examination by age and educational level. *JAMA* **1993**, *269*, 2386–2391. [CrossRef] [PubMed]

124. Polidori, M.C.; Praticó, D.; Mangialasche, F.; Mariani, E.; Aust, O.; Anlasik, T.; Mang, N.; Pientka, L.; Stahl, W.; Sies, H. High fruit and vegetable intake is positively correlated with antioxidant status and cognitive performance in healthy subjects. *J. Alzheimers Dis.* **2009**, *17*, 921–927. [CrossRef] [PubMed]

125. Sahakian, B.J.; Morris, R.G.; Evenden, J.L.; Heald, A.; Levy, R.; Philpot, M.; Robbins, T.W. A comparative study of visuospatial memory and learning in alzheimer-type dementia and parkinson's disease. *Brain* **1988**, *111*, 695–718. [CrossRef] [PubMed]

126. Weintraub, S.; Dikmen, S.S.; Heaton, R.K.; Tulsky, D.S.; Zelazo, P.D.; Bauer, P.J.; Carlozzi, N.E.; Slotkin, J.; Blitz, D.; Wallner-Allen, K. Cognition assessment using the nih toolbox. *Neurology* **2013**, *80*, S54–S64. [CrossRef] [PubMed]

127. Pipingas, A.; Harris, E.; Tournier, E.; King, R.; Kras, M.; Stough, C.K. Assessing the efficacy of nutraceutical interventions on cognitive functioning in the elderly. *Curr. Top. Nutraceutical Res.* **2010**, *8*, 79.

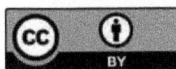

nutrients

MDPI

Article

Vitamin C Status Correlates with Markers of Metabolic and Cognitive Health in 50-Year-Olds: Findings of the CHALICE Cohort Study

John F. Pearson [1], Juliet M. Pullar [2], Renee Wilson [3], Janet K. Spittlehouse [4], Margreet C. M. Vissers [2], Paula M. L. Skidmore [5], Jinny Willis [6], Vicky A. Cameron [3] and Anitra C. Carr [2,*]

[1] Biostatistics and Computational Biology Unit, University of Otago, Christchurch 8140, New Zealand; john.pearson@otago.ac.nz
[2] Department of Pathology, University of Otago, Christchurch 8140, New Zealand; juliet.pullar@otago.ac.nz (J.M.P.); margreet.vissers@otago.ac.nz (M.C.M.V.)
[3] Department of Medicine, University of Otago, Christchurch 8140, New Zealand; renee.wilson@postgrad.otago.ac.nz (R.W.); vicky.cameron@otago.ac.nz (V.A.C.)
[4] Department of Psychological Medicine, University of Otago, Christchurch 8140, New Zealand; janet.spittlehouse@otago.ac.nz
[5] Department of Human Nutrition, University of Otago, Dunedin 9054, New Zealand; paula.skidmore@otago.ac.nz
[6] Lipid & Diabetes Research Group, Canterbury District Health Board, Christchurch 8140, New Zealand; jinny.willis@cdhb.health.nz
* Correspondence: anitra.carr@otago.ac.nz; Tel.: +64-3-364-0649

Received: 14 July 2017; Accepted: 31 July 2017; Published: 3 August 2017

Abstract: A cohort of 50-year-olds from Canterbury, New Zealand ($N = 404$), representative of midlife adults, undertook comprehensive health and dietary assessments. Fasting plasma vitamin C concentrations ($N = 369$) and dietary vitamin C intake ($N = 250$) were determined. The mean plasma vitamin C concentration was 44.2 µmol/L (95% CI 42.4, 46.0); 62% of the cohort had inadequate plasma vitamin C concentrations (i.e., <50 µmol/L), 13% of the cohort had hypovitaminosis C (i.e., <23 µmol/L), and 2.4% had plasma vitamin C concentrations indicating deficiency (i.e., <11 µmol/L). Men had a lower mean plasma vitamin C concentration than women, and a higher percentage of vitamin C inadequacy and deficiency. A higher prevalence of hypovitaminosis C and deficiency was observed in those of lower socio-economic status and in current smokers. Adults with higher vitamin C levels exhibited lower weight, BMI and waist circumference, and better measures of metabolic health, including HbA1c, insulin and triglycerides, all risk factors for type 2 diabetes. Lower levels of mild cognitive impairment were observed in those with the highest plasma vitamin C concentrations. Plasma vitamin C showed a stronger correlation with markers of metabolic health and cognitive impairment than dietary vitamin C.

Keywords: ascorbate; cognition; HbA1c; insulin; glucose; hypovitaminosis C

1. Introduction

The role of vitamin C in health and disease has been actively studied since its discovery over 80 years ago [1]. Vitamin C has a number of well-recognized biological functions, all of which depend upon its ability to act as an electron donor [2]. One of the most significant of these is its cofactor activity for a variety of enzymes with critical functions throughout the body. These include the copper-containing monooxygenases dopamine hydroxylase and peptidyl-glycine α-amidating monooxygenase [3] and the Fe (II) and 2-oxoglutarate-dependent family of dioxygenases [4]. The latter is a large and varied family, with a continually expanding membership that includes the collagen prolyl hydroxylases responsible for stabilization of the tertiary structure of collagen, the prolyl and asparaginyl hydroxylases which regulate hypoxia-inducible factors (HIF) activity, and DNA and histone demethylases involved in the epigenetic regulation of gene expression. Vitamin C also functions as a highly effective water-soluble antioxidant, protecting in vivo biomolecules from oxidation [5], and there is good evidence to suggest it is involved in the regeneration of vitamin E in vivo [6,7].

Because humans are unable to synthesize their own vitamin C, it must be obtained from the diet, principally through fruit and vegetable consumption. Inadequate dietary intake results in the potentially fatal deficiency disease, scurvy. As little as 10 mg/day vitamin C is sufficient to prevent overt scurvy [8] and, although scurvy is considered to be relatively rare in Western populations, vitamin C deficiency is the fourth most prevalent nutrient deficiency reported in the United States [9,10]. Hypovitaminosis C (defined as a plasma concentration $\leq$23 μmol/L) affects a significant proportion of the population, with estimates as large as 15–20% in the United States [9]. Similar data for the New Zealand population are lacking, although dietary vitamin C intake has been used to estimate the prevalence of inadequate intake, defined as not meeting the estimated average requirement (EAR) [11].

The classical symptoms of scurvy, such as joint pain, lassitude, bleeding and ulceration are thought to be due to the loss in activity of the vitamin C-cofactor enzymes, particularly the collagen hydroxylases. It is becoming increasingly acknowledged, however, that vitamin C is required at concentrations above those needed for the prevention of scurvy for the maintenance of good health [12,13]. For example, individuals with hypovitaminosis C are known to present with fatigue, depression and deficiencies in wound healing [14,15], suggesting a requirement for vitamin C status to be above 23 μmol/L in plasma to support these functions. There is also epidemiological evidence to support a role for vitamin C in the prevention of some chronic disease, with intakes >100 mg/day recommended [12]; these intakes will provide adequate plasma levels (i.e., >50 μmol/L) [14,16]. Although the Australasian Recommended Dietary Intake (RDI) for vitamin C is only 45 mg/day, the New Zealand Ministry of Health, in accord with other international bodies, has a suggested dietary target of ~200 mg/day vitamin C for the reduction of chronic disease risk [17]. As the many cofactor functions of vitamin C become more widely understood, epidemiological studies in areas in which its biological activity can be justified are required.

The CHALICE (Canterbury Health, Ageing and Lifecourse) study is a unique New Zealand study comprising a comprehensive database of determinants of health. It has prospectively recruited ~400 fifty-year-olds at random from the electoral roll within the Canterbury region. Participants have undergone extensive health, dietary and social assessments [18]. Here we report on the plasma vitamin C status and dietary vitamin C intake of the participants, and examine the relationships between these measures and a range of health indicators.

2. Materials and Methods

2.1. Study Population

Participants were from a random sample drawn from the New Zealand electoral roll, recruited to take part in a prospective longitudinal study of health and wellbeing (2010–2013), called the Canterbury Health, Ageing and Lifecourse (CHALICE) study (detailed in [18]). Participants had to be aged 49–51 years, intend to reside within the greater Christchurch area for at least 6 of the next 12 months, live in the community (i.e., not in a prison or a rest home) and be able to complete the assessment (e.g., speak English proficiently). Māori, the indigenous people of New Zealand, were over-sampled so that they represented 15% of the CHALICE study sample. Enrolment statistics estimate that, in 2012, 94.9% of the target population were registered to vote in the Christchurch City Council area [19]. Relative to the rest of New Zealand, the Canterbury area has a slightly higher proportion of people aged $\geq$40 years and a higher proportion of people living in the least economically deprived national quintile [20].

Ethical approval was obtained from the Upper South A Regional Ethics Committee (URA/10/03/021) and all participants provided written informed consent.

Data were collected during a 4–6 h interview, via self-completed questionnaires and lifestyle diaries, and from blood and urine tests. The full cohort was 404 participants, and the present analysis is based on the 369 participants for whom fasting plasma vitamin C measurements were obtained and a sample of 250 for whom dietary vitamin C intake was determined.

2.2. Blood Sample Collection

Fasting blood samples were collected into EDTA anticoagulant tubes and sent to Canterbury Health Laboratories, an International Accreditation New Zealand (IANZ) laboratory, for analysis of biomarkers. Additional fasting samples were centrifuged at 4000 rpm for 10 min at 4 °C to separate plasma, and the plasma stored at −80 °C for vitamin C analysis.

2.3. Sample Preparation for Vitamin C Analysis

Stored EDTA-plasma was rapidly thawed and a 500 µL aliquot was treated with an equal volume of ice-cold 0.54 M HPLC-grade perchloric acid solution (containing 100 µmol/L of the metal chelator DTPA) to precipitate protein and stabilize the vitamin C. Samples were mixed, incubated on ice for a few minutes, then centrifuged. A 100 µL aliquot of the deproteinated supernatant was treated with 10 µL of the reducing agent TCEP (100 mg/mL stock) for 2 h at 4 °C to recover any oxidized vitamin C [21]. Samples were further diluted with an equal volume of ice-cold 77 mM perchloric acid/DTPA solution for HPLC analysis.

2.4. Vitamin C HPLC Analysis

The total vitamin C content (ascorbic acid plus dehydroascorbic acid) of the samples was determined by HPLC with electrochemical detection as described previously [22]. Samples (20 µL) were separated on a Synergi 4 µ Hydro-RP 80A column 150 mm × 4.6 mm (Phenomenex NZ Ltd, Auckland, New Zealand) using a Dionex Ultimate 3000 HPLC unit (with autosampler chilled to 4 °C and column temperature set at 30 °C) and an ESA coulochem II detector (+200 mV electrode potential and 20 µA sensitivity). The mobile phase comprised 80 mM sodium acetate buffer, pH 4.8, containing DTPA (0.54 mmol/L) and freshly added ion pair reagent n-octylamine (1 µmol/L), delivered at a flow rate of 1.2 mL/min. A standard curve of sodium-L-ascorbate, standardized spectrophotometrically at 245 nm ($\varepsilon = 9860$), was freshly prepared for each HPLC run in 77 mmol/L HPLC-grade perchloric acid containing DTPA (100 µmol/L). Plasma vitamin C content is expressed as µmol/L.

Fasting plasma vitamin C concentrations were classified as follows; deficient <11 µmol/L, marginal 11–23 µmol/L, inadequate 23–50 µmol/L or adequate >50 µmol/L [13,15].

2.5. Metabolic and Heart Health Assessments

Metabolic health was assessed by body measurements and fasting blood tests. Participants' height, weight and waist circumference were taken by the study interviewer, and body mass index (BMI) calculated (kg/m^2). Fasting blood tests comprised triglycerides, high-density lipoprotein (HDL), glucose, HbA1c and insulin (Canterbury Health Laboratories).

Heart health was assessed by blood pressure and participants had their NZ cardiovascular risk score calculated. Blood pressure measurements were taken while seated. Five year cardiovascular risk (%) was derived according to the New Zealand adaptation of the Framingham risk score; the following variables are included in the calculation: age, gender, systolic blood pressure, diabetic status, smoking history, and total cholesterol to HDL ratio [23].

2.6. Dietary Intake Assessment

Participants were asked to complete the Four Day Estimated Food Diary (4DEFD) in the week after their interview; on one weekend day and three weekdays. The 4DEFD included detailed instructions on how to record portion sizes, using common household measures. The completed 4DEFD were checked by a trained nutritionist and additional information obtained from participants where necessary before the data were entered into the nutrient analysis program Kai-culator (version 1.08d, Department of Human Nutrition, University of Otago, Dunedin, New Zealand). Dietary analysis was performed on 250 of the CHALICE participants, who had dietary data entered and cleaned at the time of analysis, for whom the mean daily intake of vitamin C was calculated. Data entry was undertaken by experienced nutritionists and all diaries were further checked for accuracy by one person who also made any necessary changes, to ensure consistency of data entry.

2.7. Wellbeing, Depression and Cognition

2.7.1. Mental Wellbeing

The Warwick–Edinburgh Mental Wellbeing Scale (WEMWBS) was used to assess general wellbeing. The 14 item questionnaire aims to measure positive mental health by assessing both aspects of well-being: eudaimonic and hedonic [24].

2.7.2. Depression

During the assessment, trained interviewers used the Mini-International Neuropsychiatric Interview (MINI) for diagnosis of current and past depressive episodes using DSM IV criteria [25].

2.7.3. Cognition

Participants completed the Montreal Cognitive Assessment (MoCA) version 7.1 (original version) [26], a short screening test for mild cognitive impairment. It assesses the cognitive domains of attention and concentration, executive functions, memory, language, visuoconstructional skills, conceptual thinking, calculations, and orientation. A score of 26 or more indicates normal functioning, while a score less than 26 might indicate mild cognitive impairment. MoCA scores were excluded from the analysis if English was the second language or if a previous event (e.g., carbon monoxide poisoning) had affected cognitive ability.

2.8. Socio-Economic Status

The Economic Living Standard Index Short Form (ELSI$_{SF}$) was used to assess standard of living [27]. Developed in New Zealand, the ELSI$_{SF}$ assesses a person's consumption and personal possessions, calculating a total score by combining information from all items of the survey. The ELSI$_{SF}$ scores range from 0–31, with those who score 0–16 described as being in hardship, scores of 17–24 as comfortable and scores of 25 or above as socio-economically good or very good. The ELSI$_{SF}$ has excellent internal consistency (coefficient alpha of 0.88).

2.9. Statistical Analyses

Statistical analyses were performed using R 3.3.1 software (R Foundation for Statistical Computing, Vienna, Austria). Univariate tests on continuous variables were t-tests with Satterthwhaite's adjustment for unequal variances while Wald odds ratios and Fisher exact p-values were calculated for categorical variables. Sample characteristics were compared with census proportions using the chi squared goodness of fit test. All health measures were examined independently for association with vitamin C (plasma vitamin C concentration or dietary vitamin C intake) using linear or logistic regression models. The models fitted the dietary measure, gender (dichotomous), Māori ethnicity (dichotomous) and current smoking (dichotomous). Models were fitted on males and females separately and the whole cohort combined. Modeling assumptions were verified with no material departures observed. For each outcome, the *p* values were adjusted for multiple comparisons using the Benjamini and Yekutieli method. The nominal *p* value for statistical significance is the usual 0.05 or 5% type II error rate. All *p* < 0.1 are shown in the tables with *p* > 0.1 shown as NS (not significant). The odds of currently smoking for those in the lowest socio-economic strata was 3.8 times that of the highest strata (95% CI 1.7–9.0), *p* = 0.002. Similarly the odds of current smoking were 3.4 times higher in the least educated strata than the most educated (95% CI 1.75, 6.54), *p* = 0.0006. To prevent over fitting, socio-economic status and education were not fitted, however smoking acts as a reasonable proxy for population modeling.

3. Results

3.1. Characteristics of the Study Population

Of the full CHALICE cohort (*N* = 404), 46.8% (189) were male, with 83.7% (338) self-identifying as New Zealand European and 14.9% (60) as Māori (Table 1). The majority of the participants were in the highest ELSI$_{SF}$ category. There were 60 current smokers in the cohort.

Table 1. CHALICE participants compared with Census 2006 50–54-year-olds from same region.

		Chalice (*n*, %)		Census 2006 (%)	*p*
Gender	Female	215	53.2	50.9	NS
	Male	189	46.8	49.1	
Ethnicity	Māori	60	14.9	4.5	<0.0001
	NZ European	338	83.7	74.2	
Socio-Economic Status	Low (ELSI$_{SF}$ score 0–16)	30	7.4	8.2	NS
	Medium (ELSI$_{SF}$ score 17–24)	122	30.2	29.4	
	High (ELSI$_{SF}$ score 25–31)	252	62.4	62.5	
Education	No Qualification	53	13.1	23.9	<0.0001
	Secondary School Qualification	110	27.2	35.2	
	Post-secondary	168	41.6	25.6	
	University Degree	73	18.1	15.3	
Current Smoker		60	14.9	16.6	NS

N = 404; *p* (χ^2_{n-1}) > 0.1 shown as not significant, NS.

Table 1 compares the CHALICE participants to the New Zealand Census 2006 data for similar age and region. The CHALICE participants had higher rates of Māori ethnicity and higher qualifications than the Canterbury average (Table 1), whereas socio-economic status and smoking were within stochastic limits. This suggests the sample is reasonably representative of Canterbury 50-year-olds and hence the national cohort allowing for regional bias.

The CHALICE cohort also had typical levels of health for a community sample (Table 2). Anthropometric measures were close to those of the New Zealand population. Average metabolic and cardiac markers for the cohort were generally within the healthy range. However, the high prevalence of chronic conditions in the New Zealand population was also readily apparent.

Table 2. Health of CHALICE participants and normal ranges for the New Zealand population.

	Female				Male			
Body Measurements	**Mean**	**Min**	**Max**	**NZ Female Mean**	**Mean**	**Min**	**Max**	**NZ Male Mean**
Weight kg	78.6	49.1	149.9	74.8 (73.5–76.1)	88.4	50.8	143.8	88.0 (86.9–89.1)
BMI kg/m^2	29.1	17.4	63.4	28.1 (27.6–28.6)	28.1	19.2	48.6	28.6 (28.2–28.9)
Waist cm	92.0	63.0	144.0	86.6 (85.5–87.6)	98.3	72.5	148.0	98.4 (97.4–99.3)
Metabolism	**Mean**	**Min**	**Max**	**Healthy Range**	**Mean**	**Min**	**Max**	**Healthy Range**
Triglycerides mmol/L	1.3	0.4	11.7	<1.7	1.6	0.4	11.7	<1.7
HDL mmol/L	1.4	0.8	2.7	1.0–2.2	1.2	0.7	1.9	0.9–2.0
Glucose mmol/L	5.1	3.2	10.8	<6.1	5.4	3.7	17.9	<6.1
HbA1c mmol/L	38.2	27.0	74.0	<40	39.9	28.0	102.0	<40
Insulin pmol/L	60.9	10.0	277.0	10–80	61.2	4.0	480.0	10–80
Heart Health	**Mean**	**Min**	**Max**	**Healthy Range**	**Mean**	**Min**	**Max**	**Healthy Range**
BP (systolic) mmHg	131.1	104.0	183.7	120	134.2	97.7	185.7	120
BP (diastolic) mmHg	82.5	60.3	106.0	80	85.0	61.0	128.3	80
CVD risk score %	2.5–5	<2.5	20–25	<2.5	5–10	2.5–5	20–25	<2.5
Mental Health	**Mean**	**Min**	**Max**		**Mean**	**Min**	**Max**	
Wellbeing	53.0	16	70		52.7	30	70	
Cognition	27.1	19	30		26.6	16	30	
Current Depression *n* (%)	17 (7.9)				12 (6.3)			

BMI: body mass index, HDL: high-density lipoprotein, BP: blood pressure, CVD: Cardiovascular disease. Body measurements compared with New Zealand mean (95% confidence interval) for 45–55 age range [28]. Metabolic and heart health compared with normal healthy range [23,29,30]. Wellbeing measured by Warwick–Edinburgh scale, cognition by MoCA. Current depression is those currently clinically depressed excluding those diagnosed bipolar (*N* = 203 female, 179 male). One female has no waist measurement, three females no fasting metabolic measures, one male no fasting metabolic measures, one male glucose assay failed and two males HbA1c assay failed, otherwise data are for 215 females and 189 males.

3.2. Vitamin C Status of the Study Population

Fasting plasma vitamin C measurements were available for 369 of the CHALICE participants. The mean plasma vitamin C concentration was 44.2 µmol/L (95% CI 42.4, 46.0); 62% of the participants were below the adequate level (i.e., 50 µmol/L), and 93% of the participants were below the optimal saturating level (i.e., 70 µmol/L; Figure 1). Ten percent of the cohort had marginal vitamin C concentrations (i.e., 11–23 µmol/L), and vitamin C deficiency, defined as a plasma concentration of <11 µmol/L, was apparent in 2.4% of the cohort (Table 3).

Plasma vitamin C status was substantially lower in men than in women (*p* = 0.005), and it also varied by socio-economic status (*p* = 0.003). For example, 8% of those in the lowest socio-economic category were vitamin C deficient compared to 2.4% of the entire cohort (*n* = 369). Smoking status was also associated with plasma vitamin C status with current smokers having lower vitamin C levels (*p* < 0.001; Table 3).

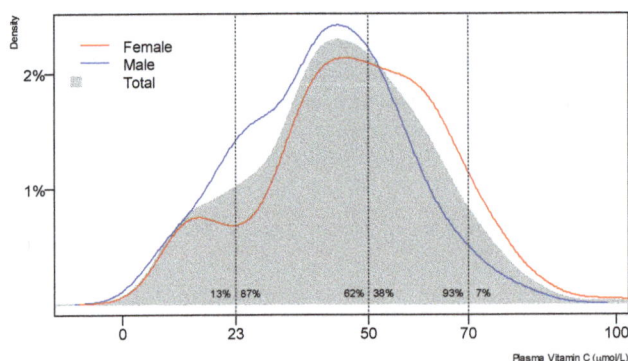

Figure 1. Density plot of plasma vitamin C. Proportion of sample at given vitamin C level; *n* = 369.

Table 3. Categories of vitamin C status.

		Plasma Vitamin C		Deficient		Marginal		Inadequate		Adequate		*p*
		Mean	95% CI	*n*	%	*n*	%	*n*	%	*n*	%	
Total		44.2	(42.4, 46.0)	9	2.4	39	10.6	183	49.6	138	37.4	
Gender	Female	47.4	(44.9, 49.9)	2	1.0	20	10.3	85	43.6	88	45.1	0.005
	Male	40.6	(38.2, 43.0)	7	4.0	19	10.9	98	56.3	50	28.7	
Ethnicity	Non Māori	44.5	(42.6, 46.4)	7	2.2	31	9.8	159	50.3	119	37.7	NS
	Māori	42.4	(37.2, 47.6)	2	3.8	8	15.1	24	45.3	19	35.8	
Socio-Economic Status	Low	36.8	(28.3, 45.3)	2	8.0	7	28.0	9	36.0	7	28.0	0.003
	Medium	43.7	(40.3, 47.1)	4	3.5	14	12.3	53	46.5	43	37.7	
	High	45.3	(43.2, 47.4)	3	1.3	18	7.8	121	52.6	88	38.3	
Education	None	38.7	(33.6, 43.9)	3	6.1	6	12.2	26	53.1	14	28.6	NS
	Secondary School	45.9	(42.1, 49.7)	1	1.0	13	12.6	49	47.6	40	38.8	
	Post-secondary	43.1	(40.6, 45.7)	5	3.3	16	10.6	75	49.7	55	36.4	
	University Degree	48.1	(44.4, 51.9)	0	0.0	4	6.1	33	50.0	29	43.9	
Tobacco	Not Current Smoker	45.9	(44.1, 47.8)	6	1.9	26	8.2	157	49.7	127	40.2	<0.001
	Current Smoker	34.1	(29.2, 38.9)	3	5.7	13	24.5	26	49.1	11	20.8	

Plasma vitamin C classified as deficient <11 µmol/L, marginal 11–23 µmol/L, inadequate 23–50 µmol/L or adequate >50 µmol/L; *n* = 369.

Study participants with and without vitamin C measurements do not differ significantly by gender, ethnicity, education, socio-economic status, smoking status, waist, weight or BMI (all *p* > 0.13), hence are treated as missing at random.

3.3. Associations of Vitamin C Status with Markers of Metabolic and Mental Health

The results of the statistical modeling with plasma vitamin C are summarized in Table 4. Higher plasma vitamin C status was associated with lower weight, BMI and waist circumference in the CHALICE cohort, even after adjustment for gender, ethnicity and current smoking. Of the other markers of metabolic health, plasma vitamin C was negatively associated with blood triglycerides, HbA1c and insulin, and positively associated with HDL levels. However, after multiple adjustment only triglycerides, HbA1c and insulin levels remained significant. No correlation was found between plasma vitamin C and the two indicators of heart health; blood pressure and cardiovascular risk score.

Table 4. Significant plasma vitamin C effects for body measures, metabolic health and mental health.

	Vitamin C <23 µmol/L (*n* = 47)		Vitamin C >23 µmol/L (*n* = 321)		*p*	*p* Adjusted
	Mean	95% CI	Mean	95% CI		
Body measurements						
Weight	90.3	(83.3, 97.4)	81.7	(79.8, 83.6)	0.024	0.004
BMI	31.4	(28.7, 34.0)	28.1	(27.5, 28.7)	0.021	<0.001
Waist	103.3	(97.6, 108.9)	93.3	(91.8, 94.8)	0.001	<0.001
Metabolism						
Triglycerides	1.8	(1.4, 2.3)	1.4	(1.3, 1.5)	0.061	0.029
HDL	1.3	(1.2, 1.3)	1.4	(1.3, 1.4)	0.033	NS
Glucose	5.6	(5.2, 6.0)	5.2	(5.0, 5.3)	0.072	0.073
HbA1c	42.2	(39.6, 44.8)	38.5	(37.7, 39.3)	0.009	0.015
Insulin	91.0	(68.4, 113.6)	56.3	(51.9, 60.8)	0.004	0.000
Heart health						
BP (systolic)	132.2	(128.0, 136.4)	132.5	(130.8, 134.2)	NS	NS
BP (diastolic)	83.6	(81.0, 86.3)	83.5	(82.4, 84.6)	NS	NS
CVD risk score	5–10%	(<2.5%, 20–25%)	2.5–5%	(3.5–5%, 5–10%)	0.057	NS
Mental Health						
Wellbeing	50.9	(48.4, 53.4)	53.0	(52.0, 53.9)	NS	NS
	n	%	*n*	%		
MCI	17	40.5	66	21.5	0.012	0.02
Current Depression	6	12.5	20	6.2	NS	NS

MCI: Mild Cognitive Impairment indicated by MoCA score <26 for those without excluding conditions. Current depression is for those without Bipolar Disorder. P values less than 0.1 shown otherwise NS: Not Significant. *p* values adjusted for gender, ethnicity and current smoking.

Mild cognitive impairment was assessed by the MoCA test. Higher plasma vitamin C status was correlated with lower mild cognitive impairment, which was maintained after adjustment for gender, ethnicity and current smoking (Table 4). A 1 µmol/L increase in plasma vitamin C was associated with 3% reduced odds of mild cognitive impairment (OR = 0.97, 95% CI = (0.96, 0.99), p = 0.004). Indeed, the odds of mild cognitive impairment were twice as high for those below 23 µmol/L plasma vitamin C (OR = 2.1, 95% CI = (1.2, 3.7), p = 0.01). Plasma vitamin C status was not associated with wellbeing or depression.

3.4. Dietary Vitamin C Intake

Dietary intake analysis was performed on 250 of the CHALICE participants. The average dietary vitamin C intake was 110 mg/day, with 12% falling below the New Zealand recommended dietary intake (RDI, Table 5). There was little effect of gender, ethnicity or socio-economic status on dietary intake. However, those with the lowest educational qualifications tended to have lower dietary vitamin C intake, although this was not quite significant. Current smokers also had a lower dietary intake of vitamin C (p < 0.001). Dietary vitamin C intake correlated somewhat less than expected with plasma levels of vitamin C, although the correlation was statistically significant (Pearson's correlation coefficient r = 0.27, p = 0.00002).

Table 5. Categories of dietary vitamin C intake.

		Dietary Vitamin C		Below RDI		RDI-Average		Above Average		p
		Mean	95% CI	n	%	n	%	n	%	
Total		109.8	(101.5, 118.1)	30	12	126	50.4	94	37.6	
Gender	Female	107.4	(96.6, 118.2)	13	9.7	73	54.5	48	35.8	NS
	Male	112.6	(99.7, 125.6)	17	14.7	53	45.7	46	39.7	
Ethnicity	Non Māori	112.0	(102.7, 121.2)	22	10.3	111	51.9	81	37.9	NS
	Māori	97.2	(79.6, 114.7)	8	22.2	15	41.7	13	36.1	
Socio-Economic Status	Low	78.8	(54.4, 103.1)	4	26.7	8	53.3	3	20.0	NS
	Medium	105.0	(90.7, 119.2)	12	15.2	36	45.6	31	39.2	
	High	115.3	(104.4, 126.1)	14	9.0	82	52.6	60	38.5	
Education	None	83.5	(64.2, 102.7)	8	28.6	13	46.4	7	25.0	0.1
	Secondary School	117.1	(98.4, 135.7)	6	10.0	32	53.3	22	36.7	
	Post-secondary	108.6	(97.1, 120.1)	11	9.9	59	53.2	41	36.9	
	University Degree	118.4	(97.6, 139.2)	5	9.8	22	43.1	24	47.1	
Tobacco	Not Current Smoker	114.1	(105.3, 122.8)	20	9.0	112	50.7	89	40.3	<0.001
	Current Smoker	77.5	(54.6, 100.5)	10	34.5	14	48.3	5	17.2	

The cut-off values for the vitamin C categories are as follows: New Zealand recommended dietary intake is 45 mg/day, the average New Zealand intake is 109 mg/day for men and 106 mg/day for women [11]; n = 250.

3.5. Associations of Dietary Vitamin C Intake with Markers of Metabolic and Mental Health

There was evidence that higher dietary intake of vitamin C was associated with lower waist circumference and insulin levels, after adjustment for gender, ethnicity and current smoking (Table 6). Glucose and HbA1c levels were inversely associated with dietary vitamin C intake in the initial models, however they did not remain so after correction for multiple comparisons. Higher dietary vitamin C intake was also associated with lower blood pressure, although there was no effect on cardiovascular risk score. There was little association between dietary vitamin C intake and mental health measures, although dietary intake was inversely associated with mild cognitive impairment in the unadjusted model.

Table 6. Significant dietary vitamin C effects based on average intake for body measures, metabolic health and heart health.

	Intake < Average (*n* = 147)		Intake > Average (*n* = 103)		*p*	*p* Adjusted
	Mean	95% CI	Mean	95% CI		
Body measurements						
Weight	82.2	(79.2, 85.3)	79.8	(76.4, 83.3)	NS	NS
BMI	28.5	(27.4, 29.6)	27.2	(26.2, 28.1)	0.08	0.063
Waist	94.6	(92.2, 97.0)	91.2	(88.5, 93.8)	0.06	0.047
Metabolism						
Triglycerides	1.4	(1.3, 1.5)	1.3	(1.1, 1.6)	NS	NS
HDL	1.4	(1.3, 1.4)	1.4	(1.3, 1.4)	NS	NS
Glucose	5.3	(5.1, 5.5)	5.0	(4.9, 5.2)	0.03	0.078
HbA1c	39.6	(38.3, 41.0)	37.8	(36.9, 38.7)	0.03	NS
Insulin	64.6	(55.5, 73.6)	52.3	(44.3, 60.3)	0.05	0.041
Heart health						
BP (systolic)	135.0	(132.5, 137.5)	130.6	(127.4, 133.8)	0.03	0.016
BP (diastolic)	85.2	(83.6, 86.7)	82.3	(80.4, 84.1)	0.02	0.007
CVD risk score	2.8	(2.6, 3.0)	2.6	(2.2, 2.9)	NS	NS
Mental Health						
Wellbeing	52.5	(51.1, 53.8)	52.9	(51.3, 54.4)	NS	NS
	n	%	*n*	%		
MCI	36	24.5	14	13.6	0.04	NS
Current Depression	13	8.8	4	3.9	NS	NS

MCI Mild Cognitive Impairment indicated by MoCA score <26 for those without excluding conditions. Current depression is for those without Bipolar Disorder. *p* values less than 0.1 shown otherwise NS: Not Significant. *p* values adjusted for gender, ethnicity and current smoking. Average is New Zealand average of 109 mg/day for men, 106 mg/day for women [11].

4. Discussion

These findings were drawn from the first phase of the CHALICE study, a longitudinal observational study of randomly selected 50-year-olds from the Canterbury region, New Zealand in 2010–2013. The comprehensive range of instruments used in the CHALICE study gives a broad picture of the cohort's health and the agreement between the study data and national demographics provides confidence that the study is representative of the health of 50-year-old New Zealanders in 2010. The cohort has typical levels of metabolic and cardiac markers, with indications of overweight/obesity and hypertension in some individuals. Our study provides new evidence that mid-life adults with higher vitamin C levels exhibited better measures of metabolic health and lower levels of mild cognitive impairment.

In New Zealand, dietary vitamin C intake has been estimated by several comprehensive national dietary surveys, including the 2008/2009 New Zealand Adult Nutrition Survey in which the mean usual adult daily intake was 108 mg based on 24 h dietary recall data [11]. This is close to the average dietary intake of 110 mg/day found in the current study. However, measuring vitamin C concentrations in the body has a number of advantages over dietary intake. It does not rely on participant's recall of their diet, and takes in all sources of the vitamin, including supplements, and the potential impact of vitamin C losses due to food processing and preparation. More particularly, it accounts for confounders of vitamin C status such as smoking, alcohol consumption, prescription medications and health conditions which may affect turnover of the vitamin [31]. The CHALICE study is the first representative study of plasma vitamin C status within the New Zealand population. Only smaller studies in specific, non-representative groups have measured plasma vitamin C concentrations within the New Zealand population [32,33].

In our study, we found that 2.4% of 50-year-olds were deficient in vitamin C (i.e., <11 µmol/L), putting them at higher risk of developing scurvy and other health effects that may be associated with very low vitamin C status. Men were at greater risk of being deficient than women, and having lower socio-economic status significantly increased risk. Smoking also increased the risk of deficiency, most likely due to increased oxidative stress causing faster turnover of the vitamin [31]. In addition, in our cohort, smokers had a lower dietary intake of vitamin C. Numerous studies have previously shown gender, socio-economic status and smoking to be important predictors of vitamin C status [9,33–37]. A recent study suggests the effect of gender on vitamin C status may be due to the differing fat free mass between men and women, meaning vitamin C is distributed throughout a higher volume in men, leading to lower vitamin C concentrations in the plasma [36].

Data from large international cohorts show similar levels of vitamin C deficiency and hypovitaminosis C to the CHALICE cohort [37,38], although the United States and lower socio-economic groups in the United Kingdom stand out as having higher rates of deficiency [9,34]. In the current study, hypovitaminosis C (i.e., <23 µmol/L) was apparent in 13% of participants, and this increased to 36% for those in the lowest socio-economic category. Symptoms such as decreased mood and energy levels may be observed with hypovitaminosis C, and are possibly related to the role of vitamin C as a cofactor in carnitine and catecholamine neurotransmitter synthesis [3,14]. A high proportion (63%) of our participants had inadequate plasma vitamin C concentrations (i.e., <50 µmol/L). Indeed, very few of our participants, only 7%, had saturating plasma vitamin C status (i.e., >70 µmol/L), implying that current Ministry of Health guidelines recommending consumption of at least five servings of vegetables and fruit per day are ineffective [39]. Since the vitamin C content of fruit and vegetables is quite variable, we suggest that it is important to highlight the consumption of high vitamin C-content fruit and/or vegetables to provide plasma saturation in this age group.

High vitamin C concentrations in the blood were associated with significantly lower weight, waist circumference and BMI, and the effect of plasma vitamin C status was significant enough to survive the correction for multiple comparisons. The association of low vitamin C with obesity in this study replicates results in the literature [35,40–44], and it is apparent that individuals with higher weight require higher intakes of vitamin C to reach adequate vitamin C status [45,46]. We also show that higher plasma vitamin C status is associated with lower circulating levels of blood triglycerides, insulin and HbA1c, associations which survive correction for gender, ethnicity and current smoking. These findings are in agreement with a number of smaller intervention studies that have found inverse relationships of vitamin C with various markers of metabolic health [47–49], although others have failed to observe an effect of intervention [50]. Dakhale and coworkers show a small decrease in HbA1c and fasting blood glucose in individuals with type 2 diabetes after vitamin C supplementation of 1 g/day for 12 weeks [51]. Observational studies also provide evidence that low vitamin C status is associated with increased risk of metabolic syndrome [52–54].

A role for vitamin C in the prevention or management of diabetes and/or metabolic syndrome has been suggested [47,51,53,54]. Obesity is a major risk factor for diabetes, and it may be that vitamin C has a role in moderating the inflammatory effect of adipose tissue. Vitamin C is thought to have anti-inflammatory activity, decreasing levels of inflammatory markers such as C-reactive protein and pro-inflammatory cytokines, although the exact mechanism(s) responsible for this are unknown [55,56]. Disorders of energy balance and metabolism are common worldwide. For example, in New Zealand, around 241,000 individuals have been diagnosed with diabetes, and significant numbers have undiagnosed diabetes, or pre-diabetes [57]. Further, among people aged over 15 years, 65% of individuals meet the criteria for overweight and obesity [58]. Diet and lifestyle factors are associated with these disorders and represent key modifiable determinants. Interestingly, in the CHALICE cohort there were no consistent significant effects identified between plasma vitamin C status and blood pressure or cardiovascular disease risk, although higher dietary vitamin C intake was associated with decreased blood pressure, an effect that has been observed previously [59].

In this study, we also demonstrate lower levels of mild cognitive impairment in those with high vitamin C status, even after adjustment for gender, ethnicity and smoking. Current smoking was a good proxy for socio-economic status and educational achievement in the model; thus, the relationship with vitamin C status survived correction for these important predictors of cognitive impairment. The odds of mild cognitive impairment were twice as high for those below 23 µmol/L plasma vitamin C concentration. Vitamin C is present at very high concentrations in the brain [60], and animal models have shown that the brain is the last organ to be depleted of the vitamin during prolonged deficiency [61], suggesting an important requirement for vitamin C in the central nervous system. A recent animal study has shown that moderate vitamin C deficiency may play a role in accelerating amyloid plaque accumulation in Alzheimer's disease, the most common form of dementia [62]. However, epidemiological studies have been inconclusive in regards to whether vitamin C status may affect cognitive decline [63,64] and Alzheimer's disease specifically [65,66]. Lu and co-workers investigated the relationship between dietary nutrients and mild cognitive impairment in 2892 elderly Chinese participants using the MoCA test, and found that vitamin C intake exhibited a significant protective effect [64]. Our study has the advantage over many in that plasma vitamin C concentrations have been measured; we were not reliant on dietary intake, which may be susceptible to problems with recall ability and the other confounders mentioned above.

In later life, dementia and disorders of cognition are highly prevalent. Even in the CHALICE sample of 50-year-olds, 15% of the sample scored below the recommended cut point on the MoCA. There is considerable interest in the effect of diet on maintaining cognitive function and delaying neuro-degenerative disease in old age. A 2015 study with 37 older healthy adults demonstrated reduced rates of cognitive decline following consumption of orange juice [67]. This was attributed to the high flavanone content of the orange juice, since flavonoids have been associated with reduced rates of cognitive decline [68,69]. However, it is possible that the vitamin C content of the orange juice may have contributed to the observed effect. In support of this premise, studies have shown that supplementation of older adults with the antioxidant vitamins C and E was able to preserve cognitive performance [70–72]. Another study, however, found no impact of antioxidant vitamin supplementation on cognition, despite improvements in markers of oxidative stress [73], demonstrating mixed results in the literature. Intervention studies often look for relatively short-term impacts on cognition instruments in response to different nutrient intakes. In contrast, the CHALICE study measured the association of plasma vitamin C status and dietary intake, more likely to be markers of longer-term lifestyle patterns, with a cognitive instrument (MoCA) as an assessment of current mild cognitive impairment.

There are several limitations to our study, notably the observational design, in which associations do not imply causation. Many factors impact on the health status of individuals and groups, including diet, exercise, temperament, behaviors, socio-economic status and genetics. These factors typically interact and correlate with each other, as they do in the CHALICE cohort, with the result that predictors of health outcomes are related (e.g., low blood pressure is associated with low BMI). We have addressed multiple testing issues with the use of corrected p values, and multi-collinearity does not affect individual models as each model only has one independent predictor, with the dichotomous covariates having limited capacity to induce collinearity. While we have focused on the associations of vitamin C with health outcomes, these associations could include the effects of unmeasured nutrients associated with vitamin C intake. Dietary vitamin C and plasma vitamin C status did not always correlate with the same health indicators. However, as detailed above, this is likely due to fasting plasma vitamin C concentration being a more accurate indicator of body status.

5. Conclusions

The CHALICE cohort of 404 individuals aged 50 years had an average vitamin C intake of ~110 mg/day, which should provide adequate plasma concentrations [14]. Despite this, a significant proportion of the participants had inadequate plasma vitamin C status. This indicates the likely effects of confounding factors, such as chronic disease, on plasma vitamin C status, and suggests that dietary interventions targeting increased consumption of fruit and vegetables, and increased vitamin C intake in particular, are required for this age group. Metabolic health markers were significantly better in participants with higher plasma vitamin C concentrations, even after correction for confounders. The association of high vitamin C concentrations with the reduction in risk of impaired cognition is intriguing and merits further investigation.

Nutrients **2017**, *9*, 831

Acknowledgments: We would like to acknowledge the participants of the CHALICE study and the CHALICE study investigators. The CHALICE study was supported by grants awarded from the Department of Internal Affairs' Lotteries Health (grant number: AP265022), Canterbury Community Trust, Otago Thyroid Research Foundation and University of Otago Foundation Trust (grant number: TL1060). Funding for the vitamin C analyses was provided by Zespri International Ltd, Mt Maunganui, New Zealand. A.C. is the recipient of a Health Research Council of New Zealand Sir Charles Hercus Health Research Fellowship.

Author Contributions: J.S. coordinated study; A.C., J.M.P. and M.V. measured vitamin C status; R.W. and P.S. calculated dietary intakes; V.C. contributed to design of cardiovascular measures; A.C., P.S. and J.F.P. conceived paper; J.F.P. analyzed data; J.M.P., A.C. and J.F.P. interpreted data and wrote paper; and M.V., P.S., J.W., J.S. and V.C. edited paper. J.F.P., J.M.P. and A.C. contributed to the work equally.

Conflicts of Interest: The authors declare no conflict of interest.

References

1. Svirbely, J.L.; Szent-Gyorgyi, A. The chemical nature of vitamin C. *Biochem. J.* **1933**, *27*, 279–285. [CrossRef] [PubMed]
2. Du, J.; Cullen, J.J.; Buettner, G.R. Ascorbic acid: Chemistry, biology and the treatment of cancer. *Biochim. Biophys. Acta* **2012**, *1826*, 443–457. [CrossRef] [PubMed]
3. England, S.; Seifter, S. The biochemical functions of ascorbic acid. *Annu. Rev. Nutr.* **1986**, *6*, 365–406. [CrossRef] [PubMed]
4. Vissers, M.C.; Kuiper, C.; Dachs, G.U. Regulation of the 2-oxoglutarate-dependent dioxygenases and implications for cancer. *Biochem. Soc. Trans.* **2014**, *42*, 945–951. [CrossRef] [PubMed]
5. Carr, A.; Frei, B. Does vitamin C act as a pro-oxidant under physiological conditions? *Faseb J.* **1999**, *13*, 1007–1024. [PubMed]
6. Bruno, R.S.; Leonard, S.W.; Atkinson, J.; Montine, T.J.; Ramakrishnan, R.; Bray, T.M.; Traber, M.G. Faster plasma vitamin E disappearance in smokers is normalized by vitamin C supplementation. *Free. Radic. Biol. Med.* **2006**, *40*, 689–697. [CrossRef] [PubMed]
7. Lin, J.Y.; Selim, M.A.; Shea, C.R.; Grichnik, J.M.; Omar, M.M.; Monteiro-Riviere, N.A.; Pinnell, S.R. UV photoprotection by combination topical antioxidants vitamin C and vitamin E. *J. Am. Acad. Dermatol.* **2003**, *48*, 866–874. [CrossRef] [PubMed]
8. Krebs, H.A. The Sheffield Experiment on the vitamin C requirement of human adults. *Proc. Nutr. Soc.* **1953**, *12*, 237–246. [CrossRef]
9. Schleicher, R.L.; Carroll, M.D.; Ford, E.S.; Lacher, D.A. Serum vitamin C and the prevalence of vitamin C deficiency in the United States: 2003–2004 National Health and Nutrition Examination Survey (NHANES). *Am. J. Clin. Nutr.* **2009**, *90*, 1252–1263. [CrossRef] [PubMed]
10. CDC's Second Nutrition Report. Available online: https://www.cdc.gov/nutritionreport/report.html (accessed on 28 June 2017).
11. A Focus on Nutrition: Key findings from the 2008/09 NZ Adult Nutrition Survey. Available online: http://www.health.govt.nz/publication/focus-nutrition-key-findings-2008-09-nz-adult-nutrition-survey (accessed on 8 June 2017).
12. Carr, A.C.; Frei, B. Toward a new recommended dietary allowance for vitamin C based on antioxidant and health effects in humans. *Am. J. Clin. Nutr.* **1999**, *69*, 1086–1107. [PubMed]
13. Lykkesfeldt, J.; Poulsen, H.E. Is vitamin C supplementation beneficial? Lessons learned from randomised controlled trials. *Br. J. Nutr.* **2010**, *103*, 1251–1259. [CrossRef] [PubMed]
14. Levine, M.; Conry-Cantilena, C.; Wang, Y.; Welch, R.W.; Washko, P.W.; Dhariwal, K.R.; Park, J.B.; Lazarev, A.; Graumlich, J.F.; King, J.; et al. Vitamin C pharmacokinetics in healthy volunteers: Evidence for a recommended dietary allowance. *Proc. Natl. Acad. Sci. USA* **1996**, *93*, 3704–3709. [CrossRef] [PubMed]
15. Jacob, R.A. Assessment of human vitamin C status. *J. Nutr.* **1990**, *120*, 1480–1485. [PubMed]
16. Tetens, I. Scientific opinion on dietary reference values for vitamin C. *EFSA. J.* **2013**, *11*, 3418–3486.
17. Nutrient Reference Values for Australia and New Zealand Executive Summary. Available online: https://www.nhmrc.gov.au/guidelines-publications/n35-n36-n37 (accessed on 7 June 2017).
18. Schluter, P.J.; Spittlehouse, J.K.; Cameron, V.A.; Chambers, S.; Gearry, R.; Jamieson, H.A.; Kennedy, M.; Lacey, C.J.; Murdoch, D.R.; Pearson, J.; et al. Canterbury Health, Ageing and Life Course (CHALICE) study: Rationale, design and methodology. *N. Z. Med. J.* **2013**, *126*, 71–85. [PubMed]

19. Enrolment Statistics: Comparison of Estimated Eligible Voting Population to Enrolled Electors for Christchurch City. Available online: http://www.elections.org.nz/councils/ages/district_60_christchurch_city.html (accessed on 12 March 2013).

20. Population of Canterbury DHB. Available online: http://www.health.govt.nz/new-zealand-health-system/my-dhb/canterbury-dhb/population-canterbury-dhb (accessed on 12 March 2013).

21. Sato, Y.; Uchiki, T.; Iwama, M.; Kishimoto, Y.; Takahashi, R.; Ishigami, A. Determination of dehydroascorbic acid in mouse tissues and plasma by using tris(2-carboxyethyl)phosphine hydrochloride as reductant in metaphosphoric acid/ethylenediaminetetraacetic acid solution. *Biol. Pharm. Bull.* **2010**, *33*, 364–369. [CrossRef] [PubMed]

22. Carr, A.C.; Pullar, J.M.; Moran, S.; Vissers, M.C. Bioavailability of vitamin C from kiwifruit in non-smoking males: Determination of 'healthy' and 'optimal' intakes. *J. Nutr. Sci.* **2012**, *1*, e14. [CrossRef] [PubMed]

23. New Zealand Primary Care Handbook 2012. Available online: http://www.health.govt.nz/publication/new-zealand-primary-care-handbook-2012 (accessed on 9 July 2017).

24. Tennant, R.; Hiller, L.; Fishwick, R.; Platt, S.; Joseph, S.; Weich, S.; Parkinson, J.; Secker, J.; Stewart-Brown, S. The Warwick-Edinburgh mental well-being scale (WEMWBS): Development and UK validation. *Health Qual. Life Outcomes* **2007**, *5*, 63. [CrossRef] [PubMed]

25. Sheehan, D.V.; Lecrubier, Y.; Sheehan, K.H.; Janavs, J.; Weiller, E.; Keskiner, A.; Schinka, J.; Knapp, E.; Sheehan, M.F.; Dunbar, G.C. The validity of the Mini International Neuropsychiatric Interview (MINI) according to the SCID-P and its reliability. *Eur. Psychiatry* **1997**, *12*, 232–241. [CrossRef]

26. Nasreddine, Z.S.; Phillips, N.A.; Bedirian, V.; Charbonneau, S.; Whitehead, V.; Collin, I.; Cummings, J.L.; Chertkow, H. The Montreal Cognitive Assessment, MoCA: A brief screening tool for mild cognitive impairment. *J. Am. Geriatr. Soc.* **2005**, *53*, 695–699. [CrossRef] [PubMed]

27. ELSI Short Form: User Manual for a Direct Measure of Living Standards. Available online: https://www.msd.govt.nz/about-msd-and-our-work/publications-resources/monitoring/living-standards/elsi-short-form.html (accessed on 7 June 2017).

28. A Portrait of Health: Key results of the 2006/07 New Zealand Health Survey. Available online: http://www.health.govt.nz/publication/portrait-health-key-results-2006-07-new-zealand-health-survey (accessed on 15 May 2017).

29. The Royal College of Pathologists of Australasia: RCPA. Available online: https://www.rcpa.edu.au/ (accessed on 9 July 2017).

30. Definition and Diagnosis of Diabetes Mellitus and Intermediate Hyperglycaemia. Available online: http://www.who.int/diabetes/publications/diagnosis_diabetes2006/en/ (accessed on 15 May 2017).

31. Kallner, A.B.; Hartmann, D.; Hornig, D.H. On the requirements of ascorbic acid in man: Steady-state turnover and body pool in smokers. *Am. J. Clin. Nutr.* **1981**, *34*, 1347–1355. [PubMed]

32. McClean, H.E.; Stewart, A.W.; Riley, C.G.; Beaven, D.W. Vitamin C status of elderly men in a residential home. *N. Z. Med. J.* **1977**, *86*, 379–382. [PubMed]

33. McClean, H.E.; Dodds, P.M.; Abernethy, M.H.; Stewart, A.W.; Beaven, D.W. Vitamin C concentration in plasma and leucocytes of men related to age and smoking habit. *N. Z. Med. J.* **1976**, *83*, 226–229. [PubMed]

34. Mosdol, A.; Erens, B.; Brunner, E.J. Estimated prevalence and predictors of vitamin C deficiency within UK's low-income population. *J. Public Health (Oxf.)* **2008**, *30*, 456–460. [CrossRef] [PubMed]

35. Galan, P.; Viteri, F.E.; Bertrais, S.; Czernichow, S.; Faure, H.; Arnaud, J.; Ruffieux, D.; Chenal, S.; Arnault, N.; Favier, A.; et al. Serum concentrations of beta-carotene, vitamins C and E, zinc and selenium are influenced by sex, age, diet, smoking status, alcohol consumption and corpulence in a general French adult population. *Eur. J. Clin. Nutr.* **2005**, *59*, 1181–1190. [CrossRef] [PubMed]

36. Jungert, A.; Neuhauser-Berthold, M. The lower vitamin C plasma concentrations in elderly men compared with elderly women can partly be attributed to a volumetric dilution effect due to differences in fat-free mass. *Br. J. Nutr.* **2015**, *113*, 859–864. [CrossRef] [PubMed]

37. Langlois, K.; Cooper, M.; Colapinto, C.K. Vitamin C status of Canadian adults: Findings from the 2012/2013 Canadian Health Measures Survey. *Health Rep.* **2016**, *27*, 3–10. [PubMed]

38. Faure, H.; Preziosi, P.; Roussel, A.M.; Bertrais, S.; Galan, P.; Hercberg, S.; Favier, A. Factors influencing blood concentration of retinol, alpha-tocopherol, vitamin C, and beta-carotene in the French participants of the SU.VI.MAX trial. *Eur. J. Clin. Nutr.* **2006**, *60*, 706–717. [CrossRef] [PubMed]

39. Eating and Activity Guidelines for New Zealand Adults. Available online: http://www.health.govt.nz/ publication/eating-and-activity-guidelines-new-zealand-adults (accessed on 7 July 2017).

40. Block, G.; Jensen, C.D.; Dalvi, T.B.; Norkus, E.P.; Hudes, M.; Crawford, P.B.; Holland, N.; Fung, E.B.; Schumacher, L.; Harmatz, P. Vitamin C treatment reduces elevated C-reactive protein. *Free Radic. Biol. Med.* **2009**, *46*, 70–77. [CrossRef] [PubMed]

41. Canoy, D.; Wareham, N.; Welch, A.; Bingham, S.; Luben, R.; Day, N.; Khaw, K.T. Plasma ascorbic acid concentrations and fat distribution in 19,068 British men and women in the European Prospective Investigation into Cancer and Nutrition Norfolk cohort study. *Am. J. Clin. Nutr.* **2005**, *82*, 1203–1209. [PubMed]

42. Garcia, O.P.; Ronquillo, D.; Caamano Mdel, C.; Camacho, M.; Long, K.Z.; Rosado, J.L. Zinc, vitamin A, and vitamin C status are associated with leptin concentrations and obesity in Mexican women: Results from a cross-sectional study. *Nutr. Metab. (Lond.)* **2012**, *9*, 59. [CrossRef] [PubMed]

43. Johnston, C.S.; Beezhold, B.L.; Mostow, B.; Swan, P.D. Plasma vitamin C is inversely related to body mass index and waist circumference but not to plasma adiponectin in nonsmoking adults. *J. Nutr.* **2007**, *137*, 1757–1762. [PubMed]

44. Moor de Burgos, A.; Wartanowicz, M.; Ziemlanski, S. Blood vitamin and lipid levels in overweight and obese women. *Eur. J. Clin. Nutr.* **1992**, *46*, 803–808. [PubMed]

45. Block, G.; Mangels, A.R.; Patterson, B.H.; Levander, O.A.; Norkus, E.P.; Taylor, P.R. Body weight and prior depletion affect plasma ascorbate levels attained on identical vitamin C intake: A controlled-diet study. *J. Am. Coll. Nutr.* **1999**, *18*, 628–637. [CrossRef] [PubMed]

46. Carr, A.C.; Pullar, J.M.; Bozonet, S.M.; Vissers, M.C. Marginal Ascorbate Status (Hypovitaminosis C) Results in an Attenuated Response to Vitamin C Supplementation. *Nutrients* **2016**, *8*, 341. [CrossRef] [PubMed]

47. Ellulu, M.S.; Rahmat, A.; Patimah, I.; Khaza'ai, H.; Abed, Y. Effect of vitamin C on inflammation and metabolic markers in hypertensive and/or diabetic obese adults: A randomized controlled trial. *Drug Des. Dev. Ther.* **2015**, *9*, 3405–3412. [CrossRef] [PubMed]

48. Chaudhari, H.V.; Dakhale, G.N.; Chaudhari, S.; Mahatme, M. The beneficial effect of vitamin C supplementation on serum lipids in type 2 diabetic patients: A randomised double blind study. *Int. J. Diabetes Metab.* **2012**, *20*, 53–58.

49. Paolisso, G.; Balbi, V.; Volpe, C.; Varricchio, G.; Gambardella, A.; Saccomanno, F.; Ammendola, S.; Varricchio, M.; D'Onofrio, F. Metabolic benefits deriving from chronic vitamin C supplementation in aged non-insulin dependent diabetics. *J. Am. Coll. Nutr.* **1995**, *14*, 387–392. [CrossRef] [PubMed]

50. Chen, H.; Karne, R.J.; Hall, G.; Campia, U.; Panza, J.A.; Cannon, R.O.; Wang, Y.; Katz, A.; Levine, M.; Quon, M.J. High-dose oral vitamin C partially replenishes vitamin C levels in patients with Type 2 diabetes and low vitamin C levels but does not improve endothelial dysfunction or insulin resistance. *Am. J. Physiol. Heart Circ. Physiol.* **2006**, *290*, H137–H145. [CrossRef] [PubMed]

51. Dakhale, G.N.; Chaudhari, H.V.; Shrivastava, M. Supplementation of vitamin C reduces blood glucose and improves glycosylated hemoglobin in type 2 diabetes mellitus: A randomized, double-blind study. *Adv. Pharmacol. Sci.* **2011**, *2011*, 195271. [CrossRef] [PubMed]

52. Godala, M.M.; Materek-Kusmierkiewicz, I.; Moczulski, D.; Rutkowski, M.; Szatko, F.; Gaszynska, E.; Tokarski, S.; Kowalski, J. Lower Plasma Levels of Antioxidant Vitamins in Patients with Metabolic Syndrome: A Case Control Study. *Adv. Clin. Exp. Med.* **2016**, *25*, 689–700. [CrossRef] [PubMed]

53. Kim, J.; Choi, Y.H. Physical activity, dietary vitamin C, and metabolic syndrome in the Korean adults: The Korea National Health and Nutrition Examination Survey 2008 to 2012. *Public Health* **2016**, *135*, 30–37. [CrossRef] [PubMed]

54. Wei, J.; Zeng, C.; Gong, Q.Y.; Li, X.X.; Lei, G.H.; Yang, T.B. Associations between Dietary Antioxidant Intake and Metabolic Syndrome. *PLoS ONE* **2015**, *10*, e0130876. [CrossRef] [PubMed]

55. Mazidi, M.; Kengne, A.P.; Mikhailidis, D. P.; Cicero, A.F.; Banach, M. Effects of selected dietary constituents on high-sensitivity C-reactive protein levels in U.S. adults. *Ann. Med.* **2017**, 1–6. [CrossRef] [PubMed]

56. Mikirova, N.; Casciari, J.; Rogers, A.; Taylor, P. Effect of high-dose intravenous vitamin C on inflammation in cancer patients. *J. Transl. Med.* **2012**, *10*, 189. [CrossRef] [PubMed]

57. Ministry of Health: Virtual Diabetes Register. Available online: http://www.health.govt.nz/our-work/ diseases-and-conditions/diabetes/about-diabetes/virtual-diabetes-register-vdr (accessed on 10 July 2017).

58. Understanding Excess Body Weight: New Zealand Health Survey. Available online: http://www.health.govt. nz/publication/understanding-excess-body-weight-new-zealand-health-survey (accessed on 12 June 2017).

59. Juraschek, S.P.; Guallar, E.; Appel, L.J.; Miller, E.R. Effects of vitamin C supplementation on blood pressure: A meta-analysis of randomized controlled trials. *Am. J. Clin. Nutr.* **2012**, *95*, 1079–1088. [CrossRef] [PubMed]
60. Hornig, D. Distribution of ascorbic acid, metabolites and analogues in man and animals. *Ann. N. Y. Acad. Sci.* **1975**, *258*, 103–118. [CrossRef] [PubMed]
61. Vissers, M.C.; Bozonet, S.M.; Pearson, J.F.; Braithwaite, L.J. Dietary ascorbate intake affects steady state tissue concentrations in vitamin C-deficient mice: Tissue deficiency after suboptimal intake and superior bioavailability from a food source (kiwifruit). *Am. J. Clin. Nutr.* **2011**, *93*, 292–301. [CrossRef] [PubMed]
62. Dixit, S.; Bernardo, A.; Walker, J.M.; Kennard, J.A.; Kim, G.Y.; Kessler, E.S.; Harrison, F.E. Vitamin C deficiency in the brain impairs cognition, increases amyloid accumulation and deposition, and oxidative stress in APP/PSEN1 and normally aging mice. *ACS Chem. Neurosci.* **2015**, *6*, 570–581. [CrossRef] [PubMed]
63. Masaki, K.H.; Losonczy, K.G.; Izmirlian, G.; Foley, D.J.; Ross, G.W.; Petrovitch, H.; Havlik, R.; White, L.R. Association of vitamin E and C supplement use with cognitive function and dementia in elderly men. *Neurology* **2000**, *54*, 1265–1272. [CrossRef] [PubMed]
64. Lu, Y.; An, Y.; Guo, J.; Zhang, X.; Wang, H.; Rong, H.; Xiao, R. Dietary Intake of Nutrients and Lifestyle Affect the Risk of Mild Cognitive Impairment in the Chinese Elderly Population: A Cross-Sectional Study. *Front. Behav. Neurosci.* **2016**, *10*, 229. [CrossRef] [PubMed]
65. Morris, M.C.; Evans, D.A.; Bienias, J.L.; Tangney, C.C.; Bennett, D.A.; Aggarwal, N.; Wilson, R.S.; Scherr, P.A. Dietary intake of antioxidant nutrients and the risk of incident Alzheimer disease in a biracial community study. *JAMA* **2002**, *287*, 3230–3237. [CrossRef] [PubMed]
66. Zandi, P.P.; Anthony, J.C.; Khachaturian, A.S.; Stone, S.V.; Gustafson, D.; Tschanz, J.T.; Norton, M.C.; Welsh-Bohmer, K.A.; Breitner, J.C. Reduced risk of Alzheimer disease in users of antioxidant vitamin supplements: The Cache County Study. *Arch. Neurol.* **2004**, *61*, 82–88. [CrossRef] [PubMed]
67. Kean, R.J.; Lamport, D.J.; Dodd, G.F.; Freeman, J.E.; Williams, C.M.; Ellis, J.A.; Butler, L.T.; Spencer, J.P. Chronic consumption of flavanone-rich orange juice is associated with cognitive benefits: An 8-wk, randomized, double-blind, placebo-controlled trial in healthy older adults. *Am. J. Clin. Nutr.* **2015**, *101*, 506–514. [CrossRef] [PubMed]
68. Letenneur, L.; Proust-Lima, C.; Le Gouge, A.; Dartigues, J.F.; Barberger-Gateau, P. Flavonoid intake and cognitive decline over a 10-year period. *Am. J. Epidemiol.* **2007**, *165*, 1364–1371. [CrossRef] [PubMed]
69. Touvier, M.; Druesne-Pecollo, N.; Kesse-Guyot, E.; Andreeva, V.A.; Fezeu, L.; Galan, P.; Hercberg, S.; Latino-Martel, P. Dual association between polyphenol intake and breast cancer risk according to alcohol consumption level: A prospective cohort study. *Breast Cancer Res. Treat* **2013**, *137*, 225–236. [CrossRef] [PubMed]
70. Smith, A.P.; Clark, R.E.; Nutt, D.J.; Haller, J.; Hayward, S.G.; Perry, K. Vitamin C, Mood and Cognitive Functioning in the Elderly. *Nutr. Neurosci.* **1999**, *2*, 249–256. [CrossRef] [PubMed]
71. Kang, J.H.; Cook, N.R.; Manson, J.E.; Buring, J.E.; Albert, C.M.; Grodstein, F. Vitamin E, vitamin C, beta carotene, and cognitive function among women with or at risk of cardiovascular disease: The Women's Antioxidant and Cardiovascular Study. *Circulation* **2009**, *119*, 2772–2780. [CrossRef] [PubMed]
72. Kesse-Guyot, E.; Fezeu, L.; Jeandel, C.; Ferry, M.; Andreeva, V.; Amieva, H.; Hercberg, S.; Galan, P. French adults' cognitive performance after daily supplementation with antioxidant vitamins and minerals at nutritional doses: A post hoc analysis of the Supplementation in Vitamins and Mineral Antioxidants (SU.VI.MAX) trial. *Am. J. Clin. Nutr.* **2011**, *94*, 892–899. [CrossRef] [PubMed]
73. Naeini, A.M.; Elmadfa, I.; Djazayery, A.; Barekatain, M.; Ghazvini, M.R.; Djalali, M.; Feizi, A. The effect of antioxidant vitamins E and C on cognitive performance of the elderly with mild cognitive impairment in Isfahan, Iran: A double-blind, randomized, placebo-controlled trial. *Eur. J. Nutr.* **2014**, *53*, 1255–1262. [CrossRef] [PubMed]

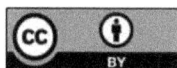

nutrients

MDPI

Article

Inadequate Vitamin C Status in Prediabetes and Type 2 Diabetes Mellitus: Associations with Glycaemic Control, Obesity, and Smoking

Renée Wilson [1], Jinny Willis [2], Richard Gearry [1], Paula Skidmore [3], Elizabeth Fleming [3], Chris Frampton [1] and Anitra Carr [4,*]

1   Department of Medicine, University of Otago, Christchurch 8011, New Zealand; renee.wilson@postgrad.otago.ac.nz (R.W.); richard.gearry@otago.ac.nz (R.G.); chris.frampton@otago.ac.nz (C.F.)
2   Lipid and Diabetes Research Group, Canterbury District Health Board, Christchurch 8011, New Zealand; jinny.willis@cdhb.health.nz
3   Department of Human Nutrition, University of Otago, Dunedin 9016, New Zealand; paula.skidmore@otago.ac.nz (P.S.); liz.fleming@otago.ac.nz (E.F.)
4   Department of Pathology, University of Otago, Christchurch 8011, New Zealand
*   Correspondence: anitra.carr@otago.ac.nz; Tel.: +64-3-364-0649

Received: 14 July 2017; Accepted: 6 September 2017; Published: 9 September 2017

Abstract: Vitamin C (ascorbate) is an essential micronutrient in humans, being required for a number of important biological functions via acting as an enzymatic cofactor and reducing agent. There is some evidence to suggest that people with type 2 diabetes mellitus (T2DM) have lower plasma vitamin C concentrations compared to those with normal glucose tolerance (NGT). The aim of this study was to investigate plasma vitamin C concentrations across the glycaemic spectrum and to explore correlations with indices of metabolic health. This is a cross-sectional observational pilot study in adults across the glycaemic spectrum from NGT to T2DM. Demographic and anthropometric data along with information on physical activity were collected and participants were asked to complete a four-day weighed food diary. Venous blood samples were collected and glycaemic indices, plasma vitamin C concentrations, hormone tests, lipid profiles, and high-sensitivity C-reactive protein (hs-CRP) were analysed. A total of 89 participants completed the study, including individuals with NGT (n = 35), prediabetes (n = 25), and T2DM managed by diet alone or on a regimen of Metformin only (n = 29). Plasma vitamin C concentrations were significantly lower in individuals with T2DM compared to those with NGT (41.2 µmol/L versus 57.4 µmol/L, p < 0.05) and a higher proportion of vitamin C deficiency (i.e. <11.0 µmol/L) was observed in both the prediabetes and T2DM groups. The results showed fasting glucose (p = 0.001), BMI (p = 0.001), smoking history (p = 0.003), and dietary vitamin C intake (p = 0.032) to be significant independent predictors of plasma vitamin C concentrations. In conclusion, these results suggest that adults with a history of smoking, prediabetes or T2DM, and/or obesity, have greater vitamin C requirements. Future research is required to investigate whether eating more vitamin C rich foods and/or taking vitamin C supplements may reduce the risk of progression to, and/or complications associated with, T2DM.

Keywords: vitamin C; glycaemic control; metabolic health; prediabetes; type 2 diabetes mellitus

1. Introduction

Type 2 diabetes mellitus (T2DM) is a complex disorder influenced by both genetic and environmental factors. It is characterized by chronic hyperglycemia, altered insulin secretion, and insulin resistance [1]. As in many Western countries, T2DM is associated with increased morbidity and mortality due to microvascular (e.g. retinopathy, nephropathy, and neuropathy) and macrovascular complications (e.g. myocardial infarction, peripheral vascular disease, and stroke) [1]. Diabetes is one of the largest global health emergencies with 415 million people between the ages of 20 and 70 worldwide estimated as having diabetes in 2015 and the prevalence is increasing [2]. T2DM accounts for at least 90% of all cases of diabetes [2]. In 2016, approximately 5% of New Zealanders were living with diabetes compared to an estimated 6.5% of people in the UK [3,4].

Research suggests that chronic low grade inflammation and oxidative stress plays a pivotal role in the development of insulin resistance and T2DM, as well as the related complications [5]. Vitamin C is an essential micronutrient with potent antioxidant properties [6]. Vitamin C can protect important biomolecules from oxidation through participating in oxidation-reduction reactions whereby it is readily oxidized to dehydroascorbic acid, which in turn is rapidly reduced back to ascorbate [7]. Vitamin C is naturally present in fruit and vegetables, is often added as a preservative to foods/beverages, and is also used as a dietary supplement [6]. As a result of being water-soluble, it has a relatively short half-life in the body due to rapid renal clearance and a regular and adequate intake is required to prevent deficiency.

Previous research suggests that people with T2DM have lower plasma vitamin C concentrations than those with normal glucose control [8–10]. There are several proposed mechanisms including: (1) increased ascorbate excretion in those with microalbuminuria, (2) blood glucose may compete with vitamin C for uptake into cells due to its structural similarity to the oxidised form (dehydroascorbic acid), and (3) increased oxidative stress may deplete antioxidant stores [8]. Recent research has indicated that the glucose-dependent inhibition of dehydroascorbic acid uptake into erythrocytes may contribute to enhanced erythrocyte fragility and could potentially contribute to complications such as diabetic microvascular angiopathy [11].

As dietary vitamin C contributes to plasma vitamin C concentrations, potential differences in the intake between those with normal glucose control and T2DM must also be considered. A prospective study of 48,850 men revealed that while the baseline consumption of fruit and vegetables was similar, men who developed T2DM increased their consumption of fruit and vegetables by 1.6 serves/week compared to an increase of 0.7 serves/week in those who remained diabetes free [12]. Therefore, it seems that people with T2DM are altering their diet in an attempt to manage their blood sugar. Indeed, clinical advice to those newly-diagnosed with T2DM focuses on improving the diet. However, the dietary changes appear to be small and, furthermore, those with T2DM appear to have a similar intake of fruit and vegetables to those without T2DM [12].

The lower plasma vitamin C concentrations reported in people with T2DM has led to a growing interest in the role that vitamin C may afford against the development of T2DM and associated complications. A prospective survey of the Dutch and Finnish cohorts within the Seven Countries Study revealed an inverse association between dietary vitamin C intake and glucose intolerance, suggesting that antioxidants such as vitamin C may play a protective role against the development of impaired glucose tolerance and T2DM [13]. Further, the European Prospective Investigation of Cancer (EPIC)-Norfolk Study of some 21,000 individuals ascertained 735 cases of T2DM after a 12 year follow-up, and demonstrated a strong inverse association between plasma vitamin C concentration and T2DM risk [14].

However, studies investigating plasma vitamin C and glycaemic control have often failed to account for factors such as smoking status and dietary vitamin C intake, which are known to impact plasma vitamin C concentrations. When dietary intake is taken into account there are conflicting results, with one study showing a low plasma vitamin C concentration in people with diabetes consuming a similar amount of dietary vitamin C to those without diabetes [15], compared to another study that reported no differences in serum vitamin C concentrations in people grouped by T2DM status after adjustment for dietary vitamin C intake [16]. Therefore, the objective of this study was to determine the association between plasma vitamin C status and glycaemic control accounting for vitamin C intake in adults.

2. Materials and Methods

2.1. Study Participants

This study was approved by the New Zealand Central Health and Disability Ethics Committee (consent no. 14/CEN/34). Written informed consent was obtained from all participants. Individuals aged ≥ 18 years meeting the inclusion criteria detailed below were recruited from General Practice, Prediabetes and Diabetes Services, Retinal Screening Services, Pharmacies, and from local advertisements. Fasting glucose cut-off values for normal glucose tolerance (NGT), prediabetes, and T2DM were based on the American Diabetes Association (ADA) criteria [1]. Those taking Metformin were also included in the T2DM group. A total of 101 individuals underwent a screening questionnaire to ascertain the eligibility for the study. Ninety participants were enrolled and 89 participants completed the study. One participant was excluded due to incomplete sample collection.

2.2. Study Design

This was a cross-sectional observational pilot study that was part of a wider study on the gut microbiota and glycaemic control. At their study appointment, participants completed demographic and physical activity questionnaires. Anthropometric data were collected including the body mass index (BMI), waist and hip circumference, and bioelectrical impedance. The completed four-day weighed food diary was reviewed and additional information was added if necessary. A venous blood sample was also collected after an overnight fast and the blood pressure was measured.

2.2.1. Inclusion Criteria

Individuals aged ≥18 years with: NGT (fasting glucose ≤5.5 mmol/L) (n = 35), prediabetes (fasting glucose ≥5.6 mmol/L) (n = 25), T2DM taking no diabetes medication (fasting glucose ≥7.0 mmol/L) or on a regimen of Metformin only (n = 29).

2.2.2. Exclusion Criteria

Individuals unable to give informed consent, those who had taken antibiotics in the last month, those with a medical history of significant gastrointestinal disease e.g. inflammatory bowel disease, those who had undergone a previous bowel resection, and individuals taking diabetes medication other than Metformin.

2.3. Demographic Information

Participants recorded their date of birth, sex, ethnicity, qualification, and smoking status. They also recorded information on current medication and supplement use.

2.4. Anthropometric Measures

Weight (kg). Participants were asked to remove their footwear and heavy outer clothing such as jackets and were weighed to the nearest 0.1 kg on calibrated Tanita scales (Model BWB-800A, Tanita Corporation, Tokyo, Japan).

Height (m). Measured once to the nearest mm using calibrated height measures.

BMI (kg/m²). Widely accepted as an appropriate population-level indicator of excess body fat [17]. BMI is calculated by weight in kilograms divided by height in metres squared.

Waist circumference and the waist-to-hip ratio are alternative anthropometric measures that also indicate whether excess body fat is centrally or peripherally located.

Waist circumference (cm). The World Health Organisation (WHO) STEPwise Approach to Surveillance (STEPS) protocol for measuring the waist circumference was used. The measurement was made at the approximate midpoint between the lower margin of the last palpable rib and the top of the iliac crest [18]. The tightness of the tape was controlled by using a Gulick II Measuring tape

(Model 67020, Country Technology Inc, Gays Mills, Wisconsin, WI, USA). Two to three measures were recorded and if the difference between the measurements exceeded 1.5 cm, a third measure was taken. The measures for each participant were averaged.

Hip circumference (cm). Measured to the nearest mm around the widest portion of the buttocks with the tape parallel to the floor using a Gulick II Measuring tape, as described above.

Waist-to-hip ratio. Calculated by dividing the waist circumference by the hip measurement.

Fat mass (%). Measured using the BIA 450 Bioimpedance Analyser (Biodynamics Corporation, Seattle, Washington, DC, USA). Patient assessments were conducted using a connection between the individual's wrist and ankle and the analyser using standard ECG sensor pad electrodes (CONMED Corporation, Utica, New York, NY, USA).

Blood Pressure. Measured using an automated blood pressure monitor (Bp TRU, BTM-300, Omron Healthcare Co., Ltd, Muko, Kyoto, Japan). The measurement was repeated if the results were outside the normal range. If there was an obvious outlier, this result was removed and the other results were averaged.

2.5. Blood Parameters

Venous blood samples were collected after a 12–hour fast.

Glycated haemoglobin (HbA1c). Determined in EDTA blood by standard methods (Bio-rad Variant HPLC, Bio-Rad, Hercules, California, CA, USA) at an International Accreditation New Zealand (IANZ) laboratory.

Glucose. Fasting glucose was measured in blood collected in fluoride oxalate venoject tubes by standard methods (Glucose Hexokinase Enzymatic Assay, Abbott c series analyser, Abbott Park, Illinois, USA) at an IANZ laboratory.

Lipid parameters. Total cholesterol (TC), HDL-cholesterol (HDL), LDL-cholesterol (LDL), and triglycerides (TG) were determined in lithium heparin blood by standard methods (Abbott c series analyser, Abbott Park, Illinois, IL, USA) at an IANZ laboratory.

High-sensitivity C-reactive protein (hs-CRP). The inflammatory marker hs-CRP was measured using end-point nephelometry at an IANZ laboratory.

Plasma vitamin C and hormones. EDTA blood was collected and centrifuged for 15 min at 1500 g at 4 °C. The plasma was stored −80 °C prior to analysis.

2.5.1. Plasma Vitamin C

Stored plasma was rapidly thawed, and acidified with perchloric acid and a metal chelator (DTPA) to precipitate the protein and stabilise the ascorbate [19]. Following centrifugation, the supernatant was treated with a reducing agent (TCEP) to recover any ascorbate that had become oxidised during the processing and storage of the samples [20]. The vitamin C concentration of the processed samples was determined using high performance liquid chromatography (HPLC) with electrochemical detection in the Department of Pathology, University of Otago Christchurch, as described previously [19].

2.5.2. Plasma Ghrelin, Leptin, and Adiponectin

Plasma hormones were determined by the Christchurch Heart Institute, Department of Medicine, University of Otago, Christchurch.

Plasma ghrelin was measured by an in-house radioimmunoassay (RIA) following extraction from plasma using Sep Pak C_{18} cartridges, as described previously [21]. The assay recognises the total circulating ghrelin (i.e. both octanoyl and non-octanoyl forms). The cross reactivities of other peptides in the assay, including vasointestinal peptide, prolactin, galanin, growth hormone releasing hormone, neuropeptide Y, brain natriuretic peptide, atrial natriuretic peptide, endothelin-1, and angiotensin II were all less than 0.03%. The RIA had a mean detection limit of 10.8 ± 0.8 pmol/L and mean ED_{50} of 136.2 ± 10.0 pmol/L over 23 consecutive assays.

Plasma leptin and adiponectin were measured using commercial enzyme-linked immunosorbent assays (ELISA) from BioVendor (Brno, Czech Republic), Research and Diagnostic products (RD191001100 Human Leptin ELISA and RD191023100 Human Adiponectin ELISA) according to the manufacturer's instructions.

2.5.3. Plasma Insulin

Plasma insulin was measured using the Roche Cobas e411 method in an IANZ laboratory. After storage at −80 °C, thawed plasma was pre-treated using 25% polyethylene glycol to precipitate any unwanted antibodies.

2.6. Dietary Intake of Vitamin C, Macronutrients, and Fibre

Participants completed a four day (non-consecutive) weighed food diary (including one weekend day) prior to their study visit. Participants received training using the Salter digital scales and on how to record the data, either at home or in the clinic, prior to the diary being completed. Once completed, the diary was also reviewed at their second study visit to add any missing information if necessary. The food diaries were entered into the nutrient analysis programme Kai-culator (version 1.08d, Department of Human Nutrition, University of Otago, Dunedin, New Zealand). Kai-culator uses the 2014 version of the New Zealand food composition database "NZ FOODfiles". The methodology for entering the diaries was developed by a dietitian and data entry was undertaken by an experienced dietitian and an experienced nutritionist who cross-checked each other's data and were overseen by an experienced nutritionist and dietitian. A further 16% of the diaries were checked again for accuracy. The Acceptable Macronutrient Distribution Ranges (AMDR) are the recommendations for the balance of protein, fat, and carbohydrate in the diet with respect to the relative contribution to dietary energy [22]. Total daily vitamin C, energy, and fibre were calculated, along with the percent energy values for fat, carbohydrate, and protein. Participants were asked to record the name of dietary supplements taken within the last month, the amount per dose, the frequency, when they started taking the supplement, and when their last dose was.

2.7. Physical Activity

Participants completed the self-administered short form version of the International Physical Activity Questionnaire (IPAQ). The questionnaire asks about physical activity over the previous seven days.

2.8. Statistical Analyses

Standard descriptive statistics including means, standard deviations, frequencies, and percentages as appropriate were used to summarise the demographic, anthropometric, and laboratory results across participants grouped by fasting glucose and T2DM treatment. Four of the laboratory measures (hs-CRP, Ghrelin, Leptin, and Adiponectin) showed a strong positive skew and were therefore $\log_e$ transformed prior to analyses. These variables are described using geometric means and 95% confidence intervals. Associations between the clinical characteristics of the cohorts grouped by fasting glucose (including those treated with Metformin) were tested using one way analysis of variance (ANOVA) and chi-squared tests as appropriate. Where significant associations were identified, these were further explored with pair-wise comparisons amongst the fasting glucose groups. The univariate associations between plasma vitamin C and demographic, anthropometric, and laboratory measures were tested using Pearson's Correlations coefficients and one way ANOVA. Significant predictors identified from these univariate analyses were then combined in a multiple regression analysis to identify significant independent associations with plasma vitamin C. The two-tailed p-value < 0.05 was taken to indicate statistical significance. All statistical analyses were undertaken using SPSS (version 24.0, IBM Corp., Armonk, New York, NY, USA).

3. Results

3.1. Participant Characteristics

The NGT group was slightly younger than the prediabetes and T2DM groups and there were more females in the NGT group and less in the T2DM group. The majority of participants were European and there were a mix of qualifications, as would be expected given the age of the participants (Table 1). There were no significant differences in physical activity between the study groups although those in the NGT and prediabetes groups had reported slightly higher levels of activity than those with T2DM.

Table 1. General characteristics of participants classified as having normal glucose tolerance (NGT) ($n = 35$), prediabetes ($n = 25$), and T2DM ($n = 29$).

Characteristics	NGT	Prediabetes	T2DM	Total
Age * (years)	55 ± 13 [a]	63 ± 9 [b]	61 ± 11 [b]	59 ± 11
Sex *				
Female % (n)	74 (26) [a]	52 (13) [ab]	35 (10) [b]	55% (49)
Male % (n)	26 (9)	48 (12)	66 (19)	45% (40)
Ethnicity				
European % (n)	86 (30)	88 (22)	97 (28)	90% (80)
Maori % (n)	9 (3)	4 (1)	3 (1)	6% (5)
Pacific Island % (n)	0 (0)	4 (1)	0 (0)	1% (1)
Asian % (n)	3 (1)	4 (1)	0 (0)	2% (2)
Other % (n)	3 (1)	0 (0)	0 (0)	1% (1)
Qualification				
No Qualification % (n)	96 (3)	20 (5)	25 (7)	17% (15)
Secondary School % (n)	20 (7)	24 (6)	32 (9)	25% (22)
Post-Secondary Certificate, Diploma or Trade Diploma % (n)	43 (15)	20 (5)	25 (7)	31% (27)
University % (n)	27 (10)	36 (9)	18 (5)	27% (24)
Physical Activity (MET min/week)	1723 ± 1687	2496 ± 3671	1320 ± 1490	1772 ± 2327
Anthropometry				
Weight * (kg)	76 ± 18 [a]	89 ± 19 [b]	96 ± 20 [b]	86 ± 21
BMI * (kg/m^2)	28 ± 6 [a]	30 ± 7 [ab]	33 ± 6 [b]	30 ± 7
Fat Mass (%)	32 ± 8	33 ± 8	35 ± 7	33 ± 8
Waist Circumference * (cm)	89 ± 16 [a]	99 ± 14 [b]	110 ± 15 [c]	99 ± 17
Waist-to-Hip Ratio *	0.9 ± 0.1 [a]	0.9 ± 0.1 [b]	1.0 ± 0.1 [b]	0.9 ± 0.1
Blood Pressure Diastolic (mmHg)	78 ± 9	83 ± 8	79 ± 9	80 ± 9
Blood Pressure Systolic * (mmHg)	125 ± 14 [a]	132 ± 14 [ab]	135 ± 15 [b]	130 ± 15
Smoking Status				
Current Smoker % (n)	7 (2)	5 (1)	3 (1)	5% (4)
Ex-smoker % (n)	28 (8)	439 (9)	38 (11)	35% (28)
Non-smoker % (n)	66 (19)	52 (11)	59 (17)	60% (47)

Values represented as mean ± SD unless stated otherwise. *All p values from ANOVA tests. Groups sharing a common subscript letter denotes the study groups that do not differ significantly from each other at the 0.05 level based on characteristics from Post Hoc analysis. Note: There was missing data from one participant for qualification (1 × T2DM), 12 participants for physical activity (7 × NGT and 5 × prediabetes), five participants for waist-to-hip ratio (2 × NGT and 3 × prediabetes), nine participants for blood pressure measures (4 × NGT and 5 × prediabetes), and 10 participants did not provide smoking status data (6 × NGT, 4 × prediabetes).

The mean BMI for the NGT and prediabetes groups reflects the international BMI cut-off points for overweight (25.00–29.99 kg/m^2) and the T2DM group were obese ($\geq$30.00 kg/m^2). The waist circumference and waist-to-hip ratio increased across the groups from NGT to T2DM along with fat mass (%), as would be expected given that obesity is a risk factor for T2DM.

3.2. Metabolic and Inflammatory Plasma Biomarkers

Glycaemic measures (fasting glucose and HbA1c), used as the basis for defining prediabetes and T2DM, increased from NGT to T2DM as expected and differed significantly between the study groups ($p < 0.05$, Table 2). Although fasting glucose was used as the basis for classifying participants in the analysis, the mean HbA1c of 35 mmol/mol for the NGT group and 40 mmol/mol for the prediabetes group were consistent with the New Zealand guidelines for the classification of diabetes based on HbA1c [23]. The mean HbA1c of 47 mmol/mol for the T2DM group is lower than the current threshold for the diagnosis of diabetes in New Zealand (50 mmol/mol) using this measure because some of the individuals in this category were treated with the biguanide oral hypoglycaemic drug, Metformin. Fasting and postprandial glucose were likely reduced in these treated individuals. The mean HbA1c for all participants was 41 mmol/mol (Table 2). While hs-CRP was inversely associated with glycaemic control, this was not significant.

Table 2. Laboratory measures of participants classified as having normal glucose tolerance (NGT) ($n = 35$), prediabetes ($n = 25$), and T2DM ($n = 29$).

Laboratory Measures	NGT	Prediabetes	T2DM	Total
Fasting Glucose * (mmol/L)	5.0 ± 0.4 [a]	6.2 ± 0.4 [b]	7.2 ± 1.3 [c]	6.0 ± 1.2
HbA1c * (mmol/mol)	35 ± 4 [a]	40 ± 5 [b]	47 ± 9 [c]	41 ± 8
hs-CRP (mg/L) Mean (95% CI)	1.2 (0.9–1.6)	1.6 (1.0–2.3)	2.1 (1.4–2.8)	1.6 (1.3–1.9)
Total Cholesterol * (mmol/L)	5.3 ± 0.9 [a]	5.9 ± 1.2 [a]	4.3 ± 1.1 [b]	5.0 ± 1.1
Cholesterol HDL * (mmol/L)	1.5 ± 0.4 [a]	1.3 ± 0.3 [b]	1.1 ± 0.2 [b]	1.3 ± 0.3
Cholesterol LDL * (Calc) (mmol/L)	3.4 ± 0.8 [a]	3.3 ± 1.0 [a]	2.5 ± 1.0 [b]	3.1 ± 1.0
Triglycerides * (mmol/L)	1.1 ± 0.4 [a]	1.3 ± 0.7 [ab]	1.4 ± 0.6 [b]	1.3 ± 0.6
Cholesterol (total/HDL) (ratio)	3.8 ± 0.8	4.2 ± 0.8	3.9 ± 1.1	4.0 ± 0.9
Fasting Insulin * (pmol/L)	53 ± 37 [a]	89 ± 53 [b]	95 ± 48 [b]	77 ± 49
Ghrelin * (pmol/L) Mean (95% CI)	171 (142–207) [a]	111 (88–140) [b]	112 (91–139) [b]	132 (117–150)
Leptin (ng/mL) Mean (95% CI)	27 (20–38)	33 (20–54)	33 (23–47)	31 (25–38)
Adiponectin * (μg/mL) Mean (95% CI)	11 (9–13) [a]	9 (7–11) [a]	7 (6–8) [b]	9 (8–10)
Plasma vitamin C * (μmol/L)	57 ± 14 [a]	48 ± 16 [b]	41 ± 18 [b]	49 ± 17

Values represented as mean ± SD unless stated otherwise. *All *p* values from ANOVA tests. Groups sharing a common subscript letter denotes the study groups that do not differ significantly from each other at the 0.05 level based on characteristics from Post Hoc analysis. Log conversion was carried out for Ghrelin, Leptin, Adiponectin, and hs-CRP. Note: There was missing data from three participants for plasma vitamin C (2 × NGT and 1 × prediabetes).

The average fasting insulin concentrations were consistent with the glycaemic measures and were significantly higher in the T2DM group compared to the NGT group. The increasing BMI across the groups was associated with the increase in leptin concentrations, and the reduction in ghrelin concentrations.

Total, HDL, and LDL cholesterol decreased from the NGT to the T2DM group, which may reflect the use of lipid lowering medications which are routinely used in individuals with T2DM.

There was a slight increase in TG across the groups, with the average for each group remaining below the recommended cut-off in New Zealand (<1.7 mmol/L). There were no significant differences in the total cholesterol/HDL ratio between groups, and each group was below the recommended cut-off in New Zealand of 4.5.

3.3. Dietary Intake of Vitamin C, Macronutrients, and Fibre

There were no significant differences in macronutrient intake and dietary vitamin C intake across the groups (Table 3). The AMDR range for protein is 15–25% of total energy, total fat 20–35% of total energy, and carbohydrate 45–65% of total energy [22]. All study groups had slightly higher average total fat intakes and slightly lower CHO intakes than recommended, but the average protein intake for all groups fell within the recommended range.

The adequate intake (AI) for dietary fibre in New Zealand and Australia is set at the median for dietary fibre intake recorded in the 1995 National Nutrition Survey of Australia (ABS 1998) and the 1997 National Nutrition Survey of New Zealand (MOH 1999) [22]. The AI is 25 g for women and 30 g for men. Although fibre intake is not reported by sex in Table 1, the average daily fibre intake for each group of 24 g, 25 g, and 27 g for the NGT, prediabetes, and T2DM groups, respectively, was similar to recommendations.

Six participants reported taking a high dose vitamin C supplement (≥500 mg vitamin C). The plasma vitamin C concentration of five of these participants ranged from 36–59 μmol/L, which reflects inadequate to adequate plasma vitamin C concentrations and suggests that they didn't take the supplement close to their study appointment. The other participant had a plasma vitamin C concentration of 74 µmol/L, which is a saturating concentration, but they also had an average dietary vitamin C intake of 194 mg/day and so this high plasma concentration could be explained by their dietary intake as 200 mg/day will saturate plasma [19].

Table 3. Dietary intake of participants classified as having normal glucose tolerance (NGT) ($n = 35$), prediabetes ($n = 25$), and T2DM ($n = 29$).

Total Daily Dietary intake	NGT	Prediabetes	T2DM	Total
Energy (KJ)	8192 ± 2336	8430 ± 2260	8033 ± 2416	8204 ± 2321
Fibre (g)	24 ± 9	25 ± 8	27 ± 9	25 ± 9
Protein (% of Energy)	17 ± 3	18 ± 4	17 ± 3	17 ± 3
Fat (% of Energy)	37 ± 6	39 ± 8	36 ± 7	37 ± 7
Carbohydrate (% of Energy)	44 ± 6	40 ± 8	44 ± 8	43 ± 7
Dietary Vitamin C Intake (mg)	103 ± 76	94 ± 58	101 ± 61	100 ± 66

Values represented as mean ± SD unless stated otherwise. Note: There was missing data from one participant for dietary information (1 × prediabetes). There were no significant differences between the study groups for any of the dietary intake measures.

3.4. Plasma Vitamin C Status and Dietary Vitamin C Intakes

A significant decrease in the mean plasma vitamin C concentration was observed between the NGT (57.4 µmol/L) and the prediabetes group (48.2 µmol/L) ($p = 0.035$) and the T2DM (41.2 µmol/L) group ($p < 0.001$) (Table 2). Furthermore, there was a much higher proportion of individuals with prediabetes and T2DM with deficient (4% and 3% respectively), marginal (14% in T2DM group), and inadequate (58% in prediabetes and 52% in T2DM group) plasma vitamin C concentrations, compared with the NGT group (3% marginal and 21% inadequate) (Figure 1).

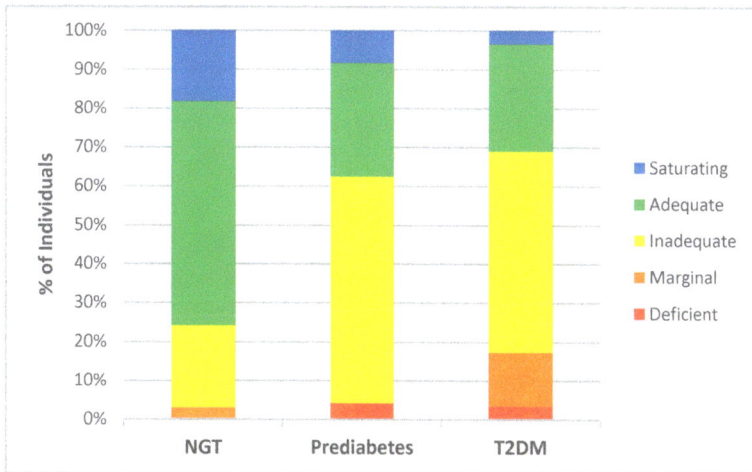

Figure 1. Plasma vitamin C status of individuals within study groups. Percentage of individuals from each study group [normal glucose tolerance (NGT), prediabetes, and type 2 diabetes mellitus (T2DM), including those taking no diabetes medication (fasting glucose ≥ 7.0 mmol/L or on a regimen of Metformin only (T2DM)], classified as having saturating (>70 µmol/L), adequate (51.0–69.9 µmol/L), inadequate (24.0–50.9 µmol/L), marginal (11.0–23.9 µmol/L), and deficient (<11.0 µmol/L) plasma vitamin C concentrations [24].

Although plasma vitamin C decreased from NGT to T2DM, there were no significant differences in dietary vitamin C concentrations between study groups determined from the four day weighed food diaries (Table 3). The majority of participants met the New Zealand recommended dietary intake

(RDI) of 45 mg/day (Figure 2). Furthermore, there were no participants in the T2DM group that had intakes below the New Zealand estimated average requirement (EAR) (30 mg/day). At the group level, it appears that most participants had an adequate fruit and vegetable intake to meet the recommended vitamin C intakes. However, few participants were reaching the New Zealand Ministry of Health's suggested dietary targets (SDT) to reduce chronic disease risk, i.e. 220 mg/day for men and 190 mg/d for women (Figure 2).

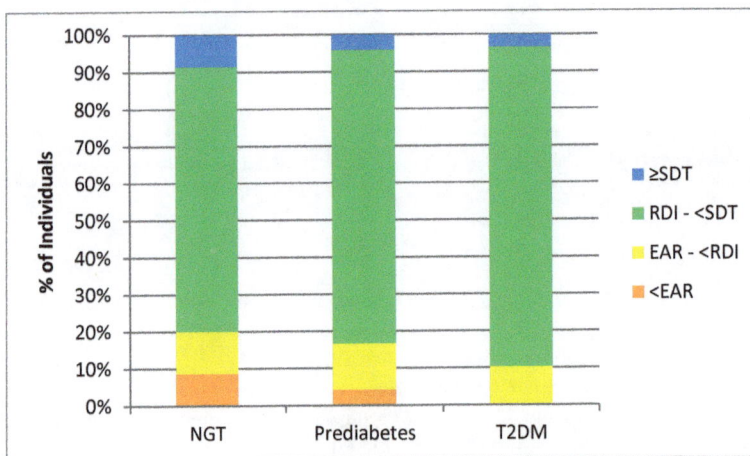

Figure 2. Individuals meeting New Zealand dietary intake recommendations for vitamin C. Percentage of individuals from each study group [normal glucose tolerance (NGT), prediabetes, and type 2 diabetes mellitus (T2DM), including those taking no diabetes medication (fasting glucose ≥7.0 mmol/L or on a regimen of Metformin only (T2DM)], meeting the estimated average requirement (EAR) (30 mg/day), recommended dietary intake (RDI) (45 mg/day), and suggested dietary target (SDT) to reduce chronic disease risk (220 mg/day for men and 190 mg/day for women) for dietary vitamin C intake using the nutrient reference values for Australia and New Zealand [22].

3.5. Plasma Vitamin C Correlations

There were no significant associations between age, gender, ethnicity, education level, and plasma vitamin C concentrations. There was a significant association between smoking history and plasma vitamin C concentration ($p = 0.035$), with current (mean 30.9 µmol/L) and ex-smokers (mean 47.3 µmol/L) having lower concentrations than non-smokers (mean 52.6 µmol/L). There was a significant linear association between vitamin C intake and plasma vitamin C concentration ($r = 0.353$, $p = 0.001$).

The three anthropometric measures (BMI, fat mass, and waist-to-hip ratio) were all significantly negatively associated with plasma vitamin C ($p < 0.05$) when conducting univariate analyses. When these three variables were included in a multiple regression, only BMI was independently negatively associated with plasma vitamin C ($p < 0.001$). Laboratory measurements (HbA1c, fasting glucose, TG, total chol/HDL chol, insulin, and hs-CRP) were negatively associated with plasma vitamin C ($p < 0.05$) and HDL chol and ghrelin were positively associated with plasma vitamin C ($p < 0.05$) in the univariate anlaysis (Table 4). When these variables were included in a multiple regression, only hs-CRP and fasting glucose were independently negatively associated with plasma vitamin C ($p < 0.05$).

A final multiple regression showed fasting glucose ($p = 0.001$), BMI ($p = 0.001$) and smoking history ($p = 0.003$) to be significant independent predictors of plasma vitamin C. Fasting glucose and BMI were negatively associated with plasma vitamin C, and current and ex-smokers had reduced plasma vitamin C concentrations compared to non-smokers. There was a strong positive association between hs-CRP concentrations and BMI ($r = 0.618$, $p < 0.001$). Accordingly, hs-CRP does not feature as an independent predictor of plasma vitamin C. Including dietary vitamin C intake in the above model (Table 5) showed that this was a significant independent predictor ($p = 0.032$) of plasma vitamin C concentrations, and BMI, fasting glucose, and smoking history remained as significant independent predictors ($R^2 = 0.43$).

Table 4. Pearson correlations of plasma vitamin C, glycaemic indices, hormones, lipids, high sensitivity C-reactive protein, and anthropometric measures.

Measure	Pearson Correlation
Fasting Glucose (mmol/L)	−0.411 ***
HbA1c (mmol/mol)	−0.334 ***
Total Cholesterol (mmol/L)	0.093
Triglycerides (mmol/L)	−0.322 **
Cholesterol (HDL)	0.295 **
Cholesterol (total/HDL)	−0.214 *
Cholesterol (LDL) calculated	0.086
Insulin (pmol/L)	−0.353 **
hs-CRP (mg/L)	−0.333 **
Ghrelin (pmol/L)	0.295 **
Leptin (ng/mL)	−0.183
Adiponectin (ng/mL)	0.202
BMI (kg/m2)	−0.446 ***
Waist-to-Hip Ratio	−0.274 *
Fat Mass (%)	−0.295 **

*** correlations significant at 0.001 level (2-tailed); ** correlations significant at the 0.01 level (2-tailed); * correlations significant at the 0.05 level (2-tailed).

Table 5. Multiple regression analysis showing significant associations with plasma vitamin C concentrations.

Measure	B	Lower 95% CI	Upper 95% CI	*p* Value
BMI	−0.9	−1.4	−0.4	0.001
Current Smoker	−21.9	−35.8	−7.9	0.003
Ex-Smoker	−4.9	−11.2	1.5	0.128
Fasting Glucose	−4.4	−7.1	−1.8	0.001
Dietary vitamin C	0.05	0.01	0.10	0.032

B: coefficient from the multiple linear regression model.

4. Discussion

4.1. Predictors of Plasma Vitamin C

This study showed fasting glucose, BMI, smoking history, and dietary vitamin C intake to be significant independent predictors of plasma vitamin C concentrations. The inverse association between fasting glucose and plasma vitamin C concentration shown in this study is in agreement with earlier studies [8–10]. In addition, the mean plasma vitamin C concentration was significantly lower in the prediabetes group (compared to the NGT group, suggesting that a reduction in plasma vitamin C concentration occurs in parallel with the decline in glucose tolerance during the progression to T2DM. It has been proposed that the uptake of dehydroascorbic acid, the oxidized form of vitamin C, by the glucose transporters (GLUTs), could be competitively inhibited by elevated blood glucose levels [25]. This could contribute to complications such as diabetic microvascular angiopathy due to erythrocyte fragility, as erythrocytes lack the sodium-dependent vitamin C transporters (SVCTs) and are dependent on the GLUTs for the uptake of vitamin C [11]. Our study also found plasma vitamin C concentration to be inversely related to BMI, which concurs with previous research [26]. Individuals with a higher weight are prone to vitamin C inadequacy and are known to require higher intakes of vitamin C in order to reach adequate plasma concentrations [27,28].

Oxidative stress is defined as a significant imbalance between the production of reactive oxygen species (ROS) and antioxidant defenses, and leads to alterations in signalling pathways and to potential tissue damage [29]. ROS activate nuclear factor κB (NFκB), a pro-inflammatory transcription factor, triggering a signalling cascade that leads to the continued synthesis of oxidative species and low-grade chronic inflammation [29]. High-sensitivity CRP, produced by the liver, reflects the presence of inflammation in the body. The concentration of hs-CRP increased with the deterioration of glycaemic control and increase in BMI. This result is consistent with the evidence suggesting that obesity can lead to chronic activation of the innate immune system and low-grade systemic inflammation and oxidative stress, which have been implicated in the development of insulin resistance and T2DM [5,30,31]. Hyperglycaemia, increased plasma concentrations of free fatty acids (FFAs), and hyperinsulinaemia have all been linked to an increased production of ROS [29,31]. Our data showed an inverse relationship between hs-CRP and plasma vitamin C. It is therefore hypothesized that lower plasma vitamin C in those with higher BMI, prediabetes, and T2DM reflects the depletion of the vitamin due to its antioxidant and anti-inflammatory activities.

Consistent with the role of vitamin C as an antioxidant, our data showed a significant inverse relationship between plasma vitamin C concentration and smoking status, with ex- and current-smokers having lower plasma vitamin C concentrations than non-smokers, which is consistent with previous research [32,33]. It has long been recognised that smokers and passive smokers have a lower vitamin C status than non-smokers partly due to poor dietary habits, but also due to the oxidizing properties of tobacco smoke, resulting in an increased turnover of vitamin C [34].

As expected, dietary vitamin C was found to be a predictor for plasma vitamin C concentration. However, when the dietary intake of the vitamin was corrected for by covariate analysis fasting glucose, BMI and smoking status remained as significant independent predictors of plasma vitamin C concentration. That is, the associations observed were not solely explained by differences in dietary intake. This result is at odds with one study that reported no differences in serum vitamin C concentrations in people grouped by diabetes status after adjustment for dietary vitamin C intake [16].

4.2. Metabolic Hormones

The average fasting insulin concentrations were consistent with the glycaemic measures and were significantly higher in the T2DM group compared to the NGT group. A higher fasting insulin concentration indicates insulin resistance, a well-known contributor to impaired glucose tolerance and T2DM. Leptin and ghrelin are two hormones that have a major influence on energy balance [35]. Leptin is a mediator of long-term regulation of energy balance, suppressing food intake and thereby inducing weight loss. Ghrelin, on the other hand, is a fast-acting hormone, seemingly playing a role in meal initiation. In obese patients, the circulating concentration of leptin is increased, whereas surprisingly, ghrelin is decreased [35]. It is now established that obese patients are leptin-resistant [35]. Indeed, in this study, the increasing BMI across the groups was associated with an increase in leptin concentrations and a reduction in ghrelin concentrations. There was an inverse relationship between insulin and leptin and plasma vitamin C, and a positive relationship between ghrelin and plasma vitamin C; however, these hormones were also associated with fasting glucose and were thus not included as independent predictors of plasma vitamin C.

4.3. Clinical Significance

As hyperglycemia is associated with increased oxidative stress, a role for antioxidants such as vitamin C in the prevention of T2DM and/or the reduction of complications is a reasonable proposition. Indeed, a recent meta-analysis of 15 randomized control trials (RCTs) investigating vitamin C supplementation and insulin resistance and biomarkers of glycaemic control (fasting glucose, HbA1c) found that doses of $\geq$200 mg/day vitamin C significantly reduced glucose concentrations in patients with T2DM, particularly if the intervention was for more than 30 days and in older individuals [36]. Furthermore, a recent 12 month RCT found that treating those with T2DM with both Metformin and vitamin C was more effective at reducing HbA1c and risk factors for diabetes-related long-term complications than treating with Metformin alone [37].

Although T2DM is not traditionally considered a risk factor for vitamin C deficiency, our research indicates that those with prediabetes or T2DM are more likely to have inadequate or deficient plasma vitamin C concentrations. This did not appear to be due to a lower dietary vitamin C intake, so dietary advice needs to emphasise the importance of consuming high vitamin C foods, aiming for an intake of at least 200 mg/day [22]. This is particularly relevant in light of the associated T2DM risk factors of higher BMI and smoking status, both of which impact vitamin C status. Further research into the possibility of a higher RDI for vitamin C for those with prediabetes and T2DM is warranted, in line with what has been recommended in some countries for smokers [38].

4.4. Study Strengths and Limitations

Our study used robust methodology for dietary intake, plasma vitamin C, and statistical analysis, and accounted for other factors that are known to impact plasma vitamin C concentration such as smoking status, dietary vitamin C intake, and supplement use. The participants with T2DM were clinically well defined and were either not treated with diabetes medication or treated with a single oral hypoglycaemic agent only (Metformin). Those taking Metformin were included in the overall analysis. When the Metformin treated cases were excluded, the correlation between fasting glucose and plasma vitamin C concentrations was similar in direction and magnitude ($n = 64$, $r = -0.477$, $p < 0.001$) to the entire cohort ($n = 86$, $r = -0.411$, $p = 0.001$). Further, the current norm is for Metformin treatment to be initiated at diagnosis, rather than after the failure of diet and lifestyle changes to optimize glucose control. As such, it will become increasingly difficult to recruit treatment-naïve individuals with T2DM to studies.

T2DM has been shown to increase the urinary excretion of vitamin C, leading to reduced plasma vitamin C concentrations in a rodent model [39]. Whether this also occurs in humans is unknown. In addition, the duration of T2DM was not reported. Indeed, many individuals have undiagnosed T2DM for a significant period of time prior to formal diagnosis, making it very difficult to interpret data on the duration of the disease. There are always limitations around the self-reporting of dietary data and supplement use, and the study cohort was relatively small with 89 participants. Our study had only one measure of plasma vitamin C per participant and so future research should ideally incorporate repeated samples to account for any temporal fluctuations. There was a limitation around the lack of detail with regards to vitamin C supplement use; however, only six participants reported taking high dose vitamin C supplements and the use was sporadic.

5. Conclusions

Our cross-sectional observational study has identified a moderate inverse relationship between plasma vitamin C and both fasting glucose and BMI in adult subjects across the glycaemic spectrum. The relationship can be explained by the depletion of vitamin C due to oxidative stress and inflammation resulting from dysglycaemia, overweight/obesity, and smoking, rather than lower dietary intakes. Further research is required to determine whether those with an increased dietary intake through fruit and vegetables and/or vitamin C supplementation have a decreased risk of progression to T2DM and/or complications associated with the metabolic syndrome and T2DM.

Acknowledgments: We would like to thank all participants for volunteering their time to take part in the study, Sharon Berry for helping take blood samples, and Angie Anderson and Lizzie Jones for food diary data entry. Rénee Wilson, Jinny Willis, Richard Gearry, and Paula Skidmore are the recipients of a Zespri International Ltd. grant. Anitra Carr is the recipient of a Health Research Council of New Zealand Sir Charles Hercus Health Research Fellowship.

Author Contributions: R.W. conducted participant recruitment and interviews; R.W., P.S., and L.F. completed the dietary analysis, A.C. vitamin C analysis, and C.F. statistical analysis; R.W., A.C., and J.W. undertook the conception and writing of the paper; R.G. and P.S. edited the paper.

Conflicts of Interest: The authors declare no conflict of interest.

References

1. American Diabetes Association. Diagnosis and classification of diabetes mellitus. *Diabetes Care* **2014**, *37*, S81–S90.
2. International Diabetes Federation. IDF diabetes atlas 2015. Available online: http://www.diabetesatlas.org. (accessed on 5 June 2017).
3. Ministry of Health. Virtual diabetes register 2017. Available online: http://www.health.govt.nz/our-work/diseases-and-conditions/diabetes/about-diabetes/virtual-diabetes-register-vdr. (accessed on 11 June 2017).
4. Primary Care Domain NHS Digital. Quality and outcomes framework-prevalence, achievements and exceptions report 2016. Available online: http://www.content.digital.nhs.uk/catalogue/PUB22266 (accessed on 25 June 2017).
5. McArdle, M.; Finucane, O.; Connaughton, R.; McMorrow, A.; Roche, H. Mechanisms of obesity-induced inflammation and insulin resistance: insights into the emerging role of nutritional strategies. *Front. Endocrinol. (Lausanne)* **2013**, *4*, 1–23. [CrossRef] [PubMed]
6. Carr, A.C.; Frei, B. Toward a new recommended dietary allowance for vitamin C based on antioxidant and health effects in humans. *Am. J. Clin. Nutr.* **1999**, *69*, 1086–1107. [PubMed]
7. Carr, A.; Frei, B. Does vitamin C act as a pro-oxidant under physiological conditions? *FASEB J.* **1999**, *13*, 1007–1024. [PubMed]
8. Will, J.C.; Byers, T. Does diabetes mellitus increase the requirement for vitamin C? *Nutr. Rev.* **1996**, *54*, 193–202. [CrossRef] [PubMed]
9. Sargeant, L.; Wareham, N.; Bingham, S.; Day, N. Vitamin C and hyperglycemia in the European prospective investigation into cancer-Norfolk (EPIC-Norfolk) study: A population-based study. *Diabetes Care.* **2000**, *23*, 726–732. [CrossRef] [PubMed]
10. Kositsawat, J.; Freeman, V.L. Vitamin C and A1c relationship in the National Health and Nutrition Examination Survey (NHANES) 2003–2006. *J. Am. Coll. Nutr.* **2011**, *30*, 477–483. [CrossRef] [PubMed]
11. Tu, H.; Li, H.; Wang, Y.; Niyyati, M.; Wang, Y.; Leshin, J.; Levine, M. Low red blood cell vitamin C concentrations induce red blood cell fragility: A link to diabetes via glucose, glucose transporters, and dehydroascorbic Acid. *EBioMedicine* **2015**, *2*, 1735–1750. [CrossRef] [PubMed]
12. Olofsson, C.; Discacciati, A.; Akesson, A.; Orsini, N.; Brismar, K.; Wolk, A. Changes in fruit, vegetable and juice consumption after the diagnosis of type 2 diabetes: A prospective study in men. *Br. J. Nutr.* **2017**, *117*, 712–719. [CrossRef] [PubMed]
13. Feskens, E.J.M.; Virtanen, S.M.; Räsänen, L.; Tuomilehto, J.; Stengård, J.; Pekkanen, J.; Nissinen, A.; Kromhout, D. Dietary factors determining diabetes and impaired glucose tolerance: A 20-year follow-up of the Finnish and Dutch cohorts of the Seven Countries Study. *Diabetes Care.* **1995**, *18*, 1104–1112. [CrossRef] [PubMed]
14. Harding, A.H.; Wareham, N.J.; Bingham, S.A.; Khaw, K.; Luben, R.; Welch, A.; Forouhi, N.G. Plasma vitamin C level, fruit and vegetable consumption, and the risk of new-onset type 2 diabetes mellitus: The European prospective investigation of cancer-Norfolk prospective study. *Arch. Intern. Med.* **2008**, *168*, 1493. [CrossRef] [PubMed]
15. Som, S.; Basu, S.; Mukherjee, D.; Deb, S.; Choudhury, P.R.; Mukherjee, S.; Chatterjee, S.N.; Chatterjee, I.B. Ascorbic acid metabolism in diabetes mellitus. *Metabolism* **1981**, *30*, 572–577. [CrossRef]
16. Will, J.; Ford, E.; Bowman, B. Serum vitamin C concentrations and diabetes: Findings from the third National Health and Nutrition Examination Survey, 1988–1994. *Am. J. Clin. Nutr.* **1999**, *70*, 49–52. [PubMed]
17. World Health Organization. Obesity: Preventing and managing the global epidemic. Report of a WHO consultation. 2000. Available online: http://www.who.int/nutrition/publications/obesity/WHO_TRS_894/en/ (accessed on 10 June 2017).
18. World Health Organization. Section 5: Collecting step 2 data: Physical measurements 2017. Available online: http://www.who.int/chp/steps/Part3_Section5.pdf?ua=1 (accessed on 19 June 2017).

19. Carr, A.C.; Pullar, J.M.; Moran, S.; Vissers, M.C. Bioavailability of vitamin C from kiwifruit in non-smoking males: Determination of 'healthy' and 'optimal' intakes. *J. Nutr. Sci.* **2012**, *1*, e14. [CrossRef] [PubMed]

20. Sato, Y.; Uchiki, T.; Iwama, M.; Kishimoto, Y.; Takahashi, R.; Ishigami, A. Determination of dehydroascorbic acid in mouse tissues and plasma by using tris(2-carboxyethyl)phosphine hydrochloride as reductant in metaphosphoric acid/ethylenediaminetetraacetic acid solution. *Biol. Pharm. Bull.* **2010**, *33*, 364–369. [CrossRef] [PubMed]

21. Bang, A.S.; Soule, S.G.; Yandle, T.G.; Richards, A.M.; Pemberton, C.J. Characterisation of proghrelin peptides in mammalian tissue and plasma. *J. Endocrinol.* **2007**, *192*, 313–323. [CrossRef] [PubMed]

22. National Health and Medical Research Council. Nutrient Reference Values for Australia and New Zealand Including Recommended Dietary Intakes Canberra: ACT: National Health and Medical Research Council. 2006. Available online: https://www.nhmrc.gov.au/_files_nhmrc/file/publications/17122_nhmrc_nrv_update-dietary_intakes-web.pdf (accessed on 12 June 2017).

23. New Zealand Society for the Study of Diabetes. NZSSD position statement on the diagnosis of, and screening for, type 2 diabetes 2011. Available online: http://www.nzssd.org.nz/HbA1c/1.%20NZSSD%20position%20statement%20on%20screening%20for%20type%202%20diabetes%20final%20Sept%202011.pdf (accessed on 20 June 2017).

24. Lykkesfeldt, J.; Poulsen, H.E. Is vitamin C supplementation beneficial? Lessons learned from randomised controlled trials. *Br. J. Nutr.* **2010**, *103*, 1251–1259. [CrossRef] [PubMed]

25. Girgis, C.; Christie-David, D.; Gunton, J. Effects of vitamins C and D in type 2 diabetes mellitus. *Nutr. Diet. Suppl.* **2015**, *7*, 21–28. [CrossRef]

26. Johnston, C.S.; Beezhold, B.L.; Mostow, B.; Swan, P.D. Plasma vitamin C is inversely related to body mass index and waist circumference but not to plasma adiponectin in nonsmoking adults. *J. Nutr.* **2007**, *137*, 1757–1762. [PubMed]

27. Block, G.; Mangels, A.R.; Patterson, B.H.; Levander, O.A.; Norkus, E.P.; Taylor, P.R. Body weight and prior depletion affect plasma ascorbate levels attained on identical Vitamin C intake: A controlled-diet study. *J. Am. Coll. Nutr.* **1999**, *18*, 628–637. [CrossRef] [PubMed]

28. Carr, A.C.; Pullar, J.M.; Bozonet, S.M.; Vissers, M.C. Marginal ascorbate status (hypovitaminosis C) results in an attenuated response to vitamin C supplementation. *Nutrients* **2016**, *8*, 341. [CrossRef] [PubMed]

29. Lamb, R.E.; Goldstein, B.J. Modulating an oxidative-inflammatory cascade: Potential new treatment strategy for improving glucose metabolism, insulin resistance, and vascular function. *Int. J. Clin. Pract.* **2008**, *62*, 1087–1095. [CrossRef] [PubMed]

30. Calle, M.C.; Fernandez, M.L. Inflammation and type 2 diabetes. *Diabetes Metab.* **2012**, *38*, 183–191. [CrossRef] [PubMed]

31. Garcia-Bailo, B.; El-Sohemy, A.; Haddad, P.S.; Arora, P.; Benzaied, F.; Karmali, M.; Badawi, A. Vitamins D, C, and E in the prevention of type 2 diabetes mellitus: Modulation of inflammation and oxidative stress. *Biologics* **2011**, *5*, 7–19. [PubMed]

32. Schectman, G.; Byrd, J.; Gruchow, H. The influence of smoking on vitamin C status in adults. *Am. J. Public Health* **1989**, *79*, 158. [CrossRef] [PubMed]

33. Pfeiffer, C.M.; Sternberg, M.R.; Schleicher, R.L.; Rybak, M.E. Dietary supplement use and smoking are important correlates of biomarkers of water-soluble vitamin status after adjusting for sociodemographic and lifestyle variables in a representative sample of U.S. adults. *J. Nutr.* **2013**, *143*, 957S–965S. [CrossRef] [PubMed]

34. Lykkesfeldt, J.; Michels, A.J.; Frei, B. Vitamin C. *Adv. Nutr.* **2014**, *5*, 16–18. [CrossRef] [PubMed]

35. Klok, M.D.; Jakobsdottir, S.; Drent, M.L. The role of leptin and ghrelin in the regulation of food intake and body weight in humans: A review. *Obes. Rev.* **2007**, *8*, 21–34. [CrossRef] [PubMed]

36. Ashor, A.W.; Werner, A.D.; Lara, J.; Willis, N.D.; Mathers, J.C.; Siervo, M. Effects of vitamin C supplementation on glycaemic control: a systematic review and meta-analysis of randomised controlled trials. *Eur. J. Clin. Nutr.* **2017**. [CrossRef] [PubMed]

37. Gillani, S.W.; Sulaiman, S.A.S.; Abdul, M.I.M.; Baig, M.R. Combined effect of metformin with ascorbic acid versus acetyl salicylic acid on diabetes-related cardiovascular complication a 12-month single blind multicenter randomized control trial. *Cardiovasc. Diabetol.* **2017**, *16*, 103. [CrossRef] [PubMed]

Nutrients **2017**, *9*, 997

38. Institute of Medicine, Panel on Dietary Antioxidants Related Compounds. *Dietary Reference Intakes for Vitamin C, Vitamin E, Selenium, and Carotenoids: A Report of the Panel on Dietary Antioxidants and Related Compounds, Subcommittees on Upper Reference Levels of Nutrients and of Interpretation and Use of Dietary Reference Intakes, and the Standing Committee on the Scientific Evaluation of Dietary Reference Intakes, Food and Nutrition Board, Institute of Medicine*; National Academy Press: Washington, DC, USA, 2000.

39. Zebrowski, E.J.; Bhatnagar, P.K. Urinary excretion pattern of ascorbic acid in streptozotocin diabetic and insulin treated rats. *Pharmacol. Res. Commun.* **1979**, *11*, 95–103. [CrossRef]

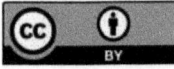

nutrients

MDPI

Article

Poor Vitamin C Status Late in Pregnancy Is Associated with Increased Risk of Complications in Type 1 Diabetic Women: A Cross-Sectional Study

Bente Juhl [1], Finn Friis Lauszus [2] and Jens Lykkesfeldt [3,*]

[1] Medical Department, Aarhus University Hospital, Nørrebrogade 44, 8000 Aarhus C, Denmark;
    bente311057@gmail.com
[2] Gynecology & Obstetrics Department, Herning Hospital, Gl. Landevej 61, 7400 Herning, Denmark;
    Finn.Friis.Lauszus@vest.rm.dk
[3] Faculty of Health and Medical Sciences, University of Copenhagen, Ridebanevej 9, Frederiksberg C,
    1870 Copenhagen, Denmark
*   Correspondence: jopl@sund.ku.dk; Tel.: +45-353-331-63

Received: 22 January 2017; Accepted: 20 February 2017; Published: 23 February 2017

Abstract: Vitamin C (vitC) is essential for normal pregnancy and fetal development and poor vitC status has been related to complications of pregnancy. We have previously shown lower vitC status in diabetic women throughout pregnancy compared to that of non-diabetic controls. Here, we evaluate the relationship between vitC status late in diabetic pregnancy in relation to fetal outcome, complications of pregnancy, diabetic characteristics, and glycemic control based on data of 47 women from the same cohort. We found a significant relationship between the maternal vitC level > or $\leq$ the 50% percentile of 26.6 µmol/L, respectively, and the umbilical cord blood vitC level (mean (SD)): 101.0 µmol/L (16.6) versus 78.5 µmol/L (27.8), $p = 0.02$; $n = 12/16$), while no relation to birth weight or Apgar score was observed. Diabetic women with complications of pregnancy had significantly lower vitC levels compared to the women without complications (mean (SD): 24.2 µmol/L (10.6) vs. 34.6 µmol/L (14.4), $p = 0.01$; $n = 19$ and 28, respectively) and the subgroup of women (about 28%) characterized by hypovitaminosis C (<23 µmol/L) had an increased relative risk of complications of pregnancy that was 2.4 fold higher than the one found in the group of women with a vitC status above this level ($p = 0.02$, 95% confidence interval 1.2–4.4). No correlation between diabetic characteristics of the pregnant women and vitC status was observed, while a negative association of maternal vitC with HbA1c at delivery was found at regression analysis ($r = -0.39$, $p < 0.01$, $n = 46$). In conclusion, our results may suggest that hypovitaminosis C in diabetic women is associated with increased risk of complications of pregnancy.

Keywords: type 1 diabetes; pregnancy; vitamin C; pregnancy outcome; pregnancy complications; cross-sectional study

---

1. Introduction

The importance of an adequate supply of micronutrients for normal pregnancy and fetal development is well established, particularly in the last trimester due to the increasing needs during the growth spurt of the fetus [1,2]. As early as 1938, Teel and co-workers described the fetus as *acting as a parasite on the mother's vitamin C pool* based on the observed gradient between maternal plasma and umbilical cord vitamin C (vitC) concentration at term, and the fact that the fetus apparently was preferentially supplied with vitC at the expense of the mother [3–5]. Subsequently, several studies have reported that pregnancy in healthy women is associated with a significant decrease in maternal vitC status during pregnancy [4,6–8], perhaps partly due to increased blood volume in pregnancy.

In experimental studies in guinea pigs, which like humans depend on an adequate supply of vitC through their diet, the offspring of vitC deficient guinea pigs have shown abnormalities of fetal bone development, with atrophy of the osteoblasts and retarded osteoid formation [9]. Macroscopic fetal, uterine, and placental hemorrhages as well as poor attachment of the placenta to the uterus were also evident in vitC deficient animals [9]. Other experimental studies have shown an association of infertility, increased incidence of premature- and stillbirths, and increased frequency of abortion with vitC deficiency [10,11]. Intrauterine growth retardation was related to insufficient vitC status in guinea pigs [10]. More recently, experimental reports from animal studies demonstrated that CNS development in particular requires high amounts of vitC and may be impaired by an inadequate maternal supply [12–15].

In humans, abortion and premature rupture of the fetal membrane are related to low levels of vitC in plasma, leucocytes, and amniotic fluid [16–24]. Abnormalities of cardiotocography (CTG) and discolored/green amniotic fluid was also associated with low vitC status at the time of delivery [25]. Furthermore, vitC deficiency may play a leading role in placental abruption [26]. Human studies suggest that poor vitC status leads to fetal oxidative stress and impaired placental implantation due to oxidative stress is thought to increase risk of preeclampsia and miscarriages [27]. Epidemiological studies have also supported an association between vitC deficiency and preeclampsia [28,29]. However recently, human intervention studies using vitC in the prevention of preeclampsia have produced conflicting results [30–32]. Another study found no effect of vitamin C on prevention of spontaneous preterm birth [33]. A recent review concluded that a general recommendation of vitC supplementation to pregnant women was not warranted, but subpopulations such as women with vitC deficiency, smokers or diabetics were not discussed [34].

Thus in diabetic animals, experimental data support the amelioration of these risks by vitC supplementation [35–38]. In one human study, borderline gestational diabetes mellitus had an increased risk of adverse health outcomes compared with women no diabetes [39]. Another human controlled intervention study in type 1 diabetes mellitus (T1DM) pregnancy found a lower risk of premature birth in women receiving vitC and E supplementation and suggested regarding preeclampsia that vitC supplementation may be beneficial in women with a low antioxidant status at baseline; no effect on preeclampsia was observed in the T1DM cohort as a whole [40]. Another study also failed to prevent preeclampsia with vitC and E supplementation in women with T1DM and even a high risk pro-angiogenic haptoglobin genotype [41].

In T1DM, vitC levels are significantly lower than in non-diabetic subjects [42,43]. This seems to be the case in the diabetic pregnancy, too, as we recently reported in a prospective study [8]. We found that the level of vitC was lower throughout pregnancy compared to the control group, and hypovitaminosis C (vitC < 23 μmol/L [44]) was found in 51% of the diabetic women at some stage during pregnancy. Here, we report our evaluation of vitC status in the same cohort of pregnant T1DM women with regard to labor data and the outcome of pregnancies.

2. Materials and Methods

All T1DM women from June 1992 to August 1994 attending the Department of Obstetrics, Aarhus University Hospital (Aarhus, Denmark), were screened for participation in the prospective study on vitC during pregnancy and compared to controls as described previously [8]. The inclusion criteria were pregestational T1DM, age >18 years, no other systemic disease than diabetes, and singleton pregnancy. Blood samples for vitC were taken when the diabetic women attended the maternity ward and were taken in a non-fasting state to avoid hypoglycemic episodes. At delivery, an umbilical blood sample for vitC was taken from the newborn. In total, 76 women with T1DM consented to participate in the prospective study [8]. Of these, 47 women had vitC measurements taken in late pregnancy within four weeks of delivery and were included in the present cross-sectional evaluation of vitC status in relation to labor data and outcome of pregnancy. If more than one sample in the 4-week interval before labor were obtained, the mean concentration of the samples was used in the analysis.

Blood samples for plasma vitC measurements were stabilized in sodium EDTA-anticoagulated vacutainer tubes containing dithiothreitol. Tubes were centrifuged and plasma was removed and deproteinized by the addition of 6% perchloric acid. The samples were kept at minus 80 degrees Celsius until analysis and assayed by HPLC using 3,4-dihydroxybenzylamine hydrobromide as internal standard [45]. A plot of the ratio of vitC to internal standard versus the concentration of 6 aqueous standards resulted in a linear curve to at least 86 μmol/L ($y = 0.16x - 0.028$, $R^2 = 0.99$). The within-day and between-day coefficient of variation was 2.6% and 3.9%, respectively, of a mean concentration of 19 μmol/L. Limit of detection and limit of quantification were 0.525 μmol/L and 1.75 μmol/L, respectively. The analytical recoveries were 111%, 104%, 102%, and 101% at vitC concentrations of 5.75, 28.75, 43.125, and 57.5 μmol/L, respectively.

We carried out predefined plasma vitC subgroup analyses according to the 50% percentile of maternal vitC level and these subgroups were used for evaluating other quantitative and qualitative data on pregnancy, labor, and neonates. This 50% percentile was chosen as we a priori had calculated, that we thereby had sufficient data to minimize a type2 error (power > 80%) on expected SDs in relation to third trimester measurements of pregnancy and in relation to labor and fetus related features as we earlier have reported in T1DM pregnancy [8].

Twenty-eight blood samples from the umbilical cords were also obtained as a surrogate measure of the level of vitC of the fetus. However umbilical cord blood was in the same level as found in the heel blood of 200 newborns [25].

The following data were recorded: Age, duration of diabetes, presence of diabetic microangiopathy, glycemic control, diurnal blood pressure, albumin excretion rate, creatinine, creatinine clearance, pregnancy and labor data, and the neonate's Apgar score at one minute, birth weight, and presence of malformations. The study was part of an evaluation of morbidity in diabetic pregnancy with respect to nephropathy and retinopathy approved by the local Ethics Committee (jr.nr.1992/2523, 1998/4147, and 2026-99). It was performed in concordance with the Helsinki II declaration and all women had given their informed consent. The collection of samples for vitC was approved by the local Ethics Committee (jr.nr. 1992/2328). Hypovitaminosis C was defined as a plasma vitC <23 μmol/L [44].

Preeclampsia was defined as systolic/diastolic blood pressure >140/90 mmHg when normo-hypertensive before week 20 and, simultaneously, albuminuria >300 mg in previously normo-albuminuric women. Pregnancy-induced hypertension was defined as hypertension without signs of preeclampsia. Preterm delivery was defined as delivery following <37 weeks of gestation.

Statistics was performed with IBM SPSS Statistics 20. Difference between two means was tested with Student's *t*-test if data followed Gaussian distribution; otherwise, Mann-Whitney's test was used. Proportional data were analyzed by χ^2 test or Fisher's Exact test. Values are given as mean ± SD if not otherwise stated. Median (25%–75% interval) indicates variable of non-Gaussian distribution and values were subjected to non-parametric testing. A two-sided $p < 0.05$ was chosen as level of significance.

3. Results

Clinical data from the pregnant diabetic women are shown in Table 1 and are also presented in subgroups according to the median value (25%–75%) of maternal plasma vitC taken within four weeks of delivery. All comparisons of baseline data and diabetic characteristics in relation to the 50% percentile of vitC (26.6 (22.0–37.2) μmol/L) were non-significant (Table 1). The range (0%–100%) of plasma vitC in the cohort was 3.1–61.0 μmol/L.

Results regarding pregnancy and fetal related features are presented in Table 2. No relationship between maternal vitC level and birth weight or Apgar score was observed. Nor was the way of delivery (acute cesarean section, elective cesarean and induced delivery; 7/19/21) associated with vitC status. Moreover, no difference was observed in the level of HbA1c in relation of the median maternal vitC of 26.6 μmol/L, but a negative association of maternal vitC with HbA1c at delivery was found at regression analysis ($r = -0.39$, $p = 0.006$, $n = 46$). The vitC levels of the umbilical cord blood correlated positively with the obtained Apgar score of the newborn ($r = 0.45$, $p = 0.011$), also when corrected for maternal vitC, HbA1c and diabetes duration ($r = 0.52$, $p = 0.025$).

Table 1. Clinical data and characteristics of the diabetic status by maternal vitamin C (vitC) within the last four weeks of pregnancy ($n = 23/24$) and of the whole cohort ($n = 47$).

	VitC > Median >26.6 µmol/L	VitC ≤ Median ≤26.6 µmol/L	*p* Value	Characteristics of the Whole Cohort
Vit C (µmol/L), $n = 23/24/47$	37.1 (28.2–61.0) [1]	22.1 (3.1–28.2)		30.1 (13.6)
Age (yr), $n = 23/24/47$	28.8 (3.7) [2]	27.7 (3.5)	0.314	27 (26–31)
Maternal weight at delivery (kg) $n = 12/11/23$	78.5 (72.3–87.5)	74.0 (68.0–86.0)	0.32	78 (70–86)
Maternal height (cm), $n = 11/11/22$	166.2 (6.2)	164.4 (8.3)	0.569	165.3 (7.2)
Diabetes duration (year), $n = 23/24/47$	15.0 (8.9)	13.2 (9.0)	0.486	14.1 (8.9)
Parity, $n = 23/24/47$	1.8 (0.8)	1.8 (0.7)	0.876	2 (1.2)
Systolic blood pressure at entry (mmHg), $n = 15/14/29$	120.1 (10.3)	120.5 (9.9)	0.641	120.0 (9.9)
Diastolic blood pressure at entry (mmHg) $n = 15/14/29$	72.1 (6.6)	70.9 (6.7)	0.673	71.2 (6.9)
Retinopathy Non/Simplex/Proliferative, $n = N/S/P$	12/8/3	12/9/3	0.881	24/17/6
BMI (kg/m^2) at delivery, $n = 11/10/21$	29.2 (3.8)	27.6 (4.4)	0.607	28.6 (4.3)
Normo-/Micro-/Macro-albuminuria $n = N/Mi/Ma$	18/4/1	20/4/0	0.581	38/8/1
HbA1c (%) at entry, $n = 22/23/45$	7.7 (1.6)	7.9 (1.2)	0.0697	7.7 (1.4)
Creatinine clearance at entry (ml/min) $n = 15/15/30$	123.3 (22.1)	116.2 (32.3)	0.869	122.1 (27.1)
Smoking, $n = $ Yes/no/unknown	6/16/1	10/14/0	0.538	16/30/1

[1] VitC levels in each subgroup is reported given as median (range); [2] Other data are listed as mean (SD), median (25%–75%) or *n*-values.

Table 2. Labor and fetus related features in relation to above or below the median level of maternal vitC in late pregnancy.

	VitC > Median >26.6 µmol/L	VitC ≤ Median ≤26.6 µmol/L	*p* Value
VitC in umbilical cord (µmol/L), $n = 12/16$	101.0 (16.6) [1]	78.5 (27.8)	0.02
Umbilical cord/maternal vitC ratio, $n = 12/16$	2.6 (2.1–2.9)	4.1 (2.8–5.1)	0.007
Apgar score at one minute, $n = 19/23$	10 (9–10)	9 (9–10)	0.56
Birth weight (g), $n = 23/24$	3867 (649)	3533 (771)	0.12
Gestations age at labor (weeks), $n = 23/24$	37.4 (1.1)	37.2 (1.5)	0.64
Normal delivery (*n*)	0	0	
Induced delivery and elective section/acute section, (*n/n*)	20/3	20/4	1.0
HbA1c at delivery (%), $n = 23/23$	6.7 (1.1)	7.2 (1.0)	0.14

[1] Data are listed as mean (SD), median (25%–75%) or *n*-values.

Hypovitaminosis C was found in 13 out of 47 diabetic women (28%) and was associated with a risk of complications of 69%, while the risk of complications was 29% in case of higher levels of vitC (Table 3). The relative risk of having complications of pregnancy was 2.4 times in case of maternal hypovitaminosis C compared to higher levels of maternal vitC ($p = 0.02$). In accordance, the diabetic women with complications of pregnancy had a significantly lower vitC status in late pregnancy compared to those without complications (mean (SD) 24.2 µmol/L (95% CI: 19.4–30) vs. 34.6 µmol/L (95% CI: 29.6–40); $p = 0.011$, $n = 19$ and 28, respectively). The type and distribution of complications are given in Table 4.

Table 3. Women with complications in subgroups according to vitC status in late pregnancy.

Complications of Pregnancy	Hypovitaminosis C [1]	Above Hypovitaminosis C Level	All Women	Fisher's Exact Test
Yes (*n*)	9	10	19	
No (*n*)	4	24	28	
Total (*n*)	13	34	47	$p = 0.02$

[1] Plasma concentration <23 µmol/L.

Table 4. The type and distribution of complications in T1DM women (n = 47). Recorded complications were prematurity, gestational hypertension, asphyxia, malformation, still birth, placental abruption, preeclampsia.

Complication	Frequency	VitC µmol/L Mean (SD)
Women with/without complications	19/47 vs. 28/47	24.2 (10.6)/34.6 (14.4)
Fetal malformation	4/47 [1]	18.1 (9.0)
Asphyxia/abnormal CTG [2]	9/47	22.9 (12.8)
Preeclampsia	5/47	25.0 (10.6)
Prematurity	5/47	20.9 (6.0)
Placental abruption	2/47	18.6 (0.9)
Still birth	2/47	30.9 (0.4)
Pregnancy-induced hypertension	2/47	30.0 (7.1)

[1] The fetal malformations consisted of two neonates with cardiac malformations with transposition and atrium septum defect and two others were related to skeletal abnormalities; [2] CTG: Cardiotocography. Abnormal CTG was diagnosed in nine women at delivery and of these, seven ended in acute cesarean section and two in induced delivery. Women may have more than one complication.

4. Discussion

The present cross-sectional study of T1DM pregnancy found an inverse relationship between vitC status and risks of complications in pregnancy. Thus, poor vitC status within four weeks of delivery was a positive predictor (69%) for complications of pregnancy, while a maternal vitC >23 µmol/L was a negative predictor (71%) for complications of pregnancy, respectively. In support of the observed relationship between maternal vitC status in late pregnancy and complications, we found a low maternal plasma vitC in case of complications of pregnancy (power of test > 80%).

The mean level of vitC was 24.2 µmol/L in the group with complications in pregnancy, thus in this normally distributed group nearly the half of the women had a level of vitC characterized as hypovitaminosis C. Much of the literature showing associations between vitC status and complications in pregnancy was conducted in pregnant experimental animals with or without induced diabetes and related to severe vitC deficiency (<11 µmol/L). This level increases the risk of developing outright scurvy, the ultimately mortal manifestation of prolonged severe vitC deficiency. However, only about 4% of the present cohort (2 patients out of 47) had severe vitC deficiency within four weeks of delivery and no clinical symptoms of scurvy were recorded in the case records of the pregnant women in this study. Therefore, it appears that the complications in diabetic pregnancy are already present at suboptimal vitC levels. In agreement, previous human studies identified a range of complications of pregnancy in non-diabetic women, the risks of which were inversely correlated with plasma vitC; this was, indeed, found over a wide concentration range above the level critical for development of scorbutic manifestations [16–27]. Thus, although higher levels of vitC are not associated with scurvy, lack of scurvy does not preclude the presence of several other negative health effects of a suboptimal vitC status, and the optimal vitC intake in humans is still a matter of considerable debate [46].

In humans, a randomized placebo-controlled intervention study with vitamin C and E in T1DM pregnancies showed no overall effect of supplementation (1000 mg vitamin C and 400 IU vitamin E (α-tocopherol) daily until delivery) on the incidence of preeclampsia [40]. However, subgroup analysis did reveal a significant positive effect of supplementation vs placebo on preeclampsia among patients who were vitC deficient at baseline (<10 µmol/L). Thus, the authors suggested that the significant benefit of supplementation on preeclampsia may be limited to women with severe vitC deficiency [40]. VitC and E supplementation also resulted in fewer preterm deliveries compared to placebo in the cohort as a whole, but the potential correlation to vitC status at entry was not explored [40]. Another study has also reported lack of effects of supplementation with vitC on the incidence of preeclampsia in high-risk T1DM women [41]. The absence of effect of vitC supplementation on preeclampsia in humans with or without diabetes may arise from the variation in the degree of plasma saturation and subsequent differential outcomes of supplementation as discussed elsewhere [47].

Another interesting result of the present study is the difference in vitC level in umbilical cord blood of newborns reflects some of the difference in the mothers' vitC level. Combined with the observation that the ratio of umbilical cord/maternal vitC favors babies born by mothers with vitC level below the median, our data collectively support the notion that the fetus is preferentially supplied with vitC at the expense of the mother [5,48]. However, as the vitC level in these babies is significantly lower than that of those born by mothers with vitC level above the median, it also suggests that such a preferential supply cannot fully compensate for poor maternal vitC status. The maternal as well the umbilical vitC measurements were conducted with sufficient data to minimize a type 2 error on conclusions (power of *t* test > 80%). Thus in this study—in spite of the fetus acting as a "parasite" as described by Teel et al. [3]—the newborns of mothers with low maternal vitC seem not to be able to obtain the same level of vitC in the umbilical cord as newborns of mothers with a higher vitC level, although their ratio is larger. This is in line with experimental data from guinea pigs showing that the preferential fetal transport may be overridden by increased needs of the mother during situations of deficiency, thereby potentially influencing the health of the offspring [13,49]. In accordance, the vitC levels of the umbilical cord blood correlated positively with the obtained Apgar score of the newborn.

Finally, no correlation between diabetic characteristics of the pregnant women and vitC status was observed, although glycemic control measured as HbA1c showed an inverse correlation with maternal vitC level. VitC is thought to be actively transported by SVCT transporters in the placenta [50]; however, it also shares the same transporters as glucose via the GLUT-mediated transport of dehydroascorbic acid (DHA; the oxidized form of vitC) [51]. Thus, it may be speculated that the degree of glycemic control and, consequently, the level of oxidative stress and ascorbate oxidation rate may affect the bioavailability of vitC in T1DM pregnant women through competitive inhibition of DHA transport as proposed by Mann and Newton already in 1975 [52] and supported by the NHANES study 2003–2006 data [53]; here an inverse relationship between vitC and HbA1c was reported in 7697 non-diabetic participants. Moreover, Tu et al. have recently proposed that impaired red cell recycling of DHA may be a key link in diabetes [54].

Limitations of the present study include the small number of participants and that the registration of complications of pregnancy was done retrospectively on the case report forms, which in some cases may be imprecise. The included T1DM patients with diabetic complications, i.e., retino- and nephropathy, could potentially influence the outcome of pregnancy. However, we did not find any relationship of these variables with vitC probably due to the small number of participants. Finally, the samples for vitC were taken in a non-fasting state to avoid hypoglycemic episodes, which may have increased the SD of the vitC measurements and, thus, the risk of type 2 error.

5. Conclusions

In conclusion, the results from this small study of a pregnant T1DM cohort suggest that hypovitaminosis C in late pregnancy may be associated with an increased risk of developing complications in pregnancy and may also, to some extent, limit the obtainable level of vitC of the fetus as measured by umbilical values in the newborn. Further investigations are needed to disclose the possible clinical significance of vitC in the diabetic pregnancy and to confirm in larger studies that a benefit of vitC supplementation exists in pregnancies characterized by hypovitaminosis C.

Acknowledgments: Jens Lykkesfeldt is partly supported by the Lifepharm Centre for In Vivo Pharmacology.

Author Contributions: Bente Juhl designed and performed the experiments; Bente Juhl, Finn Friis Lauszus, and Jens Lykkesfeldt analyzed and interpreted the data; Bente Juhl, Finn Friis Lauszus, and Jens Lykkesfeldt wrote the paper.

Conflicts of Interest: The authors declare no conflict of interest.

References

1. Christian, P. Micronutrients, birth weight, and survival. *Annu. Rev. Nutr.* **2010**, *30*, 83–104. [CrossRef] [PubMed]
2. World Health Organization (WHO). *Vitamin and Minerals Requirements in Human Nutrition*, 2nd ed.; WHO: Geneva, Switzerland, 2004; p. 341.
3. Teel, H.M.; Burke, B.S.; Draper, R. Vitamin C in human pregnancy and lactation: I Studies During pregnancy. *Am. J. Dis. Child* **1938**, *56*, 1004–1010. [CrossRef]
4. Scaife, A.R.; McNeill, G.; Campbell, D.M.; Martindale, S.; Devereux, G.; Seaton, A. Maternal intake of antioxidant vitamins in pregnancy in relation to and fetal levels at delivery. *Br. J. Nutr.* **2006**, *95*, 771–778. [CrossRef]
5. Wang, Y.Z.; Ren, W.H.; Liao, W.Q.; Zhang, G.Y. Concentrations of antioxidant vitamins in maternal and cord serum and their effect on birth outcomes. *J. Nutr. Sci. Vitam.* **2009**, *55*, 1–8. [CrossRef]
6. Mason, M.; Rivers, J.M. Plasma ascorbic levels in pregnancy. *Am. J. Obstst. Gynecol.* **1971**, *109*, 960–961. [CrossRef]
7. Vobecky, J.S.; Vobecky, J.; Shapcoot, D.; Munan, L. Vitamin C and outcome of pregnancy. *Lancet* **1974**, *303*, 630–631. [CrossRef]
8. Juhl, B.; Lauszus, F.F.; Lykkesfeldt, J. Ascorbic acid is lower during pregnancy in diabetic women compared to controls: A prospective study. *Int. J. Vit. Nutr. Res.* **2017**, *87*, 1–6. [CrossRef] [PubMed]
9. Rivers, J.M.; Lennart, K.; Cormier, A. Biochemimical and histological study of guinea pig fetal and uterine tissue in ascorbic acid deficiency. *J. Nutr.* **1970**, *100*, 217–227. [PubMed]
10. Pye, O.F.; Tayler, C.M.; Fontanares, E. The effect of different levels of ascorbic acid in the diet of guinea pigs on health, reproduction and survival. *J. Nutr.* **1961**, *73*, 236–242.
11. Kramer, M.M.; Harman, M.T.; Brill, A.K. Disturbances of reproduction and ovarian changes in the guinea pig in relation to vitamin deficiency. *Am. J. Physiol.* **1933**, *106*, 611–622.
12. Paidi, M.D.; Schjoldager, J.G.; Lykkesfeldt, J.; Tveden-Nyborg, P. Prenatal vitamin C deficiency results in differential expression of oxidative stress during late gestation in foetal guinea pig brains. *Redox Biol.* **2014**, *2*, 361–367. [CrossRef] [PubMed]
13. Schjoldager, J.G.; Tveden-Nyborg, P.; Lykkesfeldt, J. Prolonged maternal vitamin C deficiency overrides preferential fetal ascorbate transport but does not influence perinatal survival in guinea pigs. *Br. J. Nutr.* **2013**, *110*, 1573–1579. [CrossRef] [PubMed]
14. Tveden-Nyborg, P.; Vogt, L.; Schjoldager, J.G.; Jeannet, N.; Hasselholt, S.; Paidi, M.; Christen, S.; Lykkesfeldt, J. Maternal vitamin C deficiency during pregnancy persistently impairs hippocampal neurogenesis in offspring of guinea pigs. *PLoS ONE* **2012**, *7*, e48488. [CrossRef] [PubMed]
15. Tveden-Nyborg, P.; Johansen, L.K.; Hansen, Z.L.; Villumsen, C.K.; Larsen, J.O.; Lykkesfeldt, J. Vitamin C deficiency induces impaired neuronal and cognitive development in neonatal guinea pigs. *Am. J. Clin. Nutr.* **2009**, *90*, 540–546. [CrossRef] [PubMed]
16. Wideman, G.L.; Baird, G.H.; Bolding, O.T. Ascorbic acid deficiency and premature rupture of fetal membranes. *Am. J. Obstet. Gynecol.* **1964**, *88*, 592–595. [CrossRef]
17. Aplin, J.D.; Campbell, S.; Donnai, P.; Bard, J.B.L.; Allen, T.D. Importance of vitamin C in maintenance of the normal amnion: An experimental study. *Placenta* **1986**, *7*, 377–389. [CrossRef]
18. Casanueva, E.; Magana, L.; Pfeffer, F.; Baez, A. Incidence of premature rupture of membranes in pregnant women with low leucocyte levels of vitamin, C. *Eur. J. Clin. Nutr.* **1991**, *45*, 401–405. [PubMed]
19. Casanueva, E.; Polo, E.; Tejero, E.; Meza, C. Premature rupture of amniotic membranes as functional assessment of vitamin C status during pregnancy. *Ann. N. Y. Acad. Sci.* **1993**, *678*, 369–370. [CrossRef] [PubMed]
20. Barret, B.; Gunter, E.; Jenkins, J.; Wang, M. Ascorbic acid concentration in amniotic fluid in late pregnancy. *Biol. Neonate* **1991**, *60*, 333–335. [CrossRef]
21. Barret, B.M.; Sowell, A.; Gunter, E.; Wang, M. Potential role of ascorbic acid and β-carotene in the prevention of preterm rupture of fetal membranes. *Int. J. Vit. Nutr. Res.* **1994**, *64*, 192–197. [CrossRef]
22. Javert, C.T.; Stander, H.J. Plasma vitamin C and prothrombin concentrations in pregnancy and in threatened, spontaneous and habitual abortions. *J. Surg. Gynec. Obstet.* **1943**, *76*, 115–122.

23. Parry, S.; Strauss, J.F. Premature rupture of the fetal membranes. *N. Engl. J. Med.* **1998**, *338*, 663–670. [PubMed]

24. Casanueva, E.; Ripoll, C.; Tolentino, M.; Morales, R.M.; Pfeffer, F.; Vilchis, P.; Vadillo-ortega, F. Vitamin C supplementation to prevent premature rupture of the chorioamniotic membranes: A randomized trial. *Am. J. Clin. Nutr.* **2005**, *81*, 859–863. [PubMed]

25. Heinz-Erian, P.; Achmuller, M.; Berger, H.; Brabec, W.; Nirk, S.; Rufer, R. Vitamin C concentrations in maternal plasma, amniotic fluid, cord blood, in the plasma of the newborn and in colostrum, transitorial and mature breastmilk. *Padiatrie Padol.* **1987**, *22*, 163–178.

26. Clemetson, C.A.B.; Cafaro, V. Abruptio placentae. *Int. J. Gynaecol. Obstet.* **1981**, *19*, 453–460. [CrossRef]

27. Jauniaux, E.; Poston, L.; Burton, G.J. Placental-related diseases of pregnancy: Involvement of oxidative stress and implications in human evolution. *Hum. Reprod. Update* **2006**, *12*, 747–755. [CrossRef] [PubMed]

28. Mikhail, M.S.; Anyaegbunam, A.; Garfinkel, D.; Palan, P.R.; Basu, J.; Romney, S.L. Preeclampsia and antioxidant nutrients- decreased plasma levels of reduces ascorbic acid, alfa tocopherol and beta-caroten in women with preeclampsia. *Am. J. Obstet. Gynecol.* **1994**, *171*, 150–157. [CrossRef]

29. Zhang, C.; Williams, M.A.; King, I.B. Vitamin C and risk of preeclapsia—Results from dietary questionnaire and plasma assay. *Epidemiology* **2002**, *13*, 409–416. [CrossRef] [PubMed]

30. Chappell, L.C.; Seed, P.T.; Kelly, F.J.; Briley, A.; Hunt, B.J.; Charnock-Jones, D.S.; Mallet, A.; Poston, L. Vitamin C and E supplementation in women at risk of preeclapsia is associated with changes in indices of oxidative stress and placental function. *Am. J. Obstet. Gynecol.* **2002**, *187*, 777–784. [CrossRef] [PubMed]

31. Rumbold, A.R.; Crowther, C.A.; Haslan, R.R.; Dekker, G.A.; Robinson, J.S.; ACTS Study Group. Vitamin C and E and the risk of preeclapsia and perinatal complications. *N. Engl. J. Med.* **2006**, *354*, 1796–1806. [CrossRef] [PubMed]

32. Roberts, J.M.; Myatt, L.; Spongy, C.Y.; Thom, E.A.; Hauth, J.C.; Leveno, K.J.; Pearson, G.D.; Wapner, R.J.; Varner, M.W.; Mercer, B.M.; et al. Eunice Kennedy Shriver National Institute of Child Health and Human Development (NICHD) Maternal-Fetal Medicine Unit Network (MFMU) Vitamin C and E to prevent complications of pregnancy-associated hypertension. *N. Engl. J. Med.* **2010**, *362*, 1282–1291. [CrossRef] [PubMed]

33. Hauth, J.C.; Clifton, R.G.; Roberts, J.M.; Spongy, C.Y.; Myatt, L.; Leveno, K.J.; Pearson, G.D.; Varner, M.W.; Mercer, B.M.; Peaceman, A.M.; et al. Eunice Kennedy Shriver National Institute of Child Health and Human Development (NICHD) Maternal-Fetal Medicine Unit Network (MFMU). Vitamin C and E to prevent spontaneous preterm birth: A randomized controlled trial. *Obstet. Gynecol.* **2010**, *116*, 653–658. [CrossRef] [PubMed]

34. Duerbeck, N.B.; Dowling, D.D.; Duerbeck, J.M. Vitamin, C. promises not kept. *Obstet. Gynecol. Surv.* **2016**, *71*, 187–193. [CrossRef] [PubMed]

35. Dheen, S.T.; Tay, S.S.; Boran, J.; Ting, L.W.; Kumar, S.D.; Fu, J.; Ling, E.A. Recent studies on neural tube defects in embryos of diabetic pregnancy: An overview. *Curr. Med. Chem.* **2009**, *16*, 2345–2354. [CrossRef] [PubMed]

36. Cederberg, J.; Eriksson, U.K. Antioxidative treatment of pregnant diabetic rats diminished embryonic dysmorphogenesis. *Birth Defect. Res. A Clin. Mol. Teratol.* **2005**, *3*, 498–505. [CrossRef] [PubMed]

37. Cederberg, J.; Siman, C.M.; Eriksson, U.J. Combined treatment with vitamin E and C decreases oxidative stress and improves fetal outcome in experimental diabetic pregnancy. *Pediatr. Res.* **2001**, *49*, 755–762. [CrossRef] [PubMed]

38. Siman, C.M.; Eriksson, U.J. Vitamin C supplementation of the maternal diet reduces the rate of malformations in the offspring of diabetic rats. *Diabetologia* **1997**, *40*, 1416–1424. [CrossRef] [PubMed]

39. Ju, H.; Rumbold, A.R.; Willson, K.J.; Crowther, C.A. Borderline gestational diabetes mellitus and pregnancy outcomes. *BMC Pregnancy Childbirth* **2008**, *30*, 8–31. [CrossRef] [PubMed]

40. McCance, D.R.; Holmes, V.A.; Maresh, M.J.; Patterson, C.C.; Walker, J.D.; Pearson, D.W.; Young, I.S. Diabetes and Pre-eclampsia Intervention Trial (DAPIT) Study Group.Vitamins C and E for prevention of pre-eclampsia in women with type 1 diabetes (DAPIT): A randomised placebo-controlled trial. *Lancet* **2010**, *376*, 259–266. [CrossRef]

41. Weissgerber, T.L.; Gandley, R.E.; Roberts, J.M.; Patterson, C.C.; Holmes, V.A.; Young, I.S.; McCance, D.R. Diabetes and preeclampsia interventions Trial (DAPIT) study group. *BJOG* **2013**, *120*, 1192–1199. [CrossRef] [PubMed]

42. Brownlee, M. The Pathobiology of Diabetic Complications: A Unifying Mechanism. *Diabetes* **2006**, *54*, 1615–1625. [CrossRef]

43. Sinclair, A.J.; Girling, A.J.; Gray, L.; Le Guen, C.; Lunec, J.; Barnett, A.H. Disturbed handling of ascorbic acid in diabetic patients with and without microangiopathy during high dose ascorbate supplementation. *Diabetologia* **1991**, *34*, 171–175. [CrossRef] [PubMed]

44. Jacob, R.A.; Otradovec, C.L.; Russell, R.M.; Munro, H.N.; Hartz, S.C.; McGandy, R.B.; Morrow, F.D.; Sadowski, J.A. Vitamin C status and nutrient interactions in a healthy elderly population. *Am. J. Clin. Nutr.* **1988**, *48*, 1436–1442. [PubMed]

45. Lee, W.; Hamernyik, P.; Hutchinson, M.; Raisys, V.A.; Labbé, R.F. Ascorbic acid in lymphocytes: Cell preparation and liquid-chromatographic assay. *Clin. Chem.* **1982**, *28*, 2165–2169. [PubMed]

46. Frei, B.; Birlouez-Aragon, I.; Lykkesfeldt, J. Author's perspective: What is the optimum intake of vitamin C in humans? *Crit. Rev. Food Sci. Nutr.* **2012**, *52*, 815–829. [CrossRef] [PubMed]

47. Tveden-Nyborg, P.; Lykkesfeldt, J. Does vitamin C deficiency increase lifestyle-associated vascular disease progression?—Evidence based on experimental and clinical studies. *Antioxid. Redox Sign.* **2013**, *19*, 2084–2104. [CrossRef] [PubMed]

48. Jain, S.; Wise, R.; Yanamandra, K.; Dhanireddy, R.; Bocchini, J. The effect of maternal and cord-blood vitamin C, vitamin E and lipid peroxide levels on newborn birth weight. *Mol. Cell. Biochem.* **2008**, *309*, 217–221. [CrossRef] [PubMed]

49. Schjoldager, J.G.; Paidi, M.D.; Lindblad, M.M.; Birck, M.M.; Kjærgaard, A.B.; Dantzer, V.; Lykkesfeldt, J.; Tveden-Nyborg, P. Maternal vitamin C deficiency during pregnancy results in transient fetal and placental growth retardation in guinea pigs but does not affect prenatal survival. *Eur. J. Nutr.* **2015**, *54*, 667–676. [CrossRef] [PubMed]

50. Takanaga, H.; Mackenzie, B.; Hediger, M.A. Sodium-dependent ascorbic acid transporter family SLC23. *Pflug. Arch.* **2004**, *447*, 677–682. [CrossRef] [PubMed]

51. Lindblad, M.M.; Tveden-Nyborg, P.; Lykkesfeldt, J. Regulation of vitamin C homeostasis during deficiency. *Nutrients* **2013**, *5*, 2860–2879. [CrossRef] [PubMed]

52. Mann, G.V.; Newton, P. The membrane transport of ascorbic acid. *Ann. N. Y. Acad. Sci.* **1975**, *258*, 243–252. [CrossRef] [PubMed]

53. Kositsawat, J.; Freeman, V.L. Vitamin C and A1c relationship in the national health and nutrition examination Survey (NHANES) 2003–2006. *J. Am. Coll. Nutr.* **2011**, *30*, 477–483. [CrossRef] [PubMed]

54. Tu, H.; Li, H.; Wang, Y.; Niyyati, M.; Wang, Y.; Leshin, J.; Levine, M. Low red blood cell vitamin C concentrations induce red blood cell fragility: A link to diabetes via glucose, glucose transporters and dehydrascorbic acid. *EBiomedicine* **2015**, *2*, 1735–1750. [CrossRef] [PubMed]

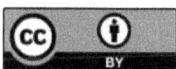

nutrients

MDPI

Review

Protective Role for Antioxidants in Acute Kidney Disease

Joanne M. Dennis and Paul K. Witting *

Redox Biology Group, Discipline of Pathology, Charles Perkins Centre, Sydney Medical School,
The University of Sydney, Sydney, NSW 2006, Australia; jo-dennis@optusnet.com.au

Received: 24 May 2017; Accepted: 4 July 2017; Published: 7 July 2017

Abstract: Acute kidney injury causes significant morbidity and mortality in the community and clinic. Various pathologies, including renal and cardiovascular disease, traumatic injury/rhabdomyolysis, sepsis, and nephrotoxicity, that cause acute kidney injury (AKI), induce general or regional decreases in renal blood flow. The ensuing renal hypoxia and ischemia promotes the formation of reactive oxygen species (ROS) such as superoxide radical anions, peroxides, and hydroxyl radicals, that can oxidatively damage biomolecules and membranes, and affect organelle function and induce renal tubule cell injury, inflammation, and vascular dysfunction. Acute kidney injury is associated with increased oxidative damage, and various endogenous and synthetic antioxidants that mitigate source and derived oxidants are beneficial in cell-based and animal studies. However, the benefit of synthetic antioxidant supplementation in human acute kidney injury and renal disease remains to be realized. The endogenous low-molecular weight, non-proteinaceous antioxidant, ascorbate (vitamin C), is a promising therapeutic in human renal injury in critical illness and nephrotoxicity. Ascorbate may exert significant protection by reducing reactive oxygen species and renal oxidative damage via its antioxidant activity, and/or by its non-antioxidant functions in maintaining hydroxylase and monooxygenase enzymes, and endothelium and vascular function. Ascorbate supplementation may be particularly important in renal injury patients with low vitamin C status.

Keywords: antioxidant; renal injury; oxidant; hypoxia; ischemia; vitamin C; endothelium

1. Introduction

Acute kidney injury (AKI, also known as acute renal failure) is an increasing healthcare challenge [1]. It is defined as a sudden reduction in renal function or glomerular filtration rate (GFR), leading to azotemia and/or insufficient urine production caused by reduced renal blood flow, and kidney damage, inflammation, or obstruction. Clinical presentation of AKI can be wide-ranging, and risk factors include peripheral artery disease, hypertension and diabetes. It is an important cause of morbidity and mortality, and a common complication of traumatic physical injury, sepsis, severe burns, and complex surgery. The socioeconomic importance of AKI is rising, as it is recognized to increase the risk of chronic or end-stage kidney disease, or adverse complications in non-renal tissues such as heart and lung [2].

The majority of AKI causes are associated with ischemia and acute hypoxia from general or regional decreases in renal blood flow. Ischemia severely limits cellular oxygen and nutrient uptake, resulting in acute tubular necrosis and inflammation that can exacerbate renal injury and cause functional changes in the kidney [3]. Ischemia and reperfusion are well-known activators of tissue damage via reactive oxygen species (ROS) [4]. Although ROS perform physiological functions, supra- or unregulated ROS accumulation can cause biomolecule oxidative damage, and perturbations in membrane, macromolecule, and organelle functionality. Detoxification or decomposition processes facilitated by endogenous antioxidants normally counterbalance oxidant production. However, pathophysiological conditions can enhance ROS production and overwhelm the availability and/or decrease endogenous antioxidant activity and promote vascular dysfunction, inflammation, and renal tubule cell cytotoxicity typically observed in the pathogenesis of acute kidney injury (AKI) [5].

Although the exact mechanism whereby ROS are generated in AKI is not defined, decreased ROS generation and oxidative damage are potential therapeutic end points. Antioxidants have the potential to intervene early in the pathogenesis of kidney injury by directly eliminating ROS or the oxidant source. Studies in renal cells, kidney tubules, and animal models of AKI, have identified reno-protective agents with antioxidant activities that mitigate renal oxidative damage (see reviews [5–8]). This review will focus on oxidative stress in AKI and the therapeutic potential of antioxidants, including the nutrient vitamin C, in experimental and human acute renal injury.

2. Oxidative Damage in Acute Renal Injury and Disease

There is considerable evidence that oxidative damage to tubular cells and renal tissue is linked to AKI. Animal studies demonstrate increased oxidative damage and decreased tissue antioxidant status after renal ischemia and/or nephrotoxicity [9,10]. Studies in critically ill or sepsis patients with kidney injury and varying degrees of renal insufficiency, show increased circulating biomarkers of protein and lipid oxidation that correlate with markers of pro-inflammatory, pro-oxidative mediators, and cytokines [11]. Moreover, uremia is associated with increased circulating carbonyl and indole compounds, with the potential to increase systemic oxidative stress [12]. Further, oxidative stress and reactive oxygen species (ROS) are thought to be driving factors in other chronic diseases such as cardiovascular disease and diabetes, that predispose to AKI or are present as co-morbidities in the same subjects [5].

Chronic reduction in renal blood flow from pre-existing medical conditions such as liver and renal disease, atherosclerosis, hypertension, diabetes, or from severe illness (traumatic injury, heart failure, sepsis, rhabdomyolysis), or localized acute blood flow insufficiency due to renal ischemia or nephrotoxicity, are responsible for the majority of AKI cases, and primarily manifest as acute obstruction that prevents urine flow [13,14]. The importance of ROS in the pathogenesis of AKI has been intensely examined because hypoxia and ischemia, that link to renal injury, can induce ROS [4] (Figure 1). The kidney is highly sensitive to hypoxia and ischemia may be unavoidable in some clinical settings such as renal transplantation. Further, inflammation and oxidative damage are closely linked in ischemia/reperfusion (I/R) injury and AKI [14], as ROS can promote immune responses and vice versa. Experimental models of AKI show that endothelium activation that promotes leukocyte recruitment and microvascular congestion, as well as altered nitric oxide (NO$^{\bullet}$) biosynthesis, mitochondrial dysfunction, and redox active iron, contribute to heightened ROS generation and oxidative damage.

2.1. Sources of ROS in Various Causes of AKI

Various patho/physiological ROS, including the free radicals superoxide anion ($O_2^{\bullet-}$) and hydroxyl radical (OH$^{\bullet}$), and the non-radical oxidants hydrogen peroxide (H_2O_2), hypochlorous acid (HOCl), and peroxynitrite (ONOO$^-$), may be relevant oxidants in AKI [5,15,16]. $O_2^{\bullet-}$ is a significant precursor of ROS such as H_2O_2, HOCl and OH$^{\bullet}$, and can react with other radicals including NO$^{\bullet}$ to form reactive nitrogen species (RNS) such as peroxynitrite. Cellular $O_2^{\bullet-}$ is produced by dysfunctional mitochondria in hypoxia, ischemia, and toxicity [3], and enzymically by plasma membrane and phagocyte NADPH oxidase (NOX). Limiting substrate or cofactors in injury or pathological conditions can uncouple nitric oxide synthase (NOS) to also generate $O_2^{\bullet-}$ [15]. ROS, including those derived from $O_2^{\bullet-}$, can induce lipid and protein oxidation observed in renal injury.

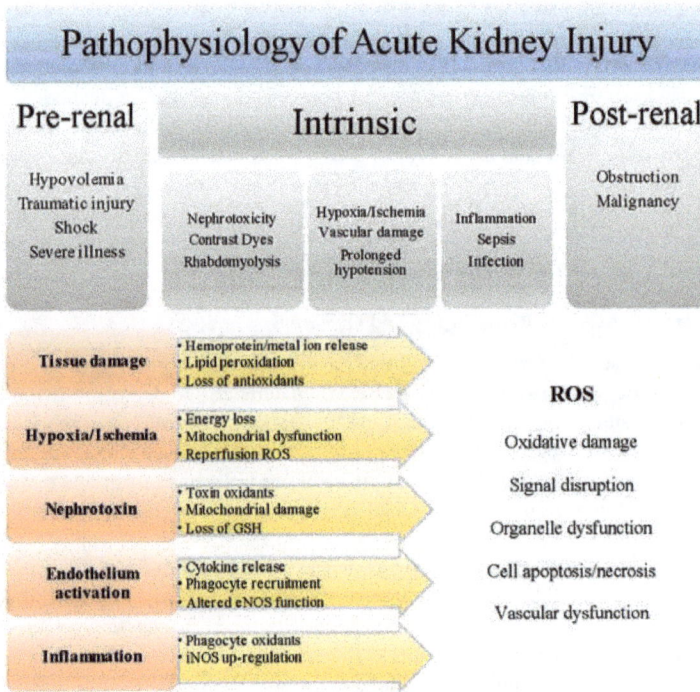

Figure 1. Increased reactive oxygen species (ROS) levels in acute kidney injury (AKI) induce renal oxidative damage and injury. Hypoxia and ischemia perturb microcirculation, cellular enzymes, and mitochondrial function, supporting production of intracellular ROS such as $O_2^{\bullet-}$ and H_2O_2, resulting in mitochondrial damage, depletion of ATP, and activation of cell death pathways. Reperfusion after ischemia also increases ROS. Ischemic injury activates endothelial cells up-regulating pro-inflammatory cytokines and recruiting phagocytes that contribute ROS via NOX and MPO. Inflammation induces ROS and iNOS, promoting peroxynitrite formation. Trauma and toxins generate oxidative stress by depleting endogenous antioxidants and increasing redox-active metal ions. Vascular dysfunction promoted by ischemia, inflammation, or toxicity, affects eNOS function, inducing ROS generation. ROS perturb kinase/phosphatase activities and transcription factor signaling pathways important in cell homeostasis. Oxidative modification of membranes and proteins disrupts cell ion and nutrient transport, energy metabolism, and organelle function, ultimately affecting kidney viability.

A causal role for ROS in ischemia-induced AKI was suggested in early studies in animal models showing significantly increased lipid peroxidation in kidney tissue after renal ischemia, which correlates with injury and tubular dysfunction [9]. Exploring this correlation further, several agents that inhibited ROS formation in vitro, including small molecular weight and enzymatic antioxidants and metal chelators, were effective in alleviating ischemic AKI [9,17]. Lipid peroxidation and DNA damage in ischemia are associated with the formation of 3-nitrotyrosine, a biomarker for ROS/RNS, suggesting that $NO^{\bullet}$, $O_2^{\bullet-}$, and/or peroxynitrite, contribute to renal oxidative damage [18,19].

ROS may also be a causative factor in sepsis-mediated AKI. The extensive immune response induces severe renal vasoconstriction, kidney endothelial cell injury, and localized tissue hypoxia that supports ROS formation. Inflammatory cytokines and ischemia also activate vascular endothelium, recruiting immune cells that produce $O_2^{\bullet-}$ via NOX, and HOCl from H_2O_2, and phagocyte myeloperoxidase (MPO) [16]. Inflammation-induced xanthine oxidase (XO) may also produce $O_2^{\bullet-}$ [3]. Decreased plasma antioxidants (vitamins C and E, and thiols), and increased lipid peroxidation, are also found together with alterations in redox regulatory genes, such as mitochondrial superoxide dismutase (SOD), NOX, endothelial nitric oxide synthase (eNOS), heme oxygenase-1 (HO-1), and tumour necrosis factor (TNF) [16]. Mitochondrial dysfunction and bio-energetic failure is also evident in sepsis and mitochondrial complex I activity that correlates with reduced glutathione (GSH) and ATP levels, and is inversely associated with shock severity in non-surviving patients [20]. Further, inducible NOS (iNOS) is up-regulated in various organs, and shock severity is associated with $NO^\bullet$ levels [20]. Enhanced vascular $NO^\bullet$ production can outcompete SOD for $O_2^{\bullet-}$, thereby promoting peroxynitrite and other ROS/RNS formation, and this may impact on vascular tone [21].

Rhabdomyolysis (RM) is a major cause of AKI in traumatic injury and severe burns. Extensive muscle myolysis releases large quantities of heme-containing myoglobin (Mb) resulting in myoglobinuria, severe renal vasoconstriction, and vascular dysfunction from obstruction by Mb-protein casts or uric acid crystals in kidney tubules [8]. Studies in animal models show that myoglobinuric damage is associated with lipid peroxidation and GSH depletion [10]. Redox active iron released from Mb may induce $OH^\bullet$ generation through degradation of low molecular weight peroxides. However, autoxidation of Mb, that is pH dependent and favored in acidosis, or oxidation of Mb by endogenous peroxides, can also generate protein-based radicals and ferric/ferryl heme, to promote radical-mediated reactions such as lipid peroxidation [22,23]. Potent vasoactive signaling molecules, e.g., isoprostanes, are found in animal models of RM, suggestive of lipid peroxidation in situ [24,25].

Nephrotoxicity accounts for a large cohort of AKI, as renal detoxification and/or filtration of various drugs exposes the kidney to a high toxin risk. AKI induced by common pharmaceuticals and radio-contrast dyes is a significant clinical problem [26]. Renal accumulation of drugs and/or metabolites can cause direct toxic effects on tubular cells, as well as microvascular inflammation and ischemia promoting ROS. Further, drug biotransformation in the kidney is performed by ROS-inducing renal enzymes, such as cytochrome P450 [10]. Antibiotics (gentamycin) and cancer therapies (cisplatin and cyclosporine A) induce kidney tissue lipid peroxidation and renal dysfunction via increased ROS formation, and iron release from renal cortical mitochondria in vitro and in vivo [10]. Drug-induced oxidative stress may also involve depletion of antioxidants, particularly the enzymic cofactor GSH, permitting unregulated ROS/RNS accumulation and renal cell injury [10,27].

2.2. Is Oxidative Stress Causally Related to Renal Dysfunction?

Outcomes from the influential study PICARD (Project to Improve Care in Acute Renal Disease), demonstrated that acute renal failure in critically ill patients was associated with significantly more oxidative stress than that observed in subjects without AKI, healthy controls, or end-stage kidney disease [11]. Thus, plasma protein thiols, employed as a surrogate measure of antioxidant capacity, were significantly decreased, and advanced protein oxidation products were significantly increased, in subjects with clinical AKI. Also, impaired renal function associated with increased plasma pro-inflammatory cytokines (IL-6, IL-8 and TNF-α), and further, cytokines and thiols were inversely related, suggesting that inflammation promotes oxidative stress in AKI. Oxidative stress may also be important in developing chronic kidney disease, as lipid peroxidation products associate with advancing disease, as does endothelial dysfunction and loss of plasma SOD, glutathione peroxidase (GPx) activity, and selenium [28].

While pre-clinical and human studies of AKI and renal insufficiency consistently associate oxidative stress/damage and renal dysfunction, there is limited direct demonstration of the role of ROS, so it is difficult to assign the latter a definitive casual role. Some recent studies have tried to address this using non-invasive in vivo imaging techniques, or more specific indicators, to track ROS formation in AKI. For example, a stable, electron paramagnetic resonance (EPR) spin probe injected into rats showed only partial recovery of kidney reducing (antioxidant) activity after renal I/R, despite improvements in renal function and tissue phospholipid oxidation, suggesting that ongoing oxidative stress depletes antioxidant reserves in renal ischemia [29].

Loss of ATP, and alterations in mitochondrial structure, are early events in AKI that contribute to bio-energetic dysfunction [3,10]. A recent study of endogenous and exogenous multi-photon imaging in vivo, assessed kidney mitochondrial redox state, structure, and function in rodents during ischemic and nephrotoxic AKI [30]. Alterations in mitochondrial NADH and proton motive force, as well as increased mitochondrial $O_2^{\bullet-}$ levels in proximal tubules and fragmented mitochondria were observed, suggesting that this organelle is a major source of ROS, and that mitochondrial dysfunction is an important early event in renal ischemia [30]. In comparison, abnormalities in renal epithelial lysosomes and brush border cells after gentamycin treatment, preceded heterogeneous and sporadic alterations in mitochondrial morphology, NADH, and proton motive force, suggesting that mitochondrial dysfunction is a relatively late event in nephrotoxic AKI [30]. This study not only provided direct visualization of ROS alongside cell damage, but also highlighted the variation in pathophysiology and roles of ROS and mitochondrial dysfunction in different causes of AKI.

Unlike pre-clinical studies, direct measurement of ROS in renal injury/disease patients is practically limited to non-invasive biomarkers. Specific and stable markers of in vivo free radical mediated-lipid oxidation, such as isoprostanes, have been utilized to show substantial lipid peroxidation in patients with RM [31], and with progression of chronic kidney disease [32]. Increased plasma F_2-isoprostanes are also found in renal failure in sepsis [33], and with postoperative AKI [34]. In the latter study, hemoprotein-induced oxidative damage was suggested to play a role in the pathogenesis of AKI. Isofurans contain a substituted tetrahydrofuran ring and are also derived from free radical-mediated lipid oxidation, but are favoured with high oxygen tension as can occur in mitochondrial dysfunction [35]. Plasma isofuran levels similarly increase in sepsis [33], and cardiopulmonary bypass [34] patients with AKI, and in chronic kidney disease [35].

3. Mitigation of Renal Oxidative Stress and Therapeutic Benefit

Whilst ROS perform important roles in cell signaling and physiological processes [36], they are clearly linked with acute and chronic renal injury. Antioxidants participate in ROS detoxification and decomposition processes to maintain redox balance in vivo, and to protect against adverse oxidation. The major endogenous antioxidants mitigate source ROS, such as $O_2^{\bullet-}$ and H_2O_2, and their reaction with other radicals [37], and can also directly interact with pertinent non-radical oxidants derived from $O_2^{\bullet-}$, such as HOCl and peroxynitrite [38]. Notable antioxidants include the vitamins C (ascorbate) and E (tocopherol family), GSH, antioxidant proteins such as SOD, catalase and GPx, and proteins that sequester metals (ferritin, metallothionein) or degrade heme (HO-1) (Nath, 2014). Exogenous and synthetic compounds may act as direct antioxidants, or may activate adaptive systems such as the nuclear factor E2-related factor (Nrf2) signaling pathway that regulates endogenous antioxidant enzymes and cytoprotective genes [39]. Antioxidants that quench ROS or boost the endogenous antioxidant pool, may be therapeutic in AKI.

3.1. Inhibition of ROS Source

A wide range of free radical scavengers, metal chelators (that inhibit redox cycling of bound metals), and inhibitors of ROS enzyme sources, decrease lipid peroxidation, DNA damage, and/or protein oxidation/nitration, and this is closely associated with improved renal function and inflammation in animal models of AKI, and related renal cell studies. These outcomes have prompted attempts to remove potential ROS sources with inhibitors, genetic knockout techniques, or antioxidants, to not only assign a mechanistic role for ROS in AKI, but also identify ROS as a target for therapeutic advantage.

3.1.1. Pro-Oxidant Metals

The role of pro-oxidant metal ions and metal-containing heme has been intensely studied in AKI, as potent ROS such as $OH^{\bullet}$ and oxidised lipids, that are vasoactive, can be formed by redox active metals in the presence of $O_2^{\bullet-}$/peroxide, and because the latter are increased in injury. Several studies affirm that metal chelators, such as desferrioxamine, are protective against oxidative damage, and renal dysfunction in animal models of nephrotoxic and injurious AKI [40–42]. These studies also show renal protection and reduced lipid oxidation afforded by so-called OH$^\bullet$ scavengers, and more specific antioxidants such as SOD, GSH, and vitamin E [10].

One source of released iron is heme-containing proteins in mitochondria or endoplasmic reticulum or Mb, the latter being released in large amounts in RM-induced AKI [10]. Other hemoproteins may also contribute to oxidative stress. For example, cytochrome P450 inhibitors modulate kidney iron levels and improve renal function and injury in both RM-mediated AKI and cisplatin nephrotoxicity in rats, suggesting that redox cycling of this enzyme is important to renal injury [43,44]. Down-regulation of cytochrome P450 2E1, using a specific transcription inhibitor, also modulates lipid peroxidation, and associates with normalising antioxidant enzymes and iron levels, and is reno-protective in RM-induced AKI in rats [45].

Maintaining Mb heme-iron in a chemically reduced (Fe^{2+}) state also appears to ameliorate AKI and renal dysfunction, and may explain the positive effects of endogenous antioxidant replacement, and also some of the action of desferrioxamine that can reduce Mb heme [23]. Further, inhibition of Mb heme redox cycling by alkalinisation [24], or inhibition of endogenous lipid peroxidation with acetaminophen, prevents isoprostane formation and renal injury associated with RM [25]. Notably, acetaminophen was effective in reducing oxidant injury and renal dysfunction when administered either pre- or post-treatment. Whether acetaminophen removes seed lipid peroxides, or also acts on renal inflammation, is not known. In any case, removing pro-oxidant forms of iron by antioxidant therapy or chelation appears to be efficacious, particularly in injurious AKI.

3.1.2. Superoxide Radical Anion and Derived ROS Sources (NOX, Mitochondrial ROS)

The available evidence indicates that SOD and other antioxidant enzymes are decreased in pre-clinical models of AKI [46], and genetic impairment of SOD increases sensitivity to AKI in ischemia [47] and chronic hypoxia [48]. Generation of $O_2^{\bullet-}$, oxidative damage, and reduced SOD and catalase activity, persist following transient renal ischemia in rodents, and associate with functional defects that promote kidney disease. Long-term treatment with a SOD mimetic (MnTMPyp) [49] or the NOX inhibitor apocyanin (which can also act as an antioxidant radical scavenger [50], alleviated oxidation parameters and reduced the functional defects in this injury model [3]. Notably, NOX gene levels did not appear to be altered, however, other pro-oxidant genes were increased, including MPO and dual oxidase I (shares homology with NOX), whereas extracellular GPx3 was chronically decreased [3]. In comparison, NOX2/4 mRNA and protein are elevated in a pre-clinical model of nephrotoxicity [51], and both total NOX activity and NOX4 protein are increased in contrast dye-induced (CI-)AKI in hypercholesterolemic rats [52]. Also, polymorphisms affecting activity in NOX p22phox subunit gene associate with oxidation biomarkers and adverse outcomes in acute renal failure patients [53].

Blockage of ROS production from $O_2^{\bullet-}$ sources such as XO, NOX, and mitochondria, alleviates animal model AKI. Allopurinol, a XO inhibitor, modulates oxidative damage and improves renal function in renal ischemia [54] and RM-induced AKI [55]. Allopurinol also reduces vascular oxidative stress and improves endothelium function in chronic kidney disease [56,57]. Apocynin, a prototypical inhibitor of NOX, is protective against renal dysfunction and lipid peroxidation [3], and loss of SOD after I/R in rats with a similar efficacy to allopurinol [58], although whether protection is due to direct inhibition of NOX or the inhibitor antioxidant activity, per se, is not clear. Treatment with a combination of apocyninan and allopurinol failed to show any further efficacy than individual drug administration [58], suggesting that a common target, i.e., ROS, was adequately quenched by either inhibitor. In another recent study in rats, apocynin normalized kidney MPO and GPx protein, reduced lipid peroxidation, and improved kidney function after renal ischemia [59].

Mitochondrial structural damage is an early, distinctive marker in AKI, and is linked to increased production of ROS and activation of cell death pathways, and an inflammatory response that potentiates ROS formation [3]. Whether mitochondrial ROS are causative or formed subsequently in AKI is not known, however, there is ongoing interest in the development of therapeutic antioxidants specifically targeted to this organelle, and several show efficacy in preclinical AKI, and are the focus of clinical trials, especially for I/R injury [60]. For example, the ubiquinone analogue MitoQ effectively protects against kidney dysfunction and oxidative damage in renal I/R [61], nephrotoxic AKI [51], and cold storage ex vivo indices of oxidative stress and kidney damage [60]. Also, mitochondrial targeted peptides thought to protect cardiolipin from cytochrome C peroxidation, show efficacy against oxidative stress, tubular cell damage, and dysfunction in renal I/R injury [60].

3.1.3. NO$^\bullet$ Derived ROS/RNS

Peroxynitrite causes oxidation and/or nitration of lipid and protein, amino acids and DNA, depletion of thiols and antioxidants, and oxidation of heme proteins. Nitration of tyrosine residues is often used as a biological marker of peroxynitrite generation, and 3-nitrotyrosine is found in ischemic, nephrotoxic and injurious AKI. However, it should be noted that several peroxidases, including MPO, provide an alternative mechanism of protein tyrosine nitration via NO$^\bullet$ oxidase activity [62]. Thus, in addition to SOD, MPO may be considered a modulator of NO$^\bullet$ signaling during inflammation [62], and this may be relevant in sepsis where the inflammation response may contribute substantial MPO. Thus, considering that iNOS and MPO are up-regulated in infection/inflammation, the observation of 3-nitrotyrosine in vivo in various causes of AKI, is probably restricted to a nonspecific indication of ROS/RNS.

An imbalance in NO$^\bullet$ and $O_2^{\bullet-}$ production during hypoxia and I/R injury may contribute to renal cell damage [18,19]. However, use of agents to globally inhibit NO$^\bullet$ production, including that from constitutive eNOS, is not reno-protective in I/R injury [63]. Interestingly, iNOS is constitutively expressed in the kidney [64], emphasizing a role for NO$^\bullet$ in normal renal function [15]. However, sustained NO$^\bullet$ release from iNOS may also be pathogenic, as mice deficient in iNOS are resistant to renal I/R injury [65]. Moreover, specific inhibition of iNOS reduces oxidative and nitrosative damage, and renal dysfunction in animal models of renal ischemia [18,66], sepsis [67,68], and nephrotoxic AKI [27].

3.2. Antioxidant Interventions; Supplementation and Up-Regulation

Several strategies for modulation of AKI using antioxidant compounds have been tested in human and animal studies [6–8]. These include increasing bioavailability by intervention with nutrient-derived and/or synthetic antioxidants, identifying new reno-protectants with antioxidant activity, and targeting of antioxidants to specific ROS cellular domains (e.g., mitochondria). Also, anti-inflammatory agents may potentially reduce ROS via stabilising endothelium function and NO$^\bullet$ bioactivity, as well as up-regulating gene responses linked to antioxidation and cytoprotection.

3.2.1. Small Molecular Weight Endogenous/Nutrient or Synthetic Antioxidants

Several small molecular weight compounds with antioxidant and ROS scavenging actions improve renal function and decrease tubular damage. For example, edaravone (3-methyl-1-phenyl-2-pyrazolin-5-one; norphenazone, MCI-186) shows efficacy in ischemia and is an approved treatment for stroke in Japan [69]. It has been widely reported to inhibit oxidative damage and lipid peroxidation in ischemia, however, it also shows anti-inflammatory properties that may be unrelated to its antioxidant activity [69]. Edaravone attenuates ROS radical generation in kidney tubular cells in vitro, and lipid peroxidation measured as aldehyde-modified proteins in vivo, and ameliorates renal dysfunction in I/R [70] and nephrotoxicity [71] in rats. Edaravone also improves survival rates in warm and cold I/R injury in rats [72] and dogs [73], and in the latter, significantly improved renal function and reduced renal tubular cell damage, lipid, and DNA oxidation [73], suggesting that it may prevent preservation injury in transplantation. Despite these positive effects, there are reports of edaravone treatment causally associated with AKI in ischemic stroke, however, this has not been validated by a recent survey [74].

N-acetylcysteine (NAc) is a synthetic derivative of cysteine and precursor of GSH, and exhibits ROS scavenging activity via its sulfhydryl group. It is protective in ischemic, nephrotoxic, and RM-induced AKI in animal models [8], and improves kidney function, renal GSH and systemic oxidative stress, and reduces renal inflammation. However, it has no effect on urinary isoprostanes, suggesting cellular activity in addition, or unrelated, to a primary antioxidation mechanism. NAc has been tested in several clinical studies of CI-AKI [75]. However, on balance, NAc shows no overall benefit in preventing or treating CI-AKI in humans, and meta-analysis of these trials highlight heterogeneity, under-reporting of negative/no benefit, and confounding serum creatinine levels as possible contributors to the neutral effect. In addition, inadequate animal models for CI-AKI may have hampered translation. Similar to CI-AKI, pre-, intra-, or post-operative use of NAc in clinical trials to preserve renal function in cardiac or abdominal aortic surgery has largely failed to show benefit [7].

Endogenous or dietary antioxidants are protective against oxidation and/or inflammation and kidney damage in AKI. For example, vitamin E and selenium (that can enhance activity of GSH-dependent antioxidant enzymes) attenuate nephrotoxicity [7]. Interestingly, Se supplementation inhibited renal oxidative damage and inflammation, yet was not reno-protective in an animal model of RM-mediated AKI [76]. Vitamin C also attenuates oxidative damage, inflammation and renal injury in several animal models, including CI-AKI [75], and other nephrotoxic AKI [7], ischemia- [5,6] and RM-induced renal injury [8,77] (and see Table 1 for results of recent vitamin C intervention studies on oxidative damage and/or antioxidant status and kidney function in animals). Loss of GSH or GSH reductase activity worsens renal function in RM [10] and renal ischemia [78]. Conversely, supplementation of GSH decreases renal cell/tubule oxidative injury [78,79] and improves renal function in AKI [80]. NAc, that can increase intracellular GSH, and the GPx mimetic ebselen, both show efficacy in AKI in animal models [3,5]. Ebselen may also be protective by scavenging peroxynitrite [5] thereby inhibiting protein modification by this potent oxidant.

Nutrients 2017, 9, 718

Table 1. Recent vitamin C intervention studies in animal models of ischemic, nephrotoxic and injurious AKI.

AKI Model	Vitamin C Dosage (mg/kg)	Renal Improvements			Proposed Mechanism	Ref.
		Oxidation/Inflammation	Antioxidants	Function/Damage		
Single Therapy						
Renal I/R in rats	250	↓ tissue lipid oxidation	↑ tissue GSH	↓ serum urea, creatinine, tubular damage, necrosis, casts	antioxidant inhibition of oxidative stress allows recovery of renal function	[81]
Renal I/R in rats	50, 100	↓ tissue lipid oxidation, $O_2^{\bullet-}$, MPO	↑ tissue GSH, nitrate/nitrite	↓ serum urea, microproteinuria, urate improved creatinine clearance, anuria	activation of NO/soluble guanylyl cyclase pathway inhibitors reverse benefit	[82]
Aortic I/R in rats	50, 100	↓ tissue lipid oxidation, iNOS, MPO, IL-6	not determined	no effect on anuria partially improved microcirculation	reduces oxidative stress and inflammation	[83]
Renal I/R in mice	57	↓ renal artery ROS	↑ tissue GSH, NO, renal artery SOD	↓ serum urea, creatinine, renal artery resistance, tubular damage improved renal artery relaxation	$O_2^{\bullet-}$ scavenging and regulation of SOD protects GSH/NO	[84]
RM in rats	20	↓ tissue lipid oxidation	↑ tissue SOD, catalase	no significant effect on urea, creatinine, GFR; trend to decrease iron accumulation, tubular necrosis, casts	ROS scavenging prevents formation of ferryl Mb	[85]
Comparative Study						
Renal I/R in rats	500	↓ tissue lipid oxidation, inflammation	↑ tissue catalase	↓ plasma urea, creatinine	Antioxidant > reno-protection than L-arginine	[86]
Renal I/R in rats	500	↓ tissue lipid oxidation, $O_2^{\bullet-}$, MPO ↓ tissue inflammation	↑ tissue GSH, catalase	↓ serum urea, urate, tubular damage, casts, microproteinuria ↑ creatinine clearance	antioxidant, decreases $O_2^{\bullet-}$ reno-protection similar to progesterone progesterone receptor antagonist reverses benefit	[87]
Remote organ I/R	100	↓ plasma & tissue lipid oxidation, inflammation	not determined	improved blood biochemistry (pO₂, bicarbonate) ↓ tubular necrosis	vascular protective effects similar to synthetic prostacyclin	[88]
Nephrotoxicity in rats	100	↓ tissue lipid oxidation, inflammation	↑ tissue catalase, GSH, nitrite, serum antioxidants	↓ urea, creatinine, tubular necrosis improvements to serum protein	ROS scavenging decreases oxidative stress comparable to vitamin E	[89]
RM in rats	100	↓ plasma/tissue specific lipid oxidation, MCP-1, kinase activity (MAPK)	normalization of total & specific tissue GPx	↓ proteinuria, plasma urate, renal casts; normalisation of epithelial brush border	oxidative stress reduction comparable to a synthetic polyphenol; renal functional improvements unrelated to antioxidation	[77]

Endogenous antioxidants act in coordinated networks to mitigate oxidative damage, and this may help explain why they are efficacious in AKI. The low-molecular weight antioxidants, α-tocopherol and ascorbate, inhibit propagation reactions, and are effective terminating antioxidants. However, they also act as co-antioxidants to spare other antioxidants and transfer radicals away from susceptible moieties [90]. GSH performs multiple ROS detoxification roles, including ROS scavenging, preventing protein thiol oxidation, as a co-factor for the GPx enzyme family that reduces peroxides and detoxifies xenobiotics via glutathione S-transferase conjugation. GSH is regenerated from its oxidation product, GSSG, by glutathione reductase and cofactor NADPH. Further, mutual maintenance of ascorbate and GSH may occur in vivo, as ascorbate can maintain intracellular GSH, GSH can overcome scurvy, and vitamin C is recycled via GSH and/or GSH or NADH-dependent enzymes [91].

In addition to endogenous antioxidants, several dietary plant polyphenols and flavonoids including curcumin, quercetin, resveratrol, and red wine polyphenols, appear to be efficacious in RM- [7,9] and ischemic AKI [6] in animal models. While several of these phytochemicals display antioxidant activity in vitro, they are well known to activate the Nrf2 signaling cascade [39] that up-regulates several antioxidant genes, including enzymes that interconnect H_2O_2 and thiol modification (e.g., GSH biosynthesis and GSH-dependent enzymes, thioredoxin, peroxiredoxin, and GPx). Nrf2 also activates transcription of HO-1, and ferritin that can mitigate AKI and renal injury [5,7]. Synthetic phenols with antioxidant activity may also act via Nrf2 to up-regulate reno-protective HO-1 (see below and [77,92]).

3.2.2. Antioxidant Enzymes

Enhancement of antioxidant enzyme activity appears to be protective in several animal models of AKI. Early studies of ischemia showed that SOD or catalase administration attenuates ROS in proximal tubule injury after hypoxia in vitro [93], and that SOD diminishes oxygen radicals in vivo after renal ischemia in rabbits [94]. Also, SOD improved renal function and reduced kidney tissue injury and cortical mitochondrial lipid peroxidation in rats [9]. Further studies confirmed that SOD reduced ROS and was cytoprotective to renal cells in vitro and in vivo (reviewed in [3,10]). Pharmacologic agents with SOD mimetic activity (Tempol, MnTMPyP) attenuate sepsis- [95,96] and ischemia-induced AKI [97,98]. Further, MnTMPyP attenuates chronic increases in ROS and oxidative damage, and a reduction in SOD associated with kidney fibrosis after ischemic AKI [49]. In animal sepsis, MnTMPyP blocked $O_2^{\bullet-}$ and peroxynitrite formation, and reversed functional kidney deficits when added 6 h post-septic insult, suggesting that antioxidant intervention is beneficial, and that halting ROS formation can ameliorate microvascular failure and renal injury [96].

Over-expression of MnSOD, but not catalase, attenuates cisplatin-induced renal epithelial cell injury in vitro [99], further suggesting that $O_2^{\bullet-}$ is important in AKI. Also, hyperglycemia that contributes to diabetic nephropathy, induces $O_2^{\bullet-}$ within mitochondria and inactivates complex III, and these changes can be alleviated by MnSOD over-expression [100]. MnSOD efficiently converts $O_2^{\bullet-}$ to H_2O_2, allowing ROS to exit the organelle. However, renal MnSOD inactivation (up to 50%) associated with increased mitochondrial $O_2^{\bullet-}$, has been demonstrated in mouse sepsis, and this can be attenuated with the mitochondria-targeted antioxidant Mito-TEMPO [101]. Further, Mito-TEMPO mitigated renal mitochondrial and circulation dysfunction, together with doubling the survival rate, and was effective when administered post-septic insult. Whether other low-molecular weight cyclic nitroxide SOD mimetics, that also show anti-inflammatory activity independent of radical quenching [102], can provide reno-protection, requires further investigation. Similarly, the SOD mimetic, Mito-CP, also targets mitochondria and protects against tubular cell dysfunction, injury, apoptosis, and inflammation in mice administered cisplatin, accompanied by reduced NOX2/4 mRNA and protein, lipid oxidation, protein nitration, and pro-inflammation markers (MPO, ICAM-1) [51]. Thus, targeting the initial toxic insult that induces mitochondrial ROS with antioxidants may prevent further ROS formation facilitated by inflammatory cell infiltration and NOX [51].

3.2.3. HO-1 and Heme Metabolism

Heme oxygenase, normally found in the reticulo-endothelial system, can be rapidly induced in various tissues as a stress (including oxidative) protein, including the kidney. It is considered an antioxidant as it metabolizes heme from various proteins, including Mb, allowing clearance and sequestration of redox-active iron (by ferritin), and its re-utilization. In addition, heme metabolism by HO-1 produces biliverdin that can be converted to the plasma antioxidant bilirubin and CO; the latter participates in cell signaling and is cytoprotective in the vasculature [103]. Both HO-1 and ferritin are induced as an adaptive response to myoglobinuria in rats injected with glycerol to induce RM, and treatment with a competitive HO-1 inhibitor worsens renal function, while HO-1 induction by hemoglobin is protective [104]. However, it is well known that exposure of cells to heme renders them sensitive to ROS, such as H_2O_2 [105]. This suggests a fine balance between adaptive and maladaptive responses to heme, where small pre-treatment doses may be protective, similar to ischemic pre-conditioning (see below), and reliant on cell signaling processes involving antioxidant, anti-inflammatory, and vascular cytoprotective pathways.

Pharmacologic and genetic manipulation of HO-1 in animal studies suggests HO-1 is protective in other causes of AKI, including nephrotoxicity, ischemia, and sepsis [7,103]. For example, inhibition of HO-1 hinders recovery of renal function in rats after renal ischemia [106]. Transgenic deficiency in HO-1 renders mice more susceptible to renal failure and injury after cisplatin treatment and, hemin addition to renal proximal tubule cells in vitro induces HO-1 and a pronounced cytoprotective effect [107]. Furthermore, HO-1 is protective in AKI following renal transplantation, and its products inhibit tubulo-glomerular feedback and thrombotic microangiopathy in sepsis [103]. Moreover, loss of proximal tubule ferritin worsens AKI [108], and HO-1 knockout mice display increased lipid and protein oxidation, and iron deposition in kidneys [109]. HO-1 also confers protective effects in specific organelles, such as mitochondria, and appears to be induced in specific renal sites aligned with the AKI insult, and targeting of HO-1 to the proximal tubule is protective in nephrotoxicity [110].

3.2.4. Maintenance of Endothelial Function

Biomarkers of endothelium dysfunction are associated with increased risk of AKI in critically ill patients, suggesting that endothelial cell activation predisposes to developing kidney injury [111]. Ischemia can drive endothelium activation by inducing chemo/cytokines that recruit immune cells and allow their transmigration, and maintaining endothelium function may be important in limiting I/R injury in AKI. For example, ICAM-1 induces leukocyte adhesion to endothelial cells, and up-regulation of inflammatory mediators causing endothelium dysfunction and administration of an ICAM-1 antibody, genetic knockout of ICAM-1, or prevention of neutrophil infiltration in mice attenuates renal ischemia-induced AKI [112]. Various anti-inflammatory agents that hinder phagocyte infiltration, NF-Kb, and fibrosis mediators, are also effective in preserving renal function in various AKI [6,8]. I/R can induce direct endothelial cell damage via ROS and/or mitochondrial dysfunction, thereby interfering with $NO^\bullet$ homeostasis and vascular function. Several positive modulators of $NO^\bullet$ via eNOS, and selective inhibition of iNOS and/or peroxynitrite formation via SOD mimetics, reverse renal dysfunction and oxidative injury in various AKI models [5,6,8].

Pre-conditioning by imposing a stress prior to subsequent injury may be effective in renal ischemic injury. As ROS are important signaling molecules, short bursts of ischemia can promote signaling cascades that protect renal cells from more prolonged I/R injury. Thus, transcription activators such as Nrf2 and hypoxia-inducible factors (HIF) up-regulate stress-response and cytoprotective genes, e.g., HO-1, and these may be integral to the protective effects observed in remote and pharmacological pre-conditioning strategies [3]. For example, pre-conditional induction of HIF protects against ischemic AKI in rodents [113]. Some antioxidants (ascorbate, SOD) can block protection afforded by ischemic pre-conditioning in the heart [114], further indicating that ROS are important signaling molecules in vivo. A role for up-regulation of renal $NO^\bullet$ production and improved vascular function via enhanced

NO• bioavailability has also been suggested, as pre-conditioning benefits are reduced in NOS-inhibited or eNOS deficient mice [115].

4. Vitamin C and Renal Protection

There is substantial interest in vitamin C (ascorbate) as a therapeutic antioxidant in renal dysfunction, and vitamin C supplementation has been shown to be protective against ischemic, injurious and toxicity-induced oxidative stress, and kidney dysfunction/AKI in animal models, and human studies of critical illness (see Figure 2, overview of proposed mechanisms of vitamin C reno-protection). Ascorbate is an essential nutrient obtained from the diet, and is a highly effective non-protein reducing agent capable of donating electrons in various enzymatic and non-enzymatic reactions [116]. In this capacity, it can undergo two consecutive one-electron oxidations to yield first ascorbyl radical, and then dehydroascorbic acid (DHA), and both of these forms are recycled to ascorbate by thiols/GSH and/or GSH, or NAD(P)H-dependent enzymes, effectively enhancing the potential protective action of ascorbate.

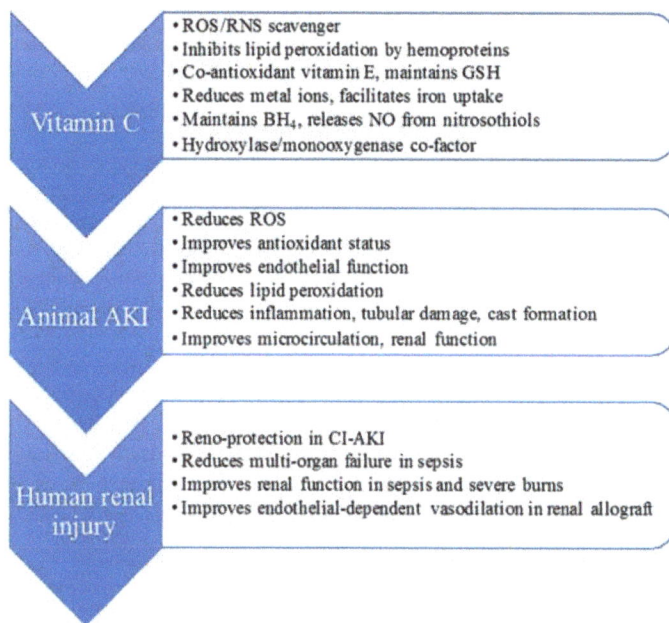

Vitamin C
- ROS/RNS scavenger
- Inhibits lipid peroxidation by hemoproteins
- Co-antioxidant vitamin E, maintains GSH
- Reduces metal ions, facilitates iron uptake
- Maintains BH$_4$, releases NO from nitrosothiols
- Hydroxylase/monooxygenase co-factor

Animal AKI
- Reduces ROS
- Improves antioxidant status
- Improves endothelial function
- Reduces lipid peroxidation
- Reduces inflammation, tubular damage, cast formation
- Improves microcirculation, renal function

Human renal injury
- Reno-protection in CI-AKI
- Reduces multi-organ failure in sepsis
- Improves renal function in sepsis and severe burns
- Improves endothelial-dependent vasodilation in renal allograft

Figure 2. Key activities of vitamin C and proposed benefit mechanisms in acute renal injury. BH4 = tetrahydrobiopterin; RNS = reactive nitrogen species; CI-AKI = chemical induced acute kidney injury

Ascorbate acts as an enzyme cofactor in several hydroxylase reactions by maintaining active-site metals in a reduced (active) state. In this regard, it is essential for functional collagen synthesis, and vitamin C deficiency adversely affects wound healing and blood vessel wall integrity, and causes scurvy. It is also a cofactor for cytoplasmic prolyl hydroxylases that control activation of HIF and up-regulation of pro-survival glycolytic and angiogenic genes [117]. In addition to these activities, vitamin C is proposed to have an important physiological role as an effective in vivo antioxidant. The basis of this is related to its low reduction potential, that allows direct interaction with a wide range of physiological ROS/RNS [118], and a large body of in vitro evidence demonstrates the effectiveness of ascorbate in inhibiting biomolecule oxidation [116].

Ascorbate is an efficient ROS/RNS scavenger in both tissue and plasma, and these non-enzymatic, antioxidant bioactivities have prompted therapeutic investigations of ascorbate in AKI and renal injury. Thus, ascorbate protects against ROS damage to protein, lipid, DNA, and carbohydrate in aqueous milieu both extra- and intra-cellularly, and in several ROS-induced pathologies [116,117]. It scavenges radicals ($O_2^{\bullet-}$, (hydro)peroxyl, nitroxide) and non-radical (HOCl, peroxynitrite) oxidants, and reduces levels of α-tocopheroxyl radical in lipids and membranes, allowing recycling of vitamin E, and inhibition of lipid peroxidation [90], and can spare GSH and protein thiols. It is also safe, with high pharmaco-economic benefit, is fast acting on systemic antioxidant status, and large quantities can be administered acutely with minimal adverse effects via various modes [117,119].

Intestinal uptake and renal re-absorption is important in ascorbate bioavailability, as humans, unlike most mammals, cannot synthesize the vitamin de novo. Circulation levels of ascorbate are tightly controlled in the micromolar range, whereas intracellular levels are much higher [120]. Ascorbate is distributed by vitamin C membrane transporters (SVCT) in nucleated cells, whereas DHA, the 2e-oxidation product of ascorbate, is transported by Na^+-independent glucose transporters (GLUT), and is rapidly reduced intracellularly. Interestingly, activation of the HIF transcription factor during ischemia also increases expression of the GLUT-1 transporter [117], and this may be a mechanism to bolster ascorbate, as well as glucose, for energy metabolism. Ascorbate oxidation can substantially increase DHA levels allowing vitamin C accumulation in various cell types, and this may be important to its antioxidant function [120]. Thus, large amounts of ascorbate can be made available during an inflammation response, e.g., phagocytic cells undergoing respiratory burst, to balance ROS production. However, genetic polymorphisms in human vitamin C transport genes affect plasma ascorbate levels, and hence disease risk and individuals with low dietary intake may be more susceptible to the effects of genetic variation [121].

Whether ascorbate performs antioxidant roles in vivo is largely unproven. Its clinical use is restricted to prevention of scurvy and promoting intestinal non-heme iron absorption, though it is currently being investigated as a pro-drug in cancer [117]. Epidemiological studies consistently show that low plasma ascorbate levels are associated with increased chronic disease risk, though vitamin C supplementation is yet to show definitive benefits [122]. Low plasma vitamin C is a risk factor for mortality and adverse cardiovascular events in hemodialysis patients [123], and AKI co-morbidities, such as diabetes, are associated with vitamin C deficiency [124]. The renal system is important in vitamin C re-absorption [125], and impairment may affect plasma ascorbate levels. Patients with renal dysfunction, such as septic, critically ill, and elderly, demonstrate low ascorbate levels [119], and bolstering vitamin C intake may prevent ROS-mediated renal damage in AKI.

4.1. Evidence for Vitamin C Efficacy in Animal Models of AKI and Proposed Actions

4.1.1. Vitamin C and Nephrotoxicity

Animal studies consistently show efficacy of vitamin C supplementation in nephrotoxic AKI by reducing ROS and inflammation damage [7]. This positive benefit on renal function is predominantly attributed to its antioxidant function and ability to reduce ROS arising from the initial toxic insult and/or secondary wave ROS induced by inflammation (Table 1). Vitamin C also appears to maintain GSH [126]. A large analysis of pre-clinical studies of aminoglycoside antibiotic-induced nephrotoxic AKI showed that both natural and synthetic compounds, including vitamin C with attributed antioxidant activity, are reno-protective [127]. Vitamin C also protects against NSAID-induced AKI in rats by improving kidney function and renal lesions, serum oxidative stress, and tissue inflammation, comparatively to vitamin E administration [89]. It is also protective against nickel-induced toxicity in mice, by improving renal function, inflammation and renal tubular degeneration, and necrosis [128]. This finding supports earlier evidence of decreased nickel-induced oxidative stress in other organ systems with ascorbate [129]. Interestingly, vitamin C supplementation reduces nickel accumulation in the kidney [128], suggesting benefit independent of ROS scavenging.

Ascorbate also improves RM-induced renal injury in animal models (Table 1). Thus, rats administered a bolus of vitamin C intraperitoneally immediately after RM induction, showed significant reductions in kidney tissue lipid peroxidation, increased antioxidant enzymes, and reduced tissue iron content and tubular necrosis [85]. Yet, no significant improvements to renal function were observed. This may be partially explained by the low dose of vitamin C chosen. However, studies in our lab have similarly demonstrated a lack of amelioration of AKI with antioxidant (synthetic polyphenol, vitamin E, selenium) supplementation in animal models of RM, despite ameliorating oxidative stress and decreasing biomarkers of inflammation, together suggesting that oxidative stress may not be causally related to renal dysfunction [76,130]. We recently compared treatment with vitamin C or the synthetic polyphenol tert-butyl-bisphenol (3,3′,5,5′-tetratert-butyl-biphenyl-4,4′-diol) in a murine model of RM-induced AKI [77]. Tert-butyl-bisphenol shows antioxidant activity similar to ascorbate, and inhibits Mb-induced renal cell dysfunction in vitro [131]. Both ascorbate and tert-butyl-bisphenol comparatively decreased plasma and kidney oxidative markers, inflammation and tissue kinase activity (Table 1) when administered alone or in combination [77]. However, only vitamin C showed potential clinical benefit and reduced proteinuria, plasma urate and renal tubule casts. This data suggests that antioxidants with enhanced water solubility, such as ascorbate, may prevent intratubule obstruction and tubular epithelial cell damage by Mb casts or urate crystals. Alternatively, ascorbate may exhibit protective activities adjunct to its ROS scavenging/antioxidant activity [77]. Vitamin C can positively affect endothelium function and exert anti-inflammatory actions, and anti-inflammation and vasoprotective therapies attenuate RM-induced AKI [8].

In addition to the above, ascorbate displays a multifunctional antioxidant role in animal models of cell-free hemoglobin exchange to prevent heme protein-mediated oxidative stress in vivo [132]. Thus, EPR spectroscopic studies show that ascorbate scavenges globin-centered radicals and reduces plasma methemoglobin (metHb, Fe^{3+}) and ferryl hemoglobin (Fe^{4+}-oxo), to remove the potential for ROS formation from peroxide/redox active heme-peroxidase reactions. Erythrocytes promote reduction of metHb by rapid recycling of ascorbate from ascorbyl radical. These antioxidant actions of ascorbate in plasma and whole blood may be relevant in reducing kidney damage when large amounts of heme proteins are released into extracellular spaces, such as in trauma and RM-induced AKI [132].

4.1.2. Vitamin C and I/R-Induced AKI

Vitamin C supplementation is also associated with improvements in I/R-induced AKI, again, largely associated with ROS scavenging and improved antioxidant status. Thus, vitamin C administration improved plasma levels of antioxidant enzymes in a model of canine renal allograft [133,134], and reduced renal lipid oxidation and reversed loss of GSH in rat renal I/R [81]. The latter study demonstrated cytoprotective and antioxidant efficacy within a short period of I/R, and with one bolus dose of vitamin C pre-ischemia, suggesting that it may be beneficial and practical in defined elective procedures, such as renal transplantation. A renal ischemic injury study in mice also showed improved kidney function and decreased tubule cell injury with vitamin C pretreatment that was associated with decreased renal lipid oxidation and improved SOD and GSH levels [84]. In this study, vitamin C also significantly improved kidney NO• levels and in vivo arterial resistance and vascular reactivity of excised renal arteries, indicating that ascorbate protects vascular function by direct ROS scavenging, and/or via up-regulation of SOD, to prevent renal injury.

Ascorbate is an electron donor for peptide alpha-amidating monooxygenases responsible for steroid and peptide hormone stability and activity. It is involved in progesterone biosynthesis [135], and progesterone shows similar antioxidant and anti-inflammatory activities to ascorbate in several diseases, including I/R-induced AKI. For example, progesterone mitigates oxidative stress and inflammation, and up-regulates antioxidant enzymes, and improves renal function in an animal model of renal I/R [87]. Interestingly, antagonism of progesterone receptors in male rats exposed to renal I/R abolished the antioxidant and anti-inflammation effects of vitamin C, suggesting the involvement of steroid receptors in ascorbate-mediated reno-protection [87].

Acute I/R injury to renal tissue from remote organ damage/surgery can be alleviated by vitamin C. Thus, renal ischemia injury in rats induced by abdominal aortic surgery that increased plasma and tissue lipid oxidation and acute inflammation, was attenuated with vitamin C, similarly, or more effectively, than a synthetic prostaglandin (PGI₂) analogue (Iloprost) [88]. PGI₂ inhibits platelet activation and is an effective vasodilator, and Iloprost is used clinically for pulmonary hypertension and ischemia. Thus, vitamin C's ability to inhibit lipid peroxidation and reduce inflammation, may prevent platelet aggregation and leukocyte adhesion [88]. Indeed, an earlier study showed that vitamin C decreases venous blood platelet activating factor (PAF) and PAF-like lipids during reperfusion after renal I/R in rabbits and rats [136]. PAF is a potent phospholipid activator of vascular and immune responses, and is up-regulated in pathological conditions, and some lipid oxidation products have PAF-like activity. The decrease in PAF activity was associated with decreased inflammation (specifically MPO activity) and DNA oxidation, and amelioration of kidney dysfunction and tubulointerstitial damage, suggesting that ascorbate can intervene in the oxidative-inflammatory response in I/R. In another study, vitamin C reduced lipid oxidation, inflammation and kidney injury, and partially improved renal oxygen delivery and consumption [83]. Despite these positive effects, vitamin C had no effect on kidney hemodynamics and urine output, reminiscent of other studies where antioxidants improve renal oxidative stress, damage or inflammation but do not improve kidney function [77].

4.1.3. Positive Effects of Vitamin C on Endothelial Function and Vascular Tone in Renal Injury

Ascorbate is vaso-protective of endothelium function, and this may be important in renal injury. Several mechanisms have been proposed, including enhancing NO• bioavailability by up-regulating eNOS, and/or increasing its activity independently of, or via, maintaining tetrahydrobiopterin (BH₄) [137]. Ascorbate may also maintain vessel integrity via scavenging ROS/antioxidant activity, preventing injury and/or inflammation, or via its other known physiological role as a co-factor of hydroxylase enzymes important in vascular structure/function [120]. Some animal AKI studies have compared the effect of L-arginine (NO donor) and vitamin C supplementation on biomarkers of lipid, DNA and protein oxidation, and kidney function, and have demonstrated superior protection afforded by vitamin C [86,138]. These improvements in renal function and oxidative stress markers in I/R-induced AKI in rats, may involve NO/soluble guanylyl cyclase (cGC), as inhibitors of this pathway (L-NAME and methylene blue) reduced the reno-protective effects of vitamin C [82]. Further, ascorbate increased tissue GSH and nitrate/nitrite levels, suggesting a preservation of NO• levels. Chemical NO• donors similarly reduce renal I/R in animal studies [6].

In addition to ischemia, vitamin C shows benefit in animal models of sepsis by improving edema, vascular tone, blood flow and pressure, platelet adhesion, coagulation, and survival [139]. The proposed mechanisms include decreased ROS/RNS, NOX, iNOS, and improved pro-inflammatory markers and GSH [119]. Vitamin C may be therapeutic in sepsis via NO• maintenance, as alleviation of septic symptoms and improved capillary blood flow observed with ascorbate injection or BH₄ superfusion is not evident in eNOS knockout mice [139]. Ascorbate can also stimulate eNOS activity in experimental sepsis via modulation of phosphorylation status, whereas other antioxidants such as NAc and trolox do not exhibit this activity [140]. Additionally, ascorbate may prevent endothelial barrier dysfunction in sepsis by modulating NOX derived ROS and peroxynitrite generation, thereby protecting the distribution of the endothelial tight junction protein occludin [140].

It is noteworthy that most mammals synthesise vitamin C de novo, and therefore, the overwhelming majority of vitamin C intervention studies that show benefit in animal AKI are performed on species (rats and mice) that are not deficient. This may suggest that endogenous levels of vitamin C are compromised in severe ischemic, nephrotoxic and/or injurious AKI, and that renal reabsorption is important in maintaining systemic vitamin C. Alternatively, vitamin C biosynthesis, that depends on adequate nutrient supply and liver function, may also be perturbed in these injury models.

4.2. Antioxidant Therapy in Human Renal Injury

AKI causes a high incidence of morbidity and mortality. Preventing AKI largely involves attempts to mitigate the inducing drug/injury/illness and renal replacement therapy (dialysis) to remove fluid overload and uremia, balance electrolytes, and correct metabolic acidosis. Addressing imbalances in nutrient-derived antioxidants, such as vitamin C, particularly after traumatic injury and in critically ill and elderly patients that show depletion of plasma antioxidants, may prevent renal injury [119,140].

Despite data showing positive benefit of antioxidants in animal models of AKI and renal injury, translation of antioxidant therapy to human studies has been of limited success. Thus, Nac has undergone several trials, but has proved largely inconclusive in alleviating CI- and other AKI [75] or chronic kidney disease [5]. It does however show some benefit in end stage renal disease and kidney transplantation. Vitamin E shows contrasting effects, either reducing chronic kidney disease risk, or displaying no benefit [5]. A clinical trial of the Nrf2 pathway enhancer bardoxolone methyl on end stage renal disease among type 2 diabetes patients and chronic kidney disease, was halted because of increased mortality (cardiovascular events) in the treatment arm [141].

4.2.1. Reno-Protection in CI-AKI

In comparison to other antioxidants, vitamin C does appear to mitigate microvascular dysfunction and renal failure in I/R and sepsis. For example, vitamin C shows promising reno-protection in AKI [5,75]. Several controlled human studies have been now been performed with vitamin C supplementation prior, during, or post contrast dye procedures, usually coronary angiography or percutaneous coronary intervention. Although some studies included patients with existing renal dysfunction, recent meta-analyses show overall benefit of vitamin C in preventing CI-AKI compared to placebo or normal saline hydration [142,143]. An exact mechanism of reno-protection by ascorbate cannot be delineated from these analyses due to lack of available biochemical data. However, it is suggested that antioxidant ROS scavenging and vascular protection may predominate, largely based on animal studies of nephrotoxic AKI, and a human study showing that vitamin C exerted a positive change in total antioxidant status immediately after drug administration, and at follow-up [144]. Although a further recent study failed to show benefit of a standard dose of intravenous vitamin C in preventing CI-AKI in patients with chronic renal insufficiency, a post hoc analysis of the data did support a reduced rate of CI-AKI in patients with mildly impaired renal function [145].

4.2.2. Benefit in Critical Illness and Sepsis

As well as providing benefit in cardiac surgery patients, vitamin C appears to benefit critically ill subjects with reduced new organ failure, ventilation, and/or time in ICU. In these studies, vitamin C was typically administered in combination with other micronutrients, vitamins E/B1, and/or selenium, so that its precise role was obscured [119,139]. However, in severe burn patients, a very high parenteral dose of vitamin C significantly reduced fluid requirements and improved urinary output, suggesting that early administration of vitamin C alone may improve morbidity in burn-induced shock [119]. Also, a recent phase I study of the safety of pharmacological doses of parenteral vitamin C, demonstrated significantly reduced multiple organ failure and pro-inflammation biomarkers in severe sepsis [146]. Low plasma vitamin C is common in patients with traumatic and critical illness, including sepsis and after cardiac surgery, and high intravenous dosages may be required to restore adequacy [119]. In a recent observational study of sepsis, early use of a combination of intravenous vitamin C, hydrocortisone, and thiamine, significantly reduced AKI, mortality, and progressive organ failure in septic patients [147]. In this study, vitamin C and hydrocortisone were proposed to act synergistically to preserve endothelium integrity and improve clinical outcomes.

Previous human studies relevant to renal injury support vitamin C producing beneficial effects on endothelium function. For example, a high intra-arterial dose of vitamin C improves endothelial-dependent vasodilatation after I/R injury and endotoxemia [148,149]. Also, vitamin C improves endothelium function and serum lipid oxidation in renal allograft transplant patients [150]. High-dose vitamin C supplementation in severe sepsis and shock may also positively benefit endogenous vasopressor synthesis via hydroxylase and monooxygenase enzymes that require ascorbate as a co-factor [151]. Vasopressors such as norepinephrine and vasopressin are important in regulating blood pressure and renal water retention in critically ill patients. An observational trial of vitamin C/hydrocortisone/thiamine supplementation in sepsis reported significant reduction in the use of vasopressors in patients receiving vitamin C [147].

Thus, in accordance with pre-clinical studies, vitamin C appears to be protective in pathologies relevant to human AKI via preserving endothelium and vascular function. Whether this benefit is attributed to direct ROS scavenging, or involves non-antioxidant functions, remains to be defined, but is important as ascorbate is a co-factor of various hydroxylase enzymes involved in vascular wall integrity and cell signaling processes. Regarding the latter, ascorbate controls HIF-1 activity by stabilizing its regulator prolyl hydroxylase, via maintaining the active site iron in a reduced (active) state. HIF-1 is a pro-survival transcription factor activated by limited oxygen, metabolic disturbance and oxidative stress, and may be important in preventing AKI via ischemic pre-conditioning [113]. However, over-activation of HIF-1 may be maladaptive in some pathologies [152] as intermittent hypoxia can mediate chronic ischemia-induced NOX expression to generate persistently elevated oxidative stress. Further, iNOS and some pro-inflammatory cytokines are activated by HIF-1 and NO$^\bullet$ can induce HIF-1 under non-limiting oxygen conditions (normoxia) such as inflammation [139,152]. Whether over-activation of HIF-1 contributes to renal injury in sepsis is largely unknown, however, ascorbate inhibits iNOS expression and activity in microvascular endothelial cells in vitro and in animal models of sepsis [140]. Thus, part of the mechanism whereby ascorbate shows efficacy in sepsis may also be via suppression of HIF-1-dependent genes.

Overall, whilst ROS and oxidative stress are closely linked to AKI, and this maybe a mechanism whereby ascorbate, as an antioxidant, intervenes, non-antioxidant bioactivities of vitamin C in immune and vascular function may contribute to its therapeutic action in renal injury and disease. Further studies are warranted to determine optimal dose and route of administration, as well as timing, e.g., in ischemic pre-conditioning, and to establish whether ascorbate supplementation is beneficial in cohorts with low vitamin C status, and if so, the precise mechanism of action.

5. Conclusions and Limitations

Despite advances in knowledge and treatment, AKI patients continue to have high mortality and morbidity, especially those with chronic medical conditions. Pre-clinical studies show that antioxidants alleviate renal injury and improve kidney function via reducing oxidative damage and/or inflammation, though several therapeutic antioxidants have largely failed to show benefit in human AKI. Vitamin C does appear to be efficacious in AKI in pathologies with endothelium dysfunction, or where low vitamin C predominates. The reno-protective effects of ascorbate may derive from its known antioxidant activity in scavenging source and derived ROS, including non-radical oxidants, and/or maintaining GSH for peroxidase activity, or BH_4 for eNOS function. Ascorbate may also preserve vascular structure and microcirculatory flow independent of antioxidant function, via maintenance of Fe^{2+} and Cu^+-containing hydroxylase and monooxygenase enzymes. The latter are essential in collagen and vasopressin synthesis central to vascular structure and functionality, and also modulate redox activated signaling pathways, such as HIF-1, down-regulating genes involved in pro-inflammation. Vitamin C shows promise as a reno-protectant in kidney injury, however, whether this is via its physiological role as an enzyme co-factor, or its recognized biochemical activity as an antioxidant, or both, remains to be fully defined.

Acknowledgments: The authors acknowledge funding from the Australian Research Council (DP0878559 and DP160102063 Discovery grants awarded to PKW).

Conflicts of Interest: The authors declare no conflict of interest.

References

1. Bellomo, R.; Kellum, J.A.; Ronco, C. Acute kidney injury. *Lancet* **2012**, *380*, 756–766. [CrossRef]
2. Coca, S.G.; Singanamala, S.; Parikh, C.R. Chronic kidney disease after acute kidney injury: A systematic review and meta-analysis. *Kidney Int.* **2012**, *81*, 442–448. [CrossRef] [PubMed]
3. Basile, D.P.; Anderson, M.D.; Sutton, T.A. Pathophysiology of acute kidney injury. *Compr. Physiol.* **2012**, *2*, 1303–1353. [PubMed]
4. McCord, J.M. Oxygen-derived free radicals in postischemic tissue injury. *N. Engl. J. Med.* **1985**, *312*, 159–163. [PubMed]
5. Ratliff, B.B.; Abdulmahdi, W.; Pawar, R.; Wolin, M.S. Oxidant mechanisms in renal injury and disease. *Antioxid. Redox Signal.* **2016**, *25*, 119–146. [CrossRef] [PubMed]
6. Chatterjee, P.K. Novel pharmacological approaches to the treatment of renal ischemia-reperfusion injury: A comprehensive review. *Naunyn Schmiedebergs Arch. Pharmacol.* **2007**, *376*, 1–43. [CrossRef] [PubMed]
7. Koyner, J.L.; Sher Ali, R.; Murray, P.T. Antioxidants. Do they have a place in the prevention or therapy of acute kidney injury? *Nephron Exp. Nephrol.* **2008**, *109*, e109–e117. [CrossRef] [PubMed]
8. Panizo, N.; Rubio-Navarro, A.; Amaro-Villalobos, J.M.; Egido, J.; Moreno, J.A. Molecular mechanisms and novel therapeutic approaches to rhabdomyolysis-induced acute kidney injury. *Kidney Blood Press. Res.* **2015**, *40*, 520–532. [CrossRef] [PubMed]
9. Paller, M.S.; Hoidal, J.R.; Ferris, T.F. Oxygen free radicals in ischemic acute renal failure in the rat. *J. Clin. Investig.* **1984**, *74*, 1156–1164. [CrossRef] [PubMed]
10. Baliga, R.; Ueda, N.; Walker, P.D.; Shah, S.V. Oxidant mechanisms in toxic acute renal failure. *Drug Metab. Rev.* **1999**, *31*, 971–997. [CrossRef] [PubMed]
11. Himmelfarb, J.; McMonagle, E.; Freedman, S.; Klenzak, J.; McMenamin, E.; Le, P.; Pupim, L.B.; Ikizler, T.A.; The, P.G. Oxidative stress is increased in critically ill patients with acute renal failure. *J. Am. Soc. Nephrol.* **2004**, *15*, 2449–2456. [CrossRef] [PubMed]
12. Himmelfarb, J.; Stenvinkel, P.; Ikizler, T.A.; Hakim, R.M. The elephant in uremia: Oxidant stress as a unifying concept of cardiovascular disease in uremia. *Kidney Int.* **2002**, *62*, 1524–1538. [CrossRef] [PubMed]
13. Thadhani, R.; Pascual, M.; Bonventre, J.V. Acute renal failure. *N. Engl. J. Med.* **1996**, *334*, 1448–1460. [CrossRef] [PubMed]
14. Bonventre, J.V.; Yang, L. Cellular pathophysiology of ischemic acute kidney injury. *J. Clin. Investig.* **2011**, *121*, 4210–4221. [CrossRef] [PubMed]
15. Araujo, M.; Welch, W.J. Oxidative stress and nitric oxide in kidney function. *Curr. Opin. Nephrol. Hypertens.* **2006**, *15*, 72–77. [CrossRef] [PubMed]
16. Andrades, M.E.; Morina, A.; Spasic, S.; Spasojevic, I. Bench-to-bedside review: Sepsis—From the redox point of view. *Crit. Care* **2011**, *15*, 230. [CrossRef] [PubMed]
17. Paller, M.S.; Hedlund, B.E. Role of iron in postischemic renal injury in the rat. *Kidney Int.* **1988**, *34*, 474–480. [CrossRef] [PubMed]
18. Noiri, E.; Nakao, A.; Uchida, K.; Tsukahara, H.; Ohno, M.; Fujita, T.; Brodsky, S.; Goligorsky, M.S. Oxidative and nitrosative stress in acute renal ischemia. *Am. J. Physiol. Ren. Physiol.* **2001**, *281*, F948–F957. [CrossRef]
19. Walker, L.M.; York, J.L.; Imam, S.Z.; Ali, S.F.; Muldrew, K.L.; Mayeux, P.R. Oxidative stress and reactive nitrogen species generation during renal ischemia. *Toxicol. Sci.* **2001**, *63*, 143–148. [CrossRef] [PubMed]
20. Brealey, D.; Brand, M.; Hargreaves, I.; Heales, S.; Land, J.; Smolenski, R.; Davies, N.A.; Cooper, C.E.; Singer, M. Association between mitochondrial dysfunction and severity and outcome of septic shock. *Lancet* **2002**, *360*, 219–223. [CrossRef]
21. Radi, R. Peroxynitrite, a stealthy biological oxidant. *J. Biol. Chem.* **2013**, *288*, 26464–26472. [CrossRef] [PubMed]
22. Witting, P.K.; Willhite, C.A.; Davies, M.J.; Stocker, R. Lipid oxidation in human low-density lipoprotein induced by metmyoglobin/H_2O_2: Involvement of alpha-tocopheroxyl and phosphatidylcholine alkoxyl radicals. *Chem. Res. Toxicol.* **1999**, *12*, 1173–1181. [CrossRef] [PubMed]
23. Reeder, B.J. The redox activity of hemoglobins: From physiologic functions to pathologic mechanisms. *Antioxid. Redox Signal.* **2010**, *13*, 1087–1123. [CrossRef] [PubMed]

24. Moore, K.P.; Holt, S.G.; Patel, R.P.; Svistunenko, D.A.; Zackert, W.; Goodier, D.; Reeder, B.J.; Clozel, M.; Anand, R.; Cooper, C.E.; et al. A causative role for redox cycling of myoglobin and its inhibition by alkalinization in the pathogenesis and treatment of rhabdomyolysis-induced renal failure. *J. Biol. Chem.* **1998**, *273*, 31731–31737. [CrossRef] [PubMed]

25. Boutaud, O.; Roberts, L.J., II. Mechanism-based therapeutic approaches to rhabdomyolysis-induced renal failure. *Free Radic. Biol. Med.* **2011**, *51*, 1062–1067. [CrossRef] [PubMed]

26. Perazella, M.A.; Moeckel, G.W. Nephrotoxicity from chemotherapeutic agents: Clinical manifestations, pathobiology, and prevention/therapy. *Semin. Nephrol.* **2010**, *30*, 570–581. [CrossRef] [PubMed]

27. Chirino, Y.I.; Pedraza-Chaverri, J. Role of oxidative and nitrosative stress in cisplatin-induced nephrotoxicity. *Exp. Toxicol. Pathol.* **2009**, *61*, 223–242. [CrossRef] [PubMed]

28. Yilmaz, M.I.; Saglam, M.; Caglar, K.; Cakir, E.; Sonmez, A.; Ozgurtas, T.; Aydin, A.; Eyileten, T.; Ozcan, O.; Acikel, C.; et al. The determinants of endothelial dysfunction in CKD: Oxidative stress and asymmetric dimethylarginine. *Am. J. Kidney Dis.* **2006**, *47*, 42–50. [CrossRef] [PubMed]

29. Hirayama, A.; Nagase, S.; Ueda, A.; Oteki, T.; Takada, K.; Obara, M.; Inoue, M.; Yoh, K.; Hirayama, K.; Koyama, A. In vivo imaging of oxidative stress in ischemia-reperfusion renal injury using electron paramagnetic resonance. *Am. J. Physiol. Ren. Physiol.* **2005**, *288*, F597–F603. [CrossRef] [PubMed]

30. Hall, A.M.; Rhodes, G.J.; Sandoval, R.M.; Corridon, P.R.; Molitoris, B.A. In vivo multiphoton imaging of mitochondrial structure and function during acute kidney injury. *Kidney Int.* **2013**, *83*, 72–83. [CrossRef] [PubMed]

31. Holt, S.; Reeder, B.; Wilson, M.; Harvey, S.; Morrow, J.D.; Roberts, L.J., II; Moore, K. Increased lipid peroxidation in patients with rhabdomyolysis. *Lancet* **1999**, *353*, 1241. [CrossRef]

32. Dounousi, E.; Papavasiliou, E.; Makedou, A.; Ioannou, K.; Katopodis, K.P.; Tselepis, A.; Siamopoulos, K.C.; Tsakiris, D. Oxidative stress is progressively enhanced with advancing stages of CKD. *Am. J. Kidney Dis.* **2006**, *48*, 752–760. [CrossRef] [PubMed]

33. Ware, L.B.; Fessel, J.P.; May, A.K.; Roberts, L.J., II. Plasma biomarkers of oxidant stress and development of organ failure in severe sepsis. *Shock* **2011**, *36*, 12–17. [CrossRef] [PubMed]

34. Billings, F.T., IV; Ball, S.K.; Roberts, L.J., II; Pretorius, M. Postoperative acute kidney injury is associated with hemoglobinemia and an enhanced oxidative stress response. *Free Radic. Biol. Med.* **2011**, *50*, 1480–1487. [CrossRef] [PubMed]

35. Gamboa, J.L.; Billings, F.T., IV; Bojanowski, M.T.; Gilliam, L.A.; Yu, C.; Roshanravan, B.; Roberts, L.J., II; Himmelfarb, J.; Ikizler, T.A.; Brown, N.J. Mitochondrial dysfunction and oxidative stress in patients with chronic kidney disease. *Physiol. Rep.* **2016**, *4*, e12780. [CrossRef] [PubMed]

36. Holmstrom, K.M.; Finkel, T. Cellular mechanisms and physiological consequences of redox-dependent signalling. *Nat. Rev. Mol. Cell. Biol.* **2014**, *15*, 411–421. [CrossRef] [PubMed]

37. Day, B.J. Antioxidant therapeutics: Pandora's box. *Free Radic. Biol. Med.* **2014**, *66*, 58–64. [CrossRef] [PubMed]

38. Winterbourn, C.C. Reconciling the chemistry and biology of reactive oxygen species. *Nat. Chem. Biol.* **2008**, *4*, 278–286. [CrossRef] [PubMed]

39. Forman, H.J.; Davies, K.J.; Ursini, F. How do nutritional antioxidants really work: Nucleophilic tone and para-hormesis versus free radical scavenging in vivo. *Free Radic. Biol. Med.* **2014**, *66*, 24–35. [CrossRef] [PubMed]

40. Shah, S.V.; Walker, P.D. Evidence suggesting a role for hydroxyl radical in glycerol-induced acute renal failure. *Am. J. Physiol.* **1988**, *255*, F438–F443. [PubMed]

41. Paller, M.S. Hemoglobin- and myoglobin-induced acute renal failure in rats: Role of iron in nephrotoxicity. *Am. J. Physiol.* **1988**, *255*, F539–F544. [PubMed]

42. Zager, R.A. Combined mannitol and deferoxamine therapy for myohemoglobinuric renal injury and oxidant tubular stress. Mechanistic and therapeutic implications. *J. Clin. Investig.* **1992**, *90*, 711–719. [CrossRef] [PubMed]

43. Baliga, R.; Zhang, Z.; Baliga, M.; Shah, S.V. Evidence for cytochrome p-450 as a source of catalytic iron in myoglobinuric acute renal failure. *Kidney Int.* **1996**, *49*, 362–369. [CrossRef] [PubMed]

44. Baliga, R.; Zhang, Z.; Baliga, M.; Ueda, N.; Shah, S.V. Role of cytochrome p-450 as a source of catalytic iron in cisplatin-induced nephrotoxicity. *Kidney Int.* **1998**, *54*, 1562–1569. [CrossRef] [PubMed]

45. Wang, Z.; Shah, S.V.; Liu, H.; Baliga, R. Inhibition of cytochrome p450 2e1 and activation of transcription factor nrf2 are renoprotective in myoglobinuric acute kidney injury. *Kidney Int.* **2014**, *86*, 338–349. [CrossRef] [PubMed]

46. Davies, S.J.; Reichardt-Pascal, S.Y.; Vaughan, D.; Russell, G.I. Differential effect of ischaemia-reperfusion injury on anti-oxidant enzyme activity in the rat kidney. *Exp. Nephrol.* **1995**, *3*, 348–354. [PubMed]

47. Yamanobe, T.; Okada, F.; Iuchi, Y.; Onuma, K.; Tomita, Y.; Fujii, J. Deterioration of ischemia/reperfusion-induced acute renal failure in sod1-deficient mice. *Free Radic. Res.* **2007**, *41*, 200–207. [CrossRef] [PubMed]

48. Son, D.; Kojima, I.; Inagi, R.; Matsumoto, M.; Fujita, T.; Nangaku, M. Chronic hypoxia aggravates renal injury via suppression of Cu/Zn-SOD: A proteomic analysis. *Am. J. Physiol. Ren. Physiol.* **2008**, *294*, F62–F72. [CrossRef] [PubMed]

49. Kim, J.; Seok, Y.M.; Jung, K.J.; Park, K.M. Reactive oxygen species/oxidative stress contributes to progression of kidney fibrosis following transient ischemic injury in mice. *Am. J. Physiol. Ren. Physiol.* **2009**, *297*, F461–F470. [CrossRef] [PubMed]

50. Heumuller, S.; Wind, S.; Barbosa-Sicard, E.; Schmidt, H.H.; Busse, R.; Schroder, K.; Brandes, R.P. Apocynin is not an inhibitor of vascular nadph oxidases but an antioxidant. *Hypertension* **2008**, *51*, 211–217. [CrossRef] [PubMed]

51. Mukhopadhyay, P.; Horvath, B.; Zsengeller, Z.; Zielonka, J.; Tanchian, G.; Holovac, E.; Kechrid, M.; Patel, V.; Stillman, I.E.; Parikh, S.M.; et al. Mitochondrial-targeted antioxidants represent a promising approach for prevention of cisplatin-induced nephropathy. *Free Radic. Biol. Med.* **2012**, *52*, 497–506. [CrossRef] [PubMed]

52. Duan, S.B.; Yang, S.K.; Zhou, Q.Y.; Pan, P.; Zhang, H.; Liu, F.; Xu, X.Q. Mitochondria-targeted peptides prevent on contrast-induced acute kidney injury in the rats with hypercholesterolemia. *Ren. Fail.* **2013**, *35*, 1124–1129. [CrossRef] [PubMed]

53. Perianayagam, M.C.; Liangos, O.; Kolyada, A.Y.; Wald, R.; MacKinnon, R.W.; Li, L.; Rao, M.; Balakrishnan, V.S.; Bonventre, J.V.; Pereira, B.J.; et al. Nadph oxidase p22phox and catalase gene variants are associated with biomarkers of oxidative stress and adverse outcomes in acute renal failure. *J. Am. Soc. Nephrol.* **2007**, *18*, 255–263. [CrossRef] [PubMed]

54. Prieto-Moure, B.; Lloris-Carsi, J.M.; Belda-Antoli, M.; Toledo-Pereyra, L.H.; Cejalvo-Lapena, D. Allopurinol protective effect of renal ischemia by downregulating TNF-alpha, IL-1beta, and IL-6 response. *J. Investig. Surg.* **2017**, *30*, 143–151. [CrossRef] [PubMed]

55. Gois, P.H.; Canale, D.; Volpini, R.A.; Ferreira, D.; Veras, M.M.; Andrade-Oliveira, V.; Camara, N.O.; Shimizu, M.H.; Seguro, A.C. Allopurinol attenuates rhabdomyolysis-associated acute kidney injury: Renal and muscular protection. *Free Radic. Biol. Med.* **2016**, *101*, 176–189. [CrossRef] [PubMed]

56. George, J.; Carr, E.; Davies, J.; Belch, J.J.; Struthers, A. High-dose allopurinol improves endothelial function by profoundly reducing vascular oxidative stress and not by lowering uric acid. *Circulation* **2006**, *114*, 2508–2516. [CrossRef] [PubMed]

57. Yelken, B.; Caliskan, Y.; Gorgulu, N.; Altun, I.; Yilmaz, A.; Yazici, H.; Oflaz, H.; Yildiz, A. Reduction of uric acid levels with allopurinol treatment improves endothelial function in patients with chronic kidney disease. *Clin. Nephrol.* **2012**, *77*, 275–282. [CrossRef] [PubMed]

58. Choi, E.K.; Jung, H.; Kwak, K.H.; Yeo, J.; Yi, S.J.; Park, C.Y.; Ryu, T.H.; Jeon, Y.H.; Park, K.M.; Lim, D.G. Effects of allopurinol and apocynin on renal ischemia-reperfusion injury in rats. *Transplant. Proc.* **2015**, *47*, 1633–1638. [CrossRef] [PubMed]

59. Altintas, R.; Polat, A.; Vardi, N.; Oguz, F.; Beytur, A.; Sagir, M.; Yildiz, A.; Parlakpinar, H. The protective effects of apocynin on kidney damage caused by renal ischemia/reperfusion. *J. Endourol.* **2013**, *27*, 617–624. [CrossRef] [PubMed]

60. Tabara, L.C.; Poveda, J.; Martin-Cleary, C.; Selgas, R.; Ortiz, A.; Sanchez-Nino, M.D. Mitochondria-targeted therapies for acute kidney injury. *Expert Rev. Mol. Med.* **2014**, *16*, e13. [CrossRef] [PubMed]

61. Dare, A.J.; Bolton, E.A.; Pettigrew, G.J.; Bradley, J.A.; Saeb-Parsy, K.; Murphy, M.P. Protection against renal ischemia-reperfusion injury in vivo by the mitochondria targeted antioxidant mitoq. *Redox Biol.* **2015**, *5*, 163–168. [CrossRef] [PubMed]

62. Eiserich, J.P.; Baldus, S.; Brennan, M.L.; Ma, W.; Zhang, C.; Tousson, A.; Castro, L.; Lusis, A.J.; Nauseef, W.M.; White, C.R.; et al. Myeloperoxidase, a leukocyte-derived vascular no oxidase. *Science* **2002**, *296*, 2391–2394. [CrossRef] [PubMed]

63. Yaqoob, M.; Edelstein, C.L.; Schrier, R.W. Role of nitric oxide and superoxide balance in hypoxia-reoxygenation proximal tubular injury. *Nephrol. Dial. Transplant.* **1996**, *11*, 1738–1742. [CrossRef] [PubMed]

64. Thomas, D.D.; Heinecke, J.L.; Ridnour, L.A.; Cheng, R.Y.; Kesarwala, A.H.; Switzer, C.H.; McVicar, D.W.; Roberts, D.D.; Glynn, S.; Fukuto, J.M.; et al. Signaling and stress: The redox landscape in NOS2 biology. *Free Radic. Biol. Med.* **2015**, *87*, 204–225. [CrossRef] [PubMed]

65. Ling, H.; Edelstein, C.; Gengaro, P.; Meng, X.; Lucia, S.; Knotek, M.; Wangsiripaisan, A.; Shi, Y.; Schrier, R. Attenuation of renal ischemia-reperfusion injury in inducible nitric oxide synthase knockout mice. *Am. J. Physiol.* **1999**, *277*, F383–F390. [PubMed]

66. Noiri, E.; Peresleni, T.; Miller, F.; Goligorsky, M.S. In vivo targeting of inducible no synthase with oligodeoxynucleotides protects rat kidney against ischemia. *J. Clin. Investig.* **1996**, *97*, 2377–2383. [CrossRef] [PubMed]

67. Wu, L.; Mayeux, P.R. Effects of the inducible nitric-oxide synthase inhibitor L-n(6)-(1-iminoethyl)-lysine on microcirculation and reactive nitrogen species generation in the kidney following lipopolysaccharide administration in mice. *J. Pharmacol. Exp. Ther.* **2007**, *320*, 1061–1067. [CrossRef] [PubMed]

68. Wu, L.; Gokden, N.; Mayeux, P.R. Evidence for the role of reactive nitrogen species in polymicrobial sepsis-induced renal peritubular capillary dysfunction and tubular injury. *J. Am. Soc. Nephrol.* **2007**, *18*, 1807–1815. [CrossRef] [PubMed]

69. Kikuchi, K.; Takeshige, N.; Miura, N.; Morimoto, Y.; Ito, T.; Tancharoen, S.; Miyata, K.; Kikuchi, C.; Iida, N.; Uchikado, H.; et al. Beyond free radical scavenging: Beneficial effects of edaravone (radicut) in various diseases (review). *Exp. Ther. Med.* **2012**, *3*, 3–8. [PubMed]

70. Doi, K.; Suzuki, Y.; Nakao, A.; Fujita, T.; Noiri, E. Radical scavenger edaravone developed for clinical use ameliorates ischemia/reperfusion injury in rat kidney. *Kidney Int.* **2004**, *65*, 1714–1723. [CrossRef] [PubMed]

71. Satoh, M.; Kashihara, N.; Fujimoto, S.; Horike, H.; Tokura, T.; Namikoshi, T.; Sasaki, T.; Makino, H. A novel free radical scavenger, edarabone, protects against cisplatin-induced acute renal damage in vitro and in vivo. *J. Pharmacol. Exp. Ther.* **2003**, *305*, 1183–1190. [CrossRef] [PubMed]

72. Matsuyama, M.; Hayama, T.; Funao, K.; Tsuchida, K.; Takemoto, Y.; Sugimura, K.; Kawahito, Y.; Sano, H.; Nakatani, T.; Yoshimura, R. Treatment with edaravone improves the survival rate in renal warm ischemia-reperfusion injury using rat model. *Transplant. Proc.* **2006**, *38*, 2199–2200. [CrossRef] [PubMed]

73. Tahara, M.; Nakayama, M.; Jin, M.B.; Fujita, M.; Suzuki, T.; Taniguchi, M.; Shimamura, T.; Furukawa, H.; Todo, S. A radical scavenger, edaravone, protects canine kidneys from ischemia-reperfusion injury after 72 hours of cold preservation and autotransplantation. *Transplantation* **2005**, *80*, 213–221. [CrossRef] [PubMed]

74. Kamouchi, M.; Sakai, H.; Kiyohara, Y.; Minematsu, K.; Hayashi, K.; Kitazono, T. Acute kidney injury and edaravone in acute ischemic stroke: The fukuoka stroke registry. *J. Stroke Cerebrovasc. Dis.* **2013**, *22*, e470–e476. [CrossRef] [PubMed]

75. Chalikias, G.; Drosos, I.; Tziakas, D.N. Prevention of contrast-induced acute kidney injury: An update. *Cardiovasc. Drugs Ther.* **2016**, *30*, 515–524. [CrossRef] [PubMed]

76. Shanu, A.; Groebler, L.; Kim, H.B.; Wood, S.; Weekley, C.M.; Aitken, J.B.; Harris, H.H.; Witting, P.K. Selenium inhibits renal oxidation and inflammation but not acute kidney injury in an animal model of rhabdomyolysis. *Antioxid. Redox Signal.* **2013**, *18*, 756–769. [CrossRef] [PubMed]

77. Groebler, L.K.; Wang, X.S.; Kim, H.B.; Shanu, A.; Hossain, F.; McMahon, A.C.; Witting, P.K. Cosupplementation with a synthetic, lipid-soluble polyphenol and vitamin C inhibits oxidative damage and improves vascular function yet does not inhibit acute renal injury in an animal model of rhabdomyolysis. *Free Radic. Biol. Med.* **2012**, *52*, 1918–1928. [CrossRef] [PubMed]

78. Paller, M.S. Renal work, glutathione and susceptibility to free radical-mediated postischemic injury. *Kidney Int.* **1988**, *33*, 843–849. [CrossRef] [PubMed]

79. Weinberg, J.M.; Davis, J.A.; Abarzua, M.; Rajan, T. Cytoprotective effects of glycine and glutathione against hypoxic injury to renal tubules. *J. Clin. Investig.* **1987**, *80*, 1446–1454. [CrossRef] [PubMed]

80. Abul-Ezz, S.R.; Walker, P.D.; Shah, S.V. Role of glutathione in an animal model of myoglobinuric acute renal failure. *Proc. Natl. Acad. Sci. USA* **1991**, *88*, 9833–9837. [CrossRef] [PubMed]

81. Korkmaz, A.; Kolankaya, D. The protective effects of ascorbic acid against renal ischemia-reperfusion injury in male rats. *Ren. Fail.* **2009**, *31*, 36–43. [CrossRef] [PubMed]

82. Koul, V.; Kaur, A.; Singh, A.P. Investigation of the role of nitric oxide/soluble guanylyl cyclase pathway in ascorbic acid-mediated protection against acute kidney injury in rats. *Mol. Cell. Biochem.* **2015**, *406*, 1–7. [CrossRef] [PubMed]

83. Ergin, B.; Zuurbier, C.J.; Bezemer, R.; Kandil, A.; Almac, E.; Demirci, C.; Ince, C. Ascorbic acid improves renal microcirculatory oxygenation in a rat model of renal I/R injury. *J. Transl. Int. Med.* **2015**, *3*, 116–125. [CrossRef] [PubMed]

84. Zhu, Y.B.; Zhang, Y.P.; Zhang, J.; Zhang, Y.B. Evaluation of vitamin C supplementation on kidney function and vascular reactivity following renal ischemic injury in mice. *Kidney Blood Press. Res.* **2016**, *41*, 460–470. [CrossRef] [PubMed]

85. Ustundag, S.; Yalcin, O.; Sen, S.; Cukur, Z.; Ciftci, S.; Demirkan, B. Experimental myoglobinuric acute renal failure: The effect of vitamin C. *Ren. Fail.* **2008**, *30*, 727–735. [CrossRef] [PubMed]

86. Mohamed Abd, E.; Lasheen, N.N. Comparative study on the protective role of vitamin C and L-arginine in experimental renal ischemia reperfusion in adult rats. *Int. J. Physiol. Pathophysiol. Pharmacol.* **2014**, *6*, 153–165. [PubMed]

87. Sandhi, J.; Singh, J.P.; Kaur, T.; Ghuman, S.S.; Singh, A.P. Involvement of progesterone receptors in ascorbic acid-mediated protection against ischemia-reperfusion-induced acute kidney injury. *J. Surg. Res.* **2014**, *187*, 278–288. [CrossRef] [PubMed]

88. Ozcan, A.V.; Sacar, M.; Aybek, H.; Bir, F.; Demir, S.; Onem, G.; Goksin, I.; Baltalarli, A.; Colakoglu, N. The effects of iloprost and vitamin C on kidney as a remote organ after ischemia/reperfusion of lower extremities. *J. Surg. Res.* **2007**, *140*, 20–26. [CrossRef] [PubMed]

89. El-Shafei, R.A.; Saleh, R.M. Pharmacological effects of vitamin C & E on diclofenac sodium intoxicated rats. *Biomed. Pharmacother.* **2016**, *84*, 314–322. [PubMed]

90. Stocker, R.; Keaney, J.F., Jr. Role of oxidative modifications in atherosclerosis. *Physiol. Rev.* **2004**, *84*, 1381–1478. [CrossRef] [PubMed]

91. Meister, A. Glutathione-ascorbic acid antioxidant system in animals. *J. Biol. Chem.* **1994**, *269*, 9397–9400. [PubMed]

92. Stocker, R. Antioxidant defenses in human blood plasma and extra-cellular fluids. *Arch. Biochem. Biophys.* **2016**, *595*, 136–139. [CrossRef] [PubMed]

93. Paller, M.S.; Neumann, T.V. Reactive oxygen species and rat renal epithelial cells during hypoxia and reoxygenation. *Kidney Int.* **1991**, *40*, 1041–1049. [CrossRef] [PubMed]

94. Nilsson, U.A.; Haraldsson, G.; Bratell, S.; Sorensen, V.; Akerlund, S.; Pettersson, S.; Schersten, T.; Jonsson, O. ESR-measurement of oxygen radicals in vivo after renal ischaemia in the rabbit. Effects of pre-treatment with superoxide dismutase and heparin. *Acta Physiol. Scand.* **1993**, *147*, 263–270. [CrossRef] [PubMed]

95. Leach, M.; Frank, S.; Olbrich, A.; Pfeilschifter, J.; Thiemermann, C. Decline in the expression of copper/zinc superoxide dismutase in the kidney of rats with endotoxic shock: Effects of the superoxide anion radical scavenger, tempol, on organ injury. *Br. J. Pharmacol.* **1998**, *125*, 817–825. [CrossRef] [PubMed]

96. Wang, Z.; Holthoff, J.H.; Seely, K.A.; Pathak, E.; Spencer, H.J., III; Gokden, N.; Mayeux, P.R. Development of oxidative stress in the peritubular capillary microenvironment mediates sepsis-induced renal microcirculatory failure and acute kidney injury. *Am. J. Pathol.* **2012**, *180*, 505–516. [CrossRef] [PubMed]

97. Chatterjee, P.K.; Cuzzocrea, S.; Brown, P.A.; Zacharowski, K.; Stewart, K.N.; Mota-Filipe, H.; Thiemermann, C. Tempol, a membrane-permeable radical scavenger, reduces oxidant stress-mediated renal dysfunction and injury in the rat. *Kidney Int.* **2000**, *58*, 658–673. [CrossRef] [PubMed]

98. Liang, H.L.; Hilton, G.; Mortensen, J.; Regner, K.; Johnson, C.P.; Nilakantan, V. Mntmpyp, a cell-permeant sod mimetic, reduces oxidative stress and apoptosis following renal ischemia-reperfusion. *Am. J. Physiol. Ren. Physiol.* **2009**, *296*, F266–F276. [CrossRef] [PubMed]

99. Davis, C.A.; Nick, H.S.; Agarwal, A. Manganese superoxide dismutase attenuates cisplatin-induced renal injury: Importance of superoxide. *J. Am. Soc. Nephrol.* **2001**, *12*, 2683–2690. [PubMed]

100. Munusamy, S.; MacMillan-Crow, L.A. Mitochondrial superoxide plays a crucial role in the development of mitochondrial dysfunction during high glucose exposure in rat renal proximal tubular cells. *Free Radic. Biol. Med.* **2009**, *46*, 1149–1157. [CrossRef] [PubMed]

101. Patil, N.K.; Parajuli, N.; MacMillan-Crow, L.A.; Mayeux, P.R. Inactivation of renal mitochondrial respiratory complexes and manganese superoxide dismutase during sepsis: Mitochondria-targeted antioxidant mitigates injury. *Am. J. Physiol. Ren. Physiol.* **2014**, *306*, F734–F743. [CrossRef] [PubMed]

102. Alrabadi, N.; Chami, B.; Kim, H.B.; Maw, A.M.; Dennis, J.M.; Witting, P.K. Hypochlorous acid generated in the heart following acute ischaemic injury promotes myocardial damage: A new target for therapeutic development. *Trends Cell Mol. Biol.* **2014**, *9*, 1–17.

103. Nath, K.A. Heme oxygenase-1 and acute kidney injury. *Curr. Opin. Nephrol. Hypertens.* **2014**, *23*, 17–24. [CrossRef] [PubMed]

104. Nath, K.A.; Balla, G.; Vercellotti, G.M.; Balla, J.; Jacob, H.S.; Levitt, M.D.; Rosenberg, M.E. Induction of heme oxygenase is a rapid, protective response in rhabdomyolysis in the rat. *J. Clin. Investig.* **1992**, *90*, 267–270. [CrossRef] [PubMed]

105. Balla, G.; Vercellotti, G.M.; Muller-Eberhard, U.; Eaton, J.; Jacob, H.S. Exposure of endothelial cells to free heme potentiates damage mediated by granulocytes and toxic oxygen species. *Lab. Investig.* **1991**, *64*, 648–655. [PubMed]

106. Shimizu, H.; Takahashi, T.; Suzuki, T.; Yamasaki, A.; Fujiwara, T.; Odaka, Y.; Hirakawa, M.; Fujita, H.; Akagi, R. Protective effect of heme oxygenase induction in ischemic acute renal failure. *Crit. Care Med.* **2000**, *28*, 809–817. [CrossRef] [PubMed]

107. Shiraishi, F.; Curtis, L.M.; Truong, L.; Poss, K.; Visner, G.A.; Madsen, K.; Nick, H.S.; Agarwal, A. Heme oxygenase-1 gene ablation or expression modulates cisplatin-induced renal tubular apoptosis. *Am. J. Physiol. Ren. Physiol.* **2000**, *278*, F726–F736.

108. Zarjou, A.; Bolisetty, S.; Joseph, R.; Traylor, A.; Apostolov, E.O.; Arosio, P.; Balla, J.; Verlander, J.; Darshan, D.; Kuhn, L.C.; et al. Proximal tubule H-ferritin mediates iron trafficking in acute kidney injury. *J. Clin. Investig.* **2013**, *123*, 4423–4434. [CrossRef] [PubMed]

109. Poss, K.D.; Tonegawa, S. Heme oxygenase 1 is required for mammalian iron reutilization. *Proc. Natl. Acad. Sci. USA* **1997**, *94*, 10919–10924. [CrossRef] [PubMed]

110. Bolisetty, S.; Traylor, A.; Joseph, R.; Zarjou, A.; Agarwal, A. Proximal tubule-targeted heme oxygenase-1 in cisplatin-induced acute kidney injury. *Am. J. Physiol. Ren. Physiol.* **2016**, *310*, F385–F394. [CrossRef] [PubMed]

111. Robinson-Cohen, C.; Katz, R.; Price, B.L.; Harju-Baker, S.; Mikacenic, C.; Himmelfarb, J.; Liles, W.C.; Wurfel, M.M. Association of markers of endothelial dysregulation Ang1 and Ang2 with acute kidney injury in critically ill patients. *Crit. Care* **2016**, *20*, 207. [CrossRef] [PubMed]

112. Kelly, K.J.; Williams, W.W., Jr.; Colvin, R.B.; Meehan, S.M.; Springer, T.A.; Gutierrez-Ramos, J.C.; Bonventre, J.V. Intercellular adhesion molecule-1-deficient mice are protected against ischemic renal injury. *J. Clin. Investig.* **1996**, *97*, 1056–1063. [CrossRef] [PubMed]

113. Bernhardt, W.M.; Campean, V.; Kany, S.; Jurgensen, J.S.; Weidemann, A.; Warnecke, C.; Arend, M.; Klaus, S.; Gunzler, V.; Amann, K.; et al. Preconditional activation of hypoxia-inducible factors ameliorates ischemic acute renal failure. *J. Am. Soc. Nephrol.* **2006**, *17*, 1970–1978. [CrossRef] [PubMed]

114. Skyschally, A.; Schulz, R.; Gres, P.; Korth, H.G.; Heusch, G. Attenuation of ischemic preconditioning in pigs by scavenging of free oxyradicals with ascorbic acid. *Am. J. Physiol. Heart Circ. Physiol.* **2003**, *284*, H698–H703. [CrossRef] [PubMed]

115. Yamasowa, H.; Shimizu, S.; Inoue, T.; Takaoka, M.; Matsumura, Y. Endothelial nitric oxide contributes to the renal protective effects of ischemic preconditioning. *J. Pharmacol. Exp. Ther.* **2005**, *312*, 153–159. [CrossRef] [PubMed]

116. Carr, A.C.; Frei, B. Toward a new recommended dietary allowance for vitamin C based on antioxidant and health effects in humans. *Am. J. Clin. Nutr.* **1999**, *69*, 1086–1107. [PubMed]

117. Du, J.; Cullen, J.J.; Buettner, G.R. Ascorbic acid: Chemistry, biology and the treatment of cancer. *Biochim. Biophys. Acta* **2012**, *1826*, 443–457. [CrossRef] [PubMed]

118. Buettner, G.R. The pecking order of free radicals and antioxidants: Lipid peroxidation, alpha-tocopherol, and ascorbate. *Arch. Biochem. Biophys.* **1993**, *300*, 535–543. [CrossRef] [PubMed]

119. Oudemans-van Straaten, H.M.; Spoelstra-de Man, A.M.; de Waard, M.C. Vitamin C revisited. *Crit. Care* **2014**, *18*, 460. [CrossRef] [PubMed]

120. May, J.M.; Harrison, F.E. Role of vitamin C in the function of the vascular endothelium. *Antioxid. Redox Signal.* **2013**, *19*, 2068–2083. [CrossRef] [PubMed]

121. Michels, A.J.; Hagen, T.M.; Frei, B. Human genetic variation influences vitamin C homeostasis by altering vitamin C transport and antioxidant enzyme function. *Annu. Rev. Nutr.* **2013**, *33*, 45–70. [CrossRef] [PubMed]

122. Lykkesfeldt, J.; Poulsen, H.E. Is vitamin C supplementation beneficial? Lessons learned from randomised controlled trials. *Br. J. Nutr.* **2010**, *103*, 1251–1259. [CrossRef] [PubMed]

123. Deicher, R.; Ziai, F.; Bieglmayer, C.; Schillinger, M.; Horl, W.H. Low total vitamin C plasma level is a risk factor for cardiovascular morbidity and mortality in hemodialysis patients. *J. Am. Soc. Nephrol.* **2005**, *16*, 1811–1818. [CrossRef] [PubMed]

124. Tu, H.; Li, H.; Wang, Y.; Niyyati, M.; Wang, Y.; Leshin, J.; Levine, M. Low red blood cell vitamin C concentrations induce red blood cell fragility: A link to diabetes via glucose, glucose transporters, and dehydroascorbic acid. *EBioMedicine* **2015**, *2*, 1735–1750. [CrossRef] [PubMed]

125. Eck, P.; Kwon, O.; Chen, S.; Mian, O.; Levine, M. The human sodium-dependent ascorbic acid transporters SLC23A1 and SLC23A2 do not mediate ascorbic acid release in the proximal renal epithelial cell. *Physiol. Rep.* **2013**, *1*, e00136. [CrossRef] [PubMed]

126. Antunes, L.M.; Darin, J.D.; Bianchi, M.D. Protective effects of vitamin C against cisplatin-induced nephrotoxicity and lipid peroxidation in adult rats: A dose-dependent study. *Pharmacol. Res.* **2000**, *41*, 405–411. [CrossRef] [PubMed]

127. Vicente-Vicente, L.; Casanova, A.G.; Hernandez-Sanchez, M.T.; Pescador, M.; Lopez-Hernandez, F.J.; Morales, A.I. A systematic meta-analysis on the efficacy of pre-clinically tested nephroprotectants at preventing aminoglycoside nephrotoxicity. *Toxicology* **2017**, *377*, 14–24. [CrossRef] [PubMed]

128. Kadi, I.E.; Dahdouh, F. Vitamin C pretreatment protects from nickel-induced acute nephrotoxicity in mice. *Arch. Ind. Hyg. Toksikol.* **2016**, *67*, 210–215. [CrossRef] [PubMed]

129. Das, K.K.; Buchner, V. Effect of nickel exposure on peripheral tissues: Role of oxidative stress in toxicity and possible protection by ascorbic acid. *Rev. Environ. Health* **2007**, *22*, 157–173. [CrossRef] [PubMed]

130. Kim, H.B.; Shanu, A.; Wood, S.; Parry, S.N.; Collet, M.; McMahon, A.; Witting, P.K. Phenolic antioxidants tert-butyl-bisphenol and vitamin E decrease oxidative stress and enhance vascular function in an animal model of rhabdomyolysis yet do not improve acute renal dysfunction. *Free Radic. Res.* **2011**, *45*, 1000–1012. [CrossRef] [PubMed]

131. Shanu, A.; Parry, S.N.; Wood, S.; Rodas, E.; Witting, P.K. The synthetic polyphenol tert-butyl-bisphenol inhibits myoglobin-induced dysfunction in cultured kidney epithelial cells. *Free Radic. Res.* **2010**, *44*, 843–853. [CrossRef] [PubMed]

132. Dunne, J.; Caron, A.; Menu, P.; Alayash, A.I.; Buehler, P.W.; Wilson, M.T.; Silaghi-Dumitrescu, R.; Faivre, B.; Cooper, C.E. Ascorbate removes key precursors to oxidative damage by cell-free haemoglobin in vitro and in vivo. *Biochem. J.* **2006**, *399*, 513–524. [CrossRef] [PubMed]

133. Lee, J.I.; Kim, M.J.; Park, C.S.; Kim, M.C. Influence of ascorbic acid on bun, creatinine, resistive index in canine renal ischemia-reperfusion injury. *J. Vet. Sci.* **2006**, *7*, 79–81. [CrossRef] [PubMed]

134. Lee, J.I.; Son, H.Y.; Kim, M.C. Attenuation of ischemia-reperfusion injury by ascorbic acid in the canine renal transplantation. *J. Vet. Sci.* **2006**, *7*, 375–379. [CrossRef] [PubMed]

135. Wilson, J.X. The physiological role of dehydroascorbic acid. *FEBS Lett.* **2002**, *527*, 5–9. [CrossRef]

136. Lloberas, N.; Torras, J.; Herrero-Fresneda, I.; Cruzado, J.M.; Riera, M.; Hurtado, I.; Grinyo, J.M. Postischemic renal oxidative stress induces inflammatory response through PAF and oxidized phospholipids. Prevention by antioxidant treatment. *FASEB J.* **2002**, *16*, 908–910. [CrossRef] [PubMed]

137. Mortensen, A.; Lykkesfeldt, J. Does vitamin C enhance nitric oxide bioavailability in a tetrahydrobiopterin-dependent manner? In vitro, in vivo and clinical studies. *Nitric Oxide* **2014**, *36*, 51–57. [CrossRef] [PubMed]

138. Miloradovic, Z.; Mihailovic-Stanojevic, N.; Grujic-Milanovic, J.; Ivanov, M.; Kuburovic, G.; Markovic-Lipkovski, J.; Jovovic, D. Comparative effects of L-arginine and vitamin C pretreatment in SHR with induced postischemic acute renal failure. *Gen. Physiol. Biophys.* **2009**, *28*, 105–111. [PubMed]

139. Wilson, J.X. Mechanism of action of vitamin C in sepsis: Ascorbate modulates redox signaling in endothelium. *Biofactors* **2009**, *35*, 5–13. [CrossRef] [PubMed]

140. Wilson, J.X. Evaluation of vitamin C for adjuvant sepsis therapy. *Antioxid. Redox Signal.* **2013**, *19*, 2129–2140. [CrossRef] [PubMed]

141. De Zeeuw, D.; Akizawa, T.; Audhya, P.; Bakris, G.L.; Chin, M.; Christ-Schmidt, H.; Goldsberry, A.; Houser, M.; Krauth, M.; Lambers Heerspink, H.J.; et al. Bardoxolone methyl in type 2 diabetes and stage 4 chronic kidney disease. *N. Engl. J. Med.* **2013**, *369*, 2492–2503. [CrossRef] [PubMed]

142. Sadat, U.; Usman, A.; Gillard, J.H.; Boyle, J.R. Does ascorbic acid protect against contrast-induced acute kidney injury in patients undergoing coronary angiography: A systematic review with meta-analysis of randomized, controlled trials. *J. Am. Coll. Cardiol.* **2013**, *62*, 2167–2175. [CrossRef] [PubMed]

143. Navarese, E.P.; Gurbel, P.A.; Andreotti, F.; Kolodziejczak, M.M.; Palmer, S.C.; Dias, S.; Buffon, A.; Kubica, J.; Kowalewski, M.; Jadczyk, T.; et al. Prevention of contrast-induced acute kidney injury in patients undergoing cardiovascular procedures—A systematic review and network meta-analysis. *PLoS ONE* **2017**, *12*, e0168726. [CrossRef] [PubMed]

144. Spargias, K.; Alexopoulos, E.; Kyrzopoulos, S.; Iokovis, P.; Greenwood, D.C.; Manginas, A.; Voudris, V.; Pavlides, G.; Buller, C.E.; Kremastinos, D.; et al. Ascorbic acid prevents contrast-mediated nephropathy in patients with renal dysfunction undergoing coronary angiography or intervention. *Circulation* **2004**, *110*, 2837–2842. [CrossRef] [PubMed]

145. Brueck, M.; Cengiz, H.; Hoeltgen, R.; Wieczorek, M.; Boedeker, R.H.; Scheibelhut, C.; Boening, A. Usefulness of *N*-acetylcysteine or ascorbic acid versus placebo to prevent contrast-induced acute kidney injury in patients undergoing elective cardiac catheterization: A single-center, prospective, randomized, double-blind, placebo-controlled trial. *J. Invasive Cardiol.* **2013**, *25*, 276–283. [PubMed]

146. Fowler, A.A., III; Syed, A.A.; Knowlson, S.; Sculthorpe, R.; Farthing, D.; DeWilde, C.; Farthing, C.A.; Larus, T.L.; Martin, E.; Brophy, D.F.; et al. Phase i safety trial of intravenous ascorbic acid in patients with severe sepsis. *J. Transl. Med.* **2014**, *12*, 32. [CrossRef] [PubMed]

147. Marik, P.E.; Khangoora, V.; Rivera, R.; Hooper, M.H.; Catravas, J. Hydrocortisone, vitamin C and thiamine for the treatment of severe sepsis and septic shock: A retrospective before–after study. *Chest* **2016**, *151*, 1229–1238. [CrossRef] [PubMed]

148. Pleiner, J.; Mittermayer, F.; Schaller, G.; MacAllister, R.J.; Wolzt, M. High doses of vitamin C reverse escherichia coli endotoxin-induced hyporeactivity to acetylcholine in the human forearm. *Circulation* **2002**, *106*, 1460–1464. [CrossRef] [PubMed]

149. Pleiner, J.; Schaller, G.; Mittermayer, F.; Marsik, C.; MacAllister, R.J.; Kapiotis, S.; Ziegler, S.; Ferlitsch, A.; Wolzt, M. Intra-arterial vitamin C prevents endothelial dysfunction caused by ischemia-reperfusion. *Atherosclerosis* **2008**, *197*, 383–391. [CrossRef] [PubMed]

150. Williams, M.J.; Sutherland, W.H.; McCormick, M.P.; de Jong, S.A.; McDonald, J.R.; Walker, R.J. Vitamin C improves endothelial dysfunction in renal allograft recipients. *Nephrol. Dial. Transplant.* **2001**, *16*, 1251–1255. [CrossRef] [PubMed]

151. Carr, A.C.; Shaw, G.M.; Fowler, A.A.; Natarajan, R. Ascorbate-dependent vasopressor synthesis: A rationale for vitamin C administration in severe sepsis and septic shock? *Crit. Care* **2015**, *19*, 418. [CrossRef] [PubMed]

152. Prabhakar, N.R.; Semenza, G.L. Adaptive and maladaptive cardiorespiratory responses to continuous and intermittent hypoxia mediated by hypoxia-inducible factors 1 and 2. *Physiol. Rev.* **2012**, *92*, 967–1003. [CrossRef] [PubMed]

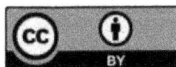

nutrients

MDPI

Article

Vitamin C Depletion and All-Cause Mortality in Renal Transplant Recipients

Camilo G. Sotomayor [1,*], Michele F. Eisenga [1], Antonio W. Gomes Neto [1], Akin Ozyilmaz [1], Rijk O. B. Gans [1], Wilhelmina H. A. de Jong [2], Dorien M. Zelle [1], Stefan P. Berger [1], Carlo A. J. M. Gaillard [1], Gerjan J. Navis [1] and Stephan J. L. Bakker [1]

[1] Department of Internal Medicine, University Medical Center Groningen, University of Groningen, Hanzeplein 1, Groningen 9700 RB, The Netherlands; m.f.eisenga@umcg.nl (M.F.E.); a.w.gomes.neto@umcg.nl (A.W.G.N.); a.ozyilmaz@umcg.nl (A.O.); r.o.b.gans@umcg.nl (R.O.B.G.); d.m.zelle@umcg.nl (D.M.Z.); s.p.berger@umcg.nl (S.P.B.); c.a.j.m.gaillard@umcg.nl (C.A.J.M.G.); g.j.navis@umcg.nl (G.J.N.); s.j.l.bakker@umcg.nl (S.J.L.B.)
[2] Department of Laboratory Medicine, University Medical Center Groningen, University of Groningen, Hanzeplein 1, Groningen 9700 RB, The Netherlands; w.h.a.de.jong@umcg.nl
* Correspondence: c.g.sotomayor.campos@umcg.nl; Tel.: +31-050-361-1564

Received: 11 April 2017; Accepted: 30 May 2017; Published: 2 June 2017

Abstract: Vitamin C may reduce inflammation and is inversely associated with mortality in the general population. We investigated the association of plasma vitamin C with all-cause mortality in renal transplant recipients (RTR); and whether this association would be mediated by inflammatory biomarkers. Vitamin C, high sensitive C-reactive protein (hs-CRP), soluble intercellular cell adhesion molecule 1 (sICAM-1), and soluble vascular cell adhesion molecule 1 (sVCAM-1) were measured in a cohort of 598 RTR. Cox regression analyses were used to analyze the association between vitamin C depletion ($\leq$28 μmol/L; 22% of RTR) and mortality. Mediation analyses were performed according to Preacher and Hayes's procedure. At a median follow-up of 7.0 (6.2–7.5) years, 131 (21%) patients died. Vitamin C depletion was univariately associated with almost two-fold higher risk of mortality (Hazard ratio (HR) 1.95; 95% confidence interval (95%CI) 1.35–2.81, $p < 0.001$). This association remained independent of potential confounders (HR 1.74; 95%CI 1.18–2.57, $p = 0.005$). Hs-CRP, sICAM-1, sVCAM-1 and a composite score of inflammatory biomarkers mediated 16%, 17%, 15%, and 32% of the association, respectively. Vitamin C depletion is frequent and independently associated with almost two-fold higher risk of mortality in RTR. It may be hypothesized that the beneficial effect of vitamin C at least partly occurs through decreasing inflammation.

Keywords: renal transplant; vitamin C; mortality; inflammation; hs-CRP

1. Introduction

Renal transplantation is currently considered the "gold standard" treatment for end-stage renal disease (ESRD) patients, since it offers superior survival, quality of life and cost-effectiveness compared to chronic dialysis treatment [1–8]. Nevertheless, survival of renal transplant recipients (RTR) is significantly lower than of age-matched controls in the general population [9].

It is worth noting that after renal transplantation a long-term ongoing inflammatory status persists [10–12]. It was recently reported that higher inflammatory status is associated with an increased risk of mortality in RTR [13]. In keeping with this finding, high sensitive C-reactive protein (hs-CRP), an established marker of inflammation, has been associated with increased risk of mortality in RTR [14,15]. It has been reported that vitamin C (ascorbic acid) is negatively correlated with C-reactive protein [16]. Both oral and high-dose intravenous vitamin C therapy reduced CRP levels and other pro-inflammatory cytokines [17–19]. Furthermore, vitamin C has been shown to be inversely associated with risk of all-cause mortality in the general population [20–24]. However, to date the role and long-term effects of vitamin C status on inflammatory biomarkers and adverse outcomes such as all-cause mortality in stable RTR remains unexplored, yet the results are of significant interest.

In this study, we aimed to investigate prospectively whether plasma vitamin C concentration and, specifically, its depletion ($\leq$28 µmol/L) [25–31] is associated with risk of all-cause mortality in RTR. In addition, we aimed to evaluate whether a putative association between vitamin C concentration and risk of all-cause mortality in RTR would be mediated by inflammatory parameters such as hs-CRP, soluble intercellular cell adhesion molecule 1 (sICAM-1) and soluble vascular cell adhesion molecule 1 (sVCAM-1).

2. Materials and Methods

2.1. Study Design

In this prospective cohort study, all adult RTR who survived with a functioning allograft beyond the first year after transplantation, and without known or apparent systemic illnesses (i.e., malignancies, opportunistic infections) were invited to participate during their next visit to the outpatient clinic. From a total of 847 eligible RTR, 606 (72%) patients signed informed consent. The group that did not sign informed consent was comparable with the group that signed informed consent with respect to age, sex, body mass index (BMI), serum creatinine, creatinine clearance, and proteinuria. Baseline data was collected between August 2001 and July 2003 at a median 5.9 (interquartile range (IQR): 2.6–11.4) years after renal transplantation. For the statistical analyses we excluded patients missing plasma vitamin C measurements (n = 8), resulting in 598 RTR eligible for analyses. Use of vitamin C supplements or multivitamin supplements containing vitamin C were documented in all RTR. The Institutional Review Board approved the study protocol (METc 2001/039). The clinical and research activities being reported are consistent with the Principles of the Declaration of Istanbul as outlined in the 'Declaration of Istanbul on Organ Trafficking and Transplant Tourism'.

The primary endpoint of this study was RTR mortality of all cause in nature. The continuous surveillance system of the outpatient program ensures up-to-date information on patient status. We contacted general practitioners or referring nephrologists in case the status of a patient was unknown. There was no loss due to follow-up.

2.2. Renal Transplant Characteristics

Relevant transplant characteristics including both donor and recipient age and gender, as well as transplant information were extracted from the Groningen Renal Transplant Database, which contains information about all renal transplantations that have been performed at the University Medical Centre Groningen since 1986. Smoking status was obtained using a self-report questionnaire. Smoking behavior was classified as never, former or current smoker. Cardiovascular disease history was considered positive if participants had a myocardial infarction, transient ischemic attack or cerebrovascular accident. Data on cumulative dose of steroids, incidence of acute rejection episodes and use of mechanistic target of rapamycin (m-TOR) inhibitors were retrieved from individual patient files. Cumulative dose of prednisolone was calculated as the sum of maintenance dose of prednisolone until inclusion and the dose of prednisolone or methylprednisolone required for treatment of acute rejection (a conversion factor of 1.25 was used to convert methylprednisolone dose to dose of prednisolone).

2.3. Measurements

Body mass index was calculated as weight in kilograms, divided by height in meters squared. Waist circumference was measured on bare skin midway between the iliac crest and the 10th rib. Blood pressure was measured as the average of three automated (Omron M4, Omron Europe B.V., Hoofddorp, The Netherlands) measurements with 1-min intervals after a 6-min rest in supine position.

Blood was drawn in the morning after an 8 to 12 h overnight fasting period, which included no medication intake. In order to measure plasma vitamin C concentration, blood was directly after phlebotomy transferred to the laboratory on ice, deproteinized and stored in the dark at –20 °C until analysis. For quantitative measurement ascorbic acid is enzymatically transformed to dehydroascorbic acid, which in turn is derivatized to 3-(1,2-dihydroxyethyl)furo-[3,4-b]quinoxaline-1-one. Then, reversed phase liquid chromatography with fluorescence detection is applied (excitation 355 nm, emission 425 nm). Serum high sensitive C-reactive protein was assessed as described before [32]. Plasma sICAM-1 and sVCAM-1 concentrations were measured by enzyme-linked immunosorbent assay kits (Diaclone Research, Besançon, France). Serum creatinine concentrations were determined using the Jaffé method (MEGA AU510, Merck Diagnostica, Darmstadt, Germany). Total cholesterol was determined using the cholesterol oxidase-phenol aminophenazone method (MEGA AU510, Merck Diagnostica, Darmstadt, Germany), and serum triglycerides were determined with the glycerol-3-phosphate oxidase-phenol aminophenazone method (MEGA AU510, Merck Diagnostica, Darmstadt, Germany). High density lipoprotein (HDL)-cholesterol was determined with the cholesterol oxidase-phenol aminophenazone method on a Technikon RA-1000 (Bayer Diagnostics, Mijdrecht, The Netherlands), and low density lipoprotein (LDL)-cholesterol was calculated using the Friedewald formula [33]. Plasma glucose was determined by the glucose-oxidase method (YSI 2300 Stat plus, Yellow Springs, OH, USA). Glycated hemoglobin (HbA1c) was determined by high performance liquid chromatography (VARIANTTM HbA1c Program with Bio-Rad CARIANT Hb Testing System, Bio-Rad, Hercules, CA, USA).

According to a strict protocol all RTR were asked to collect a 24-hour urine sample during the day before their visit to the outpatient clinic. Urine was collected under oil and chlorohexidine was added as an antiseptic agent. Proteinuria was defined as urinary protein excretion >0.5 g/24 h. Renal function was assessed by estimated Glomerular Filtration Rate (eGFR) applying the Chronic Kidney Disease Epidemiology Collaboration equation [34].

2.4. Statistical Analysis

Data were analyzed using IBM SPSS software version 23.0 (SPSS Inc., Chicago, IL, USA), STATA 12.0 (StataCorp LP, College Station, TX, USA) and R version 3.2.3. In all analyses, a 2-sided $p < 0.05$ was considered significant. Hazard ratio (HR) are reported with 95% confidence interval (CI). Continuous variables were summarized using mean (standard deviation (SD)) for normally distributed data, whereas skewed distributed variables are given as median (IQR); percentages were used to summarize categorical variables. Linear regression analyses were performed to evaluate the association of plasma vitamin C concentration with recipient-related and transplantation-related characteristics. Natural log transformation was used for analyses of variables with a skewed distribution.

A log-rank test was run to determine if there were differences in the survival distribution between plasma vitamin C status (depleted and non-depleted; $\leq$ or >28 µmol/L, respectively) of RTR. To analyze whether plasma vitamin C concentration is independently associated with mortality, we performed Cox-proportional hazards regression analyses. For these analyses plasma vitamin C concentration was used as categorical variable according to depleted or not depleted concentration [25,26,28–30]; and as continuous variable (2 base of log-transformed values to achieve a normal distribution), in order to obtain the best fitting model. First, we performed univariate Cox regression analyses. Hereafter, we adjusted for age and sex (Model 2); for eGFR, proteinuria, primary renal diseases and time since transplantation (Model 3). To avoid inclusion of too many variables for the number of events, further models were performed with additive adjustments to model 3. We performed additional adjustments for smoking status and alcohol use (Model 4); for diabetes mellitus (Model 5); and for systolic blood pressure, BMI, serum HDL cholesterol and triglycerides concentration (Model 6); and for use of calcineurin inhibitors, use of antimetabolites, use of m-TOR inhibitors, use of induction therapy, and cumulative dose of prednisolone (model 7).

As secondary analyses, we also performed classic mediation analyses according to Preacher and Hayes [35,36], which are based on logistic regression; to establish whether hs-CRP sICAM-1 and sVCAM-1 concentrations, separately and combined (sum of individual Z scores of hs-CRP + sICAM-1 + sVCAM-1), mediated the association between plasma vitamin C concentration and all-cause mortality. These analyses allow for testing significance and magnitude of mediation.

3. Results

3.1. Baseline Characteristics

A total of 598 stable RTR were included (mean age 51 ± 12 years, 54% male, 96% caucasian) at 5.9 (2.6–11.4) years after transplantation. Among them 133 (22%) RTR were vitamin C depleted. None of the patients used vitamin C supplements or multivitamin supplements containing vitamin C. Median (IQR) plasma vitamin C, hs-CRP, sICAM-1 and sVCAM-1 concentration were 44 (31–55) μmol/L, 2.0 (0.7–4.8) mg/L, 602 (514–720) ng/L, and 965 (772–1196) ng/L, respectively. Mean eGFR was 47 ± 15 mL/min/1.73 m^2, 166 (28%) participants had proteinuria. Additional baseline characteristics are shown in Table 1.

Table 1. Baseline characteristics of RTR and its association with plasma vitamin C, adjusted for age and sex.

Variables	All Patients	Vitamin C (Ln), μmol/L	
		Std. β	*p* Value
No. of patients	598	-	-
Vitamin C, μmol/L	44 (31–55)	-	-
Demographics			
Age, years	51 ± 12	−0.05 *	0.23 *
Sex (male), *n* (%)	328 (54)	−0.18 *	<0.001 *
Ethnicity (caucasian), *n* (%)	577 (96)	−0.02	0.60
Body Composition			
Body surface area, m^2	1.87 ± 0.19	−0.04	0.22
Body mass index, kg/m^2	26.0 ± 4.3	−0.08	0.06
Primary Renal Diseases		−0.02	0.61
Primary glomerulonephritis, *n* (%)	169 (28)	-	-
Glomerulonephritis due to vascular or autoimmune disease, *n* (%)	36 (6)	-	-
Tubulointerstitial nephritis and pyelonephritis, *n* (%)	92 (15)	-	-
Polycystic kidney disease, *n* (%)	106 (18)	-	-
Dysplasia and hypoplasia, *n* (%)	21 (4)	-	-
Renovascular disease, *n* (%)	32 (5)	-	-
Diabetic nephropathy, *n* (%)	22 (4)	-	-
Hereditary diseases and other, *n* (%)	117 (20)	-	-
Tobacco Use		−0.08	0.06
Never smoker, *n* (%)	214 (35)	-	-
Ex-smoker, *n* (%)	251 (42)	-	-
Current smoker, *n* (%)	131 (21)	-	-
Blood Pressure			
Systolic blood pressure, mmHg	153 ± 22	−0.11	0.004
Diastolic blood pressure, mmHg	89 ± 9	−0.11	0.01
Use of ACE-inhibitor or aII-antagonist, *n* (%)	201 (33)	0.07	0.11
Use of beta-blocker, *n* (%)	368 (61)	−0.07	0.11
Prior History of CV Disease			
History of MI, *n* (%)	48 (8)	−0.01	0.75
History of TIA/CVA, *n* (%)	32 (5)	−0.04	0.36

Table 1. *Cont.*

Variables	All Patients	Vitamin C (Ln), μmol/L	
		Std. β	*p* Value
Transplantation			
Time since transplantation, years	5.9 (2.6–11.4)	0.20	<0.001
Dialysis vintage, months		−0.14	0.001
141 (24)		-	-
1–5 years	363 (61)	-	-
>5 years	94 (16)	-	-
Deceased donor, *n* (%)	515 (86)	0.02	0.61
Immunosuppressive Therapy			
Prednisolone, mg/day	10.0 (7.5–10.0)	−0.11	0.008
Use of calcineurin inhibitors		−0.09	0.02
Cyclosporine, *n* (%)	386 (65)	-	-
Tacrolimus, *n* (%)	84 (14)	-	-
None, *n* (%)	128 (21)	-	-
Use of antimetabolites		−0.06	0.19
Azathioprine, *n* (%)	194 (32)	-	-
Mycophenolic acid, *n* (%)	247 (41)	-	-
None, (%)	157 (26)	-	-
Use of m-TOR inhibitors, *n* (%)	10 (2)	−0.10	0.02
Induction therapy		−0.20	<0.001
Anti-thymocyte globulin, *n* (%)	70 (12)	-	-
Muromonab-CD3 , *n* (%)	26 (4)	-	-
Anti-CD25 monoclonal antibodies, *n* (%)	10 (2)	-	-
None, *n* (%)	492 (82)	-	-
Acute rejection treatment		−0.13	0.03
High doses of steroids, *n* (%)	186 (31)	-	-
Other rejection therapy, *n* (%)	82 (14)	-	-
Cumulative dose of prednisolone, grams	21.3 (11.3–37.9)	0.21	<0.001
Ischemia Times			
Cold ischemia time, hours	22 (15–27)	0.01	0.75
Total warm ischemia, minutes	35 (30–45)	0.02	0.72
Renal Allograft Function			
eGFR, mL/min/1.73 m^2	47 ± 15	0.11	0.009
Urinary protein excretion, g/24 h	0.2 (0.0–0.5)	−0.06	0.22
Proteinuria (>0.5 g/24 h), *n* (%)	166 (27)	−0.11	0.006
Inflammation			
hs-CRP, mg/L	2.0 (0.7–4.8)	−0.19	<0.001
sICAM-1, ng/L	602 (514–720)	−0.17	<0.001
sVCAM-1, ng/L	965 (772–1196)	−0.16	<0.001
Lipids			
Total colesterol, mmol/L	5.6 ± 1.0	0.05	0.24
HDL colesterol, mmol/L	1.0 ± 0.3	0.11	0.004
LDL cholesterol, mmol/L	3.5 ± 0.9	0.07	0.09
Triglycerides, mmol/L	1.9 (1.4–2.6)	−0.13	0.001
Use of statins, *n* (%)	295 (49)	0.06	0.13
Oxidative Stress			
Gamma glutamate, U/L	24 (18–39)	−0.10	0.02
Alkaline phophatase, U/L	72 (57–94)	−0.21	<0.001
Uric acid, mmol/L	0.4 (0.3–0.5)	−0.08	0.05

Table 1. *Cont.*

Variables	All Patients	Vitamin C (Ln), μmol/L	
		Std. β	*p* Value
Glucose Homeostasis			
Insulin, μU/mL	11 (7–16)	−0.08	0.04
Glucose, mmol/L	4.5 (4.1–5.0)	−0.07	0.06
HbA$_{1c}$, %	6.5 ± 1.0	−0.12	0.002
Diabetes, *n* (%)	105 (17)	−0.11	0.008
Hematology			
Leukocyte count, *x* 10^9/L	8.5 ± 2.4	−0.03	0.42
Hemoglobin, mmol/L	8.5 ± 0.9	0.01	0.77
Platelets count, *x* 10^9/L	231 ± 69	−0.02	0.56

* Unadjusted. Abbreviations: ACE, angiotensin converting enzyme; CV, cardiovascular; CVA, cardiovascular accident; eGFR, estimated Glomerular Filtration Rate; HbA1c, glycated hemoglobin; HDL, high-density lipoprotein; hs-CRP, high-sensitive C reactive protein; LDL; low-density lipoprotein; m-TOR, mechanistic target of rapamycin; MI, myocardial infarction; sICAM-1, soluble intercellular cell adhesion molecule 1; sVCAM-1, soluble vascular cell adhesion molecule 1; TIA, transient ischemic attack; RTR, renal transplant recipients. Baseline characteristics normally distributed are summarized using means (SD), whereas skewed distributed variables are given as medians (IQR); percentages were used to summarize categorical variables. Multivariate linear regression analyses were performed to obtain a *p* value of potential associations of baseline characteristics of renal transplant recipients with plasma vitamin C concentration.

3.2. Association of Plasma Vitamin C Concentration with Clinical Variables

Age- and sex-adjusted plasma vitamin C concentration was associated with hs-CRP (std. β = −0.19; *p* < 0.001), sICAM-1 (std. β = −0.17; *p* < 0.001) and sVCAM-1 (std. β = −0.16; *p* < 0.001) concentrations. Moreover, alkaline phosphatase (std. β = −0.21; *p* < 0.001) and gamma glutamate (std. β = −0.10; *p* = 0.02) were associated with plasma vitamin C concentration. Furthermore, vitamin C was significantly associated with HbA1c (std. β = −0.12; *p* = 0.002), diabetes (std. β = −0.11; *p* = 0.008), and insulin concentration (std. β = −0.08; *p* = 0.04). Likewise, eGFR (std. β = 0.11; *p* = 0.009), systolic blood pressure (std. β = −0.11; *p* = 0.004) and diastolic blood pressure (std. β = −0.11; *p* = 0.01) were associated to vitamin C concentration. Dialysis vintage (std. β = −0.14; *p* = 0.001) and immunosuppressive therapy including use of calcineurin inhibitors (std. β = −0.09; *p* = 0.02), use of m-TOR inhibitors (std. β = −0.10; *p* = 0.02), induction therapy (std. β = −0.20; *p* < 0.001), acute rejection treatment (std. β = −0.13; *p* = 0.03), and cumulative dose of prednisolone (std. β = −0.21; *p* ≤ 0.001), were associated to plasma vitamin C concentration (Table 1).

3.3. Prospective Analyses

During a median follow-up of 7.0 (6.2–7.5) years, 131 (21%) patients died. 32% of plasma vitamin C depleted patients died, whereas among non-depleted patients 18% died. The survival distributions between depleted and non-depleted RTR were significantly different (log-rank test *p* < 0.001). A Kaplan-Meier curve for all-cause mortality according to plasma vitamin C status is shown in Figure 1.

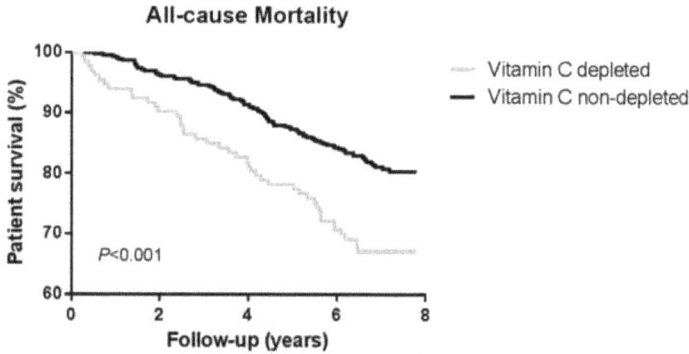

Figure 1. Kaplan-Meier curve for all-cause mortality according to plasma vitamin C status (depleted versus non-depleted) among renal transplant recipients. Vitamin C depleted: ≤28 μmol/L; Vitamin C non-depleted: >28 μmol/L.

Results of univariate and multivariate Cox-proportional hazard regression analyses are shown in Table 2. Prospective analyses of the association between vitamin C concentration with all-cause mortality showed that plasma vitamin C depleted RTR had an almost double risk of mortality (HR 1.95; 95% CI 1.35–2.81, $p < 0.001$). This association was independent of further adjustment for potential confounders, with e.g., an HR of 1.88; 95% CI 1.28–2.76, $p = 0.001$ after adjustment for age, sex, eGFR, proteinuria, primary renal disease, time since transplantation and dialysis vintage. Further adjustment for other potential confounders (i.e., smoking and alcohol status, diabetes mellitus, systolic blood pressure, BMI, HDL cholesterol and triglycerides concentration, use of calcineurin inhibitors, use of antimetabolites, use of m-TOR inhibitors, use of induction therapy, and cumulative dose of prednisolone) did not materially alter the association.

Table 2. Prospective analysis of plasma vitamin C on all-cause mortality in RTR.

	Vitamin C, Status				Vitamin C, Continuous		
	≤28 μmol/L n = 133			>28 μmol/L n = 465	2log, μmol/L n = 598		
	HR	95% CI	*p*	Reference	HR	95% CI	*p*
Model 1	1.95	1.35–2.81	<0.001	1.00	0.71	0.59–0.87	0.001
Model 2	1.92	1.33–2.77	0.001	1.00	0.74	0.61–0.90	0.002
Model 3	1.88	1.28–2.76	0.001	1.00	0.76	0.62–0.94	0.011
Model 4	1.91	1.30–2.82	0.001	1.00	0.76	0.62–0.94	0.012
Model 5	1.80	1.22–2.65	0.003	1.00	0.79	0.64–0.98	0.030
Model 6	1.70	1.15–2.52	0.008	1.00	0.79	0.63–0.98	0.030
Model 7	1.74	1.18–2.57	0.005	1.00	0.78	0.63–0.97	0.024

Abbreviations: RTR, renal transplant recipients; HR, hazard ratio; CI, confidence interval. Model 1: Univariate. Model 2: Age and sex adjusted. Model 3: Model 2 + adjustment for estimated Glomerular Filtration Rate, proteinuria, primary renal disease, time since transplantation, and dialysis vintage. Model 4: Model 3 + adjustment for smoking and alcohol use. Model 5: Model 3 + adjustment for diabetes mellitus. Model 6: Model 3 + adjustment for systolic blood pressure, body mass index, high density lipoprotein cholesterol, and triglycerides concentration. Model 7: Model 3 + adjustment for use of calcineurin inhibitors, use of antimetabolites, use of m-TOR inhibitors, use of induction therapy, and cumulative dose of prednisolone.

Vitamin C as a continuous variable was univariately associated with all-cause mortality (HR 0.71; 95% CI 0.59–0.87, $p = 0.001$), with the point estimate of the HR below 1.00 indicating that risk decreases with increasing vitamin C concentrations. In multivariable analysis, after adjustment for potential confounders the association remained, with a HR of 0.76; 95% CI 0.62–0.94, $p = 0.011$ (Table 2; Figure 2).

All-Cause Mortality

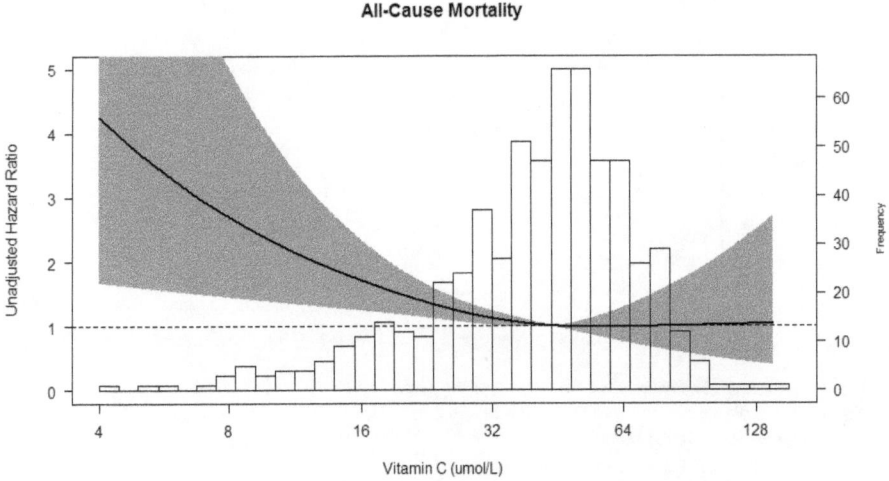

Figure 2. Association of plasma vitamin C with risk of all-cause mortality. The line in the graph represents the hazard ratio. The grey area represents the 95% confidence interval of the hazard ratio.

3.4. Mediation Analyses

In mediation analyses according to the procedures of Preacher and Hayes [35,36], hs-CRP, sICAM-1 and sVCAM-1 concentration were significant mediators (*p* value for indirect effect <0.05) in the association of vitamin C concentration with mortality. The magnitude of the mediating effects of hs-CRP, sICAM-1 and sVCAM-1 accounted 16, 17 and 15%, respectively. Furthermore, combined inflammatory biomarkers mediated 32% on the association of plasma vitamin C concentration with risk of all-cause mortality in RTR (Table 3; Figure A1).

Table 3. Mediating effects of hs-CRP, sICAM-1, sVCAM-1 separately and combined on the association of plasma Vitamin C concentration with risk of mortality in 598 RTR according to Preacher and Hayes procedure.

Potential Mediator	Effect (Path) *	Multivariate Model **	
		Coefficient (95% CI) [†]	Proportion Mediated
hs-CRP	Indirect effect (*ab* path)	−0.016 (−0.036; −0.004)	16% ***
	Total effect (*ab* + *c'* path)	−0.103 (−0.189; −0.010)	
sICAM-1	Indirect effect (*ab* path)	−0.018 (−0.043; −0.003)	17% ***
	Total effect (*ab* + *c'* path)	−0.103 (−0.194; −0.016)	
sVCAM-1	Indirect effect (*ab* path)	−0.015 (−0.040; −0.003)	15% ***
	Total effect (*ab* + *c'* path)	−0.103 (−0.200; −0.015)	
Combined inflammation	Indirect effect (*ab* path)	−0.033 (−0.065; −0.012)	32% ***
	Total effect (*ab* + *c'* path)	−0.103 (−0.191; −0.013)	

Abbreviations: hs-CRP, high sensitive C-reactive protein; sICAM-1, soluble intercellular cell adhesion molecule 1; sVCAM-1, soluble vascular cell adhesion molecule 1; RTR, renal transplant recipients; CI, confidence interval. * The coefficients of the indirect *ab* path and the total *ab* + *c'* path are standardized for the standard deviations of the potential mediators, plasma vitamin C concentration and outcomes. ** All coefficients are adjusted for age, sex, estimated Glomerular Filtration Rate, time since transplantation, primary renal disease, and proteinuria. *** The size of the significant mediated effect is calculated as the standardized indirect effect divided by the standardized total effect multiplied by 100. [†] 95% confidence intervals for the indirect and total effects were bias-corrected confidence intervals after running 2000 bootstrap samples.

4. Discussion

This study showed, first, that vitamin C depletion was common in a stable outpatient population of RTR, and that plasma vitamin C concentration was independently and inversely associated with risk of all-cause mortality in RTR. Particularly, plasma vitamin C depletion was detrimental, as depicted by an almost two fold higher risk of mortality within patients that had plasma vitamin C concentration equal or lower than 28 µmol/L [25–31]. Importantly, adjustment for several potential confounders did not alter the association. Of note, the association between vitamin C and mortality has been previously reported in the general population [20–24]; however, to our knowledge, this is the first study that examines the association of plasma vitamin C concentration with all-cause mortality in RTR and, specifically, the effect of plasma vitamin C depletion on patient survival after renal transplantation.

Further, we found that combined inflammatory biomarkers mediated the robust proportion of about one third of the association of plasma vitamin C concentration with all-cause mortality. Notwithstanding that the underlying mechanisms leading to significantly lower survival of RTR compared to age-matched controls in the general population [9] are not completely understood, it is noteworthy that a long-term ongoing inflammatory status remains after renal transplantation [10–12]. Indeed, Abedini et al. [15], reported that in a cohort of 2102 RTR, over a follow-up period of 5–6 years, hs-CRP was independently associated with all-cause mortality in RTR. Likewise, Winkelmayer et al. [14] found that, at a median follow-up of 7.8 years after renal transplantation in a cohort of 438 RTR, CRP levels of more than 5 mg/L were associated with an 83% greater mortality risk compared with lower levels of this inflammatory marker. These observations are in agreement with our findings and support the influence of low-grade ongoing inflammation on patient survival after renal transplantation. On the basis of these findings and currently available literature [10–15] one might propose that inflammation plays a major role in the underlying mechanisms leading to decreased survival after renal transplantation. Finally, taking into account that we found that vitamin C concentration was inversely associated with inflammatory biomarkers, which is in agreement with previous reports [16–19], we hypothesize that the beneficial effect of adequate vitamin C status on survival of RTR is at least partly mediated by diminishing inflammatory status.

On the basis of current findings it is expected that reduction of inflammation through vitamin C supplementation, could be an approach to encourage protection against tissue injury and improve current survival rates of RTR. A recent randomized controlled trial evaluated the effect of oral vitamin C supplementation (200 mg/day during 3 months) on inflammatory status among 100 maintenance hemodialysis patients [37]. Compared with patients that did not receive supplementation, a significant decrease of hs-CRP levels was found among the vitamin C supplemented group. Moreover, the hs-CRP levels returned to their original state after the supplementation was withdraw. In turn, Atallah et al. reported the effect of intravenous vitamin C supplementation (300 mg each dialysis session) on inflammatory parameters in hemodialysis patients. This study showed that CRP levels between baseline and 6 months were significantly decreased in the supplemented, but not in the control group [38]. Nevertheless, to our knowledge no randomized controlled trial has been reported evaluating the effect of vitamin C supplementation strategies on inflammatory biomarkers or prospective outcomes in RTR.

The strength of this study lays in its prospective design; and that it comprises a large cohort of stable RTR which were closely monitored by regular check-up in the outpatient clinic, which gives complete information on patient status. A limitation is that we did not have repeated measurements of vitamin C levels. However, it should be realized that if intra-individual variability of vitamin C is taken into account, the predictive properties become stronger. The higher the intra-individual day-to-day variation of vitamin C would be, the greater one would expect the benefit of repeated measurement for prediction of outcomes [39,40]. Moreover, as with any observational study, reversed causation or unmeasured confounding may occur, despite the substantial number of potentially confounding factors for which we adjusted. As we have no data on nutrition, we cannot exclude the possibility that the association exists as a consequence of vitamin C being a marker of poor nutrition. Finally, since this is a single center study; the predictive value of vitamin C on mortality in RTR requires to be confirmed within a multicenter study.

5. Conclusions

In conclusion, plasma vitamin C depletion is common in stable RTR, and is independently and inversely associated with all-cause mortality after renal transplantation. Since hs-CRP, sICAM-1 and sVCAM-1 were found to be important mediators in the association between vitamin C and all-cause mortality, we hypothesize that the beneficial effect of vitamin C would occur through decreasing inflammatory status. On the basis of the current findings, further research is needed to evaluate whether vitamin C supplementation could be a therapeutic strategy in order to increase survival after renal transplantation. The present study should encourage the design of multicenter, randomized, double-blind, placebo-controlled trial, aimed to test the efficacy of this novel therapeutic strategy.

Acknowledgments: This study is based on the TransplantLines Insulin Resistance and Inflammation (TxL-IRI) Biobank and Cohort Study Database, which was funded by the Dutch Kidney Foundation (grant C00.1877).

Author Contributions: C.G.S. contributed to data analysis and writing of the manuscript. M.F.E. participated in data analysis and manuscript revisions. A.W.G.N. participated in data analysis. A.O., W.H.A.d.J. and D.M.Z. participated in manuscript revisions. R.O.B.G., S.P.B. and C.A.J.M.G. contributed to the interpretation of data and manuscript revisions. G.J.N. and S.J.L.B. were responsible for the study research idea, study design and contributed to the interpretation of data and manuscript revisions.

Conflicts of Interest: The authors declare no conflict of interest.

Appendix

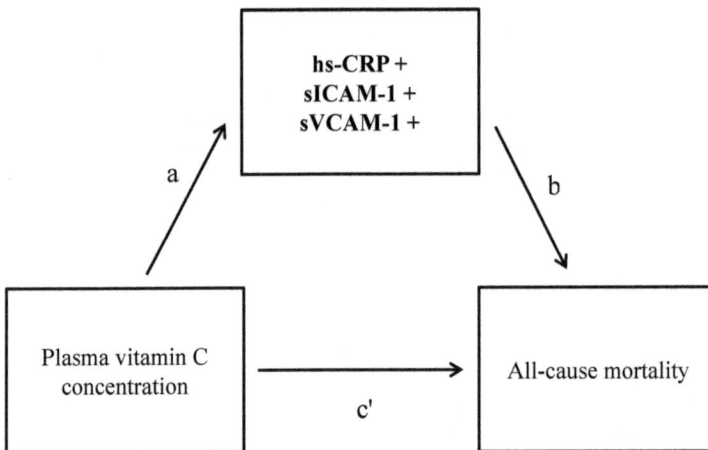

Figure A1. Mediation analysis of combined score between hs-CRP, sICAM-1 and sVCAM-1 on the association of plasma vitamin C concentration with all-cause mortality. *a*, *b* and *c* are the standardized regression coefficients between variables. The indirect effect (through a potential mediator) is calculated as $a \times b$. Total effect (*c*) is $a \times b + c'$. Magnitude of mediation is calculated as indirect effect divided by total effect.

References

1. Schippers, H.; Kalff, M.W. Cost Comparison Haemodialysis and Renal Transplantation. *HLA* **1976**, *7*, 86–90. [CrossRef]
2. Laupacis, A.; Keown, P.; Pus, N.; Krueger, H.; Ferguson, B.; Wong, C.; Muirhead, N. A Study of the Quality of Life and Cost-Utility of Renal Transplantation. *Kidney Int.* **1996**, *50*, 235–242. [CrossRef] [PubMed]
3. Jofre, R.; Lopez-Gomez, J.M.; Moreno, F.; Sanz-Guajardo, D.; Valderrabano, F. Changes in Quality of Life After Renal Transplantation. *Am. J. Kidney Dis.* **1998**, *32*, 93–100. [CrossRef] [PubMed]
4. Wolfe, R.A.; Ashby, V.B.; Milford, E.L.; Ojo, A.O.; Ettenger, R.E.; Agodoa, L.Y.C.; Held, P.J.; Port, F.K. Comparison of Mortality in all Patients on Dialysis, Patients on Dialysis Awaiting Transplantation, and Recipients of a First Cadaveric Transplant. *N. Engl. J. Med.* **1999**, *341*, 1725–1730. [CrossRef] [PubMed]
5. Fujisawa, M.; Ichikawa, Y.; Yoshiya, K.; Isotani, S.; Higuchi, A.; Nagano, S.; Arakawa, S.; Hamami, G.; Matsumoto, O.; Kamidono, S. Assessment of Health-Related Quality of Life in Renal Transplant and Hemodialysis Patients using the SF-36 Health Survey. *Urology* **2000**, *56*, 201–206. [CrossRef]
6. Oniscu, G.C.; Brown, H.; Forsythe, J.L. Impact of Cadaveric Renal Transplantation on Survival in Patients Listed for Transplantation. *J. Am. Soc. Nephrol.* **2005**, *16*, 1859–1865. [CrossRef] [PubMed]
7. Chkhotua, A.; Pantsulaia, T.; Managadze, L. The Quality of Life Analysis in Renal Transplant Recipients and Dialysis Patients. *Georgian Med. News* **2011**, *11*, 10–17. [PubMed]
8. Tonelli, M.; Wiebe, N.; Knoll, G.; Bello, A.; Browne, S.; Jadhav, D.; Klarenbach, S.; Gill, J. Systematic Review: Kidney Transplantation Compared with Dialysis in Clinically Relevant Outcomes. *Am. J. Transpl.* **2011**, *11*, 2093–2109. [CrossRef] [PubMed]
9. Oterdoom, L.H.; de Vries, A.P.; van Ree, R.M.; Gansevoort, R.T.; van Son, W.J.; van der Heide, J.J.H.; Navis, G.; de Jong, P.E.; Gans, R.O.; Bakker, S.J. N-Terminal Pro-B-Type Natriuretic Peptide and Mortality in Renal Transplant Recipients Versus the General Population. *Transplantation* **2009**, *87*, 1562–1570. [CrossRef] [PubMed]
10. Kocak, H.; Ceken, K.; Yavuz, A.; Yucel, S.; Gurkan, A.; Erdogan, O.; Ersoy, F.; Yakupoglu, G.; Demirbas, A.; Tuncer, M. Effect of Renal Transplantation on Endothelial Function in Haemodialysis Patients. *Nephrol. Dial. Transpl.* **2006**, *21*, 203–207. [CrossRef] [PubMed]
11. Turkmen, K.; Tonbul, H.Z.; Toker, A.; Gaipov, A.; Erdur, F.M.; Cicekler, H.; Anil, M.; Ozbek, O.; Selcuk, N.Y.; Yeksan, M. The Relationship between Oxidative Stress, Inflammation, and Atherosclerosis in Renal Transplant and End-Stage Renal Disease Patients. *Ren. Fail.* **2012**, *34*, 1229–1237. [CrossRef] [PubMed]
12. Ocak, N.; Dirican, M.; Ersoy, A.; Sarandol, E. Adiponectin, Leptin, Nitric Oxide, and C-Reactive Protein Levels in Kidney Transplant Recipients: Comparison with the Hemodialysis and Chronic Renal Failure. *Ren. Fail.* **2016**, *38*, 1639–1646. [CrossRef] [PubMed]
13. Cañas, L.; Iglesias, E.; Pastor, M.C.; Barallat, J.; Juega, J.; Bancu, I.; Lauzurica, R. Inflammation and Oxidation: Do they Improve After Kidney Transplantation? Relationship with Mortality After Transplantation. *Int. Urol. Nephrol.* **2017**, *49*, 533–540. [CrossRef] [PubMed]
14. Winkelmayer, W.C.; Lorenz, M.; Kramar, R.; Födinger, M.; Hörl, W.H.; Sunder-Plassmann, G. C-Reactive Protein and Body Mass Index Independently Predict Mortality in Kidney Transplant Recipients. *Am. J. Transplant.* **2004**, *4*, 1148–1154. [CrossRef] [PubMed]
15. Abedini, S.; Holme, I.; Marz, W.; Weihrauch, G.; Fellstrom, B.; Jardine, A.; Cole, E.; Maes, B.; Neumayer, H.H.; Gronhagen-Riska, C.; et al. Inflammation in Renal Transplantation. *Clin. J. Am. Soc. Nephrol.* **2009**, *4*, 1246–1254. [CrossRef] [PubMed]
16. Langlois, M.; Duprez, D.; Delanghe, J.; De Buyzere, M.; Clement, D.L. Serum Vitamin C Concentration is Low in Peripheral Arterial Disease and is Associated with Inflammation and Severity of Atherosclerosis. *Circulation* **2001**, *103*, 1863–1868. [CrossRef] [PubMed]
17. Korantzopoulos, P.; Kolettis, T.M.; Kountouris, E.; Dimitroula, V.; Karanikis, P.; Pappa, E.; Siogas, K.; Goudevenos, J.A. Oral Vitamin C Administration Reduces Early Recurrence Rates After Electrical Cardioversion of Persistent Atrial Fibrillation and Attenuates Associated Inflammation. *Int. J. Cardiol.* **2005**, *102*, 321–326. [CrossRef] [PubMed]
18. Mikirova, N.; Casciari, J.; Rogers, A.; Taylor, P. Effect of High-Dose Intravenous Vitamin C on Inflammation in Cancer Patients. *J. Transl. Med.* **2012**, *10*, 189. [CrossRef] [PubMed]

19. Mikirova, N.; Casciari, J.; Riordan, N.; Hunninghake, R. Clinical Experience with Intravenous Administration of Ascorbic Acid: Achievable Levels in Blood for Different States of Inflammation and Disease in Cancer Patients. *J. Transl. Med.* **2013**, *11*, 191. [CrossRef] [PubMed]

20. Enstrom, J.E.; Kanim, L.E.; Klein, M.A. Vitamin C Intake and Mortality among a Sample of the United States Population. *Epidemiology* **1992**, *3*, 194–202. [CrossRef] [PubMed]

21. Pandey, D.K.; Shekelle, R.; Selwyn, B.J.; Tangney, C.; Stamler, J. Dietary Vitamin C and B-Carotene and Risk of Death in Middle-Aged Men the Western Electric Study. *Am. J. Epidemiol.* **1995**, *142*, 1269–1278. [CrossRef] [PubMed]

22. Sahyoun, N.R.; Jacques, P.F.; Russell, R.M. Carotenoids, Vitamins C and E, and Mortality in an Eiderly Population. *Am. J. Epidemiol.* **1996**, *144*, 501–511. [CrossRef] [PubMed]

23. Loria, C.M.; Klag, M.J.; Caulfield, L.E.; Whelton, P.K. Vitamin C Status and Mortality in US Adults. *Am. J. Clin. Nutr.* **2000**, *72*, 139–145. [PubMed]

24. Khaw, K.; Bingham, S.; Welch, A.; Luben, R.; Wareham, N.; Oakes, S.; Day, N. Relation between Plasma Ascorbic Acid and Mortality in Men and Women in EPIC-Norfolk Prospective Study: A Prospective Population Study. *Lancet* **2001**, *357*, 657–663. [CrossRef]

25. Irwin, M.I.; Hutchins, B.K. A Conspectus of Research on Vitamin C Requirements of Man. *J. Nutr.* **1976**, *106*, 821–879. [PubMed]

26. Jacob, R.A.; Skala, J.H.; Omaye, S.T. Biochemical Indices of Human Vitamin C Status. *Am. J. Clin. Nutr.* **1987**, *46*, 818–826. [PubMed]

27. Sauberlich, H.E.; Kretsch, M.J.; Taylor, P.C.; Johnson, H.L.; Skala, J.H. Ascorbic Acid and Erythorbic Acid Metabolism in Nonpregnant Women. *Am. J. Clin. Nutr.* **1989**, *50*, 1039–1049. [PubMed]

28. Blanchard, J.; Conrad, K.A.; Watson, R.R.; Garry, P.J.; Crawley, J.D. Comparison of Plasma, Mononuclear and Polymorphonuclear Leucocyte Vitamin C Levels in Young and Elderly Women during Depletion and Supplementation. *Eur. J. Clin. Nutr.* **1989**, *43*, 97–106. [PubMed]

29. Jacob, R.A. Assessment of Human Vitamin C status12. *J. Nutr.* **1990**, *120*, 1480–1485. [PubMed]

30. Johnston, C.S.; Thompson, L.L. Vitamin C Status of an Outpatient Population. *J. Am. Coll. Nutr.* **1998**, *17*, 366–370. [CrossRef] [PubMed]

31. Johnston, C.S.; Solomon, R.E.; Corte, C. Vitamin C Depletion is Associated with Alterations in Blood Histamine and Plasma Free Carnitine in Adults. *J. Am. Coll. Nutr.* **1996**, *15*, 586–591. [CrossRef] [PubMed]

32. De Leeuw, K.; Sanders, J.S.; Stegeman, C.; Smit, A.; Kallenberg, C.G.; Bijl, M. Accelerated Atherosclerosis in Patients with Wegener's Granulomatosis. *Ann. Rheum. Dis.* **2005**, *64*, 753–759. [CrossRef] [PubMed]

33. Montoye, H.J.; Kemper, H.C.; Saris, W.H.; Washburn, R.A. *Measuring Physical Activity and Energy Expenditure*; Human Kinetics: Champaign, IL, USA, 1996.

34. Levey, A.S.; Stevens, L.A.; Schmid, C.H.; Zhang, Y.L.; Castro, A.F.; Feldman, H.I.; Kusek, J.W.; Eggers, P.; Van Lente, F.; Greene, T. A New Equation to Estimate Glomerular Filtration Rate. *Ann. Intern. Med.* **2009**, *150*, 604–612. [CrossRef] [PubMed]

35. Preacher, K.J.; Hayes, A.F. SPSS and SAS Procedures for Estimating Indirect Effects in Simple Mediation Models. *Behav. Res. Methods* **2004**, *36*, 717–731. [CrossRef]

36. Hayes, A.F. Beyond Baron and Kenny: Statistical Mediation Analysis in the New Millennium. *Commun. Monogr.* **2009**, *76*, 408–420. [CrossRef]

37. Zhang, K.; Li, Y.; Cheng, X.; Liu, L.; Bai, W.; Guo, W.; Wu, L.; Zuo, L. Cross-over study of influence of oral vitamin C supplementation on inflammatory status in maintenance hemodialysis patients. *BMC Nephrol.* **2013**, *14*, 252. [CrossRef] [PubMed]

38. Attallah, N.; Osman-Malik, Y.; Frinak, S.; Besarab, A. Effect of intravenous ascorbic acid in hemodialysis patients with EPO-hyporesponsive anemia and hyperferritinemia. *Am. J. Kidney Dis.* **2006**, *47*, 644–654. [CrossRef] [PubMed]

Nutrients **2017**, *9*, 568

39. Koenig, W.; Sund, M.; Frohlich, M.; Lowel, H.; Hutchinson, W.L.; Pepys, M.B. Refinement of the Association of Serum C-Reactive Protein Concentration and Coronary Heart Disease Risk by Correction for within-Subject Variation Over Time: The MONICA Augsburg Studies, 1984 and 1987. *Am. J. Epidemiol.* **2003**, *158*, 357–364. [CrossRef] [PubMed]

40. Danesh, J.; Wheeler, J.G.; Hirschfield, G.M.; Eda, S.; Eiriksdottir, G.; Rumley, A.; Lowe, G.D.; Pepys, M.B.; Gudnason, V. C-Reactive Protein and Other Circulating Markers of Inflammation in the Prediction of Coronary Heart Disease. *N. Engl. J. Med.* **2004**, *350*, 1387–1397. [CrossRef] [PubMed]

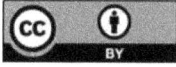

nutrients

MDPI

Review

The Roles of Vitamin C in Skin Health

Juliet M. Pullar, Anitra C. Carr and Margreet C. M. Vissers *

Department of Pathology, University of Otago, Christchurch, P.O. Box 4345, Christchurch 8140, New Zealand; juliet.pullar@otago.ac.nz (J.M.P.); anitra.carr@otago.ac.nz (A.C.C.)
* Correspondence: margreet.vissers@otago.ac.nz; Tel.: +64-3364-1524

Received: 10 July 2017; Accepted: 9 August 2017; Published: 12 August 2017

Abstract: The primary function of the skin is to act as a barrier against insults from the environment, and its unique structure reflects this. The skin is composed of two layers: the epidermal outer layer is highly cellular and provides the barrier function, and the inner dermal layer ensures strength and elasticity and gives nutritional support to the epidermis. Normal skin contains high concentrations of vitamin C, which supports important and well-known functions, stimulating collagen synthesis and assisting in antioxidant protection against UV-induced photodamage. This knowledge is often used as a rationale for the addition of vitamin C to topical applications, but the efficacy of such treatment, as opposed to optimising dietary vitamin C intake, is poorly understood. This review discusses the potential roles for vitamin C in skin health and summarises the in vitro and in vivo research to date. We compare the efficacy of nutritional intake of vitamin C versus topical application, identify the areas where lack of evidence limits our understanding of the potential benefits of vitamin C on skin health, and suggest which skin properties are most likely to benefit from improved nutritional vitamin C intake.

Keywords: ascorbate; dermis; epidermis; skin barrier function; vitamin C status; skin aging; wound healing; collagen; UV protection

1. Introduction

The skin is a multi-functional organ, the largest in the body, and its appearance generally reflects the health and efficacy of its underlying structures. It has many functions, but its fundamental role is to provide a protective interface between the external environment and an individual's tissues, providing shielding from mechanical and chemical threats, pathogens, ultraviolet radiation and even dehydration (functions reviewed in [1]). Being in constant contact with the external environment, the skin is subject to more insults than most of our other organs, and is where the first visible signs of aging occur.

The skin is composed of two main layers with quite different underlying structures—the outermost epidermis and the deeper dermis (Figure 1). The epidermis fulfils most of the barrier functions of the skin and is predominantly made up of cells, mostly keratinocytes [2]. The keratinocytes are arranged in layers throughout the epidermis; as these cells divide and proliferate away from the basal layer, which is closest to the dermis, they begin to differentiate. This process is called keratinization, and involves the production of specialized structural proteins, secretion of lipids, and the formation of a cellular envelope of cross-linked proteins. During differentiation, virtually all of the subcellular organelles disappear, including the nucleus [3,4]. The cytoplasm is also removed, although there is evidence that some enzymes remain [4]. Thus, the uppermost layer of the epidermis that interacts with the outside environment is composed of flattened metabolically 'dead' cells (the terminally differentiated keratinocytes). These cells are sealed together with lipid-rich domains, forming a water-impermeable barrier. This layer is known as the stratum corneum (Figure 1) and fulfils the primary barrier function of the epidermis, although the lower epidermal layers also contribute [5].

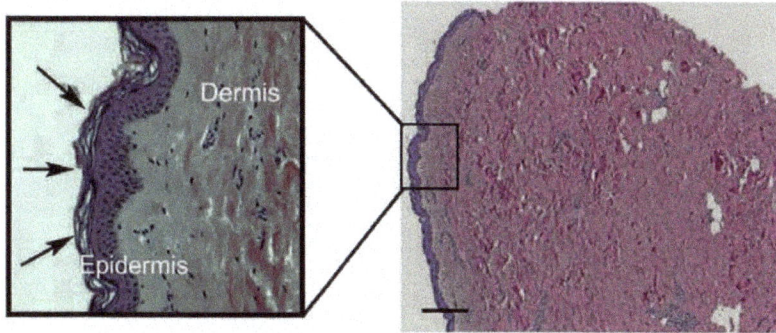

Figure 1. Micrograph of human breast skin sample, showing the full depth of the dermis (pink staining) in comparison to the thin layer of epidermis (purple staining). The scale bar indicates 200 µm. A zoomed-in image is shown within the box. The stratum corneum, the outermost layer of the epidermis, is indicated by the arrows, with its characteristic basket-weave structure. The collagen bundles in the dermis are very clear, as are the scattered purple-stained fibroblasts that generate this structure.

In contrast, the dermal skin layer provides strength and elasticity, and includes the vascular, lymphatic and neuronal systems. It is relatively acellular and is primarily made up of complex extracellular matrix proteins [6], being particularly rich in collagen fibres, which make up ~75% of the dermis dry weight (Figure 1). The major cell type present in the dermis is fibroblasts, which are heavily involved in the synthesis of many of the extracellular matrix components. Blood vessels that supply nutrients to both skin layers are also present in the dermis [1,2]. Between the two main layers is the dermal–epidermal junction, a specialised basement membrane structure that fixes the epidermis to the dermis below.

2. Role of Nutrition in Skin Health

It is accepted that nutritional status with respect to both macronutrients and micronutrients is important for skin health and appearance [7]. Evidence of this is provided by the many vitamin deficiency diseases that result in significant disorders of the skin [8]. Dermatological signs of B vitamin deficiency, for example, include a patchy red rash, seborrhoeic dermatitis and fungal skin and nail infections [9,10]. The vitamin C deficiency disease scurvy is characterised by skin fragility, bleeding gums and corkscrew hairs as well as impaired wound healing [11–18].

Nutritional status is vital for maintaining normal functioning of the skin during collagen synthesis and keratinocyte differentiation [7]. Additionally, many of the components of our antioxidant defences such as vitamins C and E and selenium are obtained from the diet, and these are likely to be important for protection against UV-induced damage [19–23].

Nutrition Issues Specific to the Skin

The epidermis is a challenged environment for nutrient delivery, as it lacks the blood vessels that normally deliver nutrients to cells. Delivery of nutrients is dependent on diffusion from the vascularized dermis [24], and this may be particularly limited for the outermost layers of the epidermis (Figure 2). Delivery is further compounded by the chemical nature of these outer epidermal layers in which there is little movement of extracellular fluid between cells due to the complex lipid/protein crosslink structure forming the skin barrier. All of this makes it likely that dietary nutrients are not easily able to reach the cells in the outermost layers of the epidermis, and these cells receive little nutrient support.

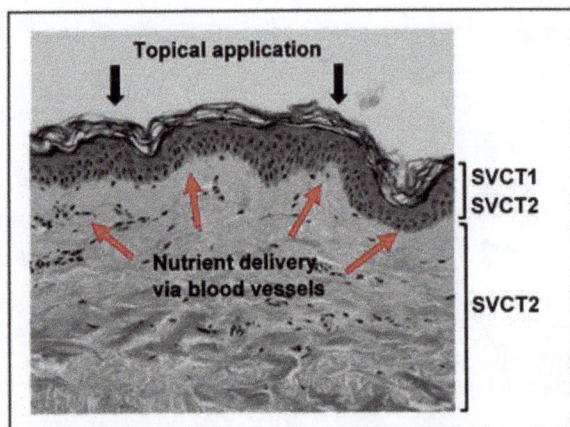

Figure 2. Delivery of nutrients to the skin. The location of the vitamin C transport proteins SVCT1 and SVCT2 are indicated. Red arrows depict nutrient flow from the blood vessels in the dermis to the epidermal layer. Nutrients delivered by topical application would need to penetrate the barrier formed by the stratum corneum.

The skin can be targeted for nutrient delivery through topical application (Figure 2). However, in this case the delivery vehicle is influential, as the stratum corneum functions as an effective aqueous barrier and prevents the passage of many substances [1]. Although some uncharged and lipid-soluble molecules can pass through the surface layer, it is unlikely that nutrients delivered via topical application would easily penetrate into the lower layers of the dermis [22]. The dermal layer functions are therefore best supported by nutrients delivered through the bloodstream.

3. Vitamin C Content of Skin

Normal skin contains high concentrations of vitamin C, with levels comparable to other body tissues and well above plasma concentrations, suggesting active accumulation from the circulation. Most of the vitamin C in the skin appears to be in intracellular compartments, with concentrations likely to be in the millimolar range [25–27]. It is transported into cells from the blood vessels present in the dermal layer. Skin vitamin C levels have not often been reported and there is considerable variation in the published levels, with a 10-fold range across a number of independent studies (Table 1). Levels are similar to that found in numerous other body organs. The variation in reported levels most likely reflects the difficulty in handling skin tissue, which is very resilient to degradation and solubilisation, but may also be due to the location of the skin sample and the age of the donor.

Table 1. Vitamin C content of human skin and a comparison with other tissues.

Tissue	Vitamin C Content (mg/100 g Wet Weight)	References
Adrenal glands	30–40	[28]
Pituitary glands	40–50	[29]
Liver	10–16	[28,30]
Spleen	10–15	[28,31]
Lungs	7	[28]
Kidneys	5–15	[30]
Heart muscle	5–15	[28,29,31]
Skeletal muscle	3–4	[29,32]
Brain	13–15	[28]
Skin-epidermis	6–64	[25–27]
Skin-dermis	3–13	[25–27]

Several reports have indicated that vitamin C levels are lower in aged or photodamaged skin [25–27]. Whether this association reflects cause or effect is unknown, but it has also been reported that excessive exposure to oxidant stress via pollutants or UV irradiation is associated with depleted vitamin C levels in the epidermal layer [33,34]. Indeed, more vitamin C is found in the epidermal layer than in the dermis, with differences of 2–5-fold between the two layers being consistently reported (Table 1 and [25,26]). Levels of vitamin C in skin are similar to the levels of other water soluble antioxidants such as glutathione [25–27,35]. There is a suggestion that vitamin C in the stratum corneum layer of the epidermis exists in a concentration gradient [36]. The lowest vitamin C concentration was present at the outer surface of the epidermis of the SKH-1 hairless mouse, a model of human skin, with a sharp increase in concentration in the deeper layers of the stratum corneum, possibly reflecting depletion in the outer cells due to chronic exposure to the environment [36].

3.1. The Bioavailability and Uptake of Vitamin C into the Skin

3.1.1. The Sodium-Dependent Vitamin C Transporters

Vitamin C uptake from the plasma and transport across the skin layers is mediated by specific sodium-dependent vitamin C transporters (SVCTs) that are present throughout the body and are also responsible for transport into other tissues. Interestingly, cells in the epidermis express both types of vitamin C transporter, SVCT1 and SVCT2 (Figure 2) [37]. This contrasts with most other tissues, which express SVCT2 only [37–39]. SVCT1 expression in the body is largely confined to the epithelial cells in the small intestine and the kidney and is associated with active inter-cellular transport of the vitamin [40,41]. The specific localisation of SVCT1 in the epidermis is of interest due to the lack of vasculature in this tissue, and suggests that the combined expression of both transporters 1 and 2 ensures effective uptake and intracellular accumulation of the vitamin. Together with the high levels of vitamin C measured in the epidermal layer, the dual expression of the SVCTs suggests a high dependency on vitamin C in this tissue.

Both transporters are hydrophobic membrane proteins that co-transport sodium, driving the uptake of vitamin C into cells. Replacement of sodium with other positively charged ions completely abolishes transport [42]. SVCT1 and SVCT2 have quite different uptake kinetics reflecting their different physiological functions. SVCT1 transports vitamin C with a low affinity but with a high capacity (K_m of 65–237 μmol/L) mediating uptake of vitamin C from the diet and re-uptake in the tubule cells in the kidney [41]. SVCT2, which is present in almost every cell in the body, is thought to be a high-affinity, low capacity transporter, with a K_m of ~20 μM meaning it can function at low concentrations of vitamin C [41]. As well as transporter affinity, vitamin C transport is regulated by the availability of the SVCT proteins on the plasma membrane.

3.1.2. Bioavailability and Uptake

Most tissues of the body respond to plasma availability of vitamin C and concentrations vary accordingly, with lower tissue levels being reported when plasma levels are below saturation [43–47]. The kinetics of uptake varies between tissues, with vitamin C levels in some organs (e.g., the brain) reaching a plateau at lower plasma vitamin C status, whereas other tissue levels (e.g., skeletal muscle) continue to increase in close association with increasing plasma supply [32,44,45,48].

Very little is known about vitamin C accumulation in the skin and there are no studies that have investigated the relationship between skin vitamin C content and nutrient intake or plasma supply. Two human studies have shown an increase in skin vitamin C content following supplementation with vitamin C, but neither contained adequate measures of plasma vitamin C levels in the participants before or after supplementation [27,49]. In one other study, vitamin C content was measured in buccal keratinocytes, as these cells are proposed to be a good model for skin keratinocytes [50]. The keratinocyte vitamin C concentration doubled upon supplementation of the participants with

3 g/day vitamin C for six weeks, a dosage that is significantly higher than the recommended daily intake and would achieve plasma saturation and likely also tissue saturation [44].

Thus it appears likely that, as with many other tissues, skin vitamin C levels respond to increases in plasma supply [27,50]. A paper by Nusgens and co-workers suggests that skin levels do not increase further once plasma saturation is reached [51]. Dietary supplementation is therefore only expected to be effective in elevating skin vitamin C in individuals who have below-saturation plasma levels prior to intervention.

3.1.3. Topical Application of Vitamin C

When plasma levels are low, some vitamin C can be delivered to the epidermal layer by topical application, although the efficacy of this is dependent on the formulation of the cream or serum used on the skin [51–55]. Vitamin C, as a water-soluble and charged molecule, is repelled by the physical barrier of the terminally differentiated epidermal cells. It is only when pH levels are below 4 and vitamin C is present as ascorbic acid that some penetration occurs [56], but whether this results in increased levels in the metabolically compromised stratum corneum is unknown. A great deal of effort has been put into the development of ascorbic acid derivatives for the purpose of topical application. Such derivatives need to ensure stabilization of the molecule from oxidation and also overcome the significant challenge of skin penetration. In addition, they must be converted to ascorbic acid in vivo in order to be effective. Whether there is a single solution to all these challenges is unclear [57]. The addition of a phosphate group confers greater stability and these derivatives may be converted to ascorbic acid in vivo, albeit at a slow rate [58], but they are poorly absorbed through the skin [56,59,60]. Ascorbyl glucoside also exhibits superior stability and can penetrate, but the rate of its in vivo conversion is not known [57,61–63]. Derivatives containing lipid-soluble moieties such as palmitate are designed to assist with delivery, and although increased uptake has been demonstrated in animals [64], they do not necessarily show improved stability and there is some doubt as to whether these derivatives are efficiently converted in vivo [57]. Recent studies suggest that encapsulation into a liospheric form may assist with transport into the lower layers of the epidermis and could result in increased uptake [65–67]. However, the most pertinent issue for the efficacy of topical application is likely to be the plasma status of the individual: if plasma levels are saturated, then it appears that topical application does not increase skin vitamin C content [51].

3.1.4. Vitamin C Deficiency

One of the most compelling arguments for a vital role for vitamin C in skin health is the association between vitamin C deficiency and the loss of a number of important skin functions. In particular, poor wound healing (associated with collagen formation), thickening of the stratum corneum and subcutaneous bleeding (due to fragility and loss of connective tissue morphology) are extreme and rapid in onset in vitamin-C-deficient individuals [11,15–18]. It is thought that similar processes occur when body stores are below optimal, although to a lesser extent [46,68].

4. Potential Functions of Vitamin C in the Skin

The high concentration of vitamin C in the skin indicates that it has a number of important biological functions that are relevant to skin health. Based on what we know about vitamin C function, attention has been focused on collagen formation and antioxidant protection; however, evidence is emerging for other activities.

4.1. The Promotion of Collagen Formation

Vitamin C acts as a co-factor for the proline and lysine hydroxylases that stabilise the collagen molecule tertiary structure, and it also promotes collagen gene expression [69–77]. In the skin, collagen formation is carried out mostly by the fibroblasts in the dermis, resulting in the generation of the basement membrane and dermal collagen matrix (Figure 3) [75,78]. The dependence of the collagen hydroxylase enzymes on vitamin C has been demonstrated in a number of studies with fibroblast cells in vitro [69,73,79], with both decreased total synthesis and decreased crosslinking when vitamin C is absent [80–82]. The activity of the hydroxylases is much more difficult to measure in vivo, as the amount of collagen synthesised may vary only a little [51,52]. Rather, animal studies with the vitamin-C-deficient GULO mouse indicate that the stability of the synthesised collagen varies with vitamin C availability, reflecting the stabilising function of the collagen crosslinks formed by the hydroxylases [76]. In addition to stabilising the collagen molecule by hydroxylation, vitamin C also stimulates collagen mRNA production by fibroblasts [78,83].

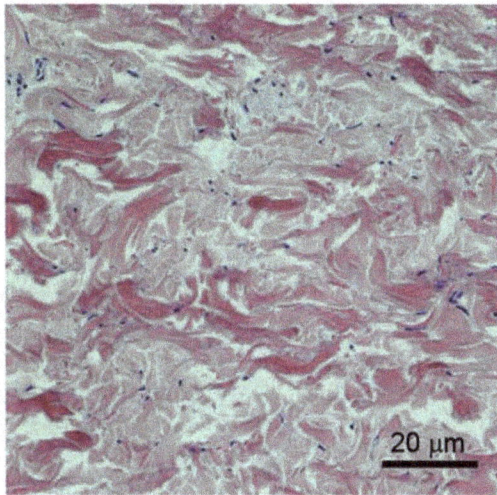

Figure 3. Structure of the dermis. Higher magnification of H&E-stained dermis, showing the irregular nature of the bundled collagen fibres (pink stained) and sparse presence of the fibroblasts (blue nuclear staining). Vitamin C present in the fibroblasts supports the synthesis of the collagen fibres.

4.2. The Ability to Scavenge Free Radicals and Dispose of Toxic Oxidants

Vitamin C is a potent antioxidant that can neutralise and remove oxidants, such as those found in environmental pollutants and after exposure to ultraviolet radiation. This activity appears to be of particular importance in the epidermis, where vitamin C is concentrated in the skin. However, vitamin C is only one player in the antioxidant arsenal that includes enzymatic defences (catalase, glutathione peroxidase and superoxide dismutase) as well as other non-enzymatic defences (vitamin E, glutathione, uric acid and other putative antioxidants such as carotenoids) [19,21,33,34,84–88]. Most intervention studies carried out to determine the capacity of antioxidants to prevent oxidative damage to skin have used a cocktail of these compounds [21,88–90]. Vitamin C is particularly effective at reducing oxidative damage to the skin when it is used in conjunction with vitamin E [21,54,89,91,92]. This is in accord with its known function as a regenerator of oxidised vitamin E, thereby effectively recycling this important lipid-soluble radical scavenger and limiting oxidative damage to cell membrane structures [92,93] (Figure 4).

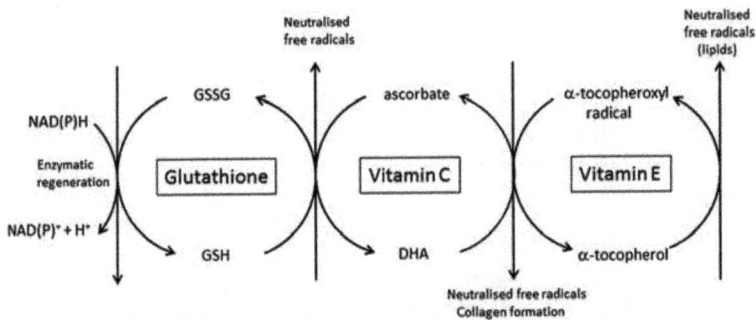

Figure 4. The central role for vitamin C and other antioxidants pertinent to the skin. The interdependence of vitamins E and C, and glutathione, in the scavenging of free radicals and regeneration of the reduced antioxidants, is shown. Vitamin E is in the lipid fraction of the cell, whereas vitamin C and glutathione are water-soluble and present in the cytosol.

4.3. Inhibition of Melanogenesis

Vitamin C derivatives, including the magnesium phosophate ascorbyl derivative, have been shown to decrease melanin synthesis both in cultured melanocytes and in vivo [94,95]. This activity has been proposed to be due to its ability to interfere with the action of tyrosinase, the rate-limiting enzyme in melanogenesis. Tyrosinase catalyses the hydroxylation of tyrosine to dihydroxyphenylalanine (DOPA), and the oxidation of DOPA to its corresponding ortho-quinone. The inhibition in melanin production by vitamin C is thought to be due to the vitamin's ability to reduce the ortho-quinones generated by tyrosinase [94], although other mechanisms are also possible [96]. Agents that decrease melanogenesis are used to treat skin hyperpigmentation in conditions such as melisma or age spots.

4.4. Interaction with Cell Signalling Pathways

In vitro studies clearly show that vitamin C can play a role in the differentiation of keratinocytes (Table 2). For example, vitamin C enhanced the differentiation of rat epidermal keratinocytes cells in an organotypic culture model [97], with markedly improved ultrastructural organisation of the stratum corneum, accompanied by enhanced barrier function. Vitamin C also increased numbers of keratohyalin granules and levels of the late differentiation marker filaggrin, which appeared to be due to altered gene expression [97]. Others have also shown that vitamin C promotes synthesis and organization of barrier lipids and increased cornified envelope formation during differentiation [98–102]. The mechanism(s) by which vitamin C modulates keratinocyte differentiation is not yet elucidated; however, it has been hypothesized to be under the control of protein kinase C and AP-1 [99].

In addition to vitamin C's ability to promote collagen synthesis [73,79], there is evidence to suggest that vitamin C increases proliferation and migration of dermal fibroblasts [78,82,102], functions vital for effective wound healing, although the underlying mechanisms driving this activity are not yet known [78]. Through the stimulation of regulatory hydroxylases, vitamin C also regulates the stabilization and activation of the hypoxia-inducible factor (HIF)-1, a metabolic sensor that controls the expression of hundreds of genes involved with cell survival and tissue remodelling, including collagenases [103–105]. Vitamin C has been shown to both stimulate [69] and inhibit elastin synthesis in cultured fibroblasts [81]. Glycosaminoglycan synthesis as part of extracellular matrix formation is also increased by vitamin C treatment [106], and it may also influence gene expression of antioxidant enzymes, including those involved in DNA repair [78]. As such, vitamin C has been shown to increase the repair of oxidatively damaged bases. [78]. The modulation of gene expression may be important for its ability to protect during UV exposure via its inhibition of pro-inflammatory cytokine secretion and apoptosis [107–109].

4.5. Modulation of Epigenetic Pathways

In addition to the gene regulatory activities listed above, vitamin C has a role in epigenetic regulation of gene expression by functioning as a co-factor for the ten-eleven translocation (TET) family of enzymes, which catalyse the removal of methylated cytosine through its hydroxylation to 5-hydroxymethylcytosine (5 hmC) [110–112]. As well as being a DNA demethylation intermediate, it appears that 5 hmC is an epigenetic mark in its own right, with transcriptional regulatory activity [113]. Aberrant epigenetic alterations are thought to have a role in cancer progression, and there is data to suggest that a loss of 5 hmC occurs during the early development and progression of melanoma [114]. Interestingly, vitamin C treatment has been shown to increase 5 hmC content in melanoma cell lines, also causing a consequent alteration in the transcriptome and a decrease in malignant phenotype [115]. Because TETs have a specific requirement for vitamin C to maintain enzyme activity [116], this provides a further mechanism by which the vitamin may affect gene expression and cell function. For example, Lin and co-workers showed that vitamin C protected against UV-induced apoptosis of an epidermal cell line via a TET-dependent mechanism, which involved increases in p21 and p16 gene expression [117].

Table 2. Summary of key in vitro studies investigating potential effects of vitamin C on the skin.

Study Description	Measured Parameters	Outcome and Comment	Reference
Effects on collagen and elastin synthesis			
Vit. C effects on collagen and elastin synthesis in human skin fibroblasts and vascular smooth muscle cells.	Monitored vit. C time of exposure and dose on collagen synthesis and gene expression, and elastin synthesis and gene regulation.	Vit. C exposure increased collagen, decreased elastin. Stabilization of collagen mRNA, lesser stability of elastin mRNA, and repression of elastin gene transcription.	[81]
Effect of vit. C on collagen synthesis and SVCT2 expression in human skin fibroblasts. Vit. C added to culture medium for 5 days.	Vit. C uptake measured into cells, collagen I and IV measured with RT-PCR and ELISA, and RT-PCR for SVCT2.	Vit. C increased collagen I and IV, and increased SVCT2 expression.	[73]
Effect of vit. C on elastin generation by fibroblasts from normal human skin, stretch-marked skin, keloids and dermal fat.	Immunohistochemistry and western blotting for detection of elastin and precursors.	50 and 200 µM vit. C increased elastin production, 800 µM inhibited. No measures of vit. C uptake into cells.	[69]
Effects on morphology, differentiation and gene expression			
Vit. C addition to cultures of rat keratinocytes (REK).	Effect on differentiation and stratum corneum formation.	Morphology showed enhanced stratum corneum structure, increased keratohyalin granules and organization of intercellular lipid lamellae in the interstices of the stratum corneum. Increased profilaggrin and filaggrin.	[97]
Effect of vit. C on human keratinocyte (HaCaT) cell line differentiation in vitro.	Measured development of cornified envelope (CE), gene expression.	CE formation and keratinocyte differentiation induced by vit. C, suggesting a role in formation of stratum corneum and barrier formation in vivo.	[99]
Effect of vit. C supplementation on gene expression in human skin fibroblasts.	Total RNA nano assay, for genetic profiling, with and without vit. C in culture medium.	Increased gene expression for DNA replication and repair and cell cycle progression. Increased mitogenic stimulation and cell motility in the context of wound healing. Faster repair of damaged DNA bases.	[78]

Table 2. *Cont.*

Study Description	Measured Parameters	Outcome and Comment	Reference
Effect of vit. C on dermal epidermal junction in skin model (keratinocytes and fibroblasts).	Keratinocyte organisation, fibroblast number, basement membrane protein deposition and mRNA expression.	Vit. C improved keratinocyte and basement membrane organisation. Increased fibroblast number, saw deposition of basement membrane proteins.	[102]
Effect of vit. C on cultured skin models—combined human epidermal keratinocytes and dermal fibroblasts.	Monitored morphology, lipid composition.	Vit. C, but not vit. E, improved epidermal morphology, ceramide production and phospholipid layer formation.	[98]
Protective effects against UV irradiation			
Effect of vit. C on UVA irradiation of primary cultures of human keratinocytes.	Vit. C added in low concentrations, monitored MDA, TBA, GSH, cell viability, IL-1, IL-6 generation.	Vit. C improved resistance to UVA, decreased MDA and TBA levels, increased GSH levels, decreased IL-1 and IL-6 levels.	[109]
Effect of vit. C uptake into human keratinocyte (HaCaT) cell line on outcome to UV irradiation.	Accumulation of vit. C in keratinocytes, antioxidant capacity by DHDCF and apoptosis induction by UV irradiation.	Keratinocytes accumulated mM levels of vit. C, increasing antioxidant status and protecting against apoptosis.	[108]
Effect of UVB on vit. C uptake into human keratinocyte cell line (HaCaT) and effects on inflammatory gene expression.	Cellular vit. C measured by HPLC, mRNA expression for chemokines, western blotting for SVCT localisation.	Vit. C uptake was increased with UVB irradiation, chemokine expression decreased with vit. C uptake.	[107]
Protective effects against ozone exposure			
Effect of antioxidant mixtures of vit. C, vit. E and ferulic acid on exposure of cultured normal human keratinocytes to ozone.	Cell viability, proliferation, HNE, protein carbonyls, Nrf2, NFkappaB activation, IL-8 generation.	Vit. C-containing mixtures inhibited toxicity. The presence of vit. E provided additional protection against HNE and protein carbonyls.	[118]
Protection of cultured skin cells against ozone exposure with vit. C, vit. E, and resveratrol. 3-D culture of human dermis—fibroblasts with collagen I + III.	Cell death, HNE levels, expression of transcription factors Nrf-2 and NfkappaB	Extensive protection against cell damage with mixtures containing vit. C. Increased expression of antioxidant proteins. Additional effect of vit. E + C. No effect with Vit. E alone.	[119]

5. Challenges to the Maintenance of Skin Health and Potential Protection by Vitamin C

During the course of a normal lifetime, the skin is exposed to a number of challenges that can affect structure, function and appearance, including:

- Deterioration due to normal aging, contributing to loss of elasticity and wrinkle formation.
- Exposure to the elements, leading to discolouration, dryness and accelerated wrinkling.
- Chemical insults including exposure to oxidising beauty and cleansing products (hair dyes, soaps, detergents, bleaches).
- Direct injury, as in wounding and burning.

Vitamin C may provide significant protection against these changes and regeneration of healthy skin following insult and injury is a goal for most of us. The following sections, and the summary in Tables 3 and 4, review the available evidence of a role for vitamin C in the maintenance of healthy skin and the prevention of damage.

5.1. Skin Aging

Like the rest of the human body, the skin is subject to changes caused by the process of natural aging. All skin layers show age-related changes in structure and functional capacity [6,120] and, as occurs in other body systems, this may result in increased susceptibility to a variety of disorders and diseases, such as the development of dermatoses and skin cancer [6,22,121,122]. As well as this, changes in the appearance of skin are often the first visible signs of aging and this can have implications for our emotional and mental wellbeing.

Aging of skin can be thought of as two distinct processes—natural or 'intrinsic' aging, caused simply by the passage of time, and environmental aging [121,123,124]. Lifestyle factors such as smoking and exposure to environmental pollutants increase the rate of environmental aging, and can have a marked impact on the function and appearance of skin [22,121–124]. Exposure to chronic ultraviolet radiation from sunlight is also a major environmental factor that prematurely damages our skin (effects are detailed in the photoaging section below) [125]. The changes due to environmental aging are usually superimposed on those that occur naturally, often making it difficult to distinguish between the two [22].

Intrinsic aging is a slow process and, in the absence of environmental aging, changes are not usually apparent until advanced age, when smooth skin with fine wrinkles, pale skin tone, reduced elasticity, and occasional exaggerated expression lines are evident [6,22,24]. There is a reduction in the thickness of the dermal layer [22], along with fewer fibroblasts and mast cells, less collagen production and reduced vascularisation [24]. Specifically, during intrinsic aging there is gradual degradation of the extracellular matrix components, particularly elastin and collagen [124,126]. The loss of elastin results in the reduction in elasticity and capacity for recoil that is observed in aging skin.

Dry skin is very common in older adults [127], largely due to a loss of glycosaminoglycans and accompanied reduction in the ability to maintain moisture levels [126,128]. The dermal-epidermal junction may also become flattened, losing surface area and leading to increased skin fragility [22], and potentially causing reduced nutrient transfer between the two layers. In general, the dermis suffers from greater age-related changes than the epidermis [1]. However, the aged epidermis shows a reduced barrier function and also reduced repair following insult [6]. Antioxidant capacity, immune function and melanin production may also be impaired in aged skin [22].

Intrinsic aging is largely unavoidable and may be largely dependent on our genetic background and other factors [129,130]. Some mitigation of these effects may be achieved by:

- Limiting exposure to environmental risk factors such as smoking, poor nutrition and chronic exposure to sunlight, which cause premature skin aging.
- Using treatments to potentially reverse skin damage, including topical or systemic treatments that help regenerate the elastic fibre system and collagen [126].

5.1.1. The Role of Vitamin C in the Prevention of Skin Aging

The ability of vitamin C to limit natural aging is difficult to distinguish from its ability to prevent the additional insults due to excessive sun exposure, smoking or environmental stress and there is very limited information available concerning a relationship between vitamin C levels and general skin deterioration. The most compelling argument for a role of vitamin C in protecting skin function comes from observations that deficiency causes obvious skin problems—early signs of scurvy, for example, include skin fragility, corkscrew hairs and poor wound healing [11–17].

Because vitamin C deficiency results in impaired function, it is assumed that increasing intake will be beneficial. However, there are no studies that have measured vitamin C levels or intake and associated aging changes [130]. Vitamin C is almost never measured in the skin and this information is needed before we can improve our understanding of what level of intake might be beneficial for skin health and protection against aging-related changes.

5.1.2. Nutritional Studies Linking Vitamin C with Skin Health

Although there is no information specific to vitamin C and aging in the skin, many studies have attempted to determine the role of nutrition more generally [85,131–133]. A recent systematic review of studies involving nutrition and appearance identified 27 studies that were either dietary intervention studies or reported dietary intakes [134]. The analysis indicated that, in the most reliable studies, intervention with a nutrient supplement (15 studies) or general foods (one study) was associated with improved measures of skin elasticity, facial wrinkling, roughness and colour [134]. Many of the nutrient interventions that showed a benefit included a high intake of fruit and vegetables, which contribute significant levels of vitamin C to the diet.

A double-blind nutrition intervention study has evaluated the effects of dietary supplementation with a fermented papaya extract, thought to have antioxidant activity [135], and an antioxidant cocktail containing 10 mg trans resveratrol, 60 µg selenium, 10 mg vitamin E and 50 mg vitamin C in a population of healthy individuals aged between 40 and 65, all with visible signs of skin aging. Following a 90-day supplementation period, skin surface, brown spots, evenness, moisture, elasticity (face), lipid peroxidation markers, superoxide dismutase activity, nitric oxide (NO) concentration, and the expression levels of key genes were measured. Notably, the intervention resulted in a measureable improvement in skin physical parameters, with a generally enhanced response from the fermented papaya extract compared with the antioxidant cocktail. Gene expression, measured by RNA extraction and RT-PCR, indicated that the papaya extract increased expression of aquaporin-3, and decreased expression of cyclophilin A and CD147. Aquaporin 3 regulates water transport across the lipid bilayer in keratinocytes and fibroblasts and therefore improves skin health [136]; cyclophilin A and the transmembrane glycoprotein CD147 negatively impact on skin DNA repair mechanisms and affect the inflammatory response, therefore negatively impacting skin health. This is an interesting study and suggests that antioxidant supplementation, including vitamin C, could benefit skin health generally. The antioxidant cocktail did not affect gene expression, and this may reflect the low concentrations of each component in the supplement, which is unlikely to influence levels in a healthy population. Although there were no direct measures to determine whether antioxidant status was actually improved in the participants, antioxidant activity was improved in the skin following intake of the papaya extract, as evidenced by decreased markers of lipid peroxidation and increased superoxide dismutase activity.

5.2. UV Radiation and Photoaging

There is mounting evidence to suggest that the most significant environmental challenge to the skin is chronic exposure to ultraviolet radiation from the sun or from tanning beds [22,90,123,137]. UV radiation damages skin through the production of reactive oxygen species, which can damage the extracellular matrix components and affect both the structure and function of cells. While the skin contains endogenous antioxidant defences, vitamins E and C and antioxidant enzymes to quench these oxidants and repair the resultant damage, these antioxidants will be consumed by repeated exposure and the skin's defences can thereby be overwhelmed [25,138–141].

Acute exposure of skin to UV radiation can cause sunburn, resulting in a large inflammatory response causing characteristic redness, swelling and heat. In addition, altered pigmentation, immune suppression and damage to the dermal extracellular matrix can occur [24,25,56,142,143]. By comparison, chronic long-term exposure to UV radiation causes premature aging of the skin, with dramatic and significant disruption to skin structure, and leads to the development of skin cancer [6,24]. Termed photoaging, the most obvious features are wrinkles, hyperpigmentation and marked changes in skin elasticity that cause skin sagging, with the skin also becoming sallow and rougher with age [123,144]. Photoaged skin is most likely to be found on the face, chest and upper surface of the arms.

Both the epidermal and dermal layers of skin are susceptible to chronic UV exposure; however, the most profound changes occur in the extracellular matrix of the dermis [24]. Changes include a significant loss of collagen fibrils within the dermis, but also specific loss of collagen anchoring fibrils at the dermal–epidermal junction [126]. Dermal glycosaminoglycan content is increased in what appear to be disorganised aggregates [126]. Elastic fibres throughout the dermis are also susceptible to UV radiation, with accumulation of disorganised elastic fibre proteins evident in severely photoaged skin. Indeed, this accumulation, termed 'solar elastosis', is considered to be a defining characteristic of severely photoaged skin [6,22,24,126]. There is also evidence of epidermal atrophy or 'wasting away' during photoaging, and of a reduction in the barrier function [6]. In addition, the epidermis can become hyperpigmented from chronic UV exposure; these lesions are known as age spots or liver spots.

Preventing exposure to UV radiation is the best means of protecting the skin from the detrimental effects of photoaging. However, avoidance is not always possible, so sunscreen is commonly used to block or reduce the amount of UV reaching the skin. However, sunscreens expose the skin to chemicals that may cause other problems such as disruption of the skin barrier function or induction of inflammation [56].

Vitamin-C-Mediated Protection against Photoaging and UV Damage

Changes to the skin due to UV exposure have much in common with the rather slower process of 'natural' aging, with one major difference being a more acute onset. It is established that vitamin C limits the damage induced by UV exposure [27,54,89,145,146]. This type of injury is directly mediated by a radical-generating process, and protection is primarily related to its antioxidant activity. This has been demonstrated with cells in vitro and in vivo, using both topical and dietary intake of vitamin C [54,139,147,148]. It appears that UV light depletes vitamin C content in the epidermis, which also indicates that it is targeted by the oxidants induced by such exposure [138,149]. Vitamin C prevents lipid peroxidation in cultured keratinocytes following UV exposure and also protects the keratinocyte from apoptosis and increases cell survival [21,99,107].

Sunburn is measured as the minimal erythemal dose (MED) in response to acute UV exposure. A number of studies have shown that supplementation with vitamin C increases the resistance of the skin to UV exposure. However, vitamin C in isolation is only minimally effective, and most studies showing a benefit use a multi-component intervention [21,50,86,90,107,150–152]. In particular, a synergy exists between vitamin C and vitamin E, with the combination being particularly effective [50]. These results indicate the need for complete oxidant scavenging and recycling as indicated in Figure 4, in order to provide effective protection from UV irradiation. This combination also decreases the inflammation induced by excessive UV exposure.

Topical application of vitamin C, in combination with vitamin E and other compounds, has also been shown to reduce injury due to UV irradiation [50,54,65,89,150,152,153]. However, the efficacy of topical vitamin C and other nutrients may depend on the pre-existing status of the skin. One study suggests that when health status is already optimal there is no absorption of vitamin C following topical application. Hence, "beauty from the inside", via nutrition, may be more effective than topical application [132].

Vitamin-C-mediated prevention of radiation injury from acute UV exposure is relatively easily demonstrated, and these studies are highlighted above. However, reversal of photoaging due to prior, chronic sun damage is much more problematic. Although there are a number of studies that claim a significant benefit from an antioxidant supplement or topical cream, interpretation of the data is confounded by the complex formulation of the interventions, with most studies using a cocktail of compounds and with the formulation of topical creams providing a moisturising effect in itself [23,61,88,154].

5.3. Dry Skin

Dry skin is a common condition typically experienced by most people at some stage in their lives. It can occur in response to a particular skin care regime, illness, medications, or due to environmental changes in temperature, air flow and humidity. The prevalence of dry skin also increases with age [127]; this was originally believed to be due to decreased water content or sebum production in the skin as we get older. However, it is now considered likely to be due to alterations in the keratinisation process and lipid content of the stratum corneum [127].

The pathogenesis of dry skin is becoming clearer and three contributing deficiencies have been identified.

- A deficiency in the skin barrier lipids, the ceramides, has been identified. These lipids are the main intercellular lipids in the stratum corneum, accounting for 40 to 50 percent of total lipids [155].
- A reduction in substances known as the natural moisturising factor (NMF) [156,157] is also thought to be involved in dry skin. These substances are found in the stratum corneum within the corneocytes, where they bind water, allowing the corneocyte to remain hydrated despite the drying effects of the environment.
- More recently, a deficiency of the skin's own moisture network in the epidermis, mediated by the newly discovered aquaporin water channels, has been suggested to play a role [131].

Treatment of dry skin involves maintenance of the lipid barrier and the natural moisturising factor components of the stratum corneum, generally through topical application (91), although nutritional support of the dermis may also be useful [135,156].

Potential for Vitamin C to Prevent Dry Skin Conditions

Cell culture studies have shown that the addition of vitamin C enhances the production of barrier lipids and induces differentiation of keratinocytes, and from these observations it has been proposed that vitamin C may be instrumental in the formation of the stratum corneum and may thereby influence the ability of the skin to protect itself from water loss [99,157]. Some studies have indicated that topical application of vitamin C may result in decreased roughness, although this may depend more on the formulation of the cream than on the vitamin C content [52,55]. Because most studies in this area involve topical application, the complex and variable effects (pH and additional compounds) of topical formulations make it difficult to come to any firm conclusion as to whether vitamin C affects skin dryness.

5.4. Wrinkles

Wrinkles are formed during chronological aging and the process is markedly accelerated by external factors such as exposure to UV radiation or smoking. The formation of wrinkles is thought to be due to changes in the lower, dermal layer of the skin [22] but little is known about the specific molecular mechanisms responsible. It is thought that loss of collagen, deterioration of collagen and elastic fibres and changes to the dermal–epidermal junction may contribute [22,120,158–160]. One hypothesis is that UV light induces cytokine production, which triggers fibroblast elastase expression causing degradation of elastic fibres, loss of elasticity and consequent wrinkle formation.

The Effect of Vitamin C on Wrinkle Formation and Reversal

The appearance of wrinkles, or fine lines in the skin, has a major impact on appearance and is therefore often a focus of intervention studies. Most have used topical applications, generally containing a mixture of vitamin C and other antioxidants or natural compounds, with varied efficacy [51,52,161]. Generally the demonstration of wrinkle decrease in these studies is less than convincing, and the technology to measure these changes is limited. More recently, improved and impartial imaging technologies such as ultrasound have been used to determine the thickness of the various skin layers [135,149]. Once again, the efficacy of topical vitamin C creams on wrinkled skin may depend on the vitamin C status of the person involved. An indication that improved vitamin C status could protect against wrinkle formation through improved collagen synthesis comes from the measured differences in wound healing and collagen synthesis in smokers, abstinent smokers and non-smokers with associated variances in plasma vitamin C status [162]. Smokers had depleted vitamin C levels compared with non-smokers; these levels could be improved by smoking cessation, with an associated improvement in wound healing and collagen formation [162].

5.5. Wound Healing

Wound healing is a complex process with three main consecutive and overlapping stages; inflammation, new tissue formation and remodelling [163]. Following vasoconstriction and fibrin clot formation to stem bleeding, inflammatory cells are recruited to the wound site. The first of these cells is the neutrophil, which clears the wound of any damaged tissue and infectious material and signals the recruitment of tissue macrophages [164]. Macrophages continue clearing damaged material and bacteria, including spent neutrophils. Crucially, they are thought to be involved in orchestrating the healing process, signalling fibroblasts to remodel tissue at the wound site and providing vital signals for re-epithelialisation and dermal repair [163,164].

Re-epithelisation restores the skin's barrier function, and occurs by a combination of migration and proliferation of the epidermal keratinocytes that reside close to the damaged area. Epidermal stem cells may also be involved in re-epithelisation [163]. In addition to the epidermal layer, the underlying dermis must also be restored. Fibroblasts from a number of sources also proliferate and move into the wound area [165], where they synthesise extracellular matrix components. These cells remove the fibrin clot from the wound area, replacing it with a more stable collagen matrix. They are also involved in wound contraction, and the reordering of collagen fibres. Proliferation of blood vessels is initiated by growth factor production by macrophages, keratinocytes and fibroblasts.

Typically, the final result of the healing process is the formation of a scar. This is an area of fibrous tissue generally made up of collagen arranged in unidirectional layers, rather than the normal basket-weave pattern. As such, the strength of skin at the repair site is never as great as the uninjured skin [163]. Variations in scar formation can occur, resulting in keloids—raised and fibrous scars—or weak thin scar tissue. At this stage no intervention has been able to prevent the formation of scar tissue although the extent of scarring may be ameliorated [166]. It is thought that nutritional support for regeneration of the skin layers is important for development of strong healthy skin [167].

Vitamin C and the Benefits for Wound Healing

Of all effects of vitamin C on skin health, its beneficial effect on wound healing is the most dramatic and reproducible. This is directly related to its co-factor activity for the synthesis of collagen, with impaired wound healing an early indicator of hypovitaminosis C [68,168]. Vitamin C turnover at wound sites, due to both local inflammation and the demands of increased collagen production, means that supplementation is useful, and both topical application and increased nutrient intake have been shown to be beneficial [166,169,170]. Supplementation with both vitamin C and vitamin E improved the rate of wound healing in children with extensive burns [171], and plasma vitamin C levels in smokers, abstaining smokers and non-smokers were positively associated with the rate of wound healing [162]. However, it would appear that the extent of the benefits of supplemented vitamin C intake is, once again, dependent upon the status of the individual at baseline, with any benefit being less apparent if nutritional intake is already adequate [167,168]. However, the complexity and poor selection of study population has often made it difficult to come to firm conclusions about the efficacy of nutritional interventions, as summarised in a meta-analysis of the effects of varied treatments on ulcer healing [172]. In a recent study, topical application of vitamin C in a silicone gel resulted in a significant reduction in permanent scar formation in an Asian population [166].

5.6. Skin Inflammatory Conditions

Inflammation in the skin underlies a number of debilitating conditions such as atopic dermatitis, psoriasis and acne, with symptoms including pain, dryness and itching. The pathology underlying these conditions is complex and involves activation of auto-immune or allergic inflammation with associated generation of cytokines and cellular dysfunction, and consequent breakdown of the skin epidermal lipid barrier [173,174]. Treatments are therefore targeted at both the underlying inflammation and the repair and maintenance of the epidermal structures. Nutrition plays an integral part in both these aspects and numerous studies have investigated the impact of dietary manipulation for alleviation of acute and chronic skin pathologies, although firm conclusions as to efficacy remain elusive [175–177]. Treatments involving supplementation with essential omega-fatty acids, lipid-soluble vitamins E and A are often employed in an attempt to assist the generation of the lipid barriers and to retain moisture in the skin [177]. Vitamin C is often used in anti-inflammatory formulations or as a component of nutrition studies but its individual efficacy has not been investigated [175–177].

Vitamin C and Skin Inflammation

Vitamin C status has been reported to be compromised in individuals with skin inflammation, with lower levels measured compared with unaffected individuals [178,179]. This may reflect increased turnover of the redox-labile vitamin C, as is seen in many inflammatory conditions [180–182], and decreased vitamin C status could be expected to impact on the numerous essential functions for which it is essential as detailed in the sections above. Recent studies have begun to provide more detailed information as to specific functional implications for suboptimal vitamin C status in inflamed skin lesions. One notable study [179] has reported significantly compromised vitamin C status in patients with atopic dermatitis, with plasma levels ranging between 6 and 31 μmol/L (optimal healthy levels > 60 μM), and an inverse relationship between plasma vitamin C and total ceramide levels in the epidermis of the affected individuals. As indicated in the sections above, ceramide is the main lipid of the stratum corneum and its synthesis involves an essential hydroxylation step catalysed by ceramide synthase, an enzyme with a co-factor requirement for vitamin C [100]. Hence the potential impact of vitamin C extends far beyond its capacity as an inflammatory antioxidant in a pathological setting.

Table 3. Skin ailments, their causes and evidence from in vitro and in vivo studies for association with vitamin C levels.

Type of Skin Damage	Cause	Skin Structure Affected	Evidence of Protection by Vitamin C	References
Sunburn	Acute and excessive UV exposure.	Cell death of all skin cells, with associated inflammation.	Improving skin vitamin C and vitamin E levels can improve resistance to UV exposure.	[21,50,86,90, 107,150–152]
Photoaging, oxidant-induced damage	Chronic UV overexposure, cigarette smoking.	Damaged collagen and elastin matrix, thinning of the epidermal layer.	Decreased signs of aging with higher fruit and vegetable intake. Protection inferred from studies with acute UV exposure.	[27,54,89,139, 145–148]
Hyperpigmentation	Chronic UV exposure and environmental stresses.	Excessive pigment formation and propagation of melanocytes in the epidermis.	Nutrition studies showing improved skin colour with higher fruit and vegetable intake.	Reviewed in [134,135]
Wrinkle formation	Natural aging, oxidative stress, UV exposure, smoking, medical treatments.	Dermal layer changes, deterioration of collagen and elastic fibres.	Lessening of wrinkle depth following vitamin C supplementation. Increased collagen formation by fibroblasts in cell culture.	[69,73,79–82, 135,149]
Skin sagging	Natural aging, oxidative stress damage, extreme weight loss.	Loss of elastin and collagen fibres, thinning of skin layers, loss of muscle tone.	Improved skin tightness in individuals with higher fruit and vegetable intake.	Reviewed in [134,135]
Loss of colour	Natural aging, UV exposure, illness.	Thinning of skin layers, loss of melanocytes or decreased melanin formation, loss of vasculature in dermis.	Improved skin tone with high fruit and vegetable intake.	Reviewed in [94,95,134,135]
Surface roughness	Chemical and UV exposure, physical abrasion, allergy and inflammation.	Stratum corneum, loss of skin moisture barrier function.	Vitamin C enhances production of barrier lipids in cell culture.	[98–102,157]

Table 3. *Cont.*

Type of Skin Damage	Cause	Skin Structure Affected	Evidence of Protection by Vitamin C	References
Dry skin	Medications, illness, extreme temperature, low humidity and wind exposure.	Stratum corneum, loss of skin barrier lipids and natural moisturising factor.	Vitamin C enhances production of barrier lipids in cell culture.	[98–102,157]
Excessive scar formation, generation of keloids	Ineffective wound healing.	Fibroblast function, collagen and elastin formation.	Supplementation improves wound healing, prevents keloid formation in vivo, enhances collagen formation by fibroblasts in vitro.	[73,79–82,166, 167]
Poor wound healing, thickening rough skin	Vitamin C deficiency.	All skin cell functions, collagen formation.	Direct association Vitamin C deficiency prevents wound healing.	[162,166,169]
Inflammatory skin lesions	Allergic and auto-inflammation.	Skin barrier integrity, underlying inflammation and swelling.	Nutrition support, decreased levels associated with loss of barrier lipid ceramide.	[179]

Table 4. Summary of key and recent in vivo studies providing evidence of vitamin C effects in the skin.

Study Description	Measured Parameters	Outcome and Comment	References
Animal Studies			
Oral Supplementation			
Dietary supplementation of pregnant female rats. Addition of 1.25 mg/mL vitamin C to drinking water for duration of gestation.	Monitored collagen and elastin content of uterosacral ligaments by histology staining and subjective assessment.	Increased collagen production in vit.-C-supplemented rats, decreased elastin loss. Implied prevention of pelvic organ prolapse and stress urinary incontinence.	[183]
Wound healing in guinea pigs following supplementation with moderate and high-dose vit. C.	Dorsal wound healing rate and strength of repair monitored.	Increased vit. C associated with faster wound recovery and strength of skin integrity. Small sample size limited stats.	[184]
Topical application			
Topical application of vit. C and vit. E-containing cream to nude mice, followed by UV irradiation.	Measured melanocyte differentiation post-irradiation. Change of skin colour—tanning, inflammation.	UVR-induced proliferation and melanogenesis of melanocytes were reduced by vit. C and E. Melanocyte population and confluence reduced when vit. C present.	[185]
Cultured skin—human keratinocytes and fibroblasts attached to collagen-glycosamino-glycan substrates, incubated for five weeks ± 0.1 mM vit. C, and then grafted to athymic mice.	Collagen IV, collagen VII and laminin 5 synthesis, epidermal barrier formation and skin graft take in athymic nude mice.	Increased cell viability and basement membrane development in vitro, better graft ability in vivo.	[157]
Human Studies			
Oral supplementation			
90-day oral supplementation with a fermented papaya preparation or an antioxidant cocktail (10 mg trans-resveratrol, 60 μg selenium, 10 mg vitamin E, 50 mg vitamin C) in 60 healthy non-smoker males and females aged 40–65 years, all with clinical signs of skin aging.	Skin surface, brown spots, skin evenness, skin moisture, elasticity (face), lipid peroxidation, superoxide dismutase levels, nitric oxide (NO) generation, and the expression levels of key genes (outer forearm sample).	Improved skin elasticity, moisture and antioxidant capacity with both fermented papaya and antioxidant cocktail. Increased effect of papaya extract and on gene expression. No baseline measures in study population. Antioxidant components of the fermented papaya unknown and direct link with vit. C not available.	[135]
Intervention with 47 men aged 30–45 given oral supplement of 54 mg or 22 mg of vit. C, 28 mg tomato extract, 27 mg grape seed extract, 210 mg of marine complex, 4 mg zinc gluconate for 180 days.	Subjective assessment of appearance and objective measures of collagen and elastin (histology and measurement in biopsy material).	Improvement in erythema, hydration, radiance, and overall appearance. Decreased intensity of general skin spots, UV spots, and brown spots, improved skin texture and appearance of pores. Increased collagen (43%–57%) and elastin (20%–31%).	[49]

Table 4. *Cont.*

Study Description	Measured Parameters	Outcome and Comment	References
Supplementation of 33 healthy men and women (aged 22–50), with placebo, 100 mg vit. C or 180 mg vit. C daily for four weeks.	EPR measurement of TEMPO scavenging in skin on arm. Raman resonance spectroscopy for skin carotenoids.	Improved oxygen radical scavenging with vit. C supplementation, dose dependency indicated and rapid response (obvious within two weeks).	[38]
Three month supplementation of 12 males and six females (21–77 y) with 2 g vit. C and 1000 IU D-alpha-tocopherol.	Measured blood vitamin levels before and after, skin resilience to UVB, detection of DNA crosslinks in skin biopsy.	Serum vit. C and vit. E doubled during intervention (implies sub-saturation at baseline). Minimal erythema dose increased with supplementation, DNA damage halved.	[20]
Investigation of antioxidant capacity in human skin before and after UV irradiation; effect of supplementation with 500 mg vit. C per day.	Measurement of erythema and antioxidant levels following UVB irradiation.	Vit. C and E levels increased, but levels not realistic (plasma vit. C 21 μM before and 26 μM after 500 mg daily). Skin MDA and glutathione content lowered, no effect on MED.	[27]
Topical application			
Topical application of vit. C cream in advance of application of hair dye product p-phenylenediamine.	Visual assessment of allergic reaction following patch application on volunteer skin (on back).	Decreased or ablation of dermatitis and allergic response due to local antioxidant action of vit. C in cream.	[170]
Clinical study applying vit. C in liposomes to human skin (abdomen), then exposure to UV irradiation.	Measured penetration through skin layers, delivery of vit. C, loss of Trolox, TNFalpha and Il-1beta.	Increased vit. C levels in epidermis and dermis with liposomes. Protection against UV increased over liposomes alone.	[67]
Microneedle skin patches to deliver vit. C into the skin assessed on areas of slight wrinkle formation (around eyes).	Global Photodamage Score by visual inspection. Skin replica analysis and skin assessment by visiometer.	Slightly improved photodamage score and lessening of wrinkles after 12 weeks of treatment with vit. C-loaded patches.	[186]
Vit. C-based solution containing Rosa moschata oil rich in vitamins A, C, E, essential fatty acids /placebo moisturizer cream applied to facial skin of 60 healthy female subjects for 40–60 days.	Ultrasound monitoring thickness of the epidermis and dermis, and low (LEP), medium (MEP), high echogenic pixels (HEP), reflecting hydration, inflammatory processes, elastin and collagen degeneration (LEP), and structure of collagen, elastin and microfibrils (MEP and LEP).	Data suggest epidermis but not the dermis increased in thickness. Increase in MEP and HEP (collagen and elastin synthesis) and decreased LEP (inflammation and collagen degeneration). No vit. C status measurements in skin of individuals.	[149]
In vivo study with 30 healthy adults. Protective effect of SPF30 sunscreen with and without anti-oxidants (vit. E, grape seed extract, ubiquinone and vit. C) against Infra-Red A irradiation on previously unexposed skin (buttock).	Skin biopsy analysis; mRNA and RT-PCR for matrix metalloprotein-1 (MMP-1) expression 24 h post irradiation.	Sunscreen plus antioxidants protected skin against MMP-1 increase, sunscreen alone did not. No indication of levels of antioxidants, or whether they were able to penetrate into skin layers. Multi-component antioxidant mix.	[153]
In vivo study of 15 healthy adults. Protective effect of vitamin C mixtures (vit. C, vit. E, ferulic acid OR vitamin C, phoretin, ferulic acid) on ozone exposure on forearms.	Skin biopsy analysis; 4-HNE and 8-iso prostaglandin levels, immunofluorescence for NF-kB p65, cyclooxygenase-2, matrix metalloprotein-9 (MMP-9), type III collagen. After 5 days of 0.8 ppm ozone for 3h/d.	Vitamin C mixture reduced ozone induced elevation in lipid peroxidation products, NF-kB p65, cyclooxygenase-2 expression and completely prevented MMP-9 induction by ozone. No indication of levels of antioxidants, or whether they were able to penetrate into skin layers. Multi-component antioxidant mix.	[187]
Test of topical silicone gel with vit. C on scar formation in a population of 80 Asian people. Gel applied for six months after operation.	Scar formation monitored by modified Vancouver Scar Scale (VSS) as well as erythema and melanin indices by spectrophotometer.	Vit. C decreased scar elevation and erythema, decreased melanin index. Improved wound healing (stitch removal).	[166]

6. Conclusions

The role of vitamin C in skin health has been under discussion since its discovery in the 1930s as the remedy for scurvy. The co-factor role for collagen hydroxylases was the first vitamin C function that was closely tied to the symptoms of scurvy and the realisation of the importance of this function for the maintenance of skin health throughout the human lifespan led to the hypothesised skin health benefit of vitamin C. In addition, the antioxidant activity of vitamin C made it an excellent candidate as a protective factor against UV irradiation. These two hypotheses have driven most of the research into the role of vitamin C and skin health to date.

The following information is available as a result of research into the role of vitamin C in skin health, and Tables 2 and 4 list a sample of key studies:

- Skin fibroblasts have an absolute dependence on vitamin C for the synthesis of collagen, and for the regulation of the collagen/elastin balance in the dermis. There is ample in vitro data with cultured cells demonstrating this dependency. In addition, vitamin C supplementation of animals has shown improved collagen synthesis in vivo.
- Skin keratinocytes have the capacity to accumulate high concentrations of vitamin C, and this in association with vitamin E affords protection against UV irradiation. This information is available from in vitro studies with cultured cells, with supportive information from animal and human studies.
- Analysis of keratinocytes in culture has shown that vitamin C influences gene expression of antioxidant enzymes, the organisation and accumulation of phospholipids, and promotes the formation of the stratum corneum and the differentiation of the epithelium in general.
- Delivery of vitamin C into the skin via topical application remains challenging. Although some human studies have suggested a beneficial effect with respect to UV irradiation protection, most effective formulations contain both vitamins C and E, plus a delivery vehicle.
- Good skin health is positively associated with fruit and vegetable intake in a number of well-executed intervention studies. The active component in the fruit and vegetables responsible for the observed benefit is unidentified, and the effect is likely to be multi-factorial, although vitamin C status is closely aligned with fruit and vegetable intake.
- Signs of aging in human skin can be ameliorated through the provision of vitamin C. A number of studies support this, although measurement of skin changes is difficult. Some studies include objective measures of collagen deposition and wrinkle depth.
- The provision of vitamin C to the skin greatly assists wound healing and minimises raised scar formation. This has been demonstrated in numerous clinical studies in humans and animals.

Acknowledgments: The writing of this review was funded by the University of Otago and Zespri International. No additional costs were obtained to publish in open access. Anitra Carr is the recipient of a Health Research Council of New Zealand Sir Charles Hercus Health Research Fellowship.

Author Contributions: Juliet Pullar and Margreet Vissers wrote the bulk of the review, with additional input and editing from Anitra Carr.

Conflicts of Interest: The authors declare no conflict of interest. Zespri International, a partial funder, had no influence on the selection of material to cover, nor on the focus and interpretation of the studies reviewed.

References

1. Weller, R.H.; John, A.; Savin, J.; Dahl, M. *The Function and Structure of Skin*, 5th ed.; Wiley-Blackwell: Massachusetts, MA, USA, 2008.
2. Patton, K.T.; Thibodeau, G.A. *Anthony's Textbook of Anatomy & Physiology*; Elsevier: Amsterdam, The Netherlands, 2012.
3. Wickett, R.R.; Visscher, M.O. Structure and function of the epidermal barrier. *Am. J. Infect. Control* **2006**, *34*, 15. [CrossRef]
4. Marks, R. The stratum corneum barrier: The final frontier. *J. Nutr.* **2004**, *134*, 2017–2021.
5. Proksch, E.; Brandner, J.M.; Jensen, J.M. The skin: An indispensable barrier. *Exp. Dermatol.* **2008**, *17*, 1063–1072. [CrossRef] [PubMed]

6. Blume-Peytavi, U.; Kottner, J.; Sterry, W.; Hodin, M.W.; Griffiths, T.W.; Watson, R.E.; Hay, R.J.; Griffiths, C.E. Age-associated skin conditions and diseases: Current perspectives and future options. *Gerontologist* **2016**, *56*, 230–242. [CrossRef] [PubMed]

7. Park, K. Role of micronutrients in skin health and function. *Biomol. Ther.* **2015**, *23*, 207–217. [CrossRef] [PubMed]

8. Boelsma, E.; Van de Vijver, L.P.; Goldbohm, R.A.; Klopping-Ketelaars, I.A.; Hendriks, H.F.; Roza, L. Human skin condition and its associations with nutrient concentrations in serum and diet. *Am. J. Clin. Nutr.* **2003**, *77*, 348–355. [PubMed]

9. Brescoll, J.; Daveluy, S. A review of vitamin B12 in dermatology. *Am. J. Clin. Dermatol.* **2015**, *16*, 27–33. [CrossRef] [PubMed]

10. Fedeles, F.; Murphy, M.; Rothe, M.J.; Grant-Kels, J.M. Nutrition and bullous skin diseases. *Clin. Dermatol.* **2010**, *28*, 627–643. [CrossRef] [PubMed]

11. Sauberlich, H.E. A History of Scurvy and Vitamin C. In *Vitamin C in Health and Disease*, 1st ed.; Packer, L., Fuchs, J., Eds.; Marcel Dekker, Inc.: New York, NY, USA, 1997; pp. 1–24.

12. Talarico, V.; Aloe, M.; Barreca, M.; Galati, M.C.; Raiola, G. Do you remember scurvy? *Clin. Ther.* **2014**, *165*, 253–256. [PubMed]

13. Alqanatish, J.T.; Alqahtani, F.; Alsewairi, W.M.; Al-kenaizan, S. Childhood scurvy: An unusual cause of refusal to walk in a child. *Pediatr. Rheumatol.* **2015**, *13*, 23. [CrossRef] [PubMed]

14. Peterkofsky, B. Ascorbate requirement for hydroxylation and secretion of procollagen: Relationship to inhibition of collagen synthesis in scurvy. *Am. J. Clin. Nutr.* **1991**, *54*, 1135–1140.

15. Ellinger, S.; Stehle, P. Efficacy of vitamin supplementation in situations with wound healing disorders: Results from clinical intervention studies. *Curr. Opin. Clin. Nutr. Metab. Care* **2009**, *12*, 588–595. [CrossRef] [PubMed]

16. Ross, R.; Benditt, E.P. Wound healing and collagen formation: II. Fine structure in experimental scurvy. *J. Cell Biol.* **1962**, *12*, 533–551. [CrossRef] [PubMed]

17. Hodges, R.E.; Baker, E.M.; Hood, J.; Sauberlich, H.E.; March, S.C. Experimental scurvy in man. *Am. J. Clin. Nutr.* **1969**, *22*, 535–548. [PubMed]

18. Hodges, R.E.; Hood, J.; Canham, J.E.; Sauberlich, H.E.; Baker, E.M. Clinical manifestations of ascorbic acid deficiency in man. *Am. J. Clin. Nutr.* **1971**, *24*, 432–443. [PubMed]

19. Evans, J.R.; Lawrenson, J.G. Antioxidant vitamin and mineral supplements for slowing the progression of age-related macular degeneration. *Cochrane Database Syst. Rev.* **2017**. [CrossRef]

20. Placzek, M.; Gaube, S.; Kerkmann, U.; Gilbertz, K.P.; Herzinger, T.; Haen, E.; Przybilla, B. Ultraviolet B-induced DNA damage in human epidermis is modified by the antioxidants ascorbic acid and D-alpha-tocopherol. *J. Investig. Dermatol* **2005**, *124*, 304–307. [CrossRef] [PubMed]

21. Stewart, M.S.; Cameron, G.S.; Pence, B.C. Antioxidant nutrients protect against UVB-induced oxidative damage to DNA of mouse keratinocytes in culture. *J. Investig. Dermatol.* **1996**, *106*, 1086–1089. [CrossRef] [PubMed]

22. Baumann, L. Skin ageing and its treatment. *J. Pathol.* **2007**, *211*, 241–251. [CrossRef] [PubMed]

23. Zussman, J.; Ahdout, J.; Kim, J. Vitamins and photoaging: Do scientific data support their use? *J. Am. Acad. Dermatol.* **2010**, *63*, 507–525. [CrossRef] [PubMed]

24. Langton, A.K.; Sherratt, M.J.; Griffiths, C.E.; Watson, R.E. A new wrinkle on old skin: The role of elastic fibres in skin ageing. *Int. J. Cosmet. Sci.* **2010**, *32*, 330–339. [CrossRef] [PubMed]

25. Rhie, G.; Shin, M.H.; Seo, J.Y.; Choi, W.W.; Cho, K.H.; Kim, K.H.; Park, K.C.; Eun, H.C.; Chung, J.H. Aging- and photoaging-dependent changes of enzymic and nonenzymic antioxidants in the epidermis and dermis of human skin in vivo. *J. Investig. Dermatol.* **2001**, *117*, 1212–1217. [CrossRef] [PubMed]

26. Shindo, Y.; Witt, E.; Han, D.; Epstein, W.; Packer, L. Enzymic and non-enzymic antioxidants in epidermis and dermis of human skin. *J. Investig. Dermatol.* **1994**, *102*, 122–124. [CrossRef] [PubMed]

27. McArdle, F.; Rhodes, L.E.; Parslew, R.; Jack, C.I.; Friedmann, P.S.; Jackson, M.J. UVR-induced oxidative stress in human skin in vivo: Effects of oral vitamin C supplementation. *Free Radic. Biol. Med.* **2002**, *33*, 1355–1362. [CrossRef]

28. Kirk, J.E. *Vitamins and Hormones*; Academic Press: New York, NY, USA, 1962; pp. 83–92.

29. Schaus, R. The vitamin C content of human pituitary, cerebral cortex, heart, and skeletal muscle and its relation to age. *Am. J. Clin. Nutr.* **1957**, *5*, 3.

30. Yavorsky, M.; Almaden, P.; King, C.G. The vitamin C content of human tissues. *J. Biol. Chem.* **1934**, *106*, 525–529.

31. Lloyd, B.B.; Sinclair, H.M. Chapter 1, pp. 369–471. In *Biochemistry and Physiology of Nutrition*; Bourne, G.H., Kidder, G.W., Eds.; Academic Press: New York, NY, USA, 1953.

32. Carr, A.C.; Bozonet, S.M.; Pullar, J.M.; Simcock, J.W.; Vissers, M.C. Human skeletal muscle ascorbate is highly responsive to changes in vitamin C intake and plasma concentrations. *Am. J. Clin. Nutr.* **2013**, *97*, 800–807. [CrossRef] [PubMed]

33. Shindo, Y.; Witt, E.; Han, D.; Packer, L. Dose-response effects of acute ultraviolet irradiation on antioxidants and molecular markers of oxidation in murine epidermis and dermis. *J. Investig. Dermatol.* **1994**, *102*, 470–475. [CrossRef] [PubMed]

34. Shindo, Y.; Witt, E.; Packer, L. Antioxidant defense mechanisms in murine epidermis and dermis and their responses to ultraviolet light. *J. Investig. Dermatol.* **1993**, *100*, 260–265. [CrossRef] [PubMed]

35. Wheeler, L.A.; Aswad, A.; Connor, M.J.; Lowe, N. Depletion of cutaneous glutathione and the induction of inflammation by 8-methoxypsoralen plus UVA radiation. *J. Investig. Dermatol.* **1986**, *87*, 658–662. [CrossRef] [PubMed]

36. Weber, S.U.; Thiele, J.J.; Cross, C.E.; Packer, L. Vitamin C, uric acid, and glutathione gradients in murine stratum corneum and their susceptibility to ozone exposure. *J. Investig. Dermatol.* **1999**, *113*, 1128–1132. [CrossRef] [PubMed]

37. Steiling, H.; Longet, K.; Moodycliffe, A.; Mansourian, R.; Bertschy, E.; Smola, H.; Mauch, C.; Williamson, G. Sodium-dependent vitamin C transporter isoforms in skin: Distribution, kinetics, and effect of UVB-induced oxidative stress. *Free Radic. Biol. Med.* **2007**, *43*, 752–762. [CrossRef] [PubMed]

38. Lauer, A.C.; Groth, N.; Haag, S.F.; Darvin, M.E.; Lademann, J.; Meinke, M.C. Dose-dependent vitamin C uptake and radical scavenging activity in human skin measured with in vivo electron paramagnetic resonance spectroscopy. *Skin Pharmacol. Physiol.* **2013**, *26*, 147–154. [CrossRef] [PubMed]

39. Mandl, J.; Szarka, A.; Banhegyi, G. Vitamin C: Update on physiology and pharmacology. *Br. J. Pharmacol.* **2009**, *157*, 1097–1110. [CrossRef] [PubMed]

40. May, J.M. The SLC23 family of ascorbate transporters: Ensuring that you get and keep your daily dose of vitamin C. *Br. J. Pharmacol.* **2011**, *164*, 1793–1801. [CrossRef] [PubMed]

41. Savini, I.; Rossi, A.; Pierro, C.; Avigliano, L.; Catani, M.V. SVCT1 and SVCT2: Key proteins for vitamin C uptake. *Amino Acids* **2008**, *34*, 347–355. [CrossRef] [PubMed]

42. Rajan, D.P.; Huang, W.; Dutta, B.; Devoe, L.D.; Leibach, F.H.; Ganapathy, V.; Prasad, P.D. Human placental sodium-dependent vitamin C transporter (SVCT2): Molecular cloning and transport function. *Biochem. Biophys. Res. Commun.* **1999**, *262*, 762–768. [CrossRef] [PubMed]

43. Levine, M.; Cantilena, C.C.; Dhariwal, K.R. In situ kinetics and ascorbic acid requirements. *World Rev. Nutr. Diet* **1993**, *72*, 114–127. [PubMed]

44. Levine, M.; Conry-Cantilena, C.; Wang, Y.; Welch, R.W.; Washko, P.W.; Dhariwal, K.R.; Park, J.B.; Lazarev, A.; Graumlich, J.F.; King, J.; et al. Vitamin C pharmacokinetics in healthy volunteers: Evidence for a recommended dietary allowance. *Proc. Natl. Acad. Sci. USA* **1996**, *93*, 3704–3709. [CrossRef] [PubMed]

45. Levine, M.; Dhariwal, K.R.; Washko, P.; Welch, R.; Wang, Y.H.; Cantilena, C.C.; Yu, R. Ascorbic acid and reaction kinetics in situ: A new approach to vitamin requirements. *J. Nutr. Sci. Vitaminol.* **1992**, *38*, 169–172. [CrossRef]

46. Levine, M.; Dhariwal, K.R.; Welch, R.W.; Wang, Y.; Park, J.B. Determination of optimal vitamin C requirements in humans. *Am. J. Clin. Nutr.* **1995**, *62*, 1347–1356.

47. Carr, A.C.; Frei, B. Toward a new recommended dietary allowance for vitamin C based on antioxidant and health effects in humans. *Am. J. Clin. Nutr.* **1999**, *69*, 1086–1107. [PubMed]

48. Carr, A.C.; Bozonet, S.M.; Pullar, J.M.; Simcock, J.W.; Vissers, M.C. A randomized steady-state bioavailability study of synthetic versus natural (kiwifruit-derived) vitamin C. *Nutrients* **2013**, *5*, 3684–3695. [CrossRef] [PubMed]

49. Costa, A.; Pereira, E.S.P.; Assumpção, E.C.; Dos Santos, F.B.C.; Ota, F.S.; De Oliveira Pereira, M.; Fidelis, M.C.; Fávaro, R.; Langen, S.S.B.; De Arruda, L.H.F.; et al. Assessment of clinical effects and safety of an oral supplement based on marine protein, vitamin C, grape seed extract, zinc, and tomato extract in the improvement of visible signs of skin aging in men. *Clin. Cosmet. Investig. Dermatol.* **2015**, *8*, 319–328. [CrossRef] [PubMed]

50. Fuchs, J.; Kern, H. Modulation of UV-light-induced skin inflammation by D-alpha-tocopherol and L-ascorbic acid: A clinical study using solar simulated radiation. *Free Radic. Biol. Med.* **1998**, *25*, 1006–1012. [CrossRef]

51. Nusgens, B.V.; Humbert, P.; Rougier, A.; Colige, A.C.; Haftek, M.; Lambert, C.A.; Richard, A.; Creidi, P.; Lapiere, C.M. Topically applied vitamin C enhances the mRNA level of collagens I and III, their processing enzymes and tissue inhibitor of matrix metalloproteinase 1 in the human dermis. *J. Investig. Dermatol.* **2001**, *116*, 853–859. [CrossRef] [PubMed]

52. Humbert, P.G.; Haftek, M.; Creidi, P.; Lapiere, C.; Nusgens, B.; Richard, A.; Schmitt, D.; Rougier, A.; Zahouani, H. Topical ascorbic acid on photoaged skin. Clinical, topographical and ultrastructural evaluation: Double-blind study vs. placebo. *Exp. Dermatol.* **2003**, *12*, 237–244. [CrossRef] [PubMed]

53. Lee, W.R.; Shen, S.C.; Kuo-Hsien, W.; Hu, C.H.; Fang, J.Y. Lasers and microdermabrasion enhance and control topical delivery of vitamin C. *J. Investig. Dermatol.* **2003**, *121*, 1118–1125. [CrossRef] [PubMed]

54. Lin, J.Y.; Selim, M.A.; Shea, C.R.; Grichnik, J.M.; Omar, M.M.; Monteiro-Riviere, N.A.; Pinnell, S.R. UV photoprotection by combination topical antioxidants vitamin C and vitamin E. *J. Am. Acad. Dermatol.* **2003**, *48*, 866–874. [CrossRef] [PubMed]

55. Sauermann, K.; Jaspers, S.; Koop, U.; Wenck, H. Topically applied vitamin C increases the density of dermal papillae in aged human skin. *BMC Dermatol.* **2004**, *4*, 13. [CrossRef] [PubMed]

56. Pinnell, S.R. Cutaneous photodamage, oxidative stress, and topical antioxidant protection. *J. Am. Acad. Dermatol.* **2003**, *48*, 1–22. [CrossRef] [PubMed]

57. Stamford, N.P.J. Stability, transdermal penetration, and cutaneous effects of ascorbic acid and its derivatives. *J. Cosmet. Dermatol.* **2012**, *11*, 310–317. [CrossRef] [PubMed]

58. Nayama, S.; Takehana, M.; Kanke, M.; Itoh, S.; Ogata, E.; Kobayashi, S. Protective effects of sodium-L-ascorbyl-2 phosphate on the development of UVB-induced damage in cultured mouse skin. *Biol. Pharm. Bull.* **1999**, *22*, 1301–1305. [CrossRef] [PubMed]

59. Kobayashi, S.; Takehana, M.; Itoh, S.; Ogata, E. Protective effect of magnesium-L-ascorbyl-2 phosphate against skin damage induced by UVB irradiation. *Photochem. Photobiol.* **1996**, *64*, 224–228. [CrossRef] [PubMed]

60. Maia Campos, P.M.; Gaspar, L.R.; Goncalves, G.M.; Pereira, L.H.; Semprini, M.; Lopes, R.A. Comparative effects of retinoic acid or glycolic acid vehiculated in different topical formulations. *Biomed. Res. Int.* **2015**, *2015*, 650316. [CrossRef] [PubMed]

61. Pinnell, S.R.; Yang, H.; Omar, M.; Monteiro-Riviere, N.; DeBuys, H.V.; Walker, L.C.; Wang, Y.; Levine, M. Topical L-ascorbic acid: Percutaneous absorption studies. *Dermatol. Surg.* **2001**, *27*, 137–142. [CrossRef] [PubMed]

62. Yamamoto, I.; Muto, N.; Murakami, K.; Akiyama, J. Collagen synthesis in human skin fibroblasts is stimulated by a stable form of ascorbate, 2-O-alpha-D-glucopyranosyl-L-ascorbic acid. *J. Nutr.* **1992**, *122*, 871–877. [PubMed]

63. Yamamoto, I.; Suga, S.; Mitoh, Y.; Tanaka, M.; Muto, N. Antiscorbutic activity of L-ascorbic acid 2-glucoside and its availability as a vitamin C supplement in normal rats and guinea pigs. *J. Pharmacobio-Dyn.* **1990**, *13*, 688–695. [CrossRef] [PubMed]

64. Jurkovic, P.; Sentjurc, M.; Gasperlin, M.; Kristl, J.; Pecar, S. Skin protection against ultraviolet induced free radicals with ascorbyl palmitate in microemulsions. *Eur. J. Pharm. Biopharm.* **2003**, *56*, 59–66. [CrossRef]

65. Wu, Y.; Zheng, X.; Xu, X.G.; Li, Y.H.; Wang, B.; Gao, X.H.; Chen, H.D.; Yatskayer, M.; Oresajo, C. Protective effects of a topical antioxidant complex containing vitamins C and E and ferulic acid against ultraviolet irradiation-induced photodamage in Chinese women. *J. Drugs Dermatol.* **2013**, *12*, 464–468. [PubMed]

66. Xu, T.H.; Chen, J.Z.; Li, Y.H.; Wu, Y.; Luo, Y.J.; Gao, X.H.; Chen, H.D. Split-face study of topical 23.8% L-ascorbic acid serum in treating photo-aged skin. *J. Drugs Dermatol.* **2012**, *11*, 51–56. [PubMed]

67. Serrano, G.; Almudever, P.; Serrano, J.M.; Milara, J.; Torrens, A.; Exposito, I.; Cortijo, J. Phosphatidylcholine liposomes as carriers to improve topical ascorbic acid treatment of skin disorders. *Clin. Cosmet. Investig. Dermatol.* **2015**, *8*, 591–599. [PubMed]

68. Carr, A.C.; Vissers, M.C. Good nutrition matters: Hypovitaminosis C associated with depressed mood and poor wound healing. *N. Z. Med. J.* **2012**, *125*, 107–109.

69. Hinek, A.; Kim, H.J.; Wang, Y.; Wang, A.; Mitts, T.F. Sodium L-ascorbate enhances elastic fibers deposition by fibroblasts from normal and pathologic human skin. *J. Dermatol. Sci.* **2014**, *75*, 173–182. [CrossRef] [PubMed]

70. Ivanov, V.; Ivanova, S.; Kalinovsky, T.; Niedzwiecki, A.; Rath, M. Inhibition of collagen synthesis by select calcium and sodium channel blockers can be mitigated by ascorbic acid and ascorbyl palmitate. *Am. J. Cardiovasc. Dis.* **2016**, *6*, 26–35. [PubMed]

71. Kivirikko, K.I.; Myllyla, R.; Pihlajaniemi, T. Protein hydroxylation: Prolyl 4-hydroxylase, an enzyme with four cosubstrates and a multifunctional subunit. *FASEB. J.* **1989**, *3*, 1609–1617. [PubMed]

72. May, J.M.; Harrison, F.E. Role of vitamin C in the function of the vascular endothelium. *Antioxid. Redox Signal.* **2013**, *19*, 2068–2083. [CrossRef] [PubMed]

73. Kishimoto, Y.; Saito, N.; Kurita, K.; Shimokado, K.; Maruyama, N.; Ishigami, A. Ascorbic acid enhances the expression of type 1 and type 4 collagen and SVCT2 in cultured human skin fibroblasts. *Biochem. Biophys. Res. Commun.* **2013**, *430*, 579–584. [CrossRef] [PubMed]

74. May, J.M.; Qu, Z.C. Transport and intracellular accumulation of vitamin C in endothelial cells: Relevance to collagen synthesis. *Arch. Biochem. Biophys.* **2005**, *434*, 178–186. [CrossRef] [PubMed]

75. Miller, R.L.; Elsas, L.J.; Priest, R.E. Ascorbate action on normal and mutant human lysyl hydroxylases from cultured dermal fibroblasts. *J. Investig. Dermatol.* **1979**, *72*, 241–247. [CrossRef] [PubMed]

76. Parsons, K.K.; Maeda, N.; Yamauchi, M.; Banes, A.J.; Koller, B.H. Ascorbic acid-independent synthesis of collagen in mice. *Am. J. Physiol. Endocrinol. Metab.* **2006**, *290*, 1131–1139. [CrossRef] [PubMed]

77. Pihlajaniemi, T.; Myllyla, R.; Kivirikko, K.I. Prolyl 4-hydroxylase and its role in collagen synthesis. *J. Hepatol.* **1991**, *13*, 2–7. [CrossRef]

78. Duarte, T.L.; Cooke, M.S.; Jones, G.D. Gene expression profiling reveals new protective roles for vitamin C in human skin cells. *Free Radic. Biol. Med.* **2009**, *46*, 78–87. [CrossRef] [PubMed]

79. Takahashi, Y.; Takahashi, S.; Shiga, Y.; Yoshimi, T.; Miura, T. Hypoxic induction of prolyl 4-hydroxylase alpha (I) in cultured cells. *J. Biol. Chem.* **2000**, *275*, 14139–14146. [CrossRef] [PubMed]

80. Geesin, J.C.; Darr, D.; Kaufman, R.; Murad, S.; Pinnell, S.R. Ascorbic acid specifically increases type I and type III procollagen messenger RNA levels in human skin fibroblast. *J. Investig. Dermatol.* **1988**, *90*, 420–424. [CrossRef] [PubMed]

81. Davidson, J.M.; LuValle, P.A.; Zoia, O.; Quaglino, D., Jr.; Giro, M. Ascorbate differentially regulates elastin and collagen biosynthesis in vascular smooth muscle cells and skin fibroblasts by pretranslational mechanisms. *J. Biol. Chem.* **1997**, *272*, 345–352. [CrossRef] [PubMed]

82. Phillips, C.L.; Combs, S.B.; Pinnell, S.R. Effects of ascorbic acid on proliferation and collagen synthesis in relation to the donor age of human dermal fibroblasts. *J. Investig. Dermatol.* **1994**, *103*, 228–232. [CrossRef] [PubMed]

83. Tajima, S.; Pinnell, S.R. Ascorbic acid preferentially enhances type I and III collagen gene transcription in human skin fibroblasts. *J. Dermatol. Sci.* **1996**, *11*, 250–253. [CrossRef]

84. Agrawal, S.; Kumar, A.; Dhali, T.K.; Majhi, S.K. Comparison of oxidant-antioxidant status in patients with vitiligo and healthy population. *Kathmandu Univ. Med. J.* **2014**, *12*, 132–136. [CrossRef]

85. Nagata, C.; Nakamura, K.; Wada, K.; Oba, S.; Hayashi, M.; Takeda, N.; Yasuda, K. Association of dietary fat, vegetables and antioxidant micronutrients with skin ageing in Japanese women. *Br. J. Nutr.* **2010**, *103*, 1493–1498. [CrossRef] [PubMed]

86. Bissett, D.L.; Chatterjee, R.; Hannon, D.P. Photoprotective effect of superoxide-scavenging antioxidants against ultraviolet radiation-induced chronic skin damage in the hairless mouse. *Photodermatol. Photoimmunol. Photomed.* **1990**, *7*, 56–62. [PubMed]

87. Shukla, A.; Rasik, A.M.; Patnaik, G.K. Depletion of reduced glutathione, ascorbic acid, vitamin E and antioxidant defence enzymes in a healing cutaneous wound. *Free Radic. Res.* **1997**, *26*, 93–101. [CrossRef] [PubMed]

88. Steenvoorden, D.P.; Van Henegouwen, G.M. The use of endogenous antioxidants to improve photoprotection. *J. Photochem. Photobiol. B* **1997**, *41*, 1–10. [CrossRef]

89. Darr, D.; Dunston, S.; Faust, H.; Pinnell, S. Effectiveness of antioxidants (vitamin C and E) with and without sunscreens as topical photoprotectants. *Acta Derm Venereol.* **1996**, *76*, 264–268. [PubMed]

90. DeBuys, H.V.; Levy, S.B.; Murray, J.C.; Madey, D.L.; Pinnell, S.R. Modern approaches to photoprotection. *Dermatol. Clin.* **2000**, *18*, 577–590. [CrossRef]

91. Dreher, F.; Gabard, B.; Schwindt, D.A.; Maibach, H.I. Topical melatonin in combination with vitamins E and C protects skin from ultraviolet-induced erythema: A human study in vivo. *Br. J. Dermatol.* **1998**, *139*, 332–339. [CrossRef] [PubMed]

92. Mukai, K. Kinetic study of the reaction of vitamin C derivatives with tocopheroxyl (vitamin E radical) and substituted phenoxyl radicals in solution. *Biochim. Biophys. Acta* **1989**, *993*, 168–173. [CrossRef]

93. Tanaka, K.; Hashimoto, T.; Tokumaru, S.; Iguchi, H.; Kojo, S. Interactions between vitamin C and vitamin E are observed in tissues of inherently scorbutic rats. *J. Nutr.* **1997**, *127*, 2060–2064. [PubMed]

94. Kameyama, K.; Sakai, C.; Kondoh, S.; Yonemoto, K.; Nishiyama, S.; Tagawa, M.; Murata, T.; Ohnuma, T.; Quigley, J.; Dorsky, A.; et al. Inhibitory effect of magnesium L-ascorbyl-2-phosphate (VC-PMG) on melanogenesis in vitro and in vivo. *J. Am. Acad. Dermatol.* **1996**, *34*, 29–33. [CrossRef]

95. Matsuda, S.; Shibayama, H.; Hisama, M.; Ohtsuki, M.; Iwaki, M. Inhibitory effects of a novel ascorbic derivative, disodium isostearyl 2-O-L-ascorbyl phosphate on melanogenesis. *Chem. Pharm. Bull.* **2008**, *56*, 292–297. [CrossRef] [PubMed]

96. Ebanks, J.P.; Wickett, R.R.; Boissy, R.E. Mechanisms regulating skin pigmentation: The rise and fall of complexion coloration. *Int. J. Mol. Sci.* **2009**, *10*, 4066–4087. [CrossRef] [PubMed]

97. Pasonen-Seppanen, S.; Suhonen, T.M.; Kirjavainen, M.; Suihko, E.; Urtti, A.; Miettinen, M.; Hyttinen, M.; Tammi, M.; Tammi, R. Vitamin C enhances differentiation of a continuous keratinocyte cell line (REK) into epidermis with normal stratum corneum ultrastructure and functional permeability barrier. *Histochem. Cell. Biol.* **2001**, *116*, 287–297. [CrossRef] [PubMed]

98. Ponec, M.; Weerheim, A.; Kempenaar, J.; Mulder, A.; Gooris, G.S.; Bouwstra, J.; Mommaas, A.M. The formation of competent barrier lipids in reconstructed human epidermis requires the presence of vitamin C. *J. Investig. Dermatol.* **1997**, *109*, 348–355. [CrossRef] [PubMed]

99. Savini, I.; Catani, M.V.; Rossi, A.; Duranti, G.; Melino, G.; Avigliano, L. Characterization of keratinocyte differentiation induced by ascorbic acid: Protein kinase C involvement and vitamin C homeostasis. *J. Investig. Dermatol.* **2002**, *118*, 372–379. [CrossRef] [PubMed]

100. Uchida, Y.; Behne, M.; Quiec, D.; Elias, P.M.; Holleran, W.M. Vitamin C stimulates sphingolipid production and markers of barrier formation in submerged human keratinocyte cultures. *J. Investig. Dermatol.* **2001**, *117*, 1307–1313. [CrossRef] [PubMed]

101. Kim, K.P.; Shin, K.O.; Park, K.; Yun, H.J.; Mann, S.; Lee, Y.M.; Cho, Y. Vitamin C stimulates epidermal ceramide production by regulating its metabolic enzymes. *Biomol. Ther.* **2015**, *23*, 525–530. [CrossRef] [PubMed]

102. Marionnet, C.; Vioux-Chagnoleau, C.; Pierrard, C.; Sok, J.; Asselineau, D.; Bernerd, F. Morphogenesis of dermal-epidermal junction in a model of reconstructed skin: Beneficial effects of vitamin C. *Exp. Dermatol.* **2006**, *15*, 625–633. [CrossRef] [PubMed]

103. Vissers, M.C.; Gunningham, S.P.; Morrison, M.J.; Dachs, G.U.; Currie, M.J. Modulation of hypoxia-inducible factor-1 alpha in cultured primary cells by intracellular ascorbate. *Free Radic. Biol. Med.* **2007**, *42*, 765–772. [CrossRef] [PubMed]

104. Vissers, M.C.; Kuiper, C.; Dachs, G.U. Regulation of the 2-oxoglutarate-dependent dioxygenases and implications for cancer. *Biochem. Soc. Trans.* **2014**, *42*, 945–951. [CrossRef] [PubMed]

105. Vissers, M.C.; Lee, W.G.; Hampton, M.B. Regulation of apoptosis by vitamin C. Specific protection of the apoptotic machinery against exposure to chlorinated oxidants. *J. Biol. Chem.* **2001**, *276*, 46835–46840. [CrossRef] [PubMed]

106. Kao, J.; Huey, G.; Kao, R.; Stern, R. Ascorbic acid stimulates production of glycosaminoglycans in cultured fibroblasts. *Exp. Mol. Pathol.* **1990**, *53*, 1–10. [CrossRef]

107. Kang, J.S.; Kim, H.N.; Jung, D.J.; Kim, J.E.; Mun, G.H.; Kim, Y.S.; Cho, D.; Shin, D.H.; Hwang, Y.I.; Lee, W.J. Regulation of UVB-induced IL-8 and MCP-1 production in skin keratinocytes by increasing vitamin C uptake via the redistribution of SVCT-1 from the cytosol to the membrane. *J. Investig. Dermatol.* **2007**, *127*, 698–706. [CrossRef] [PubMed]

108. Savini, I.; D'Angelo, I.; Ranalli, M.; Melino, G.; Avigliano, L. Ascorbic acid maintenance in HaCaT cells prevents radical formation and apoptosis by UV-B. *Free Radic. Biol. Med.* **1999**, *26*, 1172–1180. [CrossRef]

109. Tebbe, B.; Wu, S.; Geilen, C.C.; Eberle, J.; Kodelja, V.; Orfanos, C.E. L-Ascorbic acid inhibits UVA-induced lipid peroxidation and secretion of IL-1alpha and IL-6 in cultured human keratinocytes in vitro. *J. Investig. Dermatol.* **1997**, *108*, 302–306. [CrossRef] [PubMed]

110. Minor, E.A.; Court, B.L.; Young, J.I.; Wang, G. Ascorbate induces ten-eleven translocation (Tet) methylcytosine dioxygenase-mediated generation of 5-hydroxymethylcytosine. *J. Biol. Chem.* **2013**, *288*, 13669–13674. [CrossRef] [PubMed]

111. Blaschke, K.; Ebata, K.T.; Karimi, M.M.; Zepeda-Martinez, J.A.; Goyal, P.; Mahapatra, S.; Tam, A.; Laird, D.J.; Hirst, M.; Rao, A.; et al. Vitamin C induces Tet-dependent DNA demethylation and a blastocyst-like state in ES cells. *Nature* **2013**, *500*, 222–226. [CrossRef] [PubMed]

112. Yin, R.; Mao, S.Q.; Zhao, B.; Chong, Z.; Yang, Y.; Zhao, C.; Zhang, D.; Huang, H.; Gao, J.; Li, Z.; et al. Ascorbic acid enhances Tet-mediated 5-methylcytosine oxidation and promotes DNA demethylation in mammals. *J. Am. Chem. Soc.* **2013**, *135*, 10396–10403. [CrossRef] [PubMed]

113. Song, C.X.; He, C. Potential functional roles of DNA demethylation intermediates. *Trends Biochem. Sci.* **2013**, *38*, 480–484. [CrossRef] [PubMed]

114. Lian, C.G.; Xu, Y.; Ceol, C.; Wu, F.; Larson, A.; Dresser, K.; Xu, W.; Tan, L.; Hu, Y.; Zhan, Q.; et al. Loss of 5-hydroxymethylcytosine is an epigenetic hallmark of melanoma. *Cell* **2012**, *150*, 1135–1146. [CrossRef] [PubMed]

115. Gustafson, C.B.; Yang, C.; Dickson, K.M.; Shao, H.; Van Booven, D.; Harbour, J.W.; Liu, Z.J.; Wang, G. Epigenetic reprogramming of melanoma cells by vitamin C treatment. *Clin. Epigenet.* **2015**, *7*, 51. [CrossRef] [PubMed]

116. Kuiper, C.; Vissers, M.C. Ascorbate as a co-factor for Fe- and 2-oxoglutarate dependent dioxygenases: Physiological activity in tumor growth and progression. *Front. Oncol.* **2014**, *4*, 359. [CrossRef] [PubMed]

117. Lin, J.R.; Qin, H.H.; Wu, W.Y.; He, S.J.; Xu, J.H. Vitamin C protects against UV irradiation-induced apoptosis through reactivating silenced tumor suppressor genes p21 and p16 in a Tet-dependent DNA demethylation manner in human skin cancer cells. *Cancer Biother. Radiopharm.* **2014**, *29*, 257–264. [CrossRef] [PubMed]

118. Valacchi, G.; Sticozzi, C.; Belmonte, G.; Cervellati, F.; Demaude, J.; Chen, N.; Krol, Y.; Oresajo, C. Vitamin C compound mixtures prevent ozone-induced oxidative damage in human keratinocytes as initial assessment of pollution protection. *PLoS ONE* **2015**, *10*, e0131097. [CrossRef] [PubMed]

119. Valacchi, G.; Muresan, X.M.; Sticozzi, C.; Belmonte, G.; Pecorelli, A.; Cervellati, F.; Demaude, J.; Krol, Y.; Oresajo, C. Ozone-induced damage in 3D-kkin model is prevented by topical vitamin C and vitamin E compound mixtures application. *J. Dermatol. Sci.* **2016**, *82*, 209–212. [CrossRef] [PubMed]

120. Puizina-Ivic, N. Skin aging. *Acta Dermatovenerol. Alp. Pannonica Adriat.* **2008**, *17*, 47–54. [PubMed]

121. Farage, M.A.; Miller, K.W.; Elsner, P.; Maibach, H.I. Intrinsic and extrinsic factors in skin ageing: A review. *Int. J. Cosmet. Sci.* **2008**, *30*, 87–95. [CrossRef] [PubMed]

122. Fenske, N.A.; Lober, C.W. Structural and functional changes of normal aging skin. *J. Am. Acad. Dermatol.* **1986**, *15*, 571–585. [CrossRef]

123. Kang, S.; Fisher, G.J.; Voorhees, J.J. Photoaging: Pathogenesis, prevention, and treatment. *Clin. Geriatr. Med.* **2001**, *17*, 643–659. [CrossRef]

124. El-Domyati, M.; Attia, S.; Saleh, F.; Brown, D.; Birk, D.E.; Gasparro, F.; Ahmad, H.; Uitto, J. Intrinsic aging vs. photoaging: A comparative histopathological, immunohistochemical, and ultrastructural study of skin. *Exp. Dermatol.* **2002**, *11*, 398–405. [CrossRef] [PubMed]

125. Lopez-Torres, M.; Shindo, Y.; Packer, L. Effect of age on antioxidants and molecular markers of oxidative damage in murine epidermis and dermis. *J. Investig. Dermatol.* **1994**, *102*, 476–480. [CrossRef] [PubMed]

126. Naylor, E.C.; Watson, R.E.; Sherratt, M.J. Molecular aspects of skin ageing. *Maturitas* **2011**, *69*, 249–256. [CrossRef] [PubMed]

127. White-Chu, E.F.; Reddy, M. Dry skin in the elderly: Complexities of a common problem. *Clin. Dermatol.* **2011**, *29*, 37–42. [CrossRef] [PubMed]

128. Papakonstantinou, E.; Roth, M.; Karakiulakis, G. Hyaluronic acid: A key molecule in skin aging. *Derm.-Endocrinol.* **2012**, *4*, 253–258. [CrossRef] [PubMed]

129. Monnat, R.J., Jr. "...Rewritten in the skin": Clues to skin biology and aging from inherited disease. *J. Investig. Dermatol.* **2015**, *135*, 1484–1490. [CrossRef] [PubMed]

130. Rinnerthaler, M.; Bischof, J.; Streubel, M.K.; Trost, A.; Richter, K. Oxidative stress in aging human skin. *Biomolecules* **2015**, *5*, 545–589. [CrossRef] [PubMed]

131. Draelos, Z.D. Aging skin: The role of diet: Facts and controversies. *Clin. Dermatol.* **2013**, *31*, 701–706. [CrossRef] [PubMed]

132. Marini, A. Beauty from the inside. Does it really work? *Hautarzt* **2011**, *62*, 614–617. [CrossRef] [PubMed]

133. Cosgrove, M.C.; Franco, O.H.; Granger, S.P.; Murray, P.G.; Mayes, A.E. Dietary nutrient intakes and skin-aging appearance among middle-aged American women. *Am. J. Clin. Nutr.* **2007**, *86*, 1225–1231. [PubMed]

134. Pezdirc, K.; Hutchesson, M.; Whitehead, R.; Ozakinci, G.; Perrett, D.; Collins, C.E. Can dietary intake influence perception of and measured appearance? A systematic review. *Nutr. Res.* **2015**, *35*, 175–197. [CrossRef] [PubMed]

135. Bertuccelli, G.; Zerbinati, N.; Marcellino, M.; Nanda Kumar, N.S.; He, F.; Tsepakolenko, V.; Cervi, J.; Lorenzetti, A.; Marotta, F. Effect of a quality-controlled fermented nutraceutical on skin aging markers: An antioxidant-control, double-blind study. *Exp. Ther. Med.* **2016**, *11*, 909–916. [CrossRef] [PubMed]

136. Qin, H.; Zheng, X.; Zhong, X.; Shetty, A.K.; Elias, P.M.; Bollag, W.B. Aquaporin-3 in keratinocytes and skin: Its role and interaction with phospholipase D2. *Arch. Biochem. Biophys.* **2011**, *508*, 138–143. [CrossRef] [PubMed]

137. Podda, M.; Traber, M.G.; Weber, C.; Yan, L.J.; Packer, L. UV-irradiation depletes antioxidants and causes oxidative damage in a model of human skin. *Free Radic. Biol. Med.* **1998**, *24*, 55–65. [CrossRef]

138. Buettner, G.R.; Motten, A.G.; Chignell, C.E. ESR detection of endogenous ascorbyl free radical in mouse skin: Enhancement of radical production during UV irradiation following topical application of chlorpromazine. *Photochem. Photobiol.* **1987**, *46*, 161–162. [CrossRef] [PubMed]

139. Miura, K.; Green, A.C. Dietary antioxidants and melanoma: Evidence from cohort and intervention studies. *Nutr. Cancer* **2015**, *67*, 867–876. [CrossRef] [PubMed]

140. Vile, G.F.; Tyrrell, R.M. UVA radiation-induced oxidative damage to lipids and proteins in vitro and in human skin fibroblasts is dependent on iron and singlet oxygen. *Free Radic. Biol. Med.* **1995**, *18*, 721–730. [CrossRef]

141. Sander, C.S.; Chang, H.; Salzmann, S.; Muller, C.S.; Ekanayake-Mudiyanselage, S.; Elsner, P.; Thiele, J.J. Photoaging is associated with protein oxidation in human skin in vivo. *J. Investig. Dermatol.* **2002**, *118*, 618–625. [CrossRef] [PubMed]

142. Berneburg, M.; Plettenberg, H.; Krutmann, J. Photoaging of human skin. *Photodermatol. Photoimmunol. Photomed.* **2000**, *16*, 239–244. [CrossRef] [PubMed]

143. Kligman, L.H.; Kligman, A.M. The nature of photoaging: Its prevention and repair. *Photo-Dermatology* **1986**, *3*, 215–227. [PubMed]

144. Trojahn, C.; Dobos, G.; Blume-Peytavi, U.; Kottner, J. The skin barrier function: Differences between intrinsic and extrinsic aging. *G. Ital. Dermatol. Venereol.* **2015**, *150*, 687–692. [PubMed]

145. Darr, D.; Combs, S.; Dunston, S.; Manning, T.; Pinnell, S. Topical vitamin C protects porcine skin from ultraviolet radiation-induced damage. *Br. J. Dermatol.* **1992**, *127*, 247–253. [CrossRef] [PubMed]

146. Mikirova, N.A.; Ichim, T.E.; Riordan, N.H. Anti-angiogenic effect of high doses of ascorbic acid. *J. Transl. Med.* **2008**, *6*, 50. [CrossRef] [PubMed]

147. Nakamura, T.; Pinnell, S.R.; Darr, D.; Kurimoto, I.; Itami, S.; Yoshikawa, K.; Streilein, J.W. Vitamin C abrogates the deleterious effects of UVB radiation on cutaneous immunity by a mechanism that does not depend on TNF-alpha. *J. Investig. Dermatol.* **1997**, *109*, 20–24. [CrossRef] [PubMed]

148. Eberlein-Konig, B.; Placzek, M.; Przybilla, B. Protective effect against sunburn of combined systemic ascorbic acid (vitamin C) and d-alpha-tocopherol (vitamin E). *J. Am. Acad. Dermatol.* **1998**, *38*, 45–48. [CrossRef]

149. Crisan, D.; Roman, I.; Crisan, M.; Scharffetter-Kochanek, K.; Badea, R. The role of vitamin C in pushing back the boundaries of skin aging: An ultrasonographic approach. *Clin. Cosmet. Investig. Dermatol.* **2015**, *8*, 463–470. [CrossRef] [PubMed]

150. Murray, J.C.; Burch, J.A.; Streilein, R.D.; Iannacchione, M.A.; Hall, R.P.; Pinnell, S.R. A topical antioxidant solution containing vitamins C and E stabilized by ferulic acid provides protection for human skin against damage caused by ultraviolet irradiation. *J. Am. Acad. Dermatol.* **2008**, *59*, 418–425. [CrossRef] [PubMed]

151. Amber, K.T.; Shiman, M.I.; Badiavas, E.V. The use of antioxidants in radiotherapy-induced skin toxicity. *Integr. Cancer Ther.* **2014**, *13*, 38–45. [CrossRef] [PubMed]

152. Lin, F.H.; Lin, J.Y.; Gupta, R.D.; Tournas, J.A.; Burch, J.A.; Selim, M.A.; Monteiro-Riviere, N.A.; Grichnik, J.M.; Zielinski, J.; Pinnell, S.R. Ferulic acid stabilizes a solution of vitamins C and E and doubles its photoprotection of skin. *J. Investig. Dermatol.* **2005**, *125*, 826–832. [CrossRef] [PubMed]

153. Grether-Beck, S.; Marini, A.; Jaenicke, T.; Krutmann, J. Effective photoprotection of human skin against infrared A radiation by topically applied antioxidants: Results from a vehicle controlled, double-blind, randomized study. *Photochem. Photobiol.* **2015**, *91*, 248–250. [CrossRef] [PubMed]

154. Traikovich, S.S. Use of topical ascorbic acid and its effects on photodamaged skin topography. *Arch. Otolaryngol. Head Neck Surg.* **1999**, *125*, 1091–1098. [CrossRef] [PubMed]

155. Jungersted, J.M.; Hellgren, L.I.; Jemec, G.B.; Agner, T. Lipids and skin barrier function–A clinical perspective. *Contact Dermat.* **2008**, *58*, 255–262. [CrossRef] [PubMed]

156. Rawlings, A.V.; Scott, I.R.; Harding, C.R.; Bowser, P.A. Stratum corneum moisturization at the molecular level. *J. Investig. Dermatol.* **1994**, *103*, 731–741. [CrossRef] [PubMed]

157. Boyce, S.T.; Supp, A.P.; Swope, V.B.; Warden, G.D. Vitamin C regulates keratinocyte viability, epidermal barrier, and basement membrane in vitro, and reduces wound contraction after grafting of cultured skin substitutes. *J. Investig. Dermatol.* **2002**, *118*, 565–572. [CrossRef] [PubMed]

158. Craven, N.M.; Watson, R.E.; Jones, C.J.; Shuttleworth, C.A.; Kielty, C.M.; Griffiths, C.E. Clinical features of photodamaged human skin are associated with a reduction in collagen VII. *Br. J. Dermatol.* **1997**, *137*, 344–350. [CrossRef] [PubMed]

159. Sachs, D.L.; Rittie, L.; Chubb, H.A.; Orringer, J.; Fisher, G.; Voorhees, J.J. Hypo-collagenesis in photoaged skin predicts response to anti-aging cosmeceuticals. *J. Cosmet. Dermatol.* **2013**, *12*, 108–115. [CrossRef] [PubMed]

160. Contet-Audonneau, J.L.; Jeanmaire, C.; Pauly, G. A histological study of human wrinkle structures: Comparison between sun-exposed areas of the face, with or without wrinkles, and sun-protected areas. *Br. J. Dermatol.* **1999**, *140*, 1038–1047. [CrossRef] [PubMed]

161. Thomas, J.R.; Dixon, T.K.; Bhattacharyya, T.K. Effects of topicals on the aging skin process. *Facial Plast. Surg. Clin. North Am.* **2013**, *21*, 55–60. [CrossRef] [PubMed]

162. Sorensen, L.T.; Toft, B.G.; Rygaard, J.; Ladelund, S.; Paddon, M.; James, T.; Taylor, R.; Gottrup, F. Effect of smoking, smoking cessation, and nicotine patch on wound dimension, vitamin C, and systemic markers of collagen metabolism. *Surgery* **2010**, *148*, 982–990. [CrossRef] [PubMed]

163. Gurtner, G.C.; Werner, S.; Barrandon, Y.; Longaker, M.T. Wound repair and regeneration. *Nature* **2008**, *453*, 314–321. [CrossRef] [PubMed]

164. Rodero, M.P.; Khosrotehrani, K. Skin wound healing modulation by macrophages. *Int. J. Clin. Exp. Pathol.* **2010**, *3*, 643–653. [PubMed]

165. Ilina, O.; Friedl, P. Mechanisms of collective cell migration at a glance. *J. Cell Sci.* **2009**, *122*, 3203–3208. [CrossRef] [PubMed]

166. Yun, I.S.; Yoo, H.S.; Kim, Y.O.; Rah, D.K. Improved scar appearance with combined use of silicone gel and vitamin C for Asian patients: A comparative case series. *Aesthet. Plast. Surg.* **2013**, *37*, 1176–1181. [CrossRef] [PubMed]

167. Thompson, C.; Fuhrman, M.P. Nutrients and wound healing: Still searching for the magic bullet. *Nutr. Clin. Pract.* **2005**, *20*, 331–347. [CrossRef] [PubMed]

168. Young, M.E. Malnutrition and wound healing. *Heart Lung* **1988**, *17*, 60–67. [PubMed]

169. Lund, C.C.; Crandon, J.H. Ascorbic acid and human wound healing. *Ann. Surg.* **1941**, *114*, 776–790. [CrossRef] [PubMed]

170. Basketter, D.A.; White, I.R.; Kullavanijaya, P.; Tresukosol, P.; Wichaidit, M.; McFadden, J.P. Influence of vitamin C on the elicitation of allergic contact dermatitis to p-phenylenediamine. *Contact Dermat.* **2016**, *74*, 368–372. [CrossRef] [PubMed]

171. Barbosa, E.; Faintuch, J.; Machado Moreira, E.A.; Goncalves da Silva, V.R.; Lopes Pereima, M.J.; Martins Fagundes, R.L.; Filho, D.W. Supplementation of vitamin E, vitamin C, and zinc attenuates oxidative stress in burned children: A randomized, double-blind, placebo-controlled pilot study. *J. Burn Care Res.* **2009**, *30*, 859–866. [CrossRef] [PubMed]

172. Ubbink, D.T.; Santema, T.B.; Stoekenbroek, R.M. Systemic wound care: A meta-review of cochrane systematic reviews. *Surg. Technol. Int.* **2014**, *24*, 99–111. [PubMed]

173. Furue, M.; Kadono, T. "Inflammatory skin march" in atopic dermatitis and psoriasis. *Inflamm. Res.* **2017**. [CrossRef]

174. Han, H.; Roan, F.; Ziegler, S.F. The atopic march: Current insights into skin barrier dysfunction and epithelial cell-derived cytokines. *Immunol. Rev.* **2017**, *278*, 116–130. [CrossRef] [PubMed]

175. Liakou, A.I.; Theodorakis, M.J.; Melnik, B.C.; Pappas, A.; Zouboulis, C.C. Nutritional clinical studies in dermatology. *J. Drugs Dermatol.* **2013**, *12*, 1104–1109. [PubMed]

176. Rackett, S.C.; Rothe, M.J.; Grant-Kels, J.M. Diet and dermatology. The role of dietary manipulation in the prevention and treatment of cutaneous disorders. *J. Am. Acad. Dermatol.* **1993**, *29*, 447–461. [CrossRef]

177. Pappas, A.; Liakou, A.; Zouboulis, C.C. Nutrition and skin. *Rev. Endocr. Metab. Disord.* **2016**, *17*, 443–448. [CrossRef] [PubMed]

178. Leveque, N.; Robin, S.; Muret, P.; Mac-Mary, S.; Makki, S.; Berthelot, A.; Kantelip, J.P.; Humbert, P. In vivo assessment of iron and ascorbic acid in psoriatic dermis. *Acta Derm. Venereol.* **2004**, *84*, 2–5. [CrossRef] [PubMed]

179. Shin, J.; Kim, Y.J.; Kwon, O.; Kim, N.I.; Cho, Y. Associations among plasma vitamin C, epidermal ceramide and clinical severity of atopic dermatitis. *Nutr. Res. Pract.* **2016**, *10*, 398–403. [CrossRef] [PubMed]

180. Kallner, A.B.; Hartmann, D.; Hornig, D.H. On the requirements of ascorbic acid in man: Steady-state turnover and body pool in smokers. *Am. J. Clin. Nutr.* **1981**, *34*, 1347–1355. [PubMed]

181. Evans-Olders, R.; Eintracht, S.; Hoffer, L.J. Metabolic origin of hypovitaminosis C in acutely hospitalized patients. *Nutrition* **2010**, *26*, 1070–1074. [CrossRef] [PubMed]

182. Gan, R.; Eintracht, S.; Hoffer, L.J. Vitamin C deficiency in a university teaching hospital. *J. Am. Coll. Nutr.* **2008**, *27*, 428–433. [CrossRef] [PubMed]

183. Findik, R.B.; Ilkaya, F.; Guresci, S.; Guzel, H.; Karabulut, S.; Karakaya, J. Effect of vitamin C on collagen structure of cardinal and uterosacral ligaments during pregnancy. *Eur. J. Obstet. Gynecol. Reprod. Biol.* **2016**, *201*, 31–35. [CrossRef] [PubMed]

184. Silverstein, R.J.; Landsman, A.S. The effects of a moderate and high dose of vitamin C on wound healing in a controlled guinea pig model. *J. Foot Ankle Surg.* **1999**, *38*, 333–338. [CrossRef]

185. Quevedo, W.C., Jr.; Holstein, T.J.; Dyckman, J.; McDonald, C.J.; Isaacson, E.L. Inhibition of UVR-induced tanning and immunosuppression by topical applications of vitamins C and E to the skin of hairless (hr/hr) mice. *Pigment Cell Res.* **2000**, *13*, 89–98. [CrossRef] [PubMed]

186. Lee, C.; Yang, H.; Kim, S.; Kim, M.; Kang, H.; Kim, N.; An, S.; Koh, J.; Jung, H. Evaluation of the anti-wrinkle effect of an ascorbic acid-loaded dissolving microneedle patch via a double-blind, placebo-controlled clinical study. *Int. J. Cosmet. Sci.* **2016**, *38*, 375–381. [CrossRef] [PubMed]

187. Valacchi, G.; Pecorelli, A.; Belmonte, G.; Pambianchi, E.; Cervellati, F.; Lynch, S.; Krol, Y.; Oresajo, C. Protective Effects of Topical Vitamin C Compound Mixtures against Ozone-Induced Damage in Human Skin. *J. Investig. Dermatol.* **2017**, *137*, 1373–1375. [CrossRef] [PubMed]

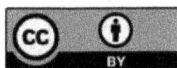

nutrients

MDPI

Article

Topical Application of Trisodium Ascorbyl 6-Palmitate 2-Phosphate Actively Supplies Ascorbate to Skin Cells in an Ascorbate Transporter-Independent Manner

Shuichi Shibuya [1], Ikuyo Sakaguchi [2], Shintaro Ito [2], Eiko Kato [3], Kenji Watanabe [1], Naotaka Izuo [1] and Takahiko Shimizu [1,*]

[1] Department of Advanced Aging Medicine, Chiba University Graduate School of Medicine, 1-8-1 Inohana, Chuo-ku, Chiba, Chiba 260-8670, Japan; s-shibuya@chiba-u.jp (S.S.); kng.wtnb@chiba-u.jp (K.W.); ntk.izuo@chiba-u.jp (N.I.)
[2] Reserch & Development Division, Club Cosmetics Co., Ltd., Ikoma, Nara 630-0222, Japan; ikuyos@clubcosmetics.co.jp (I.S.); sito@clubcosmetics.co.jp (S.I.)
[3] Functional Chemicals Division, Showa Denko K.K. Minato-ku, Tokyo 105-8518, Japan; kato.eiko.xhzqn@showadenko.com
* Correspondence: shimizut@chiba-u.jp; Tel.: +81-43-222-7171; Fax: +81-43-226-2095

Received: 2 May 2017; Accepted: 19 June 2017; Published: 22 June 2017

Abstract: Ascorbic acid (AA) possesses multiple beneficial functions, such as regulating collagen biosynthesis and redox balance in the skin. AA derivatives have been developed to overcome this compound's high fragility and to assist with AA supplementation to the skin. However, how AA derivatives are transferred into cells and converted to AA in the skin remains unclear. In the present study, we showed that AA treatment failed to increase the cellular AA level in the presence of AA transporter inhibitors, indicating an AA transporter-dependent action. In contrast, torisodium ascorbyl 6-palmitate 2-phosphate (APPS) treatment significantly enhanced the cellular AA level in skin cells despite the presence of inhibitors. In ex vivo experiments, APPS treatment also increased the AA content in a human epidermis model. Interestingly, APPS was readily metabolized and converted to AA in keratinocyte lysates via an intrinsic mechanism. Furthermore, APPS markedly repressed the intracellular superoxide generation and promoted viability associated with an enhanced AA level in *Sod1*-deficient skin cells. These findings indicate that APPS effectively restores the AA level and normalizes the redox balance in skin cells in an AA transporter-independent manner. Topical treatment of APPS is a beneficial strategy for supplying AA and improving the physiology of damaged skin.

Keywords: ascorbic acid; ascorbic acid transporter; ascorbic acid derivative; skin

1. Introduction

Ascorbic acid (AA) is a major soluble vitamin distributed in the tissues of all organisms, including animals and plants. In humans, organs such as the skin contain millimolar-order levels of AA, while plasma contains relatively low levels of AA (40–60 μM) [1,2]. Environmental factors such as lifestyle and nutrients consumed in the diet regulate the physiological kinetics of AA for maintaining organ homeostasis in the body. For example, smoking and an insufficient intake of vegetables and fruits adversely affect the AA status in the human body [3].

Accumulating evidence has shown that the chemical characteristics of AA as an electron donor play an important role in redox regulation in the human body [2,4–6]. AA also regulates many oxidase and hydroxylase activities as a cofactor to maintain cellular metabolism [4,7]. In particular, AA is an essential cofactor for post-translational modifications by lysyl oxidase and prolyl hydroxylase in collagen formation and further enhances the transcript levels of type I and III collagen genes [5,8]. AA also interferes with pigment production by interacting with copper ions at the tyrosinase activity site and reducing dopaquinone [9]. In this context, AA supplementation has been largely used to maintain the skin function and prevent skin aging in cosmetic and supplement fields worldwide.

As AA is highly fragile and not very liposoluble, allowing it to penetrate the skin and sustain its physiological function over a long period of time is difficult. To increase the stability and liposolubility of AA, various AA derivatives have been developed for dermatological application [10,11]. A phosphate group- and long hydrophobic chain-conjugated derivative, torisodium ascorbyl 6-palmitate 2-phosphate (APPS), was also developed to increase liposolubility [12]. In clinical applications, Inui and Itami have reported that topical treatment with APPS lotion for four weeks attenuated perifollicular pigmentation in female subjects [13].

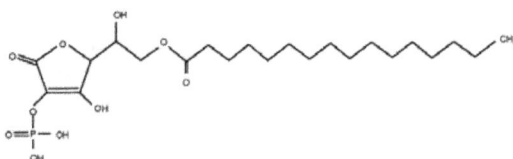

AA is incorporated into cells through two types of transporters: sodium-dependent vitamin C transporters (SVCT1 and SVCT2) and hexose transporters (GLUT1, GULT3, and GLUT4) [14]. AA and oxidized AA, known as dehydroascorbic acid (DHAA), are separately transported into the cytoplasm by SVCTs and GULTs, respectively. However, precisely how the AA derivative is transported to skin cells and converted to AA remains unclear.

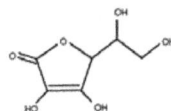

In the present study, we measured the cellular intake and transporter utilization of AA or APPS to estimate the intake efficiency of AA in skin cells. We also investigated the conversion mechanism of APPS to AA in cells. Furthermore, we investigated the redox regulation by APPS treatment in skin cells associated with oxidative damage. We then discussed the potential utility of APPS in AA supplementation and proposed an ideal protocol for applying AA derivatives to skin.

2. Materials and Methods

2.1. Materials

APPS (Figure 1) was provided by Showa Denko K.K. (Tokyo, Japan).

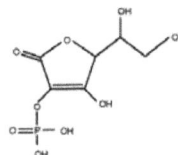

Figure 1. The structures of ascorbic acid (AA), A6Pal, APS, and APPS. L-ascorbyl 6-palmitate (A6Pal) is additionally conjugated with a long hydrophobic chain. Sodium ascorbyl 2-phosphate (APS) is additionally conjugated with a phosphate group. Torisodium ascorbyl 6-palmitate 2-phosphate (APPS) is additionally conjugated with a phosphate group and a long hydrophobic chain.

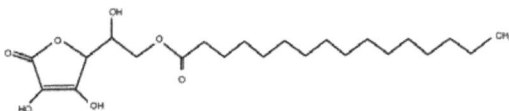

2.2. Measurement of AA Content in Skin Cells

Human fibroblasts (TIG118) were purchased from Health Science Research Resources Bank (Tokyo, Japan). TIG118 cells were maintained in DMEM (Nacalai Tesque, Kyoto, Japan) supplemented with 10% FBS (Life Technologies Corporation, Carlsbad, CA, USA), 100 units/mL of penicillin (Sigma-Aldrich, St. Louis, MO, USA), and 0.1 mg/mL of streptomycin (Sigma-Aldrich) at 37 °C in a humidified incubator with 5% CO_2. Cells were pre-incubated with or without phorbol 12-myristate 13-acetate (PMA) and glucose for 1 h to inhibit ascorbate transporters [15,16]. After pre-incubation, cells were washed three times with PBS and cultured for 1 h in culture medium with or without 10 µM AA and 10 µM APPS. Isolated cells were sonicated with 5.4% metaphosphoric acid (Wako, Osaka, Japan) to suppress oxidation. The homogenate was centrifuged at 10,000× *g* for 15 min at 4 °C, and the supernatant was then used for the assay. The AA level was measured using the Vitamin C quantitative determination Kit (SHIMA Laboratories, Tokyo, Japan) in accordance with the manufacturer's instructions (Figure 2).

2.3. A Kinetic Analysis of APPS Metabolism in Vitro

Human keratinocytes (NHEKs) were purchased from KURABO Industries (Osaka, Japan). NHEKs were cultured in HuMedia KG-2 (KURABO Industries) in accordance with the manufacturer's instructions. Cultured keratinocytes were collected and homogenized with HEPES buffer (1×10^6 cells/mL). To the homogenate was added 300 µM APPS (final concentration), and the solution was incubated at 37 °C. At each sampling point, the homogenate was centrifuged at 10,000× *g* for 15 min at 4 °C, and the supernatant was collected. Samples were filtered through a 0.22-µm membrane and measured for APPS and its metabolites (Figure 1) by high-performance liquid chromatography (HPLC) using a Shimadzu Prominence 20A system (Shimadzu Corporation, Kyoto, Japan). The separation conditions of AA, APS, A6Pal, and APPS were as follows, respectively: (1) for AA, Shodex Asahipak NH2P-50 4E column (Showa Denko K.K., Tokyo, Japan); detection wavelength, 254 nm; mobile phase, 60 mM H_3PO_4/acetonitrile (20/80); flow rate, 0.8 mL/min; (2) for APS, Shodex Asahipak NH2P-50 4E column; detection wavelength, 245 nm; mobile phase, 45 mM Na_2SO_4, 50 mM H_3PO_4/acetonitrile (80/20); flow rate, 1 mL/min; (3) for A6Pal and APPS, Shodex Silica C18P 4E column (Showa Denko K.K., Tokyo, Japan); detection wavelength, 265 nm; mobile phase, 30 mM K_2HPO_4 (pH 7.0)/tetrahydrofuran (35/65); flow rate, 0.7 mL/min. The levels of APPS and its metabolites were determined on the basis of the peak area of the standard AA curve (Figure 3A).

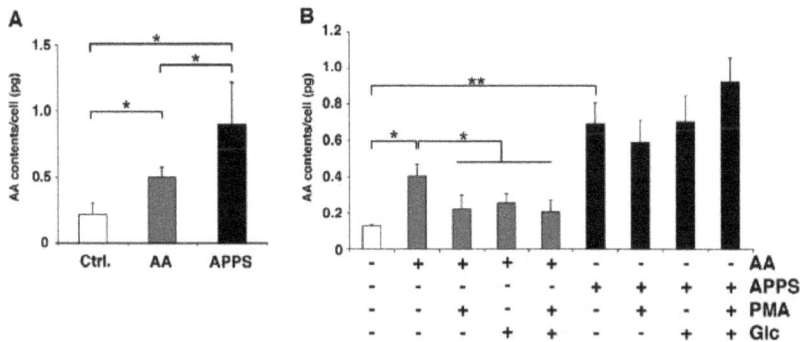

Figure 2. APPS upregulates the cellular AA level in an AA transporter-independent manner. (**A**) Intracellular ascorbic acid (AA) contents in human cells treated with 10 µM AA or 10 µM APPS for 1 h. These data represent the mean ± SE; * $p < 0.05$; (**B**) Intracellular AA contents in human cells. Human cells were pre-incubated with or without 10 µM PMA and 10 µM glucose for 1 h. After pre-incubation, cells were washed and cultured for 1h in culture medium with or without 10 µM AA and 10 µM APPS. These data represent the mean ± SEM; * $p < 0.05$ vs. no treatment control, ** $p < 0.01$ vs. no treatment control.

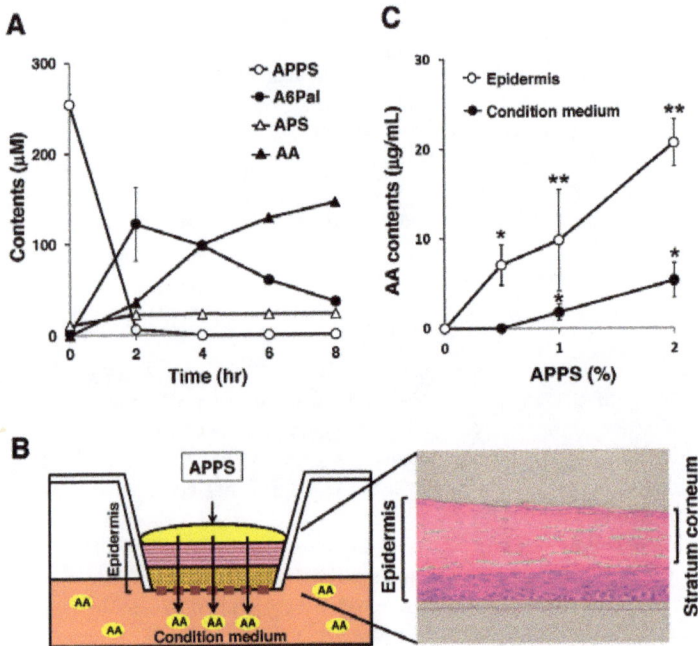

Figure 3. APPS is converted to AA by endogenous convertases. (**A**) A kinetics analysis of APPS metabolites including AA, A6Pal, and APS in keratinocyte lysates; (**B**) A human epidermal skin model (LabCyte EPI-MODEL) was used in ex vivo experiments; (**C**) AA contents in epidermis and conditioned medium in an ex vivo human epidermal skin model treated with APPS at various doses. These data represent the mean $\pm$ SEM; * $p < 0.05$ vs. no AA treatment, ** $p < 0.01$ vs. no AA treatment.

2.4. Treatment with APPS in a Human Epidermal Skin Model

A human epidermal skin model (LabCyte EPI-MODEL; J-TEC, Aichi, Japan) was cultured in accordance with the manufacturer's instructions (Figure 3B). The skin model was treated with APPS solution and cultured at 37 °C for 24 h. After incubation, skin tissues and conditioned medium were collected. Skin tissues (10 mm diameter) were homogenized with 50% ethanol (three tissues/1.5 mL) using a Biomasher (Nippi, Ibaraki, Japan). The skin homogenate was centrifuged at 15,000× *g* for 30 s at 4 °C. To the supernatant and conditioned medium was added 66% metaphosphoric acid (10 µL/200 µL supernatant), and this solution was then incubated first at 4 °C for 30 min and then with 22 mg/mL dithioerythritol (10 µL/200 µL supernatant; MP Biomedicals, LLC, Illkirch, France) at 4 °C for 30 min. The supernatant was centrifuged and filtered for a later analysis. The levels of APPS and its metabolites were measured with HPLC equipped with a Shodex Asahipak NH2P-50 4E column. The separation conditions were as follows: detection wavelength, 245 nm; mobile phase, 60 mM H_3PO_4/acetonitrile (20/80) (Figure 3C).

2.5. Measurement of AA Content in Sod1-decifient Cells

$Sod1^{+/+}$ and $Sod1^{-/-}$ dermal fibroblasts were cultured in accordance with a previous description [17]. Cells were cultured for 6 h in culture medium with or without 10 µM AA and 10 µM APPS. The AA level was measured using the Vitamin C quantitative determination Kit (SHIMA Laboratories, Tokyo, Japan) as described above (Figure 4A).

2.6. Intracellular Reactive Oxygen Species

$Sod1^{+/+}$ and $Sod1^{-/-}$ dermal fibroblasts were cultured with 10 µM AA or 10 µM APPS for 24 h in 1% O_2, followed by incubation under 20% O_2 condition for 16 h to induce oxidative stress. After treatment, the fibroblasts were stained with 10 µM dihydroethidium (DHE) fluorescent probe (Life Technologies Corporation, Carlsbad, CA, USA) and 10 µM Hoechst 33342 (Merck Millipore, Darmstadt, Germany) for 20 min under 20% O_2. The intracellular superoxide (O_2^{-}) generation was calculated as the DHE-positive area per nuclei number using fluorescent microscopy with the Leica Qwin V3 image software program (Leica Microsystems, Buffalo Grove, IL, USA).

2.7. Cell Viability and Proliferation Assay

$Sod1^{+/+}$ and $Sod1^{-/-}$ skin cells were cultured, and the number of cells was directly counted as described previously [17]. The collected medium was centrifuged at 400× *g* for 5 min at 4 °C, and the supernatant was used for the subsequent assays. The lactate dehydrogenase (LDH) level was measured using the LDH cytotoxicity assay kit (Cayman Chemical Company, Ann Arbor, MI, USA) in accordance with the manufacturer's instructions.

2.8. Statistical Analyses

The statistical analyses were performed using Student's *t*-test for comparisons between two groups and Tukey's test for comparisons among three groups. Differences between the data were considered significant when the p values were less than 0.05. All data are expressed as the mean ± standard error of the mean (SEM).

3. Results

3.1. APPS Positively Increases the Intracellular AA Contents in an AA Transporter-Independent Manner

AA has been largely used in cosmetics to maintain the skin function because of its beneficial effects, such as antioxidation and regulation of collagen biosynthesis. However, its high fragility as well as low liposolubility limit its penetration into the skin and physiological action. A number of AA derivatives have been developed to overcome these disadvantages [10,11]. One such derivative, APPS, was generated through the conjugation of a phosphate group and a long hydrophobic chain (Figure 1).

In order to evaluate the permeability of AA, we treated human skin cells with AA or APPS and biochemically measured the cellular AA contents (Figure 2A). APPS treatment for 1 h significantly increased the cellular AA levels by 4.1-fold compared to the control skin, whereas AA treatment increased them only by 2.3-fold (Figure 2A). AA is usually transported into cells through AA transporters, such as SVCTs and GLUTs [18,19]. To investigate the transporter utilization of APPS and AA, we pre-treated human skin cells with PMA and glucose as AA transport inhibitors. As shown in Figure 2B, PMA and glucose markedly inhibited the uptake of AA with only AA addition alone. In contrast, APPS treatment sustained high levels of cellular AA in fibroblasts in the presence of both PMA and glucose (Figure 2B). These results demonstrated that APPS supplementation effectively and stably enhanced the intracellular AA contents in an AA transporter-independent manner.

3.2. Topical APPS is Effectively Converted to AA in Skin Cells

Next, to investigate the conversion mechanism of APPS to AA in skin cells, we incubated APPS in homogenates of human keratinocytes and monitored the dynamics of APPS and other metabolites, including AA, L-ascorbyl 6-palmitate (A6Pal), and sodium ascorbyl 2-phosphate (APS) (Figure 1). As expected, the APPS contents were rapidly reduced at 2 h after incubation (Figure 3A). In contrast, the contents of A6Pal, a metabolite with phosphate group cleavage, were increased at 2 h after incubation and gradually decreased until 8 h (Figure 3A). Concomitantly, the AA contents were gradually increased in a time-dependent manner (Figure 3A). Interestingly, the APS contents were not altered in the homogenates (Figure 3A). Indeed, potent phosphatase and esterase activities have been detected in human as well as rodent skin tissue [20–23]. Taken together, these present and previous findings suggest that endogenous phosphatases first cleave the phosphate group of APPS followed by intrinsic esterases to release the palmitate group of A6Pal, resulting in the production of AA in the conversion process.

To estimate the permeability of APPS, we applied APPS to our human epidermis models, which consist of a stratum corneum layer on keratinocyte culture (Figure 3B). Skin tissues without APPS treatment possessed AA contents below detection limit. When we treated the model with APPS for 24 h, the AA contents in the tissue was significantly increased in a dose-dependent manner (Figure 3C), suggesting that APPS was converted to AA in the tissue. Furthermore, the AA contents in the conditioned medium at the bottom of the dish were also significantly increased in cases of high-dose treatment (Figure 3C). These results indicated that APPS is effectively converted to AA and transferred into skin cells.

3.3. APPS Attenuates Cellular Oxidative Damage in Skin

SOD1, a major antioxidant enzyme in cytoplasm, plays an important role in maintaining the cellular redox balance. SOD1 loss significantly exhibited low viability associated with enhanced intracellular reactive oxygen species and cellular damage [24–32]. Interestingly, we failed to detect trace levels of cellular AA in $Sod1^{-/-}$ cells, indicating impairment of the AA-glutathione cycle and redox balance (Figure 4A). APPS and AA treatment enhanced the cellular AA level in both $Sod1^{-/-}$ and $Sod1^{+/+}$ skin cells (Figure 4A). Pre-treatment with APPS and AA completely suppressed the O_2^- generation in $Sod1^{-/-}$ cells, resulting in production at the same level as in the $Sod1^{+/+}$ cells (Figure 4B). APPS treatment also improved the viability and promoted proliferation associated with the suppression of cellular damage (Figure 4C). These findings showed that APPS ameliorates cellular damage by increasing the cellular AA level in damaged skin cells.

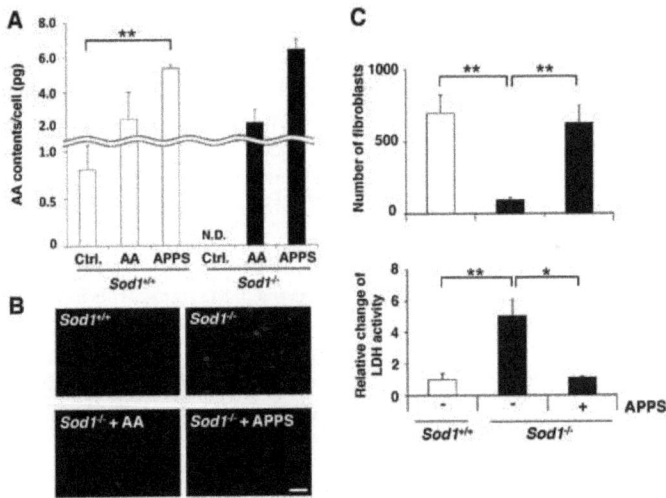

Figure 4. APPS elevates the cellular AA levels and attenuates cellular damage in skin cells. (**A**) Intracellular AA contents in $Sod1^{+/+}$ and $Sod1^{-/-}$ cells treated with 10 μM AA or 10 μM APPS for 6 h; (**B**) For the measurement of intracellular reactive oxygen species, cultured $Sod1^{+/+}$ and $Sod1^{-/-}$ cells treated with 10 μM AA or 10 μM APPS for 24 h were stained with dihydroethidium. The scale bar represents 100 μm; (**C**) The viability and proliferation of $Sod1^{+/+}$ and $Sod1^{-/-}$ cells with or without 10 μM APPS treatment for 96 h were analyzed. The lactate dehydrogenase activity in the conditioned medium used to culture the $Sod1^{+/+}$ and $Sod1^{-/-}$ skin cells for 96 h was measured. These data represent the mean ± SEM; * $p < 0.05$, ** $p < 0.01$.

4. Discussion

4.1. APPS is Effectively Converted to AA by Cellular Convertases, Resulting in AA Transport into the Cytoplasm of Skin Cells in an AA Transporter-Independent Manner

Since skin innately includes relatively high levels of AA (approximately 50-fold that of plasma) [1,2], the skin AA level generally depends on and is maintained by AA transport activity rather than concentration-directed diffusion. In the present study, we showed that APPS treatment effectively supplied AA to the cytoplasm in skin cells compared to AA treatment in vitro (Figure 2A). APPS, but not AA, significantly increased the intracellular AA level even though both SVCTs and GLUTs were inhibited (Figure 2B). This preferential capacity of APPS is due to an AA transporter-independent action. As shown in Figure 3A, the addition of APPS to cell lysate rapidly increased the content of A6Pal, but not APS, and then gradually increased the AA content. We also found that APPS efficiently penetrated and converted AA in epidermal cells, leading to passed through AA in the conditioned medium in a three-dimensional epidermis model (Figure 3C). Since skin cells possess high phosphatase and esterase activity [20–23], endogenous cellular convertases can cleave the phosphate and palmitate groups of APPS.

Glatz et al. reported that fatty acids, including palmitate, can directly traverse the plasma membrane and that albumin proteins located at the outer cell surface may play an additional role in the delivery of fatty acids into the cytoplasm in cells [33,34]. These multiple transport mechanisms of fatty acid may help facilitate the permeability of skin cells to APPS, leading to its conversion to AA by endogenous cellular enzymes, such as phosphatases and esterases.

4.2. APPS Improves the AA Level and Skin Function by Regulating Redox Balance

In the present study, in vitro experiments showed that the supply of AA by APPS treatment effectively increased the cellular AA level and suppressed the O_2^- generation associated with improved viability in $Sod1^{-/-}$ cells, resulting in physiological redox level (Figure 4A,B). We also showed that treatment with APPS significantly promoted the proliferation and migration of $Sod1^{-/-}$ skin cells associated with the suppression of LDH activity (Figure 4C). Du et al. reported that APPS treatment improved viability of PC12 cells treated with hydrogen peroxide [12], suggesting that APPS treatment protect cells from various types of oxidative damage. AA highly reacts with oxygen and O_2^-, resulting in oxidized AA forms such as mono-DHAA and DHAA [35,36]. Mono-DHAA and DHAA serve as AA radicals to capture electrons and can also be recycled back into AA by direct reduction in the AA-glutathione cycle [37]. Under highly oxidative conditions, mono-DHAA and DHAA are further degraded via hydrolysis or oxidation to 2,3-diketogulonic acid with no AA potency [38]. These results suggest that AA supplementation by APPS may increase AA recycling via these systems, resulting in improvement in the redox balance in damaged skin, such as under conditions of *Sod1* deficiency.

Long chain fatty acids, including palmitate, are required for the lipid synthesis in skin to maintain tissue homeostasis [39]. Kim et al. reported that ultraviolet (UV) irradiation and aging stress caused a reduction in the contents of palmitate, eicosatrienoic acid, and other fatty acid in skin [40]. Treatment with eicosatrienoic acid downregulated the expression of MMP1 in human keratinocytes irradiated by UV [40]. Palmitoleic acid, metabolites from palmitate, also inhibited the gene expression of *Mmp9* and RANKL-induced NF-κB activation in murine macrophages [41]. These results suggest that fatty acid supplementation to the skin may act as a regulator of skin homeostasis. In this context, palmitate cleaved from APPS in the skin might also protect skin cells from exogenous insults, such as pro-oxidants and UV.

4.3. Topical Application of APPS for Damaged Skin

The SVCT function is obligatorily dependent on a favorable inward gradient for Na^+, which in turn is sustained by the continuous extrusion of Na^+ by ATP-dependent Na^+/K^+-ATPase [42,43]. Indeed, the replacement of Na^+ with K^+, Li^+, or choline almost completely abolishes the AA uptake [42,44].

Furthermore, SVCT2 is modulated by Ca^{2+} and Mg^{2+} ions, which switch the transporter from an inactive to an active form [45]. We previously reported that *Sod1* deficiency induced age-related skin atrophy and a reduction in the AA contents in skin [25]. We also provided evidence that $Sod1^{-/-}$ skin cells showed aberrantly increased intracellular Ca^{2+} levels (data not shown) and loss of mitochondrial membrane potential associated with ATP depletion [46], indicating alteration of intracellular Ca^{2+} and ATP utilization in skin. We previously demonstrated that the topical treatment of APPS completely cured atrophy and oxidative damage in $Sod1^{-/-}$ skins [17,27]. Taken together, these findings also implied that APPS thus appears to be useful for the supply of AA to the skin and also for the mitigation of oxidative damage via penetration mechanisms independent from AA transporters. Topical treatment of APPS is a beneficial strategy for supplying AA and improving the physiology of damaged skin.

Acknowledgments: We thank Yusuke Ozawa, Toshihiko Toda, and Kinue Iizuka (Chiba University) for their valuable technical assistance.

Author Contributions: S.S. and T.S. designed the study. S.S. and T.S. wrote the manuscript. S.S., I.S., S.I. and E.K. performed the study. S.S., I.S., S.I. and E.K. analyzed the data. K.W. and N.I. edited the article. T.S. coordinated and directed the project.

Conflicts of Interest: This research was supported by funds from Club Cosmetics Company (Nara, Japan) and Showa Denko Company (Tokyo, Japan). The APPS was provided by Showa Denko (Tokyo, Japan). This does not alter the authors' adherence to all *Nutrients* policies on sharing data and materials.

References

1. Levine, M.; Wang, Y.; Padayatty, S.J.; Morrow, J. A new recommended dietary allowance of vitamin C for healthy young women. *Proc. Natl. Acad. Sci. USA* **2001**, *98*, 9842–9846. [CrossRef] [PubMed]

2. Harrison, F.E.; May, J.M. Vitamin C function in the brain: Vital role of the ascorbate transporter SVCT2. *Free Radic. Biol. Med.* **2009**, *46*, 719–730. [CrossRef] [PubMed]

3. Loria, C.M.; Klag, M.J.; Caulfield, L.E.; Whelton, P.K. Vitamin C status and mortality in US adults. *Am. J. Clin. Nutr.* **2000**, *72*, 139–145. [PubMed]

4. Padayatty, S.J.; Katz, A.; Wang, Y.; Eck, P.; Kwon, O.; Lee, J.H.; Chen, S.; Corpe, C.; Dutta, A.; Dutta, S.K.; et al. Vitamin C as an antioxidant: Evaluation of its role in disease prevention. *J. Am. Coll. Nutr.* **2003**, *22*, 18–35. [CrossRef] [PubMed]

5. Du, J.; Cullen, J.J.; Buettner, G.R. Ascorbic acid: Chemistry, biology and the treatment of cancer. *Biochim. Biophys. Acta* **2012**, *1826*, 443–457. [CrossRef] [PubMed]

6. Petruk, G.; Raiola, A.; Del Giudice, R.; Barone, A.; Frusciante, L.; Rigano, M.M.; Monti, D.M. An ascorbic acid-enriched tomato genotype to fight UVA-induced oxidative stress in normal human keratinocytes. *J. Photochem. Photobiol.* **2016**, *163*, 284–289. [CrossRef] [PubMed]

7. Saito, K.; Hosoi, E.; Ishigami, A.; Yokoyama, T. Vitamin C and physical performance in the elderly. In *Oxidative Stress and Dietary Antioxidants*; Preedy, V.R., Ed.; Academic Press: New York, NY, USA, 2014; pp. 119–128.

8. Duarte, T.L.; Almeida, I.F. Vitamin C, gene expression and skin health. In *Handbook of Diet, Nutrition and the Skin*; Preedy, V.R., Ed.; Wageningen Academic Publishers: Wageningen, The Netherlands, 2012; pp. 115–128.

9. Rendon, M.I.; Gaviria, J.I. Review of skin-lightening agents. *Dermatol. Surg.* **2005**, *31*, 886–889. [CrossRef] [PubMed]

10. Lupo, M.P. Antioxidants and vitamins in cosmetics. *Clin. Dermatol.* **2001**, *19*, 467–473. [CrossRef]

11. Palma, S.; Manzo, R.; Lo Nostro, P.; Allemandi, D. Nanostructures from alkyl vitamin C derivatives (ASCn): Properties and potential platform for drug delivery. *Int. J. Pharm.* **2007**, *345*, 26–34. [CrossRef] [PubMed]

12. Du, C.B.; Liu, J.W.; Su, W.; Ren, Y.H.; Wei, D.Z. The protective effect of ascorbic acid derivative on PC12 cells: Involvement of its ROS scavenging ability. *Life Sci.* **2003**, *74*, 771–780. [CrossRef] [PubMed]

13. Inui, S.; Itami, S. Perifollicular pigmentation is the first target for topical vitamin C derivative ascorbyl 2-phosphate 6-palmitate (APPS): Randomized, single-blinded, placebo-controlled study. *J. Dermatol.* **2007**, *34*, 221–223. [CrossRef] [PubMed]

14. Tian, W.; Wang, Y.; Xu, Y.; Guo, X.; Wang, B.; Sun, L.; Liu, L.; Cui, F.; Zhuang, Q.; Bao, X.; et al. The hypoxia-inducible factor renders cancer cells more sensitive to vitamin C-induced toxicity. *J. Biol. Chem.* **2014**, *289*, 3339–3351. [CrossRef] [PubMed]

15. Liang, W.J.; Johnson, D.; Ma, L.S.; Jarvis, S.M.; Wei-Jun, L. Regulation of the human vitamin C transporters expressed in COS-1 cells by protein kinase C. *Am. J. Physiol. Cell Physiol.* **2002**, *283*, C1696–C1704. [CrossRef] [PubMed]

16. McNulty, A.L.; Stabler, T.V.; Vail, T.P.; McDaniel, G.E.; Kraus, V.B. Dehydroascorbate transport in human chondrocytes is regulated by hypoxia and is a physiologically relevant source of ascorbic acid in the joint. *Arthritis Rheum.* **2005**, *52*, 2676–2685. [CrossRef] [PubMed]

17. Shibuya, S.; Ozawa, Y.; Toda, T.; Watanabe, K.; Tometsuka, C.; Ogura, T.; Koyama, Y.; Shimizu, T. Collagen peptide and vitamin C additively attenuate age-related skin atrophy in *Sod1*-deficient mice. *Biosci. Biotechnol. Biochem.* **2014**, *78*, 1212–1220. [CrossRef] [PubMed]

18. Tsukaguchi, H.; Tokui, T.; Mackenzie, B.; Berger, U.V.; Chen, X.Z.; Wang, Y.; Brubaker, R.F.; Hediger, M.A. A family of mammalian Na^+-dependent L-ascorbic acid transporters. *Nature* **1999**, *399*, 70–75. [PubMed]

19. Rumsey, S.C.; Kwon, O.; Xu, G.W.; Burant, C.F.; Simpson, I.; Levine, M. Glucose transporter isoforms GLUT1 and GLUT3 transport dehydroascorbic acid. *J. Biol. Chem.* **1997**, *272*, 18982–18989. [CrossRef] [PubMed]

20. Partanen, S. Histochemically demonstrable acid phosphotyrosine phosphatase activity in human tissues. *Eur. J. Histochem.* **1998**, *42*, 171–181. [PubMed]

21. Jewell, C.; Ackermann, C.; Payne, N.A.; Fate, G.; Voorman, R.; Williams, F.M. Specificity of procaine and ester hydrolysis by human, minipig, and rat skin and liver. *Drug Metab. Dispos.* **2007**, *35*, 2015–2022. [CrossRef] [PubMed]

22. Jewell, C.; Prusakiewicz, J.J.; Ackermann, C.; Payne, N.A.; Fate, G.; Williams, F.M. The distribution of esterases in the skin of the minipig. *Toxicol. Lett.* **2007**, *173*, 118–123. [CrossRef] [PubMed]

23. Prusakiewicz, J.J.; Ackermann, C.; Voorman, R. Comparison of skin esterase activities from different species. *Pharm. Res.* **2006**, *23*, 1517–1524. [CrossRef] [PubMed]

24. Shibuya, S.; Nojiri, H.; Morikawa, D.; Koyama, H.; Shimizu, T. Protective effects of vitamin C on age-related bone and skin phenotypes caused by intracellular reactive oxygen species. In *Oxidative Stress and Dietary Antioxidants*; Preedy, V.R., Ed.; Academic Press: New York, NY, USA, 2014; pp. 137–144.

25. Shibuya, S.; Ozawa, Y.; Watanabe, K.; Izuo, N.; Toda, T.; Yokote, K.; Shimizu, T. Palladium and platinum nanoparticles attenuate aging-like skin atrophy via antioxidant activity in mice. *PLoS ONE* **2014**, *9*, e109288. [CrossRef] [PubMed]

26. Watanabe, K.; Shibuya, S.; Ozawa, Y.; Nojiri, H.; Izuo, N.; Yokote, K.; Shimizu, T. Superoxide dismutase 1 loss disturbs intracellular redox signaling, resulting in global age-related pathological changes. *BioMed Res. Int.* **2014**, *2014*, 140165. [CrossRef] [PubMed]

27. Murakami, K.; Inagaki, J.; Saito, M.; Ikeda, Y.; Tsuda, C.; Noda, Y.; Kawakami, S.; Shirasawa, T.; Shimizu, T. Skin atrophy in cytoplasmic SOD-deficient mice and its complete recovery using a vitamin C derivative. *Biochem. Biophys. Res. Commun.* **2009**, *382*, 457–461. [CrossRef] [PubMed]

28. Murakami, K.; Murata, N.; Noda, Y.; Tahara, S.; Kaneko, T.; Kinoshita, N.; Hatsuta, H.; Murayama, S.; Barnham, K.J.; Irie, K.; et al. SOD1 (copper/zinc superoxide dismutase) deficiency drives amyloid beta protein oligomerization and memory loss in mouse model of Alzheimer disease. *J. Biol. Chem.* **2011**, *286*, 44557–44568. [CrossRef] [PubMed]

29. Murakami, K.; Murata, N.; Ozawa, Y.; Kinoshita, N.; Irie, K.; Shirasawa, T.; Shimizu, T. Vitamin C restores behavioral deficits and amyloid-beta oligomerization without affecting plaque formation in a mouse model of Alzheimer's disease. *J. Alzheimer's Dis.* **2011**, *26*, 7–18.

30. Nojiri, H.; Saita, Y.; Morikawa, D.; Kobayashi, K.; Tsuda, C.; Miyazaki, T.; Saito, M.; Marumo, K.; Yonezawa, I.; Kaneko, K.; et al. Cytoplasmic superoxide causes bone fragility owing to low-turnover osteoporosis and impaired collagen cross-linking. *J. Bone Miner. Res.* **2011**, *26*, 2682–2694. [CrossRef] [PubMed]

31. Morikawa, D.; Nojiri, H.; Saita, Y.; Kobayashi, K.; Watanabe, K.; Ozawa, Y.; Koike, M.; Asou, Y.; Takaku, T.; Kaneko, K.; et al. Cytoplasmic reactive oxygen species and SOD1 regulate bone mass during mechanical unloading. *J. Bone Miner. Res.* **2013**, *28*, 2368–2380. [CrossRef] [PubMed]

32. Morikawa, D.; Itoigawa, Y.; Nojiri, H.; Sano, H.; Itoi, E.; Saijo, Y.; Kaneko, K.; Shimizu, T. Contribution of oxidative stress to the degeneration of rotator cuff entheses. *J. Shoulder Elb. Surg.* **2014**, *23*, 628–635. [CrossRef] [PubMed]

33. Glatz, J.F.; Luiken, J.J.; van Nieuwenhoven, F.A.; Van der Vusse, G.J. Molecular mechanism of cellular uptake and intracellular translocation of fatty acids. *Prostaglandins Leukot. Essent. Fatty Acids* **1997**, *57*, 3–9. [CrossRef]

34. Glatz, J.F. Lipids and lipid binding proteins: A perfect match. *Prostaglandins Leukot. Essent. Fatty Acids* **2015**, *93*, 45–49. [CrossRef] [PubMed]

35. Nishikimi, M. Oxidation of ascorbic acid with superoxide anion generated by the xanthine-xanthine oxidase system. *Biochem. Biophys. Res. Commun.* **1975**, *63*, 463–468. [CrossRef]

36. Bielski, B.H.; Richter, H.W.; Chan, P.C. Some properties of the ascorbate free radical. *Ann. N. Y. Acad. Sci.* **1975**, *258*, 231–237. [CrossRef] [PubMed]

37. Wells, W.W.; Xu, D.P. Dehydroascorbate reduction. *J. Bioenerg. Biomembr.* **1994**, *26*, 369–377. [CrossRef] [PubMed]

38. Gibbons, E.; Allwood, M.C.; Neal, T.; Hardy, G. Degradation of dehydroascorbic acid in parenteral nutrition mixtures. *J. Pharm. Biomed. Anal.* **2001**, *25*, 605–611. [CrossRef]

39. Nakamura, M.T.; Yudell, B.E.; Loor, J.J. Regulation of energy metabolism by long-chain fatty acids. *Prog. Lipid. Res.* **2014**, *53*, 124–144. [CrossRef] [PubMed]

40. Kim, E.J.; Kim, M.K.; Jin, X.J.; Oh, J.H.; Kim, J.E.; Chung, J.H. Skin aging and photoaging alter fatty acids composition, including 11,14,17-eicosatrienoic acid, in the epidermis of human skin. *J. Korean Med. Sci.* **2010**, *25*, 980–983. [CrossRef] [PubMed]

41. Van Heerden, B.; Kasonga, A.; Kruger, M.C.; Coetzee, M. Palmitoleic acid inhibits RANKL-induced osteoclastogenesis and bone resorption by suppressing NF-κB and MAPK signalling pathways. *Nutrients* **2017**, *9*, 441. [CrossRef] [PubMed]

42. Castro, M.; Caprile, T.; Astuya, A.; Millan, C.; Reinicke, K.; Vera, J.C.; Vasquez, O.; Aguayo, L.G.; Nualart, F. High-affinity sodium-vitamin C co-transporters (SVCT) expression in embryonic mouse neurons. *J. Neurochem.* **2001**, *78*, 815–823. [CrossRef] [PubMed]

43. Garcia, M.D.L.; Salazar, K.; Millan, C.; Rodriguez, F.; Montecinos, H.; Caprile, T.; Silva, C.; Cortes, C.; Reinicke, K.; Vera, J.C.; et al. Sodium vitamin C cotransporter SVCT2 is expressed in hypothalamic glial cells. *Glia* **2005**, *50*, 32–47. [CrossRef] [PubMed]

44. Rajan, D.P.; Huang, W.; Dutta, B.; Devoe, L.D.; Leibach, F.H.; Ganapathy, V.; Prasad, P.D. Human placental sodium-dependent vitamin C transporter (SVCT2): Molecular cloning and transport function. *Biochem. Biophys. Res. Commun.* **1999**, *262*, 762–768. [CrossRef] [PubMed]

45. Godoy, A.; Ormazabal, V.; Moraga-Cid, G.; Zuniga, F.A.; Sotomayor, P.; Barra, V.; Vasquez, O.; Montecinos, V.; Mardones, L.; Guzman, C.; et al. Mechanistic insights and functional determinants of the transport cycle of the ascorbic acid transporter SVCT2. Activation by sodium and absolute dependence on bivalent cations. *J. Biol. Chem.* **2007**, *282*, 615–624. [CrossRef] [PubMed]

46. Watanabe, K.; Shibuya, S.; Koyama, H.; Ozawa, Y.; Toda, T.; Yokote, K.; Shimizu, T. *Sod1* loss induces intrinsic superoxide accumulation leading to p53-mediated growth arrest and apoptosis. *Int. J. Mol. Sci.* **2013**, *14*, 10998–11010. [CrossRef] [PubMed]

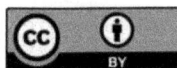

nutrients

MDPI

Article

Emerging Evidence on Neutrophil Motility Supporting Its Usefulness to Define Vitamin C Intake Requirements

Volker Elste *, Barbara Troesch, Manfred Eggersdorfer and Peter Weber

DSM Nutritional Products AG, Human Nutrition and Health, P.O. 3255, CH-4002 Basel, Switzerland; barbara.troesch@dsm.com (B.T.); manfred.eggersdorfer@dsm.com (M.E.); peter.weber@dsm.com (P.W.)
* Correspondence: volker.elste@dsm.com; Tel.: +41-61-815-81-79; Fax: +41-61-815-81-50

Received: 14 March 2017; Accepted: 10 May 2017; Published: 16 May 2017

Abstract: Establishing intake recommendations for vitamin C remains a challenge, as no suitable functional parameter has yet been agreed upon. In this report, we review the emerging evidence on neutrophil motility as a possible marker of vitamin C requirements and put the results in perspective with other approaches. A recent in vitro study showed that adequate levels of vitamin C were needed for this function to work optimally when measured as chemotaxis and chemokinesis. In a human study, neutrophil motility was optimal at intakes $\geq$250 mg/day. Interestingly, a Cochrane review showed a significant reduction in the duration of episodes of common cold with regular vitamin C intakes in a similar range. Additionally, it was shown that at a plasma level of 75 μmol/L, which is reached with vitamin C intakes $\geq$200 mg/day, incidences of cardiovascular disease were lowest. This evidence would suggest that daily intakes of 200 mg vitamin C might be advisable for the general adult population, which can be achieved by means of a diverse diet. However, additional studies are warranted to investigate the usefulness of neutrophil motility as a marker of vitamin C requirements.

Keywords: vitamin C; ascorbic acid; dietary reference value; immune function; neutrophil motility

1. Introduction

Vitamin C is an essential micronutrient. As humans cannot produce it, the daily amount needed to ensure an adequate intake is defined in dietary reference values established in many countries around the globe. The guiding principle for the definition of dietary reference values for vitamin C, as for other essential micronutrients, has changed in the past few decades from only preventing deficiency syndromes to maintaining or even improving human health and ultimately reducing the risk of non-communicable diseases [1]. Scurvy—the clinical manifestation of vitamin C deficiency—develops when intake is below 10 mg/day for a prolonged period [2]. While it takes very little vitamin C to prevent an overt deficiency, the challenge is to define the daily intake required to maintain adequate health given the many metabolic processes that vitamin C is involved in.

The role of vitamin C in the human immune defense in particular is a widely researched field. However, the heterogeneity of study designs and the variability or even inconsistency of outcomes make it difficult to use these data as the basis for daily reference values. In the past, they were consequently deemed insufficient to reliably estimate the vitamin C requirement for apparently healthy individuals. The fact that vitamin C is actively accumulated in the leukocytes resulting in an up to 20 times higher concentration in neutrophils than in the plasma underscores its important role in immune defense. Agencies such as the Institute of Medicine (IOM) in North America used the near-maximal neutrophil concentration with minimal urinary loss to derive vitamin C reference values [1]. In that approach, the vitamin C intake required to near saturate the vitamin C concentration in neutrophils was employed to define the daily reference values.

Recently, additional evidence has emerged on the functional capacity of neutrophils relative to vitamin C concentration in vitro [3] and intakes in humans [4]. It is the aim of this contribution to review the potential of neutrophil motility as a possible marker for defining intake requirements for vitamin C in light of these recent findings. We will also discuss the current levels of vitamin C intakes and how to achieve appropriate intakes.

2. Physiologic Functions of Vitamin C in Human Health

Vitamin C can be in the form of L-ascorbic acid and the oxidized form L-dehydroascorbic acid, and both are essential for a range of vital functions (Figure 1). Humans, as well as some other species such as monkeys, guinea pigs, some fish species, and birds, have lost L-gulonolactone oxidase, the enzyme catalyzing the last step in the synthesis of vitamin C, which makes them dependent on ample amounts of vitamin C from the diet [5,6].

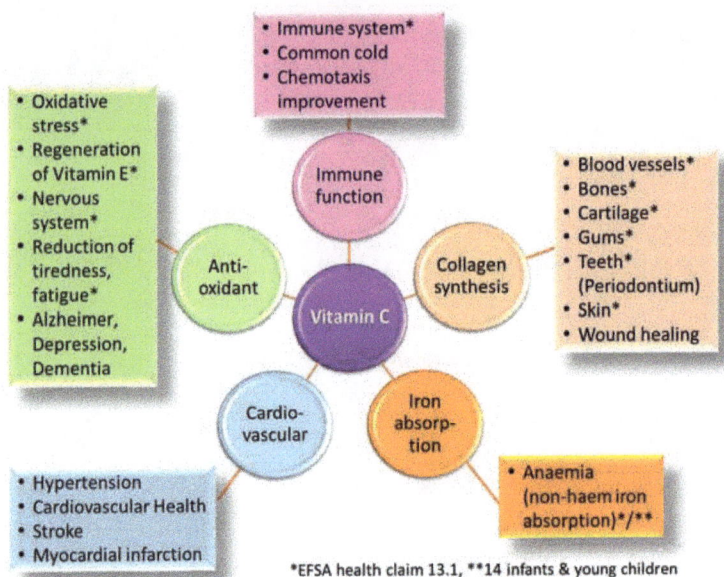

Figure 1. Summary of the functions of vitamin C and established health claims by European Food Safety Authority (EFSA), Article 13.1 and 14.

Thanks to its reducing power, vitamin C mainly functions either as an antioxidant [7] or as a cofactor in enzymatic reactions [5]. As an antioxidant, it scavenges free radicals such as reactive oxygen species and reactive nitrogen species, turning them into less reactive molecules [8]. Through this mechanism, vitamin C protects proteins, lipids, and nucleic acids, and thus the body in general, from oxidative damage. Due to its antioxidant function, it contributes, for instance, to the protection of skin from UV irradiation [9,10] and is able to recycle other antioxidants such as vitamin E [11–13]. By doing so, it helps prevent low density lipoprotein (LDL) oxidation and protects cell lipids from peroxidation [12], thus it is essential for the proper function of the endothelium. In addition, vitamin C increases the bioavailability of non-hem iron by reducing it to the ferrous form, the only form which can be absorbed in the intestine [14,15]. It also increases iron solubility in the stomach and duodenum and reduces the likelihood of iron being affected by inhibitors of iron absorption [16].

As an essential cofactor of iron- and copper-dependent enzymes, vitamin C is involved as an electron donor in a range of catalytic redox-reactions [5]: It helps catalyze the synthesis of L-carnitine from L-lysine, which plays an important role in energy production via ß-oxidation in mitochondria [17–19]. However, in this reaction, its essentiality is discussed controversially, as it may be replaced by glutathione [20]. The synthesis of the catecholamine noradrenaline, a hormone and neurotransmitter, from dopamine by the enzyme dopamine β-monooxygenase also requires vitamin C [21]. Furthermore, the alpha-amidating monooxygenase needs it to increase the stability and activity of peptide hormones such as oxytocin and vasopressin [22]. Vitamin C also plays a role in the synthesis of hypoxia-inducible factor-1 alpha [23], and it is involved in tyrosine metabolism [24].

The vitamin C-dependent enzymes proline-hydroxylases and the lysine hydroxylase are essential for the synthesis of the proteoglycan collagen, which is the main molecule in connective tissues found for example in bone, periodontium, cartilage, skin, ligaments, tendons, and blood vessels [25,26]. Impaired collagen formation due to low vitamin C intake for several weeks leads to the typical symptoms of scurvy such as bleeding gums with the loss of teeth, malformation of bones, and weak blood vessels. This ultimately results in vasomotor instability and open wounds. For the formation and remodeling of bones, not only minerals are needed but also the organic matrix which contains up to 90% collagen produced in osteoblasts. Vitamin C deficiency will lead to bone loss or reduction in bone formation [27–29]. In addition, for wound healing, adequate amounts of vitamin C are needed because it is essential for fibroblast maturation, for the formation of cross-links between collagen fibers, and for angiogenesis [30,31], and thus it also has positive effects on pressure ulcers and burns [32].

Furthermore, vitamin C is a cofactor for the rate-limiting enzyme in bile acid synthesis, which may also enhance the expression of LDL receptors on hepatocytes, thus reducing LDL blood levels [33,34]. A recent review showed significant reductions in blood lipids after vitamin C supplementation in sub-populations with dyslipidemia or low vitamin C status at baseline [35]. This is in line with its positive impact towards a healthy cardiovascular system, reducing the prevalence of coronary heart disease [34] and stroke [36]. Its antioxidant effects reduce oxidative stress and enhance endothelial function through its effects on nitric oxide preservation and generation. Nitric oxide is a signaling molecule that activates endothelial and smooth muscle cells, which increases vasodilation, thus reducing blood pressure and preventing cardiovascular disease (CVD) [37]. Recent meta-analyses support this [38,39], showing that vitamin C improves endothelial function. Antihypertensive effects of vitamin C, particularly by reducing systolic blood pressure, have been shown in short-term trials [40]. Based on this evidence, it was concluded that vitamin C may be a useful nutritional intervention for the secondary prevention of CVD [2].

Furthermore, vitamin C plays an essential role in immune function, which is impaired by insufficient supply and re-established through supplementation [41,42]. It exerts its effect via the promotion of T-cell maturation by modulating the epigenetic regulation of gene expression as a cofactor of dioxygenases [43]. For the circulating immune cells, the importance of vitamin C is highlighted by the preferential uptake via active transport by the sodium-dependent vitamin C transporter located in their cell membranes, resulting in vitamin C concentrations from 20 to 60 times higher than in the surrounding plasma [44,45]. It is assumed that the high vitamin C concentration protects neutrophils from the reactive oxygen species (ROS) they generate to kill pathogens such as bacteria and viruses. Subsequently, extracellularly accumulated L-dehydroascorbic acid is rapidly transported back by glucose transporters and recycled to L-ascorbic acid [5]. Furthermore, it could be shown that vitamin C improves the immune function by influencing chemotaxis (CT) and chemokinesis (CK) of neutrophil leukocytes [46]. The enhancement in leukocyte motility by ascorbic acid goes along with its ability to assemble microtubule organelles [47]. These findings are supported by the observation that the vitamin C level is affected in people with infections, chronic diseases [48], and higher oxidative stress, as they lead to higher metabolic losses: e.g., during common cold [49] and in smokers, a 40% higher turnover is seen [50]. The multiple functions of vitamin C are also reflected by EFSA health claims (Figure 1).

3. Approaches Used to Define Vitamin C Requirements

Currently, the recommended intakes for adults tend to vary for the genders, but they also depend on the agency issuing them (Table 1). Moreover, most have additional allowances for periods of elevated needs, typically pregnancy and lactation [1,51–58]. In some recommendations, smokers are also advised to increase their intakes because their vitamin C status is lower than in non-smokers most likely due to the oxidative potential of the inhaled smoke [1,56,59]. Even though some differences exist in the data used to evaluate dietary requirements and the rationale applied in interpreting them, dietary reference values no longer simply aim at preventing overt deficiencies. They are meant to define intakes associated with optimal health for the majority of individuals—typically 95% to 97.5% of a specific age and gender group.

Table 1. Examples for a wide range of recommended daily intakes for vitamin C in adults (≥19 years) in different countries and regions.

Country	Men (mg)	Women (mg)
Germany, Austria, and Switzerland [56,59]	110	95
United States [1]	90	75
United Kingdom [52]	40	40
Australia and New Zealand [54]	45	45
Japan [58]	100	100
Philippines [55]	75	70
Singapore [57]	105	85
South Africa [51]	90	90
FAO/WHO [53]	45	45

FAO: Food and Agriculture Organization of the United Nations; WHO: World Health Organization

The first physiological marker used to define intake recommendations was the symptoms of scurvy. These could be prevented with daily intakes of around 10 mg, which led, with the inclusion of a safety margin of 30 to 50 mg, to the first set of recommendations for vitamin C of 60 mg per day [60,61]. However, even 20 years ago, this approach was challenged with the argument that a lack of overt deficiency did not necessarily indicate the adequacy of intake [61]. It was therefore suggested that recommended intakes should be at a level that assures optimal functioning of all processes requiring vitamin C, but still sufficiently below those known to provoke adverse effects [60,61]. As a consequence, bodies such as IoM and EFSA defined new levels of adequate intakes [1,56,62]. Moreover, they discussed potential biological markers of physiological functions, such as health outcomes associated with vitamin C intake. However, it was concluded that these were insufficiently established, and consequently the recommendations were still based on indicators of vitamin C status.

EFSA determined the Average Requirement (AR) for healthy adults based on the vitamin C intake that balanced losses as metabolic and urinary losses and the quantity of vitamin C required for the replacement of these losses to metabolic losses and maintained fasting plasma ascorbate concentrations at about 50 µmol/L. This led them to propose daily vitamin C intakes such as the Population Reference Intake (PRI) of 110 mg and 95 mg for healthy adult men and women, respectively [62]. The German-speaking countries adapted their joint reference values to the EFSA recommendations [57]. IoM chose a slightly different approach by using the near-maximal neutrophil concentration with minimal urinary excretion of ascorbate to provide antioxidant protection, which led them to define a Recommended Daily Allowances (RDA) of 90 mg for adult men and 75 mg for adult women [1]. However, both IoM and EFSA highlighted the need to establish an accurate, specific, and easily measurable functional marker for vitamin C (e.g., IoM [1]).

Given the range of functions vitamin C has in the human body, there are many putative functional markers. However, their lack of specificity was one of the main reasons why they were deemed unsuitable as a basis to define vitamin C intake recommendations [63]: Assessing hepatic enzyme systems by measuring cholesterol concentration and detoxification has been proposed [64], but it is influenced by a range of factors and is therefore not specific enough to define vitamin C status. The same applies to measuring DNA oxidation as an indicator of DNA damage [63]. Collagen turnover measured as hydroxyproline excretion was another potential candidate [65]. Unfortunately, the high inter- and intra-individual variation in the response to varying vitamin C intakes reduces its usefulness as a biomarker to define intake recommendations [66]. Given the inverse relationship between vitamin C and blood pressure, this has been discussed as a putative physiological biomarker, but again, it is not sufficiently specific for vitamin C status [67–69]. Furthermore, the urinary excretion of vitamin C has been proposed as a sign of adequate intake. However, this is not a functional marker and reflects only one aspect of vitamin C plasma homeostasis. It could be shown that the bioavailability is complete for 200 mg vitamin C as a single dose [45]. These examples show that a putative marker needs to be reasonably specific to vitamin C status, sensitive to changes in intake within the relevant range, and reliably measurable.

4. New Insights Support Reassessment of Current Vitamin C RDAs

Recently published data might be able to shed some light on the question of suitable indicators and consequently enable us to define more appropriate recommendations for daily intakes. The effect of vitamin C on motility in neutrophils seems to be a promising candidate for such a marker [70]. In the following paragraphs, we review the suitability for the use of this marker and how it fits with the well-established knowledge.

Neutrophils are the most abundant type of leukocytes (40% to 75%) and play an important role in the innate immune system [71]. The cells are highly motile and are able to migrate from the blood into the affected tissues in a process initiated and orchestrated by chemoattractants such as pathogen-derived products or host-derived factors [72]. Chemotaxis (CT) and chemokinesis (CK) describe this movement: while the former is directional, the later consists of random movement [70]. Neutrophils contain high concentrations of vitamin C compared to plasma levels [45], and it is thought that they function best if adequate amounts of vitamin C are available [47]. It has, for example, been shown that inadequate intakes could impair CT in guinea pig leukocytes [73]. The underlying mechanism is thought to be the ability of vitamin C to promote the assembly of microtubule organelles [47].

Similar effects could be shown in a recent in vitro study investigating the impact of vitamin C on CT and CK in cell cultures [3]. It showed that extracellular vitamin C significantly increased CT in vitamin C-preloaded peripheral blood leukocytes, which predominantly consist of neutrophils [3]. Furthermore, vitamin C at physiological concentrations also affected CK, indicating that vitamin C enhances directional and random migration at concentrations comparable to those observed in plasma [3]. This could be seen as a further indication that neutrophil function could be a suitable functional marker to define vitamin C intake. Nevertheless, previous clinical studies investigating the role of vitamin C on neutrophil chemotaxis showed inconsistent effects, and they did not allow for the estimation of the vitamin C requirement for apparently healthy individuals reliably [1]. Therefore, further well designed human studies are warranted.

The findings of the in vitro studies are corroborated by a human study investigating the effect of vitamin C supplementation on the function of neutrophils [4]: Healthy young men with suboptimal plasma vitamin C status (<50 µmol/L) were supplemented with vitamin C rich kiwi fruits (~260 mg/day vitamin C) for four weeks. This is in line with the postulation that such studies should use the baseline vitamin status below a defined threshold as inclusion criteria [74]. Despite the relatively small sample size of 12 participants, the plasma and neutrophil vitamin C content as well as chemotaxis of neutrophils and superoxide generation increased significantly [4].

These results suggest that supplementation of vitamin C from kiwi fruits is associated with the improvement of important neutrophil functions and consequently enhanced immunity. Given the study design, it cannot be excluded that other components of the kiwi fruits contributed to this effect. This needs to be confirmed with an intervention using vitamin C supplements at different doses and a placebo group including more subjects to prove which is the right dose. However, based on the results from the in vitro study, it is very likely that vitamin C was the active compound. While neutrophil saturation was already reached at intakes of 100 mg/day [45], it seems that for optimal maturation and functioning of these cells, intakes of ≥200 mg/day result in additional benefits [3,4]. This is supported by the results from a study showing that intakes of ~110 mg (~60 mg from the diet plus ~53 mg vitamin C from one-half kiwifruit) resulted in saturated neutrophil levels, but not saturated plasma levels. [75]. When they increased the dose of kiwi fruit to two per day with a total vitamin C intake of around 210 mg, plasma vitamin C levels, as well as urinary excretion, further increased [76]. This is thought to be sufficient to achieve a plasma level of ≥70 µmol/L, which should be reached to ensure optimal immune function by the neutrophil leucocytes. Moreover, this is also within the range where the human sodium-dependent vitamin C transporter 2, which is responsible for the uptake of vitamin C into target tissues, is at maximum velocity [77]. In addition, this level of intake enables optimal vitamin C supply in all stages of the neutrophil development and therefore ensures maximal functions of these short-lived immune cells. Importantly, intakes ≥200 mg/day were not associated with any adverse outcomes [45] and are well within the range of <2000 mg/day, which are considered safe by IoM [1]. EFSA considers that supplemental daily doses of vitamin C up to about 1 g are not associated with adverse gastrointestinal effects, and an increased risk of kidney stones was not found in individuals with habitual intakes of 1.5 g/day [78].

For healthy young women, the intakes required for plasma and plasma saturation were slightly lower (100 to 200 mg/day) [79]. However, the authors of this subsequent pharmacokinetics study still concluded that vitamin C intakes of 200 mg from foods are probably required, as bioavailability might be lower from whole fruits and vegetables compared to supplements [79]. Further studies in women are needed to assess the optimal dose of the vitamin for neutrophil function. Moreover, the requirements might also increase with age and possibly body weight as well, given the increased level of inflammation and consequently oxidative stress accompanying both [80,81]. To adapt the recommendation to different groups requires further evaluations.

5. The Improvement of Neutrophil Function by Vitamin C in a Broader Human Health Perspective

5.1. Common Cold

Given its importance for the immune system, improved vitamin C status can be expected to translate into clinical endpoints when faced with infections. This was assessed in a recent Cochrane review investigating the effect of vitamin C intake on the common cold in adults and children [82]. In this meta-analysis, no significant effect of supplementation with between 200 mg and 2000 mg of vitamin C daily on the incidence of common cold was found. However, as is often the case in nutritional randomized controlled trials, the placebo group did not have zero intake of vitamin C, as the participants' diets provide potentially significant amounts of the nutrient in question [83]. Therefore, it is crucial to enroll subjects with hypovitaminosis (plasma vitamin C <50 µmol/L) for such trials [74] to be able to work with an approximation of an actual placebo group. Moreover, in a few studies, the 'placebo' groups also received 50 to 70 mg/day vitamin C for ethical reasons [82]. The fact that in a subgroup analysis of persons with 'acute physical activity' and consequently, higher requirements, vitamin C supplementation reduced the number of incidents by half (Risk Ratio 0.48, 95% Confidence Interval 0.35 to 0.64) supports this interpretation. Interestingly, this was not the case in those with long-term physical stress.

Despite these limitations, it was found that vitamin C supplementation of ≥200 mg significantly reduced the duration of common cold symptoms: In children, the effect was reduced by ~14% and in adults, it was reduced by nearly 8% [82]. Interestingly, it was found that in children, it increased to 18% if only studies supplementing ≥1000 mg were included. This might indicate that during an acute infection, higher intakes could be beneficial—even though this effect was not seen in adults. Neutrophils are under increased oxidative stress during an infection, and it has been shown that vitamin C concentrations greatly increase when they are activated (see the review by Padayatty and Levine [5]). Moreover, supplementation led to a modest but significant reduction in the days that the participants missed from work or school due to the common cold.

On average, episodes of common colds last around 10 days [84] and children tend to have 3 to 5 per year, while for adults it is 1 to 2. Consequently, it can be estimated that an adequate supply with vitamin C can reduce the days spent being ill by 4 to 6 and 1 to 2 for children and adults, respectively (see Figure 2). In addition, the meta-analysis reported a reduction in the severity of the common cold thanks to supplementation with vitamin C, even though the interpretation of this is difficult due to the wide range of the definitions of 'severity' used in the various studies [82].

The findings of studies starting vitamin C supplementation only after the onset of symptoms of common cold were equivocal [82]. This is not surprising, considering that neutrophils are crucial in recognizing an infection and initiating an immune response to fight it. They should therefore already be functioning well before a cold is caught. Given their short half-life, only regular intake at adequate levels can ensure that sufficient mature neutrophils are produced. Marginal vitamin C levels, on the other hand, reduce the CT and CK of the neutrophils, which leads to a slowed immune response.

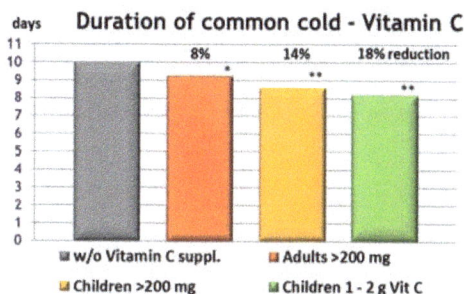

Figure 2. Duration of the common cold. Effect of regular, prophylactic supplementation of vitamin C ($\geq$200 mg/day) on the duration of the common cold, assuming a 10-day illness in adults * (17 trials, 8%; $p = 0.0002$) and in children ** (total 14 trials, 14% for $\geq$200 mg/day and 10 trials, 18% for 1 to 2 g/day; $p < 0.0001$), adapted from Hemila and Chalker, 2013 [82].

5.2. Non-Communicable Diseases

Vitamin C is thought to play an important role in the prevention of non-communicable diseases such as CVD and cancer [48,85]. One difficulty is that randomized controlled trials are not necessarily suitable for detecting such a relationship between a nutrient and a disease [83]. One review found that none of the available studies used low plasma vitamin C concentrations as inclusion criteria, and that the participants of a large majority of these trials (34 out of 35) were unlikely to show a benefit given their baseline plasma concentrations [74].

The link between inadequate vitamin C intake and non-communicable disease is best documented for CVD (for a detailed review of the evidence, see Frei et al., 2012 [85] and Moser et al., 2016 [86]). Given that atherosclerosis is an inflammatory disease [87], it seems likely that vitamin C plays an important role in protecting against it: Vitamin C depletion is thought to increase the susceptibility of LDL cholesterol to oxidation, a risk factor for CVD [88]. However, it is now equally recognized that reactive oxygen species formed by the inflammatory response in an existing atherosclerotic lesion may in turn reduce vitamin C antioxidant levels [87]. A recent review of epidemiologic studies supports the finding that endothelial function and lipid profiles, especially in subjects with low plasma levels, are improved by vitamin C. This is in line with large prospective studies that have shown an inverse relationship between plasma vitamin C status and the risk of CVD [88–92]. Also, Langlois and colleagues [93] showed a relationship between vitamin C concentration and the severity of atherosclerosis and inflammation in peripheral artery disease patients. Moreover, there is evidence from a meta-analysis of randomized controlled trials that vitamin C supplementation has a beneficial effect on blood pressure [40]. Furthermore, sub-group analysis of a recent meta-analysis revealed that vitamin C supplementation reduced LDL cholesterol in healthy participants and, triglycerides are reduced and HDL cholesterol is significantly increased in diabetics. Furthermore, greater effects of vitamin C supplementation in lowering total cholesterol and triglycerides could be shown in those with higher concentrations of these lipids at baseline and the HDL cholesterol increase was greater in participants with lower baseline plasma concentrations of vitamin C, while the overall effects were not significant [39].

Frei [85] argues that the scientific evidence from metabolic, pharmacokinetic, epidemiologic, and intervention studies strongly advocates for an increase of the recommended daily intake to ≥200 mg/day to minimize the risk of negative health effects. Moreover, if the vitamin C content of a healthy, balanced diet in line with guidelines to prevent non-communicable diseases is estimated, it adds up to values slightly above 200 mg/day [94]. Even though these findings relate to different functions of vitamin C, they indicate optimal intakes in a range similar to that suggested by neutrophil motility, thereby strengthening the proposed recommendations. In addition, even though fraught with the same problems as for the other health outcomes, there is some evidence that maintaining healthy vitamin C levels might offer some protection against age-related cognitive decline and Alzheimer's disease [95]. This is not surprising, in the light of the mounting evidence for the role of CVD [96] and oxidative stress in the development of Alzheimer's disease [97]. Given the number of people affected by hypertension, CVD, dementia, and cancer, defining recommendations with the highest risk reduction for these diseases is of paramount importance.

6. Vitamin C Status in the General Population

Proposing to increase the dietary intake recommendations for vitamin C raises the question of whether and how these can be achieved by the general population. Based on the typical food-based dietary recommendations, even the increased intakes of ≥200 mg/day should in theory not cause a problem: Many countries translated the WHO recommendation of ≥400 g of fruits and vegetables, excluding potatoes, cassava, and other tubers, per day [98] into at least five daily servings of such foods. As many of these fruits and vegetables provide significant amounts of vitamin C per average serving (see Table 2), it is feasible to supply ≥200 mg/day of the vitamin via a balanced diet. This is particularly the case if at least one item with high vitamin C levels (e.g., orange juice) is included in the daily diet and preparation techniques such as steam cooking are used that reduce the loss of vitamin C [99]. In addition, other foods also contribute important amounts: A relatively recent German dietary survey reported that the main dietary sources for vitamin C were fruits and fruit products, non-alcoholic beverages, and vegetables [100]. However, potatoes, meat, and meat products such as sausages, as well as dairy products contributed to an important, but lesser, degree [100].

A study in Greece showed that adults who did not meet the recommended daily intakes for fruits or vegetables had a higher risk of inadequate vitamin C intakes [101]. Not surprisingly, those who complied with this specific dietary recommendation tended to have adequate amounts in their diet [101]. In line with this, a study in Switzerland compared vitamin C intakes in omnivores, vegetarians, and vegans, and found mean intakes of 94 mg/day, 158 mg/day, and 239 mg/day, respectively [102]. The corresponding plasma C levels were ~55 μmol/L, ~69 μmol/L, and ~72 μmol/L, respectively. This ties in nicely with the estimate that intakes of ≥200 mg/day achieve plasma levels in the desirable range of >70 μmol/L [45]. Even though the data on foods consumed was not reported in the Swiss study, it can be assumed that the increased intakes of fruits and vegetables in vegetarians and vegans reported elsewhere [103] is reflected in this data.

However, people tend not to follow food-based dietary advice and tend to eat too much of what they should reduce and not enough of the foods that they are encouraged to eat [104]. This is no different in the case of fruits and vegetables, as seen in a recent study: 58% to 88% of adults around the world did not consume the recommended five servings per day [105]. A recent survey from Switzerland showed that only 13% consume the recommended five servings per day [106]. This is in line with an earlier study, which reported that less than 25% of the general adult population in low- and middle-income countries actually followed the recommendation of five portions of fruits and vegetables per day [107]. On the bright side, data from France shows an increase in the consumption of fresh fruits and vegetables, accompanied by a parallel increase in vitamin C intakes, albeit from comparatively low levels (mean intakes for adults <100 mg/day) [108].

Table 2. Composition of a range of raw fruits and vegetables (data from the U.S. Department of Agriculture [109]).

Food	Content per 100 g (mg)	Unit	Content per Unit (mg)
Vegetables			
Red pepper	128	1 piece (119 g)	152
Green pepper	80	1 piece (119 g)	96
Broccoli	89	1 cup [1] (91 g)	81
Brussels sprouts	85	1 cup [1] (88 g)	75
Cabbage	37	1 cup [1] (89 g)	33
Cauliflower	48	1 cup [1] (107 g)	52
Tomato	14	1 piece (123 g)	17
Green peas	40	1 cup [1] (145 g)	58
Fruits			
Orange	53	1 piece (96 g)	70
Kiwi	93	1 piece (69 g)	64
Mango	36	1 piece [2] (336 g)	122
Strawberry	59	1 cup [1] (144 g)	85
Cantaloupe melon	37	1 wedge (69 g)	25
Grapefruit	33	1 piece (118 g)	39

[1] 1 cup ≈ 2.4 dL; [2] without refuse.

This puts the French into the middle range of intakes within Europe: The European Nutrition and Health Survey reports mean vitamin C intakes ranging from ~60 mg to ~153 mg [110]. However, the informative value of mean intakes is limited when assessing the adequacy of intake of a population: despite the comparatively high mean intake reported for Germany (153 mg/day for adults) [110], half the adult population has vitamin C intake below 100 mg/day, which was the recommendation at the time of the survey [59,111,112]. Using a lower level of 60 mg/day and 50 mg/day for men and women, respectively, the European survey reports on 8% to 40% of adults with inadequate intakes [113], and similar rates were reported in the U.S. [114]. Unfortunately, for many countries, only the information on mean intakes is available. However, as the mean intakes are in a similar range as those reported in the surveys referred to above, it can be assumed that a similar problem exists in many—also affluent—parts of the world: In Japan, median intakes of 60 mg and 100 to 115 mg were reported for the age group of 15 to 49 and ≥50 years, respectively [115]. Similarly, mean intakes in South Korea were 116 mg in men and 105 mg in women [116].

Dietary supplements also play an important role in the provision of vitamin C: supplement users across all age groups were found to have higher serum concentrations and lower risk of deficiency than non-users [117]. In the U.S., the proportion of the general population (aged ≥2 years) with intakes below the *Estimated Average Requirement* for vitamin C decreased from 46% to 25% if fortified foods and supplements were taken into account [118]. However, supplement use in Europe is less common, and there is a strong north-to-south gradient, with >40% and 5%, respectively, consuming some type of dietary supplement [113]. Still, in Germany, vitamin C supplements are those used most frequently, and around 10% reported taking them [111]. Similarly, it was among the three most commonly used supplements in a study across Europe [119], and supplements can therefore be assumed to play an important role as dietary sources for the vitamin.

The contribution of different foods to vitamin C intake depends on a range of factors such as variety, maturity of the fruit or vegetable when harvested, and the climate where it grew [120–122], but also on the processing technique involved [63,109]. This makes it difficult to extrapolate the actual status from dietary intake data. However, serum vitamin C concentrations—a more direct marker of vitamin C status—show a similar picture: An analysis in Canada classified 14% of adults as vitamin

C deficient and a further 33% as having sub-optimal serum levels [123]. In the U.S., similar rates for vitamin C deficiency were measured when serum levels were reported in the 1988 to 1994 survey [124], but the prevalence was found to decrease to around 7% in 2003 to 2004 [2]. However, given that persons on low incomes were at increased risk of deficiency [2], it is very likely that the economic crisis, and the consequent increase in poverty and food insecurity [125], has reversed this trend. Moreover, there was a trend towards lower levels for obese persons, which reached significance for women, but not for men [2]. Given the dramatic increase in the prevalence of obesity reported [126], this is worrying, even though it is not clear whether there is a causal link.

In summary, it can be said that the available evidence indicates that even in affluent societies, a significant proportion of the population does not achieve adequate vitamin C status, even as defined by the current recommendations. Increasing the recommended intake to levels more in line with our current understanding of optimal status will further increase the gap between actual intakes and what is regarded as being compatible with optimal health. This might increase the motivation to optimize vitamin C intake either by food fortification or the use of supplements.

7. Conclusions

In light of the many functions that vitamin C has in the body, a range of putative biomarkers were proposed, but they have been rejected due to shortcomings such as lack of specificity (See above). Up to now, no functional biomarker was identified that could be used as a basis to define the dietary intake recommendations for vitamin C. Even though scientific bodies such as IoM argued that such an indicator is needed when they revised their recommendations, they concluded that none have been identified yet [1]. Based on the findings of an in vitro [3] and a human intervention study [4], we propose to investigate further neutrophil motility as such a functional marker.

Combined with the established knowledge from pharmacokinetic, observational, and intervention studies, they indicate that current recommended intakes are set too low and that an increase to $\geq$200 mg/day would be beneficial for the functioning of the immune system. The importance of vitamin C for the immune system was also recognized by the EFSA Panel on Dietetic Products, Nutrition, and Allergies by granting the health claim that vitamin C contributes to a normal function of the immune system [127]. Moreover, such intakes are sufficient to keep plasma vitamin C levels at >70 μmol/L—the range which is associated with plasma saturation [45], but also with reduced risk of CVD [74].

Further well-designed studies in humans are needed to validate neutrophil motility as a functional marker of vitamin C sufficiency and immune function. Moreover, existing questions on the essentiality of adequate vitamin C intakes in the prevention of a range of non-communicable diseases such as CVD, but also cancer and dementia, need to be resolved. This requires large prospective cohort studies, but also randomized controlled trials in participants with low baseline plasma vitamin C levels. In addition to the general population, studies should also address sub-populations, which might have elevated needs due to their genotype or other characteristics, such as obesity, smoking, or increased physical activity.

Even though $\geq$200 mg/day vitamin C could be achieved via a balanced diet in line with the guidelines for the prevention of non-communicable diseases, significant proportions of the population do not achieve even the current recommendations. Consequently, methods need to be found to increase vitamin C intake in the general population—ideally via increased intakes of fruits and vegetables, given the benefits of such foods beyond their vitamin C content. However, as changing people's food habits is notoriously difficult, fortified foods or supplements might provide a more realistic solution at least in the short term.

Acknowledgments: The cost of this publication was covered by DSM Nutritional Products Ltd., Kaiseraugst, Switzerland.

Author Contributions: All authors defined the scope of the publication; Volker Elste and Barbara Troesch wrote the paper; all authors had primary responsibility for the final content.

Conflicts of Interest: All authors are employed by DSM Nutritional Products Ltd., a bulk producer of vitamins.

References

1. Institute of Medicine. *Dietary Reference Intakes of Vitamin C, Vitamin E, Selenium, and Carotenoids*; National Academic Press: Washington, DC, USA, 2000; ISBN: 978-0-309-06935-9.
2. Schleicher, R.L.; Carroll, M.D.; Ford, E.S.; Lacher, D.A. Serum vitamin C and the prevalence of vitamin C deficiency in the United States: 2003–2004 National health and nutrition examination survey (NHANES). *Am. J. Clin. Nutr.* **2009**, *90*, 1252–1263. [CrossRef] [PubMed]
3. Schwager, J.; Bompard, A.; Weber, P.; Raederstorff, D. Ascorbic acid modulates cell migration in differentiated HL-60 cells and peripheral blood leukocytes. *Mol. Nutr. Food Res.* **2015**, *59*, 1513–1523. [CrossRef] [PubMed]
4. Bozonet, S.M.; Carr, A.C.; Pullar, J.M.; Vissers, M.C. Enhanced human neutrophil vitamin C status, chemotaxis and oxidant generation following dietary supplementation with vitamin C-rich sungold kiwifruit. *Nutrients* **2015**, *7*, 2574–2588. [CrossRef] [PubMed]
5. Padayatty, S.J.; Levine, M. Vitamin c: The known, the unknown, and goldilocks. *Oral Dis.* **2016**, *22*, 463–493. [CrossRef] [PubMed]
6. Linster, C.L.; Van Schaftingen, E. Vitamin c. Biosynthesis, recycling and degradation in mammals. *FEBS J.* **2007**, *274*, 1–22. [CrossRef] [PubMed]
7. Buettner, G.R.; Jurkiewicz, B.A. Catalytic metals, ascorbate and free radicals: Combinations to avoid. *Radiat. Res.* **1996**, *145*, 532–541. [CrossRef] [PubMed]
8. Valko, M.; Leibfritz, D.; Moncol, J.; Cronin, M.T.; Mazur, M.; Telser, J. Free radicals and antioxidants in normal physiological functions and human disease. *Int. J. Biochem. Cell Biol.* **2007**, *39*, 44–84. [CrossRef] [PubMed]
9. Swindells, K.; Rhodes, L.E. Influence of oral antioxidants on ultraviolet radiation-induced skin damage in humans. *Photodermatol. Photoimmunol. Photomed.* **2004**, *20*, 297–304. [CrossRef] [PubMed]
10. Eberlein-Konig, B.; Placzek, M.; Przybilla, B. Protective effect against sunburn of combined systemic ascorbic acid (vitamin C) and d-alpha-tocopherol (vitamin E). *J. Am. Acad. Dermatol.* **1998**, *38*, 45–48. [CrossRef]
11. Buettner, G.R. The pecking order of free radicals and antioxidants: Lipid peroxidation, alpha-tocopherol, and ascorbate. *Arch. Biochem. Biophys.* **1993**, *300*, 535–543. [CrossRef] [PubMed]
12. Sharma, M.K.; Buettner, G.R. Interaction of vitamin C and vitamin E during free radical stress in plasma: An esr study. *Free Radic. Biol. Med.* **1993**, *14*, 649–653. [CrossRef]
13. Benzie, I.; Strain, J.J. Effect of vitamin C supplementation on concentrations of vitamins C and E in fasting plasma. *Asia Pac. J. Clin. Nutr.* **1999**, *8*, 207–210. [CrossRef] [PubMed]
14. Forth, W.; Rummel, W. Iron absorption. *Physiol. Rev.* **1973**, *53*, 724–792. [PubMed]
15. Lynch, S.R.; Cook, J.D. Interaction of vitamin C and iron. *Ann. N. Y. Acad. Sci.* **1980**, *355*, 32–44. [CrossRef] [PubMed]
16. Scheers, N.; Andlid, T.; Alminger, M.; Sandberg, A.S. Determination of Fe^{2+} and Fe^{3+} in aqueous solutions containing food chelators by differential pulse anodic stripping voltammetry. *Electroanalysis* **2010**, *22*, 1090–1096. [CrossRef]
17. Fritz, I.B. Carnitine and its role in fatty acid metabolism. *Adv. Lipid Res.* **1963**, *1*, 285–334. [PubMed]
18. Fritz, I.B.; Yue, K.T. Long-chain carnitine acyltransferase and the role of acylcarnitine derivatives in the catalytic increase of fatty acid oxidation induced by carnitine. *J. Lipid Res.* **1963**, *4*, 279–288. [PubMed]
19. Ramsay, R.R.; Gandour, R.D.; van der Leij, F.R. Molecular enzymology of carnitine transfer and transport. *Biochim. Biophys. Acta* **2001**, *1546*, 21–43. [CrossRef]
20. Furusawa, H.; Sato, Y.; Tanaka, Y.; Inai, Y.; Amano, A.; Iwama, M.; Kondo, Y.; Handa, S.; Murata, A.; Nishikimi, M.; et al. Vitamin C is not essential for carnitine biosynthesis in vivo: Verification in vitamin C-depleted senescence marker protein-30/gluconolactonase knockout mice. *Biol. Pharm. Bull.* **2008**, *31*, 1673–1679. [CrossRef] [PubMed]
21. Rush, R.A.; Geffen, L.B. Dopamine beta-hydroxylase in health and disease. *Crit. Rev. Clin. Lab. Sci.* **1980**, *12*, 241–277. [CrossRef] [PubMed]
22. Prigge, S.T.; Kolhekar, A.S.; Eipper, B.A.; Mains, R.E.; Amzel, L.M. Substrate-mediated electron transfer in peptidylglycine alpha-hydroxylating monooxygenase. *Nat. Struct. Biol.* **1999**, *6*, 976–983. [CrossRef] [PubMed]

23. Dengler, V.L.; Galbraith, M.D.; Espinosa, J.M. Transcriptional regulation by hypoxia inducible factors. *Crit. Rev. Biochem. Mol. Biol.* **2014**, *49*, 1–15. [CrossRef] [PubMed]

24. Lindblad, B.; Lindstedt, G.; Lindstedt, S. The mechanism of enzymic formation of homogentisate from *p*-hydroxyphenylpyruvate. *J. Am. Chem. Soc.* **1970**, *92*, 7446–7449. [CrossRef] [PubMed]

25. Kukkola, L.; Hieta, R.; Kivirikko, K.I.; Myllyharju, J. Identification and characterization of a third human, rat, and mouse collagen prolyl 4-hydroxylase isoenzyme. *J. Biol. Chem.* **2003**, *278*, 47685–47693. [CrossRef] [PubMed]

26. Prockop, D.J.; Kivirikko, K.I. Collagens: Molecular biology, diseases, and potentials for therapy. *Annu. Rev. Biochem.* **1995**, *64*, 403–434. [CrossRef] [PubMed]

27. Aghajanian, P.; Hall, S.; Wongworawat, M.D.; Mohan, S. The roles and mechanisms of actions of vitamin C in bone: New developments. *J. Bone Miner. Res.* **2015**, *30*, 1945–1955. [CrossRef] [PubMed]

28. Hasegawa, T.; Li, M.; Hara, K.; Sasaki, M.; Tabata, C.; de Freitas, P.H.; Hongo, H.; Suzuki, R.; Kobayashi, M.; Inoue, K.; et al. Morphological assessment of bone mineralization in tibial metaphyses of ascorbic acid-deficient ods rats. *Biomed. Res.* **2011**, *32*, 259–269. [CrossRef] [PubMed]

29. Masse, P.G.; Jougleux, J.L.; Tranchant, C.C.; Dosy, J.; Caissie, M.; Coburn, S.P. Enhancement of calcium/vitamin D supplement efficacy by administering concomitantly three key nutrients essential to bone collagen matrix for the treatment of osteopenia in middle-aged women: A one-year follow-up. *J. Clin. Biochem. Nutr.* **2010**, *46*, 20–29. [CrossRef] [PubMed]

30. Blass, S.C.; Goost, H.; Tolba, R.H.; Stoffel-Wagner, B.; Kabir, K.; Burger, C.; Stehle, P.; Ellinger, S. Time to wound closure in trauma patients with disorders in wound healing is shortened by supplements containing antioxidant micronutrients and glutamine: A prct. *Clin. Nutr.* **2012**, *31*, 469–475. [CrossRef] [PubMed]

31. Thompson, C.; Fuhrman, M.P. Nutrients and wound healing: Still searching for the magic bullet. *Nutr. Clin. Pract.* **2005**, *20*, 331–347. [CrossRef] [PubMed]

32. Stechmiller, J.K. Understanding the role of nutrition and wound healing. *Nutr. Clin. Pract.* **2010**, *25*, 61–68. [CrossRef] [PubMed]

33. McRae, M.P. Vitamin C supplementation lowers serum low-density lipoprotein cholesterol and triglycerides: A meta-analysis of 13 randomized controlled trials. *J. Chiropr. Med.* **2008**, *7*, 48–58. [CrossRef] [PubMed]

34. Hallfrisch, J.; Singh, V.N.; Muller, D.C.; Baldwin, H.; Bannon, M.E.; Andres, R. High plasma vitamin C associated with high plasma HDL- and HDL2 cholesterol. *Am. J. Clin. Nutr.* **1994**, *60*, 100–105. [PubMed]

35. Ashor, A.W.; Siervo, M.; van der Velde, F.; Willis, N.D.; Mathers, J.C. Systematic review and meta-analysis of randomised controlled trials testing the effects of vitamin C supplementation on blood lipids. *Clin. Nutr.* **2016**, *35*, 626–637. [CrossRef] [PubMed]

36. Simon, J.A.; Hudes, E.S.; Browner, W.S. Serum ascorbic acid and cardiovascular disease prevalence in US. Adults. *Epidemiology.* **1998**, *9*, 316–321. [CrossRef] [PubMed]

37. May, J.M.; Harrison, F.E. Role of vitamin C in the function of the vascular endothelium. *Antioxid. Redox Signal.* **2013**, *19*, 2068–2083. [CrossRef] [PubMed]

38. Ashor, A.W.; Lara, J.; Mathers, J.C.; Siervo, M. Effect of vitamin C on endothelial function in health and disease: A systematic review and meta-analysis of randomised controlled trials. *Atherosclerosis* **2014**, *235*, 9–20. [CrossRef] [PubMed]

39. Ashor, A.W.; Siervo, M.; Lara, J.; Oggioni, C.; Afshar, S.; Mathers, J.C. Effect of vitamin C and vitamin E supplementation on endothelial function: A systematic review and meta-analysis of randomised controlled trials. *Br. J. Nutr.* **2015**, *113*, 1182–1194. [CrossRef] [PubMed]

40. Juraschek, S.P.; Guallar, E.; Appel, L.J.; Miller, E.R., 3rd. Effects of vitamin C supplementation on blood pressure: A meta-analysis of randomized controlled trials. *Am. J. Clin. Nutr.* **2012**, *95*, 1079–1088. [CrossRef] [PubMed]

41. Wintergerst, E.S.; Maggini, S.; Hornig, D.H. Immune-enhancing role of vitamin C and zinc and effect on clinical conditions. *Ann. Nutr. Metab.* **2006**, *50*, 85–94. [CrossRef] [PubMed]

42. Pike, J.; Chandra, R.K. Effect of vitamin and trace element supplementation on immune indices in healthy elderly. *Int. J. Vitam. Nutr. Res.* **1995**, *65*, 117–121. [PubMed]

43. Manning, J.; Mitchell, B.; Appadurai, D.A.; Shakya, A.; Pierce, L.J.; Wang, H.; Nganga, V.; Swanson, P.C.; May, J.M.; Tantin, D.; et al. Vitamin C promotes maturation of t-cells. *Antioxid. Redox Signal.* **2013**, *19*, 2054–2067. [CrossRef] [PubMed]

44. Washko, P.; Rotrosen, D.; Levine, M. Ascorbic acid transport and accumulation in human neutrophils. *J. Biol. Chem.* **1989**, *264*, 18996–19002. [PubMed]

45. Levine, M.; Conry-Cantilena, C.; Wang, Y.; Welch, R.W.; Washko, P.W.; Dhariwal, K.R.; Park, J.B.; Lazarev, A.; Graumlich, J.F.; King, J.; et al. Vitamin C pharmacokinetics in healthy volunteers: Evidence for a recommended dietary allowance. *Proc. Natl. Acad. Sci. USA* **1996**, *93*, 3704–3709. [CrossRef] [PubMed]

46. Vohra, K.; Khan, A.J.; Telang, V.; Rosenfeld, W.; Evans, H.E. Improvement of neutrophil migration by systemic vitamin c in neonates. *J. Perinatol.* **1990**, *10*, 134–136. [PubMed]

47. Boxer, L.A.; Vanderbilt, B.; Bonsib, S.; Jersild, R.; Yang, H.H.; Baehner, R.L. Enhancement of chemotactic response and microtubule assembly in human leukocytes by ascorbic acid. *J. Cell. Physiol.* **1979**, *100*, 119–126. [CrossRef] [PubMed]

48. Carr, A.C.; Frei, B. Toward a new recommended dietary allowance for vitamin C based on antioxidant and health effects in humans. *Am. J. Clin. Nutr.* **1999**, *69*, 1086–1107. [PubMed]

49. Hume, R.; Weyers, E. Changes in leucocyte ascorbic acid during the common cold. *Scott. Med. J.* **1973**, *18*, 3–7. [CrossRef] [PubMed]

50. Lykkesfeldt, J.; Loft, S.; Nielsen, J.B.; Poulsen, H.E. Ascorbic acid and dehydroascorbic acid as biomarkers of oxidative stress caused by smoking. *Am. J. Clin. Nutr.* **1997**, *65*, 959–963. [PubMed]

51. The Nutrition Information Centre of the University of Stellenbosch. Available online: http://www.sun.ac.za/english/faculty/healthsciences/nicus/Pages/Vitamin-C.aspx (accessed on 5 October 2016).

52. Department of Health. *Dietary Reference Values for Food, Energy and Nutrients for the United Kingdom in Report on Health and Social Subjects*; Department of Health: London, UK, 1991.

53. Food and Agriculture Organization; World Health Organization. *Human Vitamin and Mineral Requirements*; Training Materials for Agricultural Planning; Food and Agriculture Organization: Bangkok, Thailand, 2002.

54. Australian National Health and Medical Research Council; New Zealand Ministry of Health. Nutrient Reference Values for Australia and New Zealand. Available online: https://www.nrv.gov.au/nutrients/vitamin-c (accessed on 16 November 2016).

55. Barba, C.V.; Cabrera, M.I. Recommended energy and nutrient intakes for Filipinos 2002. *Asia Pac. J. Clin. Nutr.* **2008**, *17* (Suppl. 2), 399–404. [CrossRef] [PubMed]

56. German Nutrition Society. New reference values for vitamin C intake. *Ann. Nutr. Metab.* **2015**, *67*, 13–20. [CrossRef]

57. Health Promotion Board. Recommended Dietary Allowances. Available online: http://www.hpb.gov.sg/HOPPortal/health-article/2652 (accessed on 23 October 2016).

58. National Institute of Health and Nutrition. Dietary Reference Intakes for Japanese (2015). Available online: http://www.mhlw.go.jp/file/06-Seisakujouhou-10900000-Kenkoukyoku/overview.pdf (accessed on 1 November 2016).

59. Deutsche Gesellschaft für Ernährung; Österreichische Gesellschaft für Ernährung; Schweizerische Gesellschaft für Ernährung; Schweizerische Vereinigung für Ernährung. *Referenzwerte für die Nährstoffzufuhr*; Umschau Verlag: Frankfurt, Germany, 2008.

60. Levine, M.; Dhariwal, K.R.; Washko, P.W.; Welch, R.W.; Wang, Y. Cellular functions of ascorbic acid: A means to determine vitamin c requirements. *Asia Pac. J. Clin. Nutr.* **1993**, *2* (Suppl. 1), 5–13. [PubMed]

61. Levine, M.; Dhariwal, K.R.; Welch, R.W.; Wang, Y.; Park, J.B. Determination of optimal vitamin C requirements in humans. *Am. J. Clin. Nutr.* **1995**, *62* (Suppl. 6), 1347S–1356S. [PubMed]

62. EFSA NDA Panel. Scientific opinion on dietary reference values for Vitamin C. *EFSA J.* **2013**. [CrossRef]

63. Benzie, I.F. Vitamin C: Prospective functional markers for defining optimal nutritional status. *Proc. Nutr. Soc.* **1999**, *58*, 469–476. [CrossRef] [PubMed]

64. Ginter, E. Ascorbic acid in cholesterol metabolism and in detoxification of xenobiotic substances: Problem of optimum vitamin C intake. *Nutrition* **1989**, *5*, 369–374. [CrossRef] [PubMed]

65. Bates, C.J. Proline and hydroxyproline excretion and vitamin C status in elderly human subjects. *Clin. Sci. Mol. Med.* **1977**, *52*, 535–543. [CrossRef] [PubMed]

66. Hevia, P.; Omaye, S.T.; Jacob, R.A. Urinary hydroxyproline excretion and vitamin C status in healthy young men. *Am. J. Clin. Nutr.* **1990**, *51*, 644–648. [PubMed]

67. Rodrigo, R.; Prat, H.; Passalacqua, W.; Araya, J.; Bachler, J.P. Decrease in oxidative stress through supplementation of vitamins C and E is associated with a reduction in blood pressure in patients with essential hypertension. *Clin. Sci. (Lond.)* **2008**, *114*, 625–634. [CrossRef] [PubMed]

68. Bendich, A.; Langseth, L. The health effects of vitamin c supplementation: A review. *J. Am. Coll. Nutr.* **1995**, *14*, 124–136. [CrossRef] [PubMed]

69. Weber, P.; Bendich, A.; Schalch, W. Vitamin C and human health—A review of recent data relevant to human requirements. *Int. J. Vitam. Nutr. Res.* **1996**, *66*, 19–30. [PubMed]

70. Petrie, R.J.; Doyle, A.D.; Yamada, K.M. Random versus directionally persistent cell migration. *Nat. Rev. Mol. Cell Biol.* **2009**, *10*, 538–549. [CrossRef] [PubMed]

71. Amulic, B.; Cazalet, C.; Hayes, G.L.; Metzler, K.D.; Zychlinsky, A. Neutrophil function: From mechanisms to disease. *Annu. Rev. Immunol.* **2012**, *30*, 459–489. [CrossRef] [PubMed]

72. Foxman, E.F.; Campbell, J.J.; Butcher, E.C. Multistep navigation and the combinatorial control of leukocyte chemotaxis. *J. Cell Biol.* **1997**, *139*, 1349–1360. [CrossRef] [PubMed]

73. Johnston, C.S.; Huang, S. Effect of ascorbic acid nutriture on blood histamine and neutrophil chemotaxis in guinea pigs. *J. Nutr.* **1991**, *121*, 126–130. [PubMed]

74. Lykkesfeldt, J.; Poulsen, H.E. Is vitamin c supplementation beneficial? Lessons learned from randomised controlled trials. *Br. J. Nutr.* **2010**, *103*, 1251–1259. [CrossRef] [PubMed]

75. Carr, A.C.; Bozonet, S.M.; Pullar, J.M.; Simcock, J.W.; Vissers, M.C. Human skeletal muscle ascorbate is highly responsive to changes in vitamin c intake and plasma concentrations. *Am. J. Clin. Nutr.* **2013**, *97*, 800–807. [CrossRef] [PubMed]

76. Carr, A.C.; Pullar, J.M.; Moran, S.; Vissers, M.C.M. Bioavailability of vitamin C from kiwifruit in non-smoking males: Determination of 'healthy' and 'optimal' intakes. *J. Nutr. Sci.* **2012**, *1*, e14. [CrossRef] [PubMed]

77. Savini, I.; Rossi, A.; Pierro, C.; Avigliano, L.; Catani, M.V. Svct1 and Svct2: Key proteins for vitamin C uptake. *Amino Acid* **2008**, *34*, 347–355. [CrossRef] [PubMed]

78. Scientific Committee on Food; Scientific Panel on Dietetic Products, Nutrition and Allergies. *Tolerable Upper Intake Levels for Vitamins and Minerals*; European Food Safety Authority: Parma, Italy, 2006; ISBN: 92-9199-014-0.

79. Levine, M.; Wang, Y.; Padayatty, S.J.; Morrow, J. A new recommended dietary allowance of vitamin C for healthy young women. *Proc. Natl. Acad. Sci. USA* **2001**, *98*, 9842–9846. [CrossRef] [PubMed]

80. Mehmood, Z.-T.-N.H.; Papandreou, D. An updated mini review of vitamin D and obesity: Adipogenesis and inflammation state. *Open Access Maced. J. Med. Sci.* **2016**, *4*, 526–532. [CrossRef] [PubMed]

81. Khatami, M. Inflammation, aging, and cancer: Tumoricidal versus tumorigenesis of immunity. *Cell Biochem. Biophys.* **2009**, *55*, 55–79. [CrossRef] [PubMed]

82. Hemila, H.; Chalker, E. Vitamin C for preventing and treating the common cold. *Cochrane Database Syst. Rev.* **2013**, *1*. [CrossRef]

83. Moser, U. Vitamins—Wrong approaches. *Int. J. Vitam. Nutr. Res.* **2012**, *82*, 327–332. [CrossRef] [PubMed]

84. Thompson, M.; Vodicka, T.A.; Blair, P.S.; Buckley, D.I.; Heneghan, C.; Hay, A.D.; Team, T.P. Duration of symptoms of respiratory tract infections in children: Systematic review. *BMJ* **2013**, *347*, f7027. [CrossRef] [PubMed]

85. Frei, B. Authors perspective—What is the optimum intake of Vitamin C. *Crit. Rev. Food. Sci. Nutr.* **2012**, *52*, 815–829. [CrossRef] [PubMed]

86. Moser, M.A.; Chun, O.K. Vitamin C and heart health: A review based on findings from epidemiologic studies. *Int. J. Mol. Sci.* **2016**, *17*. [CrossRef] [PubMed]

87. Ross, R. Atherosclerosis—An inflammatory disease. *N. Engl. J. Med.* **1999**, *340*, 115–126. [CrossRef]

88. Nyyssonen, K.; Parviainen, M.T.; Salonen, R.; Tuomilehto, J.; Salonen, J.T. Vitamin C deficiency and risk of myocardial infarction: Prospective population study of men from eastern Finland. *BMJ* **1997**, *314*, 634–638. [CrossRef] [PubMed]

89. Khaw, K.T.; Bingham, S.; Welch, A.; Luben, R.; Wareham, N.; Oakes, S.; Day, N. Relation between plasma ascorbic acid and mortality in men and women in epic-norfolk prospective study: A prospective population study. European prospective investigation into cancer and nutrition. *Lancet* **2001**, *357*, 657–663. [CrossRef]

90. Singh, R.B.; Ghosh, S.; Niaz, M.A.; Singh, R.; Beegum, R.; Chibo, H.; Shoumin, Z.; Postiglione, A. Dietary intake, plasma levels of antioxidant vitamins, and oxidative stress in relation to coronary artery disease in elderly subjects. *Am. J. Cardiol.* **1995**, *76*, 1233–1238. [CrossRef]

91. Eichholzer, M.; Stahelin, H.B.; Gey, K.F. Inverse correlation between essential antioxidants in plasma and subsequent risk to develop cancer, ischemic heart disease and stroke respectively: 12-Year follow-up of the prospective Basel study. *EXS* **1992**, *62*, 398–410. [CrossRef] [PubMed]

92. Sahyoun, N.R.; Jacques, P.F.; Russell, R.M. Carotenoids, vitamins C and E, and mortality in an elderly population. *Am. J. Epidemiol.* **1996**, *144*, 501–511. [CrossRef] [PubMed]

93. Langlois, M.; Duprez, D.; Delanghe, J.; De Buyzere, M.; Clement, D.L. Serum vitamin C concentration is low in peripheral arterial disease and is associated with inflammation and severity of atherosclerosis. *Circulation* **2001**, *103*, 1863–1868. [CrossRef] [PubMed]

94. Lachance, P.; Langseth, L. The rda concept: Time for a change? *Nutr. Rev.* **1994**, *52*, 266–270. [CrossRef] [PubMed]

95. Harrison, F.E. A critical review of vitamin C for the prevention of age-related cognitive decline and Alzheimer's disease. *J. Alzheimer's Dis.* **2012**, *29*, 711–726. [CrossRef]

96. De Bruijn, R.F.A.G.; Ikram, M.A. Cardiovascular risk factors and future risk of alzheimer's disease. *BMC Med.* **2014**, *12*, 130. [CrossRef] [PubMed]

97. Tramutola, A.; Lanzillotta, C.; Perluigi, M.; Butterfield, D.A. Oxidative stress, protein modification and alzheimer disease. *Brain Res. Bull.* **2016**, *6*. [CrossRef] [PubMed]

98. World Health Organization. *Diet, Nutrition and the Prevention of Chronic Diseases*; Report of a Joint WHO/FAO Consultation; World Health Organization: Geneva, Switzerland, 2003; ISBN: 92 4 120916 X.

99. Birlouez-Aragon, I.; Saavedra, G.; Tessier, F.J.; Galinier, A.; Ait-Ameur, L.; Lacoste, F.; Niamba, C.-N.; Alt, N.; Somoza, V.; Lecerf, J.-M. A diet based on high-heat-treated foods promotes risk factors for diabetes mellitus and cardiovascular diseases. *Am. J. Clin. Nutr.* **2010**, *91*, 1220–1226. [CrossRef]

100. Max Rubner-Institut. Nationale Verzehrsstudie II. Ergebnisbericht, Teil 2. Available online: http://www.was-esse-ich.de/uploads/media/NVSII_Abschlussbericht_Teil_2.pdf (accessed on 2 July 2011).

101. Manios, Y.; Moschonis, G.; Grammatikaki, E.; Mavrogianni, C.; van den Heuvel, E.G.H.M.; Bos, R.; Singh-Povel, C. Food group and micronutrient intake adequacy among children, adults and elderly women in greece. *Nutrients* **2015**, *7*, 1841–1858. [CrossRef] [PubMed]

102. Schupbach, R.; Wegmuller, R.; Berguerand, C.; Bui, M.; Herter-Aeberli, I. Micronutrient status and intake in omnivores, vegetarians and vegans in Switzerland. *Eur. J. Nutr.* **2017**, *56*, 283–293. [CrossRef] [PubMed]

103. Clarys, P.; Deliens, T.; Huybrechts, I.; Deriemaeker, P.; Vanaelst, B.; De Keyzer, W.; Hebbelinck, M.; Mullie, P. Comparison of nutritional quality of the vegan, vegetarian, semi-vegetarian, pesco-vegetarian and omnivorous diet. *Nutrients* **2014**, *6*, 1318–1332. [CrossRef] [PubMed]

104. Krebs-Smith, S.M.; Guenther, P.M.; Subar, A.F.; Kirkpatrick, S.I.; Dodd, K.W. Americans do not meet federal dietary recommendations. *J. Nutr.* **2010**, *140*, 1832–1838. [CrossRef] [PubMed]

105. Murphy, M.M.; Barraj, L.M.; Spungen, J.H.; Herman, D.R.; Randolph, R.K. Global assessment of select phytonutrient intakes by level of fruit and vegetable consumption. *Br. J. Nutr.* **2014**, *112*, 1004–1018. [CrossRef] [PubMed]

106. Bundesamt für Lebensmittelsicherheit und Veterinärwesen. Zu viel Gewicht, zu Wenig Früchte und Gemüse. Available online: https://www.blv.admin.ch/blv/de/home/dokumentation/nsb-news-list.msg-id-64373.html (accessed on 11 November 2016).

107. Hall, J.N.; Moore, S.; Harper, S.B.; Lynch, J.W. Global variability in fruit and vegetable consumption. *Am. J. Prev. Med.* **2009**, *36*, 402–409. [CrossRef] [PubMed]

108. Dubuisson, C.; Lioret, S.; Touvier, M.; Dufour, A.; Calamassi-Tran, G.; Volatier, J.-L.; Lafay, L. Trends in food and nutritional intakes of french adults from 1999 to 2007: Results from the inca surveys. *Br. J. Nutr.* **2010**, *103*, 1035–1048. [CrossRef] [PubMed]

109. US Department of Agriculture; Agricultural Research Service; Nutrient Data Laboratory. *USDA National Nutrient Database for Standard Reference, Release 28*; Version Current; September 2015. Available online: http://www.ars.usda.gov/nea/bhnrc/ndl (accessed on 4 April 2016).

110. Elmadfa, I.; Meyer, A.; Nowak, V.; Hasenegger, V.; Putz, P.; Verstraeten, R.; Remaut-DeWinter, A.M.; Kolsteren, P.; Dostalova, J.; Dlouhy, P.; et al. *European Nutrition and Health Report 2009*, 2010/02/06 ed.; Karger: Basel, Switzerland, 2009; Volume 62. [CrossRef]

111. Deutsche Gesellschaft für Ernährung e. V. *12. Ernährungsbericht 2012*; Deutsche Gesellschaft für Ernährung e. V.: Bonn, Germany, 2012.

112. Deutsche Gesellschaft für Ernährung e. V. *Ernährungsbericht 2008*; Deutsche Gesellschaft für Ernährung e. V.: Bonn, Germany, 2008.

113. Roman Vinas, B.; Ribas Barba, L.; Ngo, J.; Gurinovic, M.; Novakovic, R.; Cavelaars, A.; de Groot, L.C.; Van't Veer, P.; Matthys, C.; Serra Majem, L. Projected prevalence of inadequate nutrient intakes in Europe. *Ann. Nutr. Metab.* **2011**, *59*, 84–95. [CrossRef] [PubMed]

114. Troesch, B.; Hoeft, B.; McBurney, M.; Eggersdorfer, M.; Weber, P. Dietary surveys indicate vitamin intakes below recommendations are common in representative western countries. *Br. J. Nutr.* **2012**, *108*, 692–698. [CrossRef] [PubMed]

115. Ministry of Health Labour and Welfare. *The Japan National Health and Nutrition Survey 2008*; Ministry of Health Labour and Welfare: Tokyo, Japan, 2008.

116. Kim, J.; Choi, Y.-H. Physical activity, dietary vitamin C, and metabolic syndrome in the Korean adults: The Korea national health and nutrition examination survey 2008 to 2012. *Public Health* **2016**, *135*, 30–37. [CrossRef] [PubMed]

117. Bailey, R.L.; Fulgoni, V.L.; Keast, D.R.; Dwyer, J.T. Dietary supplement use is associated with higher intakes of minerals from food sources. *Am. J. Clin. Nutr.* **2011**, *94*, 1376–1381. [CrossRef] [PubMed]

118. Fulgoni, V.L.; Keast, D.R.; Bailey, R.L.; Dwyer, J. Foods, fortificants, and supplements: Where do Americans get their nutrients? *J. Nutr.* **2011**, *141*, 1847–1854. [CrossRef] [PubMed]

119. Skeie, G.; Braaten, T.; Hjartåker, A.; Lentjes, M.; Amiano, P.; Jakszyn, P.; Pala, V.; Palanca, A.; Niekerk, E.M.; Verhagen, H.; et al. Use of dietary supplements in the European prospective investigation into cancer and nutrition calibration study. *Eur. J. Clin. Nutr.* **2009**, *63*, S226–S238. [CrossRef] [PubMed]

120. Nagy, S. Vitamin C contents of citrus fruit and their products: A review. *J. Agric. Food Chem.* **1980**, *28*, 8–18. [CrossRef] [PubMed]

121. Vanderslice, J.T.; Higgs, D.J. Vitamin C content of foods: Sample variability. *Am. J. Clin. Nutr.* **1991**, *54*, 1323S–1327S. [PubMed]

122. Marti, N.; Mena, P.; Canovas, J.A.; Micol, V.; Saura, D. Vitamin C and the role of citrus juices as functional food. *Nat. Prod. Commun.* **2009**, *4*, 677–700. [PubMed]

123. Cahill, L.; Corey, P.N.; El-Sohemy, A. Vitamin C deficiency in a population of young Canadian adults. *Am. J. Epidemiol.* **2009**, *170*, 464–471. [CrossRef] [PubMed]

124. Hampl, J.S.; Taylor, C.A.; Johnston, C.S. Vitamin C deficiency and depletion in the United States: The third national health and nutrition examination survey, 1988 to 1994. *Am. J. Public Health* **2004**, *94*, 870–875. [CrossRef] [PubMed]

125. Coleman-Jensen, A.; Nord, M.; Singh, A. *Household Food Security in the United States in 2012*; U.S. Department of Agriculture, Economic Research Service: Washington, DC, USA, 2013.

126. World Health Organization. Fact Sheet No. 311: Obesity and Overweight. Available online: http://www.who.int/mediacentre/factsheets/fs311/en/ (accessed on 2 May 2014).

127. EFSA NDA Panel. Scientific opinion on the substantiation of health claims related to vitamin C and protection of DNA, proteins and lipids from oxidative damage (ID 129, 138, 143, 148), antioxidant function of lutein (ID 146), maintenance of vision (ID 141, 142), collagen formation (ID 130, 131, 136, 137, 149), function of the nervous system (ID 133), function of the immune system (ID 134), function of the immune system during and after extreme physical exercise (ID 144), non-haem iron absorption (ID 132, 147), energy-yielding metabolism (ID 135), and relief in case of irritation in the upper respiratory tract (ID 1714, 1715) pursuant to article 13(1) of regulation (EC) No. 1924/2006. *EFSA J.* **2009**, *7*, 1226. [CrossRef]

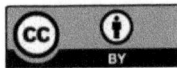

MDPI

St. Alban-Anlage 66

4052 Basel

Switzerland

Tel. +41 61 683 77 34

Fax +41 61 302 89 18

www.mdpi.com

Nutrients Editorial Office

E-mail: nutrients@mdpi.com

www.mdpi.com/journal/nutrients

www.ingramcontent.com/pod-product-compliance
Lightning Source LLC
Chambersburg PA
CBHW051718210326
41597CB00032B/5527